FROM THE EXPERTS IN ENDOCRINOL

ENDO 2019
MEET-THE-PROFESSOR

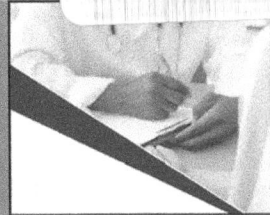

REFERENCE EDITION

ENDOCRINE
CASE MANAGEMENT

ENDO 2019

ENDOCRINE
SOCIETY

ENDOCRINE
SOCIETY

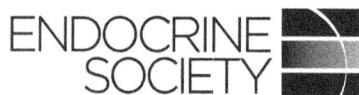

2055 L Street, NW, Suite 600
Washington, DC 20036
www.endocrine.org

Other Publications:
https://www.endocrine.org/publications

The Endocrine Society is the world's largest, oldest, and most active organization working to advance the clinical practice of endocrinology and hormone research. Founded in 1916, the Society now has more than 18,000 global members across a range of disciplines.

The Society has earned an international reputation for excellence in the quality of its peer-reviewed journals, educational resources, meetings, and programs that improve public health through the practice and science of endocrinology.

Clinical Practice Chair, ENDO 2019
Susan A. Sherman, MD

ISBN: 978-1-879225-63-3
eISBN: 978-1-879225-46-6
Library of Congress Control Number: 2019951614

On the Cover: © Shutterstock. Doctor consulting with patient in a hospital. (By New Africa).

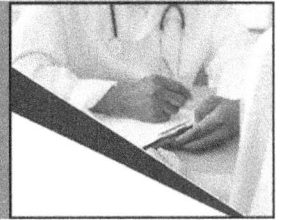

ENDO 2019
CONTENTS

ENDO 2019
FACULTY

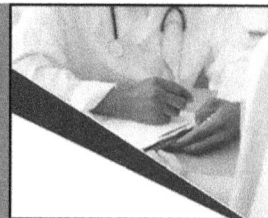

2019 MEET-THE-PROFESSOR CASE MANAGEMENT FACULTY

Jasna Aleksova, MBBS, BMedSci
Monash Health Melbourne
Australia

Bradley D. Anawalt, MD
University of Washington

Katherine Araque, MD
National Institutes of Health

Wiebke Arlt, MD, DSc
University of Birmingham
United Kingdom

Richard J. Auchus, MD, PhD
University of Michigan

Ricardo Azziz, MD, MPH, MBA
State University of New York

Linda A. Barbour, MSPH, MD
University of Colorado School of Medicine

Andrew J. Bauer, MD
The Children's Hospital of Philadelphia

Carolyn B. Becker, MD
Brigham and Women's Hospital

Sarah L. Berga, MD
University of Utah School of Medicine

Daniel H. Bessesen, MD
University of Colorado School of Medicine

Petter M. Bjornstad, MD
University of Colorado School of Medicine

Henry B. Burch, MD
National Institutes of Health

Marcelle I. Cedars, MD
University of California, San Francisco

Herbert Chen, MD
University of Alabama, Birmingham

Ellen L. Connor, MD
University of Wisconsin
American Family Children's Hospital

Marc-Andre Cornier, MD
University of Colorado School of Medicine

Wouter W. de Herder, MD, PhD
Erasmus Medical Center
Netherlands

Laura E. Dichtel, MD
Massachusetts General Hospital

William T. Donahoo, MD
University of Florida

Andrea Dunaif, MD
Icahn School of Medicine at Mount Sinai

Peter R. Ebeling, MD
Monash University
Australia

Robert Eckel, MD
University of Colorado Anschutz Medical Campus

Azeez Farooki, MD
Memorial Sloan Kettering Cancer Center

Sergio Fazio, MD, PhD
Oregon Health and Science University

Patricia Y. Fechner, MD
Seattle Children's Hospital

Kenneth Feingold, MD
University of California, San Francisco

James W. Findling, MD
Medical College of Wisconsin

Maria Fleseriu, MD
Oregon Health and Science University

Stephen Franks, MBBS, MD
Imperial College London
United Kingdom

Sheila M. Fraser, MBChB, MD
Leeds Teaching Hospitals NHS Trust
United Kingdom

Andrea Giustina, MD
San Raffaele Vita-Salute University
Italy

Jacqueline N. Gutmann, MD
RMA of Philadelphia
Thomas Jefferson University

Bryan Haugen, MD
University of Colorado School of Medicine

Camilo Jimenez, MD
University of Texas MD Anderson Cancer Center

Jacqueline Jonklaas, MD, PhD
Georgetown University Medical Center

Jens O. Jorgensen, MD, PhD
Aarhus University Hospital
Denmark

Laurence Katznelson, MD
Stanford University

Janice M. Kerr, MD
University of Colorado Health Science Center

Joanna Klubo-Gwiezdzinska, MD, PhD, MHSc
National Institutes of Health
National Institute of Diabetes and Digestive
    and Kidney Diseases

Helen M. Lawler, MD
University of Colorado, Denver

Kevin O. Lillehei, MD
University of Colorado Anschutz Medical Campus

Daria Lizneva, MD, PhD
Icahn School of Medicine at Mount Sinai

Naim Maalouf, MD
University of Texas Southwestern Medical Center

Susan J. Mandel, MD, MPH
Perelman School of Medicine
University of Pennsylvania

Michael Mannstadt, MD
Massachusetts General Hospital
Harvard Medical School

Sarah E. Mayson, MD
University of Colorado School of Medicine

Shlomo Melmed, MD
Cedars-Sinai Medical Center

Deborah P. Merke, MD, MS
National Institutes of Health

Mark E. Molitch, MD
Northwestern University
Feinberg Medical School

Lynnette K. Nieman, MD
National Institutes of Health

Asha Pathak, MD
Cedars-Sinai Medical Center

Anne Peters, MD
University of Southern California

Daniel A. Pryma, MD
University of Pennsylvania Perelman School of Medicine

Melissa S. Putman, MD
Boston Children's Hospital

Stephen M. Rosenthal, MD
University California, San Francisco

Micol S. Rothman, MD
University of Colorado, Denver

Joshua D. Safer, MD
Mount Sinai Health System
Icahn School of Medicine at Mount Sinai

Marzieh Salehi, MD, MS
University of Texas Health at San Antonio

Desmond Schatz, MD
University of Florida College of Medicine

Dolores M. Shoback, MD
University of California, San Francisco
VA Medical Center

Jennifer A. Sipos, MD
The Ohio State University

Julie A. Sosa, MD, MA
University of California, San Francisco

Robert C. Stanton, MD
Joslin Diabetes Center
Beth Israel Deaconess Medical Center
Harvard Medical School

Paul M. Stewart, MD
University of Leeds
United Kingdom

Cynthia A. Stuenkel, MD
University of California, San Diego

Dennis M. Styne, MD
University of California, Davis

Tamara J. Vokes, MD
University of Chicago

Steven G. Waguespack, MD
University of Texas MD Anderson Cancer Center

Nelson B. Watts, MD
Mercy Health

Kelly L. Wentworth, MD
University of California, San Francisco

Margaret E. Wierman, MD
University of Colorado School of Medicine

Michael W. Yeh, MD
University of California, Los Angeles

William F. Young, Jr., MD, MSc
Mayo Clinic

Philip S. Zeitler, MD, PhD
Children's Hospital Colorado
University of Colorado

ANNUAL MEETING STEERING COMMITTEE CLINICAL CHAIRS

Gregory A. Brent, MD, ENDO 2019 Chair
VA Greater LA Healthcare

Susan A. Sherman, MD, Clinical Practice Chair
Aurora Medical Associates, PC

Ghada El-Hajj Fuleihan, MD, MPH, Clinical Science Chair
American University of Beirut

Annual Meeting Steering Committee Clinical Peer Reviewers
Eliot Brinton, MD; Francesco S. Celi, MD; Mark S. Cooper, MD, PhD, FRCP, FRACP; Ann Danoff, MD; Dawn B. Davis, MD, PhD; Marie B. Demay, MD; Matthew T. Drake, MD, PhD; Maralyn R. Druce, MD, PhD; Richard A. Feelders, MD, PhD; Lauren M. Fishbein, MD, PhD; Larry A. Fox, MD; Megan R. Haymart, MD; Anders Juul, MD, PhD, DMSC; Bassil Kublaoui, MD; Margareta D. Pisarska, MD; Peter Kopp, MD; Nicola Napoli, MD, PhD; Sally Radovick, MD; Jennifer A. Sipos, MD; Adrian V. Vella, MD, FRCP; Selma F. Witchel, MD

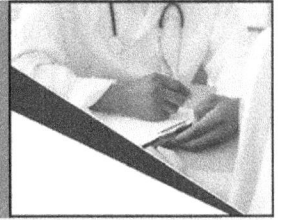

OVERVIEW

The *Meet-The-Professor Case Management* reference book is intended primarily for consultation relating to endocrinology. As a reference book, educational credits are not available. For information on educational products that include educational credit, please visit endocrine.org/store.

LEARNING OBJECTIVES

Meet-The-Professor Case Management will allow learners to assess their knowledge of all aspects of endocrinology, diabetes, and metabolism.

Upon completion of this educational activity, learners will be able to:

- Recognize clinical manifestations of endocrine and metabolic disorders and select among current options for diagnosis, management, and therapy.
- Identify risk factors for endocrine and metabolic disorders and develop strategies for prevention.
- Evaluate endocrine and metabolic manifestations of systemic disorders.
- Use existing resources pertaining to clinical guidelines and treatment recommendations for endocrine and related metabolic disorders to guide diagnosis and treatment.

TARGET AUDIENCE

Meet-The-Professor Case Management provides case-based education to clinicians interested in improving patient care.

STATEMENT OF INDEPENDENCE

The Endocrine Society has a policy of ensuring that the content and quality of this educational activity are balanced, independent, objective, and scientifically rigorous. The scientific content of this activity was developed under the supervision of the Endocrine Society's Annual Meeting Steering Committee.

DISCLOSURE POLICY

The faculty, committee members, and staff who are in position to control the content of this activity are required to disclose to the Endocrine Society and to learners any relevant financial relationship(s) of the individual or spouse/partner that have occurred within the last 12 months with any commercial interest(s) whose products or services are related to the content. Financial relationships are defined by remuneration in any amount from the commercial interest(s) in the form of grants; research support; consulting fees; salary; ownership interest (eg, stocks, stock options, or ownership interest excluding diversified mutual funds); honoraria or other payments for participation in speakers' bureaus, advisory boards, or boards of directors; or other financial benefits. The intent of this disclosure is not to prevent planners with relevant financial relationships from planning or delivering content, but rather to provide learners with information that allows them to make their own judgments of whether these financial relationships may have influenced the educational activity with regard to exposition or conclusion. The Endocrine Society has reviewed all disclosures and resolved or managed all identified conflicts of interest, as applicable.

The following faculty reported relevant financial relationship(s) as of January 1, 2019: The following faculty reported relevant financial relationships, as identified below: **Bradley D. Anawalt, MD**, Other; Self; Up to Date Author. **Wiebke Arlt, MD, DSc**, Consulting Fee; Self; Diurnal, Spruce Bioscience, Consultant. Research Investigator; Self; Diurnal, Research Investigator (PI) for clinical studies. **Richard J. Auchus, MD, PhD**, Consulting Fee; Self; US Anti-Doping Agency. **Ricardo Azziz, MD, MPH, MBA**, Consulting Fee; Self; Medtronic Minimed, Fractyl Laboratories, Up to Date, Ansh labs, Latitude Capital. Grant Recipient; Self; Ferring Pharmaceuticals. Stock Owner; Self; Global (Martin) PET Imaging. **Andrew J. Bauer, MD**, Advisory Board Member; Self; IBSA Pharma Inc. **Carolyn B. Becker, MD**, Other; Self; Up to Date. **Sarah L. Berga, MD**, Advisory Board Member; Self; AMAG. Research Investigator; Self; Ferring Pharmaceuticals. Other; Self; Salem Academy and College, Up to Date. **Daniel H. Bessesen, MD**, Other; Self; Enteromedics. **Petter M. Bjornstad, MD**, Speaker; Self; Horizon Pharma. Other; Self; Boehringer Ingelheim. **Marcelle I. Cedars, MD**, Research Funding; Self; Ferring Pharmaceuticals. **Marc-Andre Cornier, MD**, Grant Recipient; Self; Regeneron Pharmaceuticals. **Wouter W. de Herder, MD, PhD**, Advisory Board Member; Self; Novartis Pharmaceuticals, Ipsen. Grant Recipient; Self; Ipsen. **Peter R. Ebeling, MD**, Advisory Board Member; Self; Amgen Inc, Alexion Pharmaceuticals, Inc. Grant Recipient; Self; Amgen Inc, Eli Lilly & Company, Novartis Pharmaceuticals, Alexion Pharmaceuticals, Inc. Speaker; Self; Amgen Inc, Eli Lilly & Company. **Robert Eckel, MD**, Advisory Board Member; Self; Sanofi-Aventis, Regeneron Pharmaceuticals, Merck, Novo Nordisk. **Azeez Farooki, MD**, Consultant; Self; Amgen. **Sergio Fazio, MD, PhD**, Consulting Fee; Self; Kowa, Akcea Therapeutics, Amgen Inc, Aegerion Pharmaceuticals. **Kenneth Feingold, MD**, Advisory Board Member; Self; Regeneron Pharmaceuticals, Amarin. Speaker; Self; Merck & Co., Regeneron Pharmaceuticals, Sanofi. **Andrea Giustina, MD**, Consulting Fee; Self; Ipsen, Novartis Pharmaceuticals, Pfizer, Inc. **Jens O Jorgensen, MD, PhD**, Advisory Board Member; Self; Pfizer, Inc., Novo Nordisk, Ipsen. Grant Recipient; Self; Merck, Novartis Pharmaceuticals. Research Investigator; Self; Pfizer, Inc.. Speaker; Self; Novartis Pharmaceuticals, Ipsen, Pfizer, Inc., Sandoz. **Laurence Katznelson, MD**, Advisory Board Member; Self; Pfizer, Inc. Research Investigator; Self; Novartis Pharmaceuticals. **Helen M. Lawler, MD**, Consulting Fee; Self; Decision Resources Group Consulting. Research Investigator; Self; XOMA, Eiger BioPharmaceuticals, Xeris Pharmaceuticals,Inc. **Michael Mannstadt, MD**, Advisory Board Member; Self; Shire. Consulting Fee; Self; Ascendis. Employee; Spouse; Radius Health, Inc. **Sarah E. Mayson, MD**, Research Investigator; Self; Rosetta

Genomics, CBLPath. **Mark E. Molitch, MD**, Advisory Board Member; Self; Sanofi. Consulting Fee; Self; Merck, Pfizer, Inc.. Grant Recipient; Self; Bayer, Inc., Novartis Pharmaceuticals, Jansen Pharmaceuticals. **Lynnette K. Nieman, MD**, Research Investigator; Self; HRA Pharmaceuticals. **Anne Peters, MD**, Advisory Board Member; Self; Abbott Laboratories, Eli Lilly & Company, Lexicon Pharmaceuticals, Inc., Mannkind Corporation, Merck, Novo Nordisk, Sanofi. Grant Recipient; Self; AstraZeneca, Mannkind Corporation, Dexcom. Speaker; Self; Novo Nordisk. **Daniel A. Pryma, MD**, Advisory Board Member; Self; 511 Pharma. Consulting Fee; Self; Progenics, Actinium Pharmaceuticals, Nordic nanovector. Research Investigator; Self; Siemens, Progenics, 511 Pharma. **Stephen M. Rosenthal, MD**, Advisory Board Member; Self; Endo Pharmaceuticals. **Joshua D. Safer, MD**, Advisory Board Member; Self; Endo Pharmaceuticals. Employee; Spouse; Parexel. **Julie A. Sosa, MD, MA**, Other; Self; Member, Data Monitoring Committee of the Medullary Thyroid Cancer Consortium Registry supported by GlaxoSmithKline, Novo Nordisk, Astra Zeneca, Eli Lilly. **Robert C. Stanton, MD**, Advisory Board Member; Self; Jansen Pharmaceuticals, Global Renal Advisory Board. **Tamara J. Vokes, MD**, Advisory Board Member; Self; Radius Health, Inc, Shire. Consulting Fee; Self; Radius Health, Inc, Shire. Research Investigator; Self; Radius Health, Inc, Shire. Speaker; Self; Radius Health, Inc, Shire. **Nelson B. Watts, MD**, Advisory Board Member; Self; Amgen Inc, Amgen. Consulting Fee; Self; Abbvie, Sanofi. Speaker; Self; Amgen Inc, Radius Health, Inc. **Philip S. Zeitler, MD, PhD**, Consulting Fee; Self; Merck, Novo Nordisk, Boehringer Ingelheim, Janssen Research & Development Company.

The following faculty reported no relevant financial relationships as of January 1, 2019: **Jasna Aleksova, MBBS, BMedSci; Katherine Araque, MD; Linda A. Barbour, MSPH, MD; Henry B. Burch, MD; Herbert Chen, MD; Ellen L. Connor, MD; Laura E. Dichtel, MD; William T. Donahoo, MD; Andrea Dunaif, MD; Patricia Y. Fechner, MD; James W. Findling, MD; Maria Fleseriu, MD; Stephen Franks, MBBS, MD; Sheila M. Fraser, MBChB, MD; Jacqueline N. Gutmann, MD; Bryan Haugen, MD; Camilo Jimenez, MD; Jacqueline Jonklaas, MD, PhD; Janice M. Kerr, MD; Joanna Klubo-Gwiezdzinska, MD, PhD, MHSc; Kevin O. Lillehei, MD; Daria Lizneva, MD, PhD; Naim Maalouf, MD; Susan J. Mandel, MD, MPH; Asha Pathak, MD; Melissa S. Putman, MD; Micol S. Rothman, MD; Marzieh Salehi, MD, MS; Desmond Schatz, MD; Dolores M. Shoback, MD; Jennifer A. Sipos, MD; Paul M. Stewart, MD; Cynthia A. Stuenkel, MD; Dennis M. Styne, MD; Steven G. Waguespack, MD; Kelly L. Wentworth, MD; Margaret E. Wierman, MD; Michael W. Yeh, MD; William F. Young, Jr., MD, MSc.**

The following AMSC peer reviewers reported relevant financial relationship(s) as of January 1, 2019: **Eliot Brinton, MD**, Advisor and Speaker: Akcea, Amarin, Amgen, Kowa, Merck, Regeneron, Sanofi-Aventis and an Advisor, Balchem, PTS Diagnostics; Speaker, Boehringer-Ingelheim, Novo Nordisk. **Francesco S. Celi, MD, MHSc**, Advisory Board Member, LioTriDev, IBSA. **Dawn B. Davis, MD, PhD**, Site PI for clinical trial, Eiger Pharmaceuticals. **Marie B. Demay, MD**, (Spouse) CMO - Syros Pharmaceuticals. **Maralyn R. Druce, MD, PhD**, Advisory Board Member – Specific Consultations, Ipsen. **Richard A. Feelders, MD, PhD**, Research Grant Recipient, Novartis, Ipsen. **Anders Juul, MD, PhD, DMSC**, Speakers Bureau, Novo Nordisk, Pfizer, Ferring, Merck, Bayer, Sponsor and PI of a clinical multicenter trial (NESGAS), Department research grant, Ferring, Department funding to participate in the clinical trial (PORIYA), Co-

investigator in a Ferring-sponsored clinical trial, Department grantee, Diurnal, and Principal investigator for participation in a multicenter study (RCT) on long-acting hydrocortisone (Chronocort) in CAH. **Nicola Napoli, MD, PhD**, European Advisory Board Member, UCB, Eli Lilly, Consultant, Amgen, Lilly. **Sally Radovick, MD**, Consultant regarding GH Treatment, CVS Caremark; retail pharmacy and health care company. **Jennifer A. Sipos, MD**, Advisory Board Consultant and Speaker, Genzyme. **Adrian V. Vella, MD, FRCP**, Principal Investigator, Novo Nordisk, Investigator, XOMA (multi-center study), Member of Advisory Board, VTV Therapeutics, Bristol Myers Squibb.

The following AMSC peer reviewers reported no relevant financial relationships as of January 1, 2019: **Gregory A. Brent, MD; Mark S. Cooper, MD, PhD; Ann Danoff, MD; Matthew T. Drake, MD, PhD; Ghada El-Hajj Fuleihan, MD, MPH; Lauren M. Fishbein, MD, PhD; Larry A. Fox, MD; Megan R. Haymart, MD; Peter Kopp, MD; Bassil Kublaoui, MD, PhD; Margareta D. Pisarska, MD; Susan A. Sherman, MD; Selma F. Witchel, MD.**

The Endocrine Society staff associated with the development of content for this activity reported no relevant financial relationships.

DISCLAIMERS

The information presented in this activity represents the opinion of the faculty and is not necessarily the official position of the Endocrine Society.

USE OF PROFESSIONAL JUDGMENT:

The educational content in this enduring activity relates to basic principles of diagnosis and therapy and does not substitute for individual patient assessment based on the health care provider's examination of the patient and consideration of laboratory data and other factors unique to the patient. Standards in medicine change as new data become available.

DRUGS AND DOSAGES:

When prescribing medications, the physician is advised to check the product information sheet accompanying each drug to verify conditions of use and to identify any changes in drug dosage schedule or contraindications.

POLICY ON UNLABELED/OFF-LABEL USE

The Endocrine Society has determined that disclosure of unlabeled/off-label or investigational use of commercial product(s) is informative for audiences and therefore requires this information to be disclosed to the learners at the beginning of the presentation. Uses of specific therapeutic agents, devices, and other products discussed in this educational activity may not be the same as those indicated in product labeling approved by the Food and Drug Administration (FDA). The Endocrine Society requires that any discussions of such "off-label" use be based on scientific research that conforms to generally accepted standards of experimental design, data collection, and data analysis. Before recommending or prescribing any therapeutic agent or device, learners should review the complete prescribing information, including indications, contraindications, warnings, precautions, and adverse events.

ACKNOWLEDGMENT OF COMMERCIAL SUPPORT

PUBLICATION DATE: February 2019

This activity is not supported by an educational grant or other funds from any commercial supporter.

ENDO 2019
TOPIC INDEX

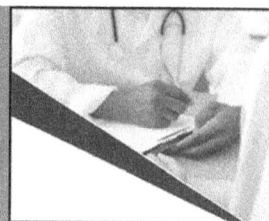

ADIPOSE TISSUE, APPETITE, AND OBESITY

ADRENAL

BONE AND MINERAL METABOLISM

CARDIOVASCULAR ENDOCRINOLOGY

DIABETES MELLITUS AND GLUCOSE METABOLISM

NEUROENDOCRINOLOGY AND PITUITARY

PEDIATRIC ENDOCRINOLOGY

REPRODUCTIVE ENDOCRINOLOGY

THYROID

MISCELLANEOUS

ENDO 2019
SPEAKER HANDOUT INDEX

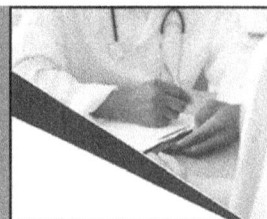

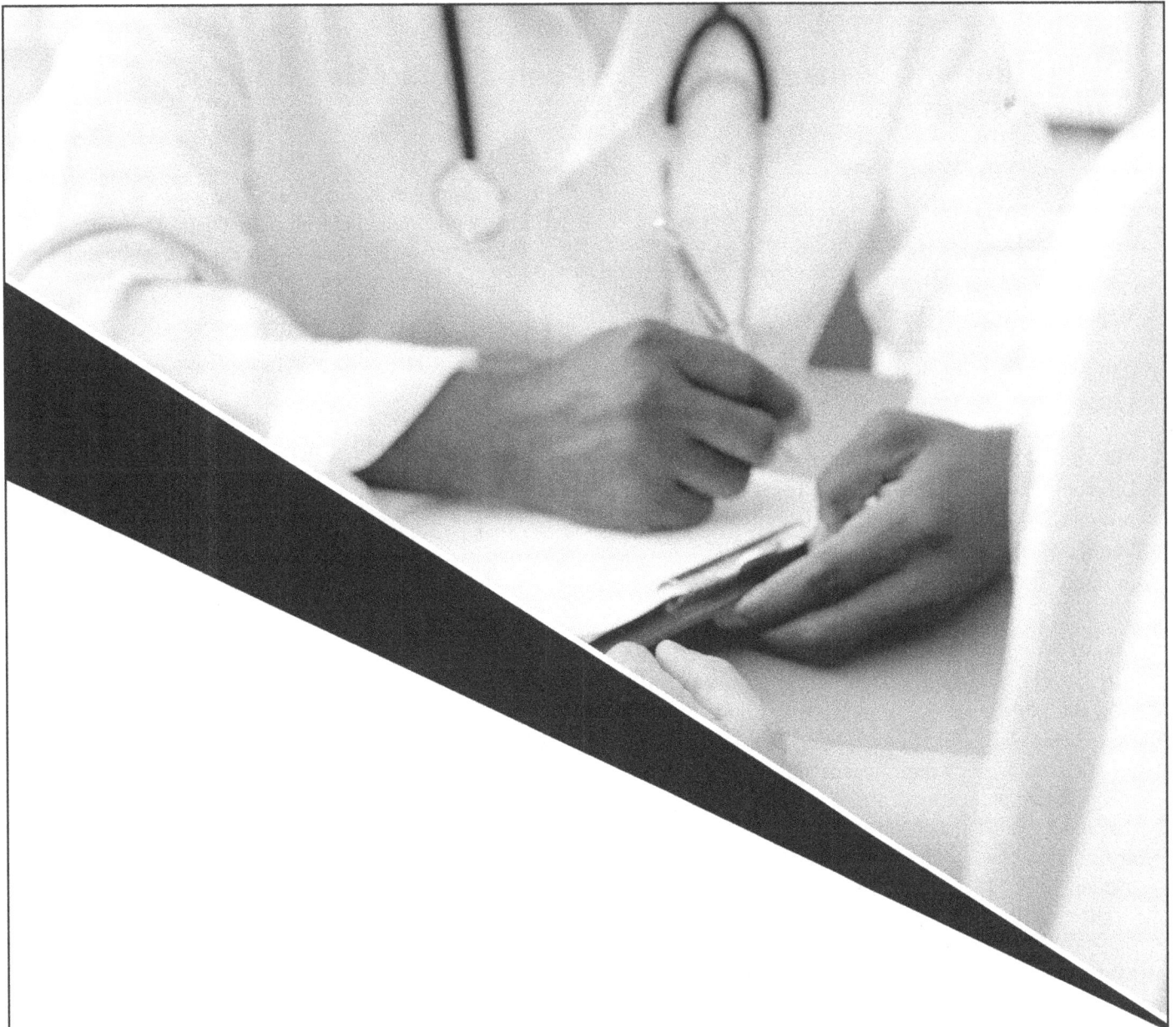

ADIPOSE TISSUE, APPETITE, AND OBESITY

Evaluation and Management of Hypoglycemia After Gastric Bypass Surgery

M01
Presented, March 23–26, 2019

Helen M. Lawler, MD. Department of Medicine, Division of Endocrinology, Metabolism, and Diabetes, University of Colorado School of Medicine, Aurora, Colorado 80045, E-mail: helen.lawler@ucdenver.edu

Marzieh Salehi, MD, MS. Department of Medicine, Division of Diabetes, University of Texas Health at San Antonio, San Antonio, Texas 78229; and South Texas Veteran Health Care System, Audie Murphy Hospital, San Antonio, Texas 78229, E-mail: salehi@uthscsa.edu

SIGNIFICANCE OF THE CLINICAL PROBLEM

Bariatric surgery induces a robust and durable weight loss and improves glucose tolerance in patients with type 2 diabetes (1). Altered glucose metabolism after Roux-en-Y gastric bypass (RYGB) surgery is partly independent of weight loss. With the increased popularity of RYGB, it has become recognized that a subgroup of individuals develop postprandial hypoglycemia associated with augmented insulin and glucagon-like peptide 1 (GLP-1) secretion several years after RYGB (2, 3).

The exact prevalence of this devastating late complication of RYGB is unknown and probably underreported. Evidence suggests that the rate of hospitalization due to hypoglycemia or its surrogates (syncope and seizure) is higher by twofold to sevenfold in patients with RYGB compared with the general population; however, the overall reported incidence is relatively small (<1%) (4, 5). Affected individuals have a substantial decline in quality of life due to inability to maintain employment, drive, and perform their daily routines. Thus, it is critical to correctly diagnose hypoglycemia after RYGB and offer available treatment options. Hypoglycemia has also been reported after sleeve gastrectomy, but the prevalence and glucose profile characteristics for this condition are largely unknown. In this section, we focus on RYGB-related hypoglycemia [postbariatric hypoglycemia (PBH)].

BARRIERS TO OPTIMAL PRACTICE

- Public and medical community awareness of this condition is lacking. Many patients with PBH do not associate their symptoms with RYGB, leading to several years of delay in diagnosis.
- Diagnosis of PBH is complex and requires documentation of Whipple's triad to differentiate this condition from asymptomatic hypoglycemia or postprandial symptoms caused by dumping with normal glucose levels.
- Current available therapies are limited and unlikely to eliminate hypoglycemia in severe cases of PBH.

LEARNING OBJECTIVES

As a result of participating in this session, learners should be able to:
- Recognize how to diagnose PBH
- Differentiate PBH from other etiologies causing hypoglycemia
- Learn mechanisms involved in the development of PBH
- Understand the current therapeutic options for treating this condition

STRATEGIES FOR DIAGNOSIS, THERAPY, AND/OR MANAGEMENT

Hypoglycemia is defined as low glucose levels (whole blood glucose < 50 mg/dL and plasma glucose < 54 mg/dL) associated with hypoglycemic symptoms that are relieved shortly after carbohydrate administration (Whipple's triad) (6–8). Hypoglycemic symptoms are categorized into those initiated by glucose deprivation of the central nervous system (neuroglycopenic) or activation of the autonomic nervous system (autonomic). Neuroglycopenic symptoms include impaired cognitive function, confusion, slurred speech, seizure, and loss of consciousness. Autonomic symptoms manifest as shakiness, palpitation, anxiety, sweating, hunger, and paresthesia. Hypoglycemia after RYGB is exclusively postprandial (1 to 3 hours) and manifests at least 6 to 12 months after surgery, unlike postprandial symptoms caused by dumping syndrome, which develop at the time of reinstatement of regular food immediately after surgery. Accordingly, confirmation of Whipple's triad is critical to differentiating PBH from conditions such as postprandial symptoms consistent with hypoglycemia associated with normal glucose (dumping) or those with asymptomatic low blood glucose levels (7–9).

Therefore, history and physical examination remain an essential part of evaluation. Detailed records of symptoms, diet, and activity provide important information regarding the severity and relationship to fasting and food intake. If the onset of hypoglycemia occurs <6 months after surgery, the patient is ill appearing, or fasting hypoglycemia is present, other causes of hypoglycemia such as insulinoma, hormone deficiencies, critical illness, malnutrition, medication side effect, autoimmune hypoglycemia, and non–islet cell tumors should be evaluated (Fig. 1) (8).

Documenting Whipple's triad with self-monitoring of blood glucose during symptoms is recommended. However, if this is not obtainable, a provocative test of a mixed meal containing

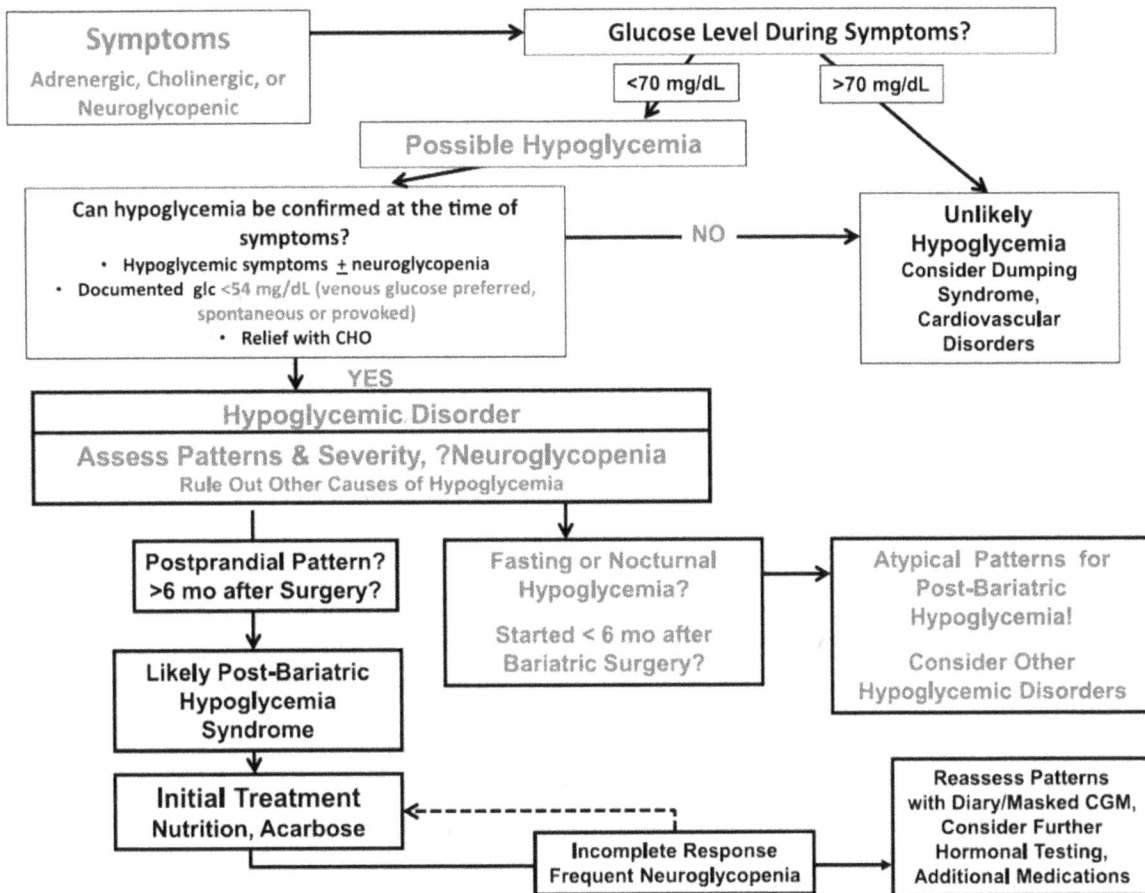

Figure 1. Suggested evaluation and treatment of PBH. Reproduced with permission from Salehi M, Vella A, McLaughlin T, Patti ME. Hypoglycemia after gastric bypass surgery: current concepts and controversies. *J Clin Endocrinol Metab.* 2018;103:2815–2826.

protein, fat, and carbohydrate can be performed to confirm hypoglycemia. Although various test meals have been used without being standardized regarding texture or energy distribution, there is no indication to use an oral glucose tolerance test to evaluate postprandial hypoglycemia in surgical or nonsurgical individuals. Continuous glucose monitoring can provide information regarding patterns of glucose excursion (both peak and nadir levels) in a free-living setting, although the sensitivity of detecting hypoglycemia is not optimal (9).

Although the underlying pathophysiology of PBH is not completely understood, changes in glucose tolerance in patients with RYGB have been attributed to rapid appearance of ingested glucose into circulation associated with greater secretion of insulin and insulinotropic gut peptide, GLP-1 (Fig. 2) (8). Patients with post-RYGB hypoglycemia have greater insulin and GLP-1 secretion along with more enhanced systemic glucose appearance compared with those without hypoglycemia after RYGB (10). Blocking the GLP-1 receptor has been shown to correct hypoglycemia during meal studies in affected subjects (10, 11). Evidence also indicates that postprandial hyperinsulinemia in patients with post-RYGB hypoglycemia is partly attributed to lower insulin clearance as well as diminished β-cell secretory suppression during

hypoglycemia. Moreover, affected patients have an impaired counter-regulatory response, such as glucagon response to hypoglycemia (12).

Because rapid nutrient transit time from bypassing the foregut is the culprit, the main goal of treatment, to date, is to reduce postprandial glucose appearance. Dietary modification remains the cornerstone of treatment of PBH; data regarding the effectiveness of recommended options are based on case reports rather than well-designed studies (Fig. 3) (8). The goal of dietary modification is to lessen glycemic peaks and subsequent insulin surges by avoiding simple carbohydrates and high glycemic index foods as well as adding protein and fat to every meal and snack where complex carbohydrates are limited to 30 and 15 g, respectively (8). In addition to reducing carbohydrate intake, manipulation of carbohydrate composition (*e.g.,* using fructose instead of nonfructose carbohydrates) has been shown to narrow glucose excursion and prevent hypoglycemia in patients with PBH (13). Uncooked starch has also been used to prevent hypoglycemia in this population based on findings from studies in nonsurgical patients with diabetes (14).

To treat hypoglycemia, oral carbohydrates (10 to 15 g) are recommended. Based on anecdotal observation, many patients use complex carbohydrates or a combination of glucose mixed

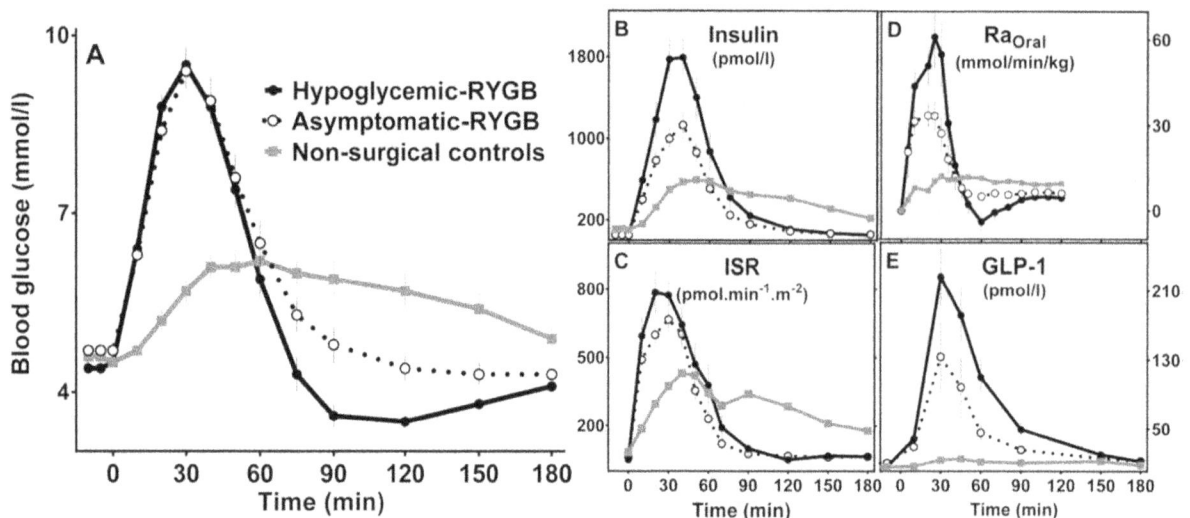

Figure 2. Glycemic and hormonal patterns during fasting and after a mixed meal tolerance test. (A) Blood glucose, (B) plasma insulin, and (C) insulin secretory response (ISR) to meal ingestion. (D) Systemic appearance of ingested glucose (Ra$_{Oral}$) and (E) circulating GLP-1 levels during mixed meal in RYGB subjects with (black ● and solid line) and without (black ○ and dashed line) hypoglycemia and nonsurgical controls (gray ■ and solid line). Panels A–C reproduced with permission from Salehi M, Gastaldelli A, D'Alessio DA. Altered islet function and insulin clearance cause hyperinsulinemia in gastric bypass patients with symptoms of postprandial hypoglycemia. _J Clin Endocrinol Metab._ 2014;99:2008–2017. Panels D and E adapted with permission from Salehi M, Gastaldelli A, D'Alessio DA. Blockade of glucagon-like peptide 1 receptor corrects postprandial hypoglycemia after gastric bypass. _Gastroenterology._ 2014;146:669–680.

with fat and protein rather than glucose tablets to avoid rebound hypoglycemia (yo-yo effect) (8). Yet, for episodes occurring after acarbose intake, glucose tablets are recommended (4). Patients are encouraged to always have a glucometer and rescue therapy on hand. A glucagon prescription is also provided; in severe neuroglycopenia when oral glucose intake is not feasible, glucagon administration is recommended (9).

Currently, there is no FDA-approved pharmacotherapy for PBH. Acarbose, an α-glucosidase inhibitor, inhibits carbohydrate absorption and is recommended as part of initial treatment along with dietary modification or as the next step

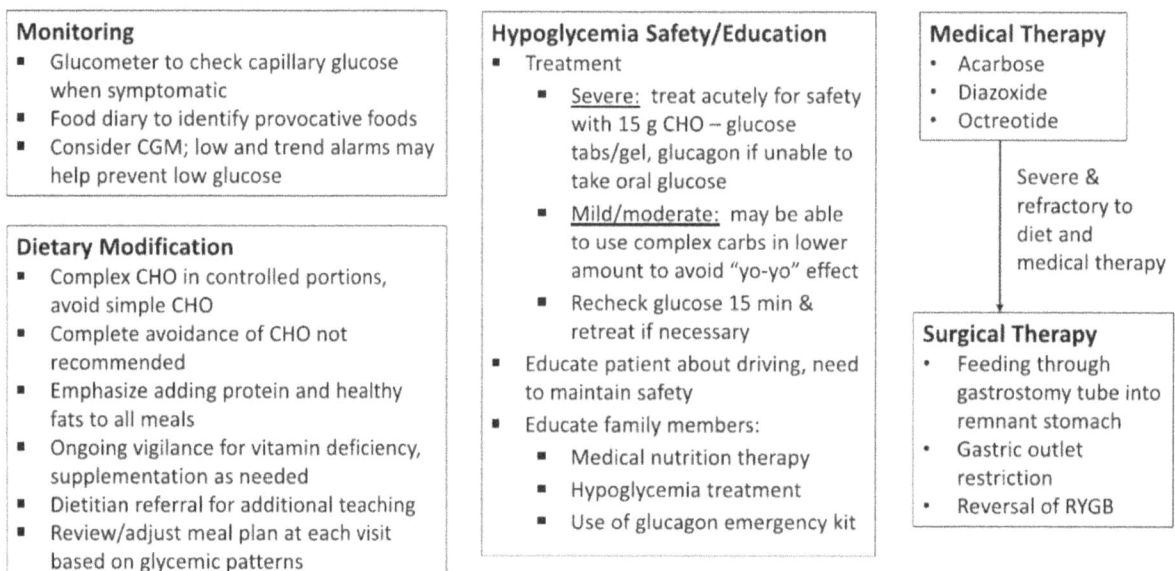

Monitoring
- Glucometer to check capillary glucose when symptomatic
- Food diary to identify provocative foods
- Consider CGM; low and trend alarms may help prevent low glucose

Dietary Modification
- Complex CHO in controlled portions, avoid simple CHO
- Complete avoidance of CHO not recommended
- Emphasize adding protein and healthy fats to all meals
- Ongoing vigilance for vitamin deficiency, supplementation as needed
- Dietitian referral for additional teaching
- Review/adjust meal plan at each visit based on glycemic patterns

Hypoglycemia Safety/Education
- Treatment
  - Severe: treat acutely for safety with 15 g CHO – glucose tabs/gel, glucagon if unable to take oral glucose
  - Mild/moderate: may be able to use complex carbs in lower amount to avoid "yo-yo" effect
  - Recheck glucose 15 min & retreat if necessary
- Educate patient about driving, need to maintain safety
- Educate family members:
  - Medical nutrition therapy
  - Hypoglycemia treatment
  - Use of glucagon emergency kit

Medical Therapy
- Acarbose
- Diazoxide
- Octreotide

Severe & refractory to diet and medical therapy

Surgical Therapy
- Feeding through gastrostomy tube into remnant stomach
- Gastric outlet restriction
- Reversal of RYGB

Figure 3. To date, recommended approach to treating PBH. Reproduced with permission from Salehi M, Vella A, McLaughlin T, Patti ME. Hypoglycemia after gastric bypass surgery: current concepts and controversies. _J Clin Endocrinol Metab._ 2018;103:2815–2826.

for patients with PBH for whom dietary modification alone has failed (1). Gastrointestinal side effects are common where slow up-titration to assist with tolerance is recommended. Acarbose 25 mg before carbohydrate-containing meals daily can slowly be increased to a maximum dose of 100 mg with three to four meals daily (2). In patients for whom acarbose fails, small studies have shown efficacy in treating PBH with somatostatin analogs because binding to somatostatin receptor subtypes 2 and 5 reduces insulin and GLP-1 secretion. Octreotide is initiated at 25 to 50 μg subcutaneously before meals. Side effects (*e.g.*, diarrhea, bile stone formation, and QT prolongation) and high cost are limiting factors (10). Case reports have also shown efficacy of diazoxide 50 to 100 mg twice daily in treating PBH. Diazoxide inhibits insulin release by opening adenosine triphosphate–sensitive potassium channels of pancreatic β-cells. Side effects include hyperglycemia, headaches, edema, fluid retention, hirsutism, and hypotension (7). In addition, case reports with small numbers of patients indicated a reduction in hypoglycemia due to PBH with calcium channel blockers and GLP-1 agonists. Clinical trials investigating the safety and durability of preventing hypoglycemia with a GLP-1 receptor antagonist, exendin-(9-39), are underway (11). The use of glucagon delivered via a pump based on sensor glucose data from a continuous glucose monitor is also being investigated as a potential treatment of PBH (12).

Some surgical interventions have been tried for treatment of patients with severe PBH for whom dietary modification and pharmacotherapy have failed (8). Placement of a gastrostomy tube into the remnant stomach aiming for reversing nutrient transport to the presurgical state, have been used to narrow glucose excursion in these individuals. Tube feeds are given continuously, overnight, or via bolus with no oral intake of carbohydrates, although oral intake of protein and fats are permitted. Long-term effectiveness of this intervention is not known, and patients are often reluctant to commit to permanent tubes given reduced quality of life. A small study showed that slowing the rapid nutrient transport by surgical restoration of gastric restriction improved PBH; however, acid reflux and nausea are potential side effects. In severe cases of PBH, gastric bypass reversal may be pursued; however, hypoglycemia may persist and weight regain may occur. Complete or distal pancreatectomy has fallen out of favor due to high morbidity and lack of resolution or recurrence of hypoglycemia.

MAIN CONCLUSIONS
- PBH is defined as postprandial neuroglycopenia with documented plasma glucose < 54 mg/dL (whole blood glucose < 50 mg/dL) occurring at least 6 to 12 months after bariatric surgery. Whipple's triad must be confirmed.
- Fasting hypoglycemia is atypical in PBH, and if present, other possible etiologies of hypoglycemia should be considered and evaluated.

- To date, the foremost part of treating PBH is dietary modification with elimination of simple carbohydrates and addition of fat and protein to all meals and snacks.
- Acarbose is recommended as initial pharmacotherapy in addition to dietary modification or as the next step for those for whom dietary modification alone has failed.
- Surgical options include tube feeds through a gastrostomy tube into the remnant stomach, surgical restoration of gastric restriction, and gastric bypass reversal. Distal or complete pancreatectomy is no longer recommended.

CASES AND DISCUSSION
Case 1
A 42-year-old well-appearing woman who underwent a laparoscopic RYGB 3 years ago for a body mass index of 45 kg/m^2 and maximum weight of 305 lbs presents with new onset of episodes of slurred speech, confusion, headache, and diaphoresis occurring approximately 2 to 3 hours after eating. She has experienced three episodes weekly over the last 2 months. She denies fasting symptoms.

Question 1
What is the initial step in evaluation?
- A. Order a 72-hour inpatient fast
- B. Rule out pheochromocytoma
- C. Confirm Whipple's triad
- D. Place a referral for her to see a neurologist

Question 2
The patient was given a glucometer and has documented hypoglycemic symptoms, both autonomic and neuroglycopenic, associated with capillary glucose values ranging from 60 to 70 mg/dL, occurring 1 to 3 hours postprandially. What is the next step?
- A. Order a 72-hour inpatient fast
- B. Order an 8:00 AM cortisol level
- C. Order an oral glucose tolerance test
- D. Order a mixed meal test

Question 3
During a mixed meal study, her plasma glucose dropped to 50 mg/dL in 90 minutes and was associated with palpitations, weakness, drowsiness, and some blurred vision. What would be the best option to treat her along with rechecking her glucose in 15 minutes?
- A. Fifteen grams oral carbohydrate (such as peanut butter crackers or glucose tablet/gel)
- B. Fifty grams oral carbohydrate (glucose tabs/gel)
- C. Intravenous infusion of dextrose 50%
- D. Wait and do nothing

Question 4
What treatment options would you recommend?
- A. Acarbose

B. Dietary modification
C. Neither
D. Both

Answers
Question 1 (Answer C)
While obtaining patient history, it is important to collect information regarding timing of symptoms in relation to food consumption. The patient should be given a glucometer to check blood glucose levels when neuroglycopenic symptoms occur. Documentation of symptoms, glucose values, and timing and the type of food consumed in a patient diary can help clarify the diagnosis and identify prandial status. It is critical to initially confirm Whipple's triad (low plasma glucose associated with hypoglycemic symptoms resolving after carbohydrate ingestion).

Question 2 (Answer D)
It is often not practical to obtain documentation of Whipple's triad during free living or clinic visits. Thus, provocation testing using mixed meal can be used if feasible. An oral glucose tolerance test has no role in evaluating postprandial hypoglycemia. Oral glucose ingestion after RYGB elicits postprandial symptoms related to dumping. Also, evidence suggests that 10% of normal healthy individuals without previous gastrointestinal surgeries develop glucose levels < 50 mg/dL during an oral glucose tolerance test. Although the significance of asymptomatic hypoglycemia during glucose ingestion is not understood, the likelihood of developing this condition during an oral glucose tolerance test should be much greater in those with a bypassed foregut. Mixed meal tests, with various carbohydrate amounts from 40 to 75 g, have been used in different clinical settings. If fasting hypoglycemia is present, adrenal insufficiency should be ruled out with an 8:00 AM cortisol level, and a 72-hour inpatient fast should be arranged to evaluate for an insulinoma. Other causes of hypoglycemia to consider, if atypical symptoms are present or if the patient is ill appearing, include critical illness, malnutrition, non–islet cell tumors, autoimmune hypoglycemia, and hypoglycemia due to a medication side effect.

Question 3 (Answer A)
When patients develop hypoglycemia, administration of oral carbohydrate 10 to 15 g with or without fat/protein is recommended. A high dose of oral carbohydrate will produce a glucose yo-yo effect leading to rebound hypoglycemia; therefore, it is recommended that treatment be initiated with a small amount of carbohydrate and repeated if needed based on rechecked glucose level.

Question 4 (Answer D)
Dietary modification is recommended as the cornerstone for treating PBH. Patients should avoid simple carbohydrates and high glycemic index foods including white bread, pineapple, bagels, *etc.* Complex carbohydrates are advised to be limited to ≤30 g per meal and ≤15 g per snack and should be consumed with protein and/or a healthy fat. Patients are also reminded to not drink fluids with meals, chew thoroughly, and eat slowly because this may help slow nutrient transport. Also, acarbose can be started with dietary modification at 25 mg before each meal and gradually titrated to the maximum dose of 100 mg before each meal up to four times daily.

Case 2
A 35-year-old woman was hospitalized after a syncopal episode while shopping at the grocery store. She was found with a blood glucose level of 40 mg/dL by emergency medical services, and treatment with glucose infusion resolved her symptoms immediately. History indicated that she had RYGB 6 months ago without any complications. She has lost approximately 100 lbs since surgery, but she appears to be well without any other pertinent findings on examination. Her pregnancy test is negative.

Question 1
What will you do next?
    A. Perform a mixed meal test
    B. Order a 72-hour inpatient fast
    C. Carefully review medications
    D. Evaluate cortisol axis activity
    E. All of the above

Answer
Question 1 (Answer E)
Albeit rare, fasting hypoglycemia caused by insulinoma or other etiologies has been reported after bariatric surgery. In a well-appearing patient with dominant fasting hypoglycemia (occurring >5 hours after previous meal ingestion), which manifests within the first 6 to 12 months after surgery, insulinoma should be excluded (15) in addition to carefully evaluating medications and conditions contributing to hypoglycemia. Lack of information about fasting vs prandial hypoglycemia in this patient also warrants evaluation of prandial glucose to check for any possible postprandial glucose abnormalities.

Case 3
A 53-year-old woman underwent laparoscopic RYGB 4 years ago for a body mass index of 40 kg/m^2 and a maximum weight of 290 lbs. She was diagnosed with PBH 3 months ago based on Whipple's triad criteria. She met with a nutritionist and has eliminated high-glycemic foods from her diet, limited complex carbohydrates to 30 g per meal, and added protein and fat to all meals. She could not tolerate taking >25 mg acarbose once or twice daily. She continued to experience hypoglycemia, with neuroglycopenic symptoms occurring 1 to 2 hours after meals, approximately four to five times per week.

Question 1
What is the next available therapeutic option?
    A. Advise that she eliminate all carbohydrates from her diet
    B. Stop acarbose and start diazoxide

C. Stop acarbose and start octreotide

D. Either B or C

Question 2

She would like to try octreotide, which was initiated at 25 μg subcutaneously before meals. What electrocardiographic abnormality has been seen with this drug?

A. A short PR interval

B. An Osborne wave

C. Prolonged QRS complex

D. QT prolongation

Question 3

She continues to have debilitating episodes of neuroglycopenia despite dietary adherence and attempted pharmacotherapy (treatment with acarbose, octreotide, and diazoxide failed). She is interested in surgical options for treating her PBH. What option should not be considered?

A. Placement of a feeding gastrostomy tube into the remnant stomach

B. Surgical restoration of gastric restriction

C. Reversal of the gastric bypass

D. Distal or partial pancreatectomy

Answers

Question 1 (Answer D)

Eliminating all carbohydrates is not advisable because hypoglycemia may worsen due to decreased glycogen stores and a potential diminished glucagon response. Diazoxide or octreotide can be considered as next steps in the treatment of PBH.

Question 2 (Answer D)

Somatostatin analog therapy can cause QT prolongation. An electrocardiogram may be obtained at baseline before initiating therapy and during therapy for monitoring, if indicated.

Question 3 (Answer D)

Options include placement of a feeding gastrostomy tube into the remnant stomach, surgical restoration of gastric restriction, and reversal of the gastric bypass. Distal or partial pancreatectomy is no longer recommended due to high morbidity risk and lack of effectiveness.

References

1. Schauer PR, Bhatt DL, Kashyap SR. Bariatric surgery or intensive medical therapy for diabetes after 5 years. *N Engl J Med.* 2017; **376**(20):1997.

2. Goldfine AB, Mun EC, Devine E, Bernier R, Baz-Hecht M, Jones DB, Schneider BE, Holst JJ, Patti ME. Patients with neuroglycopenia after gastric bypass surgery have exaggerated incretin and insulin secretory responses to a mixed meal. *J Clin Endocrinol Metab.* 2007; **92**(12):4678–4685.

3. Salehi M, Gastaldelli A, D'Alessio DA. Altered islet function and insulin clearance cause hyperinsulinemia in gastric bypass patients with symptoms of postprandial hypoglycemia. *J Clin Endocrinol Metab.* 2014;**99**(6):2008–2017.

4. Marsk R, Jonas E, Rasmussen F, Näslund E. Nationwide cohort study of post-gastric bypass hypoglycaemia including 5,040 patients undergoing surgery for obesity in 1986-2006 in Sweden. *Diabetologia.* 2010;**53**(11):2307–2311.

5. Lee CJ, Wood GC, Lazo M, Brown TT, Clark JM, Still C, Benotti P. Risk of post-gastric bypass surgery hypoglycemia in nondiabetic individuals: a single center experience. *Obesity (Silver Spring).* 2016;**24**(6): 1342–1348.

6. Whipple AO. The surgical therapy of hyperinsulinism. *Journal International de Chirurgie.* 1938;**3**:237–376.

7. Cryer PE, Axelrod L, Grossman AB, Heller SR, Montori VM, Seaquist ER, Service FJ; Endocrine Society. Evaluation and management of adult hypoglycemic disorders: an Endocrine Society Clinical Practice Guideline. *J Clin Endocrinol Metab.* 2009;**94**(3):709–728.

8. Salehi M, Vella A, McLaughlin T, Patti ME. Hypoglycemia after gastric bypass surgery: current concepts and controversies. *J Clin Endocrinol Metab.* 2018;**103**(8):2815–2826.

9. Yaqub A, Smith EP, Salehi M. Hyperinsulinemic hypoglycemia after gastric bypass surgery: what's up and what's down? [published online ahead of print 13 October 2017] *Int J Obes (Lond).* doi:10.1038/ijo.2017.257.

10. Salehi M, Gastaldelli A, D'Alessio DA. Blockade of glucagon-like peptide 1 receptor corrects postprandial hypoglycemia after gastric bypass. *Gastroenterology.* 2014;**146**(3):669–680e2.

11. Craig CM, Liu LF, Deacon CF, Holst JJ, McLaughlin TL. Critical role for GLP-1 in symptomatic post-bariatric hypoglycaemia. *Diabetologia.* 2017;**60**(3):531–540.

12. Salehi M, Woods SC, D'Alessio DA. Gastric bypass alters both glucose-dependent and glucose-independent regulation of islet hormone secretion. *Obesity (Silver Spring).* 2015;**23**(10):2046–2052.

13. Bantle AE, Wang Q, Bantle JP. Post-gastric bypass hyperinsulinemic hypoglycemia: fructose is a carbohydrate which can be safely consumed. *J Clin Endocrinol Metab.* 2015;**100**(8): 3097–3102.

14. Axelsen M, Wesslau C, Lönnroth P, Arvidsson Lenner R, Smith U. Bedtime uncooked cornstarch supplement prevents nocturnal hypoglycaemia in intensively treated type 1 diabetes subjects. *J Intern Med.* 1999;**245**(3):229–236.

15. Mulla CM, Storino A, Yee EU, Lautz D, Sawnhey MS, Moser AJ, Patti ME. Insulinoma after bariatric surgery: diagnostic dilemma and therapeutic approaches. *Obes Surg.* 2016;**26**(4):874–881.

Obesity Therapeutics

M13
Presented, March 23–26, 2019

Daniel Bessesen, MD. Department of Medicine, Division of Endocrinology, University of Colorado School of Medicine, Aurora, Colorado 80045, E-mail: daniel.bessesen@ucdenver.edu

SIGNIFICANCE OF THE PROBLEM

An estimated 39.6% of adults and 18.5% of children and adolescents in the United States are obese (1). A recent study of 195 countries around the world found in 2015 that a total of 603 million adults were obese. Since 1980, the worldwide prevalence of obesity has doubled in more than 70 countries. Another analysis of data from around the world, representing more than 19.2 million adults, concluded that by 2025 6% of men and 9% of women will have a body mass index (BMI) > 40 kg/m^2 (2). Type 2 diabetes and other chronic metabolic diseases will follow the epidemic of obesity over time, creating strain on health care services and increasing costs (3, 4). Obesity increases health care costs to patients and employers and reduces productivity.

High-intensity behavioral treatment of obesity has increasingly become the standard of care. Five medications are now US Food and Drug Administration (FDA) approved for treatment of obesity, including four drugs approved since 2012. Most patients have insurance coverage for bariatric surgery; however, treatment of obesity still faces many challenges. Many clinicians and health system leaders continue to view obesity as a lifestyle choice, rather than a chronic progressive metabolic disease. Medications to treat obesity remain excluded from most insurance formularies. Weight bias remains prevalent in health care and society.

BARRIERS TO OPTIMAL PRACTICE

- Many endocrinologists feel uncomfortable discussing weight loss options with their patients.
- There are so many weight loss options, it is difficult to have a comprehensive discussion about all options in the brief time available in most clinical encounters.
- Many weight loss treatments are not covered by insurance and cost is a substantial barrier to use for many patients.

LEARNING OBJECTIVES

As a result of participating in this session, learners should be able to:

- Advise patients about current dietary strategies and endoscopic treatments for weight loss
- Feel comfortable discussing currently available weight loss medications with their patients
- Describe the benefits and risks of commonly performed weight loss surgeries

GENERAL APPROACH TO DISCUSSING TREATMENT OPTIONS WITH THE PATIENT WITH OBESITY

When a patient asks about treatment options, a good way to start the discussion is to say that there are several options available: continue with current efforts, do more to reduce food intake and increase activity, try a weight loss medication, or consider weight loss surgery. It may be most efficient to focus the conversation in clinic on the treatment options in which the patient is most interested. The goal is to provide information on the time and investment that will be needed with each treatment option and what may be the likely benefits.

LIFESTYLE TREATMENT OF OBESITY
Dietary Modification

Patients with obesity should seek to create a negative energy balance by reducing calorie intake by 500 to 1000 calories per day. This should lead to an initial weight loss of 1 to 2 pounds per week. Ideally, the reduction in calorie intake should be accompanied by a gradual increase in physical activity. Calorie restriction is the principal method for inducing weight loss, because most patients find it easier to reduce their food intake by 500 to 1000 kcal/d than to increase their energy expenditure by an equivalent amount. For example, to achieve a 500-kcal/d energy deficit, a patient can either eliminate two 20-ounce sugar-sweetened drinks or walk 5 miles. Patients and clinicians can set a daily calorie target needed to lose weight by using easily accessible equations to estimate daily energy expenditure (*e.g.*, Harris-Benedict or Mifflin St. Jeor), then subtracting 500 to 1000 kcal from this value. The clinician should remember that persons who are overweight and obese significantly underestimate caloric intake in free-living environments. Therefore, men and women who weigh <250 pounds are commonly prescribed 1200 to 1500 kcal/d, whereas those weighing ≥250 pounds are prescribed 1500 to 1800 kcal/d as a starting point. Calorie targets are then adjusted on the basis of observed weight loss.

Patients often ask about the best dietary approach for weight loss. Most evidence suggests that eating plans that differ in macronutrient content produce similar amounts of long-term weight loss. A meta-analysis of randomized trials (48 randomized controlled trials; n = 7286) showed that all structured eating plans were more effective at 6 and 12 months compared with no diet. This study also reported that low-carbohydrate diets (*e.g.*, Atkins™, South Beach, or Zone®) produced slightly greater weight loss in the first 6 months (2 to 3 kg) compared with more moderate macronutrient plans (55% to 60% carbohydrate), but differences between eating plans were small at ≥12 months (5). A unifying feature of several popular diets is the consumption of foods that are low in energy density (number of calories per weight of food) and high in dietary fiber. Thus, an eating plan that includes high-quality lean protein sources, vegetables and fruits, and some healthy fats (*e.g.*, nuts or avocados) and that limits the intake of refined carbohydrate foods should be the initial choice for most patients. Patient preference should be incorporated into this general approach. A patient may choose to follow meal plans ranging from vegetarian all the way to a very-low-carbohydrate ketogenic diet (keto). Patients should be informed that, because of adaptations to weight loss (reductions in energy expenditure and increases in appetite), weight will plateau despite continued efforts at the diet. Published studies suggest that dietary adherence, self-monitoring, and attendance at treatment visits are more important than diet composition in determining success in weight loss.

Meal-Replacement Diets and Commercial Diet Programs

A meal replacement is defined as a shake or bar that has approximately 200 calories, at least 15 to 20 g of protein, ≤5 g of sugar, and ≥5 g of fiber and that is supplemented with essential vitamins and minerals. Meal replacements facilitate portion control and calorie counting and can be helpful for patients who do not have adequate time for food preparation. Data from randomized trials suggest that provision of a calorie target that includes replacing two meals per day (partial meal replacement strategy) with a meal replacement leads to greater weight loss compared with provision of the same calorie target using only conventional foods (6). Low-calorie commercial diets (full meal replacement strategy, 1000 to 1200 kcal/d) and other commercial programs, such as Weight Watchers®, Jenny Craig®, or Nutrisystem®, also can provide significant weight loss and are options that can be suggested if a provider does not have access to nutritional counseling in their office (7).

Intermittent Fasting

Intermittent fasting has increased in popularity as an alternative to the traditional approach of daily caloric restriction. The advantage of this approach is that patients can look forward to several days per week of normal or unrestricted eating, rather than having to face the daily symptom of hunger. At least three randomized trials (8–10) have shown that intermittent fasting or modified fasting produces weight loss similar to that of conventional daily energy restriction. One of the three trials (10) included only patients with type 2 diabetes and showed a similar impact of daily and intermittent energy restriction on glycemic control.

Role of Exercise in Weight Loss and Maintenance

Regular exercise has many important health benefits; however, exercise alone or the addition of exercise to calorie restriction adds only 1 to 3 kg of additional weight loss. Data from randomized controlled trials and observational studies suggest that exercise is more important for maintenance of weight loss, rather than for the induction of initial weight loss. Within a set amount of exercise minutes per week, the combination of aerobic and resistance training has greater health benefits compared with doing only one form of exercise. Available data suggest that more exercise is needed to maintain weight loss (300 min/wk of moderate to vigorous activity) than is needed for general health promotion (150 min/wk).

PHARMACOTHERAPY FOR OBESITY

Endocrinologists can help their patients prevent weight gain by reviewing concurrent medications (11). Medications used to treat inflammatory conditions, psychiatric disorders, diabetes, and other conditions may be associated with weight gain. Clinicians can consider substituting medications used to treat these conditions with alternatives that are weight neutral or that promote weight loss. A systematic review of randomized trials that included weight change as a secondary end point found that tricyclic antidepressants, sulfonylureas, and thiazolidinediones, as well as some atypical antidepressants, were associated with weight gain. Conversely, drugs that were associated with weight loss included metformin, glucagon-like peptide-1 agonists, SGLT2 inhibitors, topiramate, zonisamide, and bupropion (12).

The Current Six Widely Used Medications Approved by the FDA For Weight Loss
Phentermine

Phentermine is one of a group of older sympathomimetic agents that includes diethylpropion, phendimetrazine, and benzphetamine. It is listed by the FDA as schedule IV, was approved for short-term use (generally accepted to be <12 weeks) in the United States in 1959, and is available in Australia but not in Europe. Phentermine is the most widely prescribed antiobesity medication in the United States, accounting for >70% of prescriptions (13). It has been available in 15-, 30-, and 37.5-mg doses and an 8-mg preparation was approved by the FDA in September 2016. Given that long-term efficacy of antiobesity medications requires long-term use, is it reasonable to prescribe phentermine chronically without long-term safety data? In some areas of the United States, this practice is explicitly forbidden by regulatory agencies and in these areas the answer is clearly no. In places where no clear regulatory guidance exists, the Endocrine Society Pharmacotherapy Guidelines provide suggestions about specific circumstances in which long-term prescribing of phentermine might be reasonable (11). Alternatively, phentermine can be dosed intermittently (14). Prescribing phentermine intermittently or chronically is off label and this should be explicitly explained to patients. Phentermine is the least expensive antiobesity medication.

Orlistat

The safety record of orlistat is excellent and, as a result, it is even available without a prescription at a 60-mg dose. It is available in the United States, the European Union, and Australia. A related compound, cetilistat, is approved in Japan. Orlistat is not widely prescribed, in part, because of the modest placebo subtracted weight loss it provides as well as the gastrointestinal adverse effects that are the result of its mechanism of action. For a patient with cardiovascular disease, psychiatric illness, or one who wants a medication with the best long-term safety record, orlistat may be the preferred agent as orlistat is the safest of the currently available antiobesity medications.

Phentermine/Topiramate ER

Topiramate has been FDA approved for seizures since 1996 and for migraine prevention since 2004. The combination of low doses of each medication provides a greater degree of weight loss with fewer adverse effects than that observed with either drug used alone, whereas the combination has a number of adverse effects, including numbness and tingling and, in some people, changes in mentation. The main concern with this combination is the risk of oral clefts in infants exposed to topiramate *in utero*. For this reason, women of childbearing age should use a reliable form of contraception and should be monitored to ensure they do not become pregnant while using this combination. Topiramate has also been rarely associated with the development of acute angle closure glaucoma. Phentermine/topiramate ER is the most effective antiobesity medication currently available.

Lorcaserin

Fenfluramine and dexfenfluramine were previously available antiobesity medications that increased central serotonin release. These drugs were removed from the market in 1997 because of their association with cardiac valvulopathy and primary pulmonary hypertension. Lorcaserin was developed as an agonist of the serotonin 2C receptor, which is only expressed in the brain, thereby avoiding the risk of valvular heart disease. In studies of more than 2400 participants exposed to the drug for 1 year evaluated with ECG, no evidence of valvular heart disease was seen. In 2016, the FDA approved a once-daily 20-mg extended release formulation. Given the success of the combination of phentermine with fenfluramine in weight loss, it might be expected that the combination of lorcaserin and phentermine will have greater efficacy than either drug alone. A recent 12-week trial reported a 7.2% weight loss with this combination (15). Clinicians should not prescribe this combination until long-term safety has been demonstrated. Recent data demonstrate the cardiovascular safety of lorcaserin (16) and the ability of this agent to reduce the progression of prediabetes to frank diabetes (17). Lorcaserin is the most well-tolerated antiobesity medication currently available (18).

Bupropion/Naltrexone

Bupropion was approved in 1985 for depression and it remains one of the most widely prescribed antidepressants. It is the antidepressant that is least likely to produce weight gain. It is also approved for smoking cessation. Naltrexone was approved in 1984 for the treatment of opioid dependence and is also approved for the treatment of alcohol dependence. Like a number of currently available weight loss agents, this combination is associated with an increase in pulse. Because of the concern that this increase in pulse could increase cardiovascular disease risk, the FDA mandated a placebo-controlled, noninferiority trial to demonstrate cardiovascular safety (Light study) (19). Unfortunately, a planned interim analysis was inappropriately released to the public in March 2015 while the trial was still ongoing, which resulted in the premature termination of the study. Bupropion/naltrexone is intermediate in both efficacy and adverse effects.

Liraglutide 3 mg

Glucagon-like peptide-1 receptor agonists have become a mainstay in the treatment of type 2 diabetes. They not only reduce glucose levels but increase satiety, slow gastric emptying, and reduce weight in a dose=dependent manner (20). In an initial dose ranging study, the greatest weight loss was observed at a dose of 3 mg/d (21). Liraglutide 3 mg is approved as an antiobesity medication in the United States, the European Union, and Australia. There is evidence of diabetes prevention, beneficial effects in nonalcoholic steatohepatitis (22), and some evidence of cardioprotection (23). Recently, results of a 3-year follow-up demonstrated continued weight loss maintenance (24). There is concern about the potential risk of pancreatitis, although 3-year follow-up data suggest that the risk of gallbladder disease is probably greater. Medullary carcinoma of the thyroid was seen in preclinical studies, but has not been observed in humans. Liraglutide is intermediate in both efficacy and adverse effects, but is the most costly of available agents.

There have been a number of recent reviews and meta-analyses of antiobesity medications (25, 26). The recent systematic review and meta-analysis by Khera and colleagues (18) is particularly helpful. The authors performed a network meta-analysis and presented surface under the cumulative rankings results on both efficacy and adverse effects. These results support the conclusions that orlistat and lorcaserin are less effective and have fewer adverse effects, that phentermine/topiramate ER is the most effective of available agents, and that naltrexone/bupropion and liraglutide are intermediate in effectiveness but have more adverse effects than orlistat and lorcaserin.

ENDOSCOPIC AND GASTROINTESTINAL TREATMENTS FOR WEIGHT LOSS

Over the last 5 years, a number of weight loss treatments have become available that fill the treatment efficacy gap between pharmacotherapy and weight loss surgery. These treatments are typically done endoscopically, although some do not require endoscopy, and produce 12% to 16% weight loss (27). The ReShape Duo Integraged Balloon System (ReShape Medical, San Clemente, CA), the Orbera Balloon (Apollo Endosurgery, Austin, TX), and the Obalon Balloon System (Obalon Therapeutics, Carlsbad, CA) are gastric balloon systems approved for use by the FDA. In addition, Orbera, previously known as the BioInterics Balloon or BIB, has been used in clinical practice around the world for more than 20 years. Both the ReShape and Orbera balloons are made of silicone and filled with fluid and are placed and removed endoscopically, whereas the Obalon balloons are filled with a nitrogen mix gas. Obalon balloons are also swallowed and then removed endoscopically. Weight loss in clinical practice is higher than that observed in multicenter randomized controlled trials and ranges between 12% and 16% total body weight loss at 1 year.

Serious adverse event rates were higher for the Orbera balloon (10%) and the ReShape system (10.6%) compared with the Obalon device (0.5%). However, 75% of serious adverse events in the Orbera and ReShape trials were a result of hospital admissions for nausea, vomiting, abdominal pain, or early device removal after placement and resolved without additional complications within 3 to 7 days of device placement. Patients in these early trials did not receive a comprehensive medical regimen to control nausea and vomiting, which has been found to be important to avoid these complications. Other serious adverse events in the ReShape trial included one esophageal mucosal tear, one contained esophageal perforation, one bleeding gastric ulcer, and one aspiration pneumonitis. In the Orbera trial, serious adverse events included one gastric outlet obstruction with diffuse gastritis, one gastric perforation with sepsis, one aspiration pneumonia, two esophageal tears, one laryngospasm, and one infected balloon. Only one serious adverse event was reported in the Obalon trial, a bleeding gastric ulcer in a patient concomitantly taking nonsteroidal anti-inflammatory drugs against study protocol.

The AspireAssist System (Aspire Bariatrics, King of Prussia, PA) was approved by the FDA in June 2016 for patients with a BMI between 35 and 55 kg/m^2. Aspiration therapy has at least two mechanisms contributing to weight loss—aspiration of calories and behavior changes—that result in decreased overall food intake. Careful evaluation with the Eating Disorder Examination—an interview assessment of disordered attitudes and behaviors related to eating, body shape, and weight with items designed to diagnose eating disorders—found no evidence of worsening eating behaviors or compensatory eating in either the US pilot trial (28) or US pivotal trial (29). Weight loss in the US pilot trial was 18.6% total body weight loss and 14.2% for participants who completed 1 year of therapy in the US pivotal trial. Serious adverse events observed included abdominal pain after placement, peritonitis, internal ulceration, and aspiration tube–associated fungal colonization.

Weight Loss Surgery

Bariatric (weight loss) surgery is indicated for patients with a body mass index of ≥40 kg/m^2 or for those with a BMI of ≥35 kg/m^2 and at least one serious weight-related comorbid condition, such as type 2 diabetes, obstructive sleep apnea, or osteoarthritis of the hip or knee (30). Before undergoing surgery, patients ideally should have made sustained attempts at weight loss with high-intensity lifestyle modification programs, structured meal plans, and/or pharmacotherapy (31). Patients should be well informed of the risks and benefits of weight loss surgery, including the small probability of long-term adverse outcomes. In addition, patients must be informed of the need for regular follow-up to monitor weight and nutritional status, as well as to take specialized vitamin supplements for life. The 30-day mortality rate for bariatric surgery is <0.1% and is comparable to that observed with laparoscopic cholecystectomy (32, 33). Rates of major adverse events at 30 days were 5.0% for bypass and 2.6% for sleeve. These included pulmonary embolism, surgical site infections, anastomotic leaks and problems with nausea, vomiting, and dehydration.

The vast majority of surgical procedures in the United States are now sleeve gastrectomy or gastric bypass. As a result of smaller weight losses, need for adjustment, and potential for mechanical complications, the laparoscopic gastric band is now rarely performed. Roux-en-Y gastric bypass results in restricted food intake, partial malabsorption, and changes in appetite-regulating hormones (e.g., ghrelin), as well as change in bile acids and gut microbiota, all of which are thought to contribute to weight loss (34). In sleeve gastrectomy, approximately 75% of the stomach is resected, but the remainder of the intestinal tract remains intact. Weight loss is achieved principally by food restriction, although the removal of endocrine-rich gastric tissue may also contribute to weight loss.

Roux-en-Y gastric bypass surgery is somewhat more effective than sleeve gastrectomy in both weight loss and improvements in glucose control in patients with type 2 diabetes. In an analysis of administrative data from 41 health systems in the United States (gastric bypass, n = 32,208; sleeve gastrectomy, n = 29,693), weight losses at 1 year were 31.2% and 25.2% of initial weight for bypass and sleeve, respectively. Weight losses at 5 years were 25.5% and 18.8% of initial weight, respectively (35). The SLEEVEPASS trial, conducted in Finland, randomly assigned 240 patients with severe obesity (mean BMI, 45.9 kg/m^2) to laparoscopic sleeve gastrectomy or gastric bypass. Percent excess weight loss at 5 years was 49% in the gastric sleeve group and 57% in the gastric bypass group. These weight losses corresponded to reductions in BMI of 10.8 and 13 units, respectively. No differences were observed in health-related quality of life or in major complications. No patient died of a surgical complication during the 5 years of the trial (36).

Whereas glucose levels initially improve dramatically in many patients with type 2 diabetes, there is a gradual increase in HbA_{1c} levels over the 5 years after surgery. In the STAMPEDE randomized trial, 150 patients with type 2 diabetes were randomly assigned to intensive medical treatment or bariatric surgery (sleeve gastrectomy or gastric bypass). After 5 years, weight loss was 21% to 23% of initial weight in the surgically treated group *vs.* 5% of initial weight in the intensive medical treatment group. Five percent of patients in the medical treatment group achieved the primary outcome of the study—an HbA_{1c} of <6%—compared with 29% in the surgically treated group (37).

Epidemiologic and prospective nonrandomized data demonstrate an initial increase in mortality rates in the immediate postoperative period, followed by a progressive reduction in mortality in surgical patients compared with patients with severe obesity who do not undergo weight loss surgery (38, 39).

The longest available follow-up data from weight loss surgery in a US population come from the Longitudinal Assessment of Bariatric Surgery study. Seven-year outcomes were reported recently and showed a weight loss of 28.4% of initial weight for gastric bypass, including a 3.9% gain from nadir at year 3 (40).

Complications of Bariatric Surgery

The most common early complications of bariatric surgery are nausea, vomiting, thromboembolic disease, anastomotic leak (gastric sleeve), bleeding, or obstruction. Nutritional deficiencies (*e.g.*, iron or vitamin D) can occur over the long term but can be prevented with routine monitoring, the consumption of a balanced diet, and the lifetime use of specialized bariatric multivitamins. Anastomotic ulcer or stenosis can occur as an early or late complication in patients undergoing gastric bypass. Nonsteroidal anti-inflammatory medications, as well as nicotine use in any form, are probably contraindicated for life after gastric bypass as a result of ulcer risk. Uncommon but feared complications of surgery include a small but definite increase in both alcohol misuse and suicide (41, 42). In addition, gastric bypass patients are at risk for post–gastric bypass hypoglycemia (43).

Long-Term Follow-Up After Bariatric Surgery

Patients undergoing weight loss surgery must be prepared to undertake regular follow-up—several times in the first year, then at least annually—indefinitely after bariatric surgery with the goal of maintaining their weight losses and good nutritional status. In addition to screening for micronutrient deficiencies, the American Society for Metabolic and Bariatric Surgery recommends screening for osteoporosis at 2 years

after surgery in gastric bypass patients (44). Increased physical activity after bariatric surgery helps to preserve lean body mass and leads to better long-term weight loss. Prescription medications for weight loss may help some patients who do not meet weight loss goals after surgery.

SUMMARY

Obesity is a serious and growing health problem in the United States and around the world. In clinical care, a focus on lifestyle change in patients who are open to and motivated to make changes is the most practical treatment strategy. We now have a number of antiobesity medications that have been carefully reviewed by regulatory agencies and judged to be safe and effective. These medications are not widely prescribed. This situation may reflect the shadow of a long history of adverse events associated with older agents and perhaps an unwillingness of many physicians to think of obesity as a biologic condition, one for which medications are an appropriate form of therapy. This view, however, is not in step with the large body of data in animals and humans clearly demonstrating the biologic underpinnings of obesity and the significant physiologic processes that promote weight regain once a person has lost weight. Admittedly, currently available antiobesity medications are not as effective as we would like and they do have adverse effects; however, it is troubling that only 1% to 2% of eligible patients receive a prescription for one of these agents. Authoritative guidelines formulated by multiple expert panels support the use of these medications. Extensive safety and efficacy data exist for newer agents. If adherence to pharmacotherapy guidelines in diabetes, hypertension, or hyperlipidemia were this low, action would be taken.

Weight loss surgery is the most effective treatment approach for obesity. Many endocrinologists are becoming more comfortable discussing this option with their patients and are developing an approach to referral. Endoscopic therapies are not widely available and questions remain about the long-term usefulness of these approaches. However, for patients who are not ready to have weight loss surgery and who have not achieved their goals with lifestyle and medications, a discussion about these treatments with an experienced gastroenterologist may be useful. The goal is not to have all obese patients take an antiobesity medication or undergo weight loss surgery. It seems reasonable, though, to expect all physicians to be able to have a thoughtful, informed conversation with their patients about the risks and benefits of these treatment approaches when asked. Patients who struggle with their weight deserve a productive conversation about weight loss treatment options with a provider who can inform them of the benefits and risks in an effort to help the patient make informed decisions about his or her weight loss treatment options. Endocrinologists are well positioned to provide this type of clinical care.

CASES
Case 1
A 45-year-old man comes to see you for help losing weight. He has a history of hypertension, anxiety/depression, and degenerative arthritis. He is currently on hydrochlorothiazide 25 mg/d, metoprolol 25 mg two times per day, and paroxetine 20 mg/d. His BMI is 32 kg/m^2 and his blood pressure is 131/78 mm Hg. He does not think that his diet is a problem and wants to start an exercise program to lose weight. He is also curious about weight loss medications.

What Weight Loss Treatments Do You Discuss With Him?
Given his BMI and weight-associated health problems, it would be appropriate to discuss lifestyle changes (appropriate for all patients who are overweight or obese) and weight loss medications (appropriate for people with BMI of >30 kg/m^2 or >27 kg/m^2 with a weight-related comorbidity) (31). It would not be appropriate to discuss weight loss surgery (appropriate for those with BMI of >40 kg/m^2 or >35 kg/m^2 with a weight-related comorbidity). Whereas lifestyle is the foundation for any weight loss program—and you can tell him that—there is no standard definition for what level of lifestyle commitment is needed before it is appropriate to prescribe weight loss medications. I typically say that the person, at a minimum, should try some initial diet steps, such as dietary self-monitoring, before starting a weight loss medication, but if the patient says he is already doing everything he can with their diet, I typically go ahead and discuss the pros and cons of medications.

What Would You Tell Him About His Idea to Exercise?
Studies have shown that exercise alone typically results in 2% weight loss, although there is substantial individual variation. Some people lose more weight and some gain weight. I typically say that exercise is great for health but, in general, is not a good way to lose weight (https://health.gov/paguidelines/second-edition/report/). Rather, it seems to be important in maintaining a reduced weight once the weight is lost. I tell patients that, if their primary goal is weight loss, the first thing to focus on is reducing food intake.

Are There Any Changes You Can Make to His Medications to Help With His Weight Loss Attempts?
Both metoprolol and paroxetine have been shown to promote weight gain. There are a number of alternative medications that will not have this problem. Angiotensin-converting enzyme inhibitors and calcium channel blockers are blood pressure–lowering medications with little weight loss effect. If a β-blocker is needed, carvedilol and nebivolol have been shown to result in less weight gain than metoprolol (11). Bupropion is the antidepressant medication with the least effect on weight, and in studies done in patients with obesity it

has been found to even produce weight loss. I typically have patients discuss changes in their psychiatric medications with the provider who initially prescribed the drug as that individual may have had a compelling reason to prescribe it.

What Would You Tell Him About Changing His Diet?
I used to take a 24-hour diet recall history; however, this takes several minutes and often I am not sure that I found clear targets for intervention. My go-to question now is, "Is there something in your diet that you think is a problem or is contributing to your weight problem?" Most people have an answer to this question and it gets right to the thing that they have already identified as a problem in their own mind. Whereas questions about fast foods, sugar-sweetened beverages, snacking, sweets, and chips can be helpful, the initial issue is whether the person sees any problems with his or her diet and does he or she have any energy to make changes. If the patient only sees barriers, the first suggestion I make is that he or she monitor everything he or she eats and drinks for a week and to look for opportunities for change. If the patient is not willing to do this, I typically say, "It looks like you don't have much energy for making changes in your diet and so maybe accepting your weight where it is might be the best choice for right now." If he is interested in making changes, I would try to get him engaged in a formal program. I know a range of programs in my area and have information to share with my patients about these programs from Diabetes Prevention Program–based programs, Weight Watchers® and more formal group behavioral programs, and low-calorie diet meal replacement programs.

What Would You Tell Him About Weight Loss Medications?
Some patients think that if a physician would only prescribe a weight loss medication to "get them started," they could lose a substantial amount of weight. Others are curious about weight loss medications but have a certain level of skepticism. I feel that my job is to provide objective information, to the best of my ability in the limited time that I have, about the risks and benefits of weight loss medications. I typically start by saying that, "These medicines do help people lose more weight than diet alone and they are approved by the FDA." I then say that the amount of weight that is lost is typically 5% to 10%—and I give them the number of pounds that this would mean for them—over the first 3 to 4 months and that after that weight tends to plateau. Second, I mention that, like medications for other chronic health problems, such as high blood pressure, diabetes, or high cholesterol, these medicines only work as long as a person takes them, and so if the person loses weight on the medicine and then stops it, weight is typically regained. I tell the person that they likely will need to be open to long-term treatment if the medicines work. Third, I say that weight loss medications are typically not covered by insurance, so

they likely need to be willing to pay for the medicine. I give a range of costs from $20 to $200 per month and see if this is realistic for them. If they say yes, I give them a list of the medications with what, for me, is the single most prominent feature (Orlistat: the safest; lorcaserin: fewest adverse effects; phentermine/topiramate: most effective; naltrexone/bupropion and liraglutide: intermediate in adverse effects and effectiveness). I encourage them to read about each (I have handouts on each that we give to patients), look into what the cost will be for them (look into coupons and prices at different pharmacies), and then get back to me about whether they want to try one. I say you can try it for a few months to see if you have any adverse effects and if you think it is helping. Then you can decide whether to use the medication long term.

Case 2
A 34-year-old woman comes to see you at wits end about her weight. Her peak lifetime nonpregnant BMI was 45 kg/m², and with diet, exercise, and phentermine her BMI has fallen to 41 kg/m². She has degenerative arthritis, type 2 diabetes, and obstructive sleep apnea. She has heard about weight loss surgery but believes that it is not a long-term solution because "everyone regains the weight." She is also worried about being hungry and not being able to eat. She is worried that the surgical risk for her will be high. She wonders if there are any other options.

What Other Options Do You Discuss With Her?
A low-calorie diet (1000 kcal/d) using a full meal replacement program can give 14% to 16% weight loss (45). Endoscopic approaches to weight loss, including balloons or an aspiration tube, will typically provide 12% to 18% weight loss. If you are interested in advising patients about these options in your area, you will need to do some homework to see what programs are available locally and whether you are comfortable sending people to these programs. With each of these options, there are concerns about long-term sustainability. Meal replacement programs are a terrific option for people who need a moderate amount of weight loss for a particular target event (an imaging study or surgery). Meal replacements can be used as a long-term intermittent strategy. Endoscopic procedures, in my opinion, are too new to really know just how they fit into the overall armamentarium of options. I do refer patients for evaluation for these procedures because I have an experienced clinician in my area that I trust to provide patients with good information about these options.

What Do You Tell Her About the Risks and Benefits of Weight Loss Surgery?
Like many patients, this woman has ideas about weight loss surgery that are not supported by available evidence. Surgical mortality when the surgery is performed in experienced centers is 0.2% (46). This is lower than that seen with hip replacement operations and similar to that observed with laparoscopic cholecystectomy. Observation of patients who underwent weight loss surgery in the Swedish Obese Subjects study is more than 20 years and shows the durability of the weight loss. A recent study from Utah with >90% follow-up showed maintenance of a 27% weight loss at 12 years (47). Another study of 65,093 patients age 20 to 79 years with BMI of ≥35 kg/m² who had bariatric procedures performed in typical clinical environments (41 practice sites) showed similar outcomes (35). Patients who succeed at losing weight after a weight loss surgical procedure typically say that they are not hungry. One patient told me, "I don't think I ever knew what it is like to feel full until I had this surgery." I commonly ask people after weight loss surgery what they think about how much they ate before the surgery. They often say, "I can't believe how much I used to eat." I ask why they don't eat that much now and they typically will say, "I am just not interested."

Do You Encourage Her to Have Weight Loss Surgery?
I feel that my job is not to tell people what the best choice is for them, but rather to provide them with information that will help them make the best decision for themselves. For a person like this, I typically suggest he or she find a surgical program near him using the online tool available from the American Society of Metabolic and Bariatric Surgery (https://asmbs.org/patients/find-a-provider). The person inputs in his home location and the Web site directs him to surgeons in the area. Ideally, you will be able to help patients find a surgeon in whom you have confidence. The person can then attend an information session and potentially a patient support group that will allow him to speak directly with individuals who have had the surgery. This kind of interaction is often much more helpful than anything you can say about the surgery. I will typically tell a person like this that, "I am not saying you need to have surgery, and going to an information session and/or a support group does not mean you are going to have surgery; however, it seems like you really want to do something about your weight and getting more information will help you make the best decision for yourself about your options."

References
1. Hales CM, Carroll MD, Fryar CD, Ogden CL. Prevalence of obesity among adults and youth: United States, 2015-2016. *NCHS Data Brief.* 2017;**2017**(288):1–8.
2. NCD Risk Factor Collaboration (NCD-RisC). Trends in adult body-mass index in 200 countries from 1975 to 2014: A pooled analysis of 1698 population-based measurement studies with 19·2 million participants. *Lancet.* 2016;**387**(10026):1377–1396.
3. Van Gaal LF, Mertens IL, De Block CE. Mechanisms linking obesity with cardiovascular disease. *Nature.* 2006;**444**(7121):875–880.
4. Apovian CM. The clinical and economic consequences of obesity. *Am J Manag Care.* 2013;**19**(Suppl):S219–S228.
5. Johnston BC, Kanters S, Bandayrel K, Wu P, Naji F, Siemieniuk RA, Ball GD, Busse JW, Thorlund K, Guyatt G, Jansen JP, Mills EJ. Comparison of weight loss among named diet programs in overweight and obese adults: A meta-analysis. *JAMA.* 2014;**312**(9):923–933.

6. Heymsfield SB, van Mierlo CA, van der Knaap HC, Heo M, Frier HI. Weight management using a meal replacement strategy: Meta and pooling analysis from six studies. *Int J Obes Relat Metab Disord.* 2003; **27**(5):537–549.

7. Gudzune KA, Doshi RS, Mehta AK, Chaudhry ZW, Jacobs DK, Vakil RM, Lee CJ, Bleich SN, Clark JM. Efficacy of commercial weight-loss programs: An updated systematic review. *Ann Intern Med.* 2015; **162**(7):501–512.

8. Catenacci VA, Pan Z, Ostendorf D, Brannon S, Gozansky WS, Mattson MP, Martin B, MacLean PS, Melanson EL, Troy Donahoo W. A randomized pilot study comparing zero-calorie alternate-day fasting to daily caloric restriction in adults with obesity. *Obesity (Silver Spring).* 2016;**24**(9):1874–1883.

9. Trepanowski JF, Kroeger CM, Barnosky A, Klempel MC, Bhutani S, Hoddy KK, Gabel K, Freels S, Rigdon J, Rood J, Ravussin E, Varady KA. Effect of alternate-day fasting on weight loss, weight maintenance, and cardioprotection among metabolically healthy obese adults: A randomized clinical trial. *JAMA Intern Med.* 2017;**177**(7):930–938.

10. Carter S, Clifton PM, Keogh JB. Effect of intermittent compared with continuous energy restricted diet on glycemic control in patients with type 2 diabetes: A randomized noninferiority trial. *JAMA Netw Open.* 2018;**1**(3):e180756.

11. Apovian CM, Aronne LJ, Bessesen DH, McDonnell ME, Murad MH, Pagotto U, Ryan DH, Still CD, for the Endocrine Society. Pharmacological management of obesity: An Endocrine Society clinical practice guideline. *J Clin Endocrinol Metab.* 2015;**100**(2):342–362.

12. Domecq JP, Prutsky G, Leppin A, Sonbol MB, Altayar O, Undavalli C, Wang Z, Elraiyah T, Brito JP, Mauck KF, Lababidi MH, Prokop LJ, Asi N, Wei J, Fidahussein S, Montori VM, Murad MH. Clinical review: Drugs commonly associated with weight change: A systematic review and meta-analysis. *J Clin Endocrinol Metab.* 2015;**100**(2):363–370.

13. Thomas CE, Mauer EA, Shukla AP, Rathi S, Aronne LJ. Low adoption of weight loss medications: A comparison of prescribing patterns of antiobesity pharmacotherapies and SGLT2s. *Obesity (Silver Spring).* 2016;**24**(9):1955–1961.

14. Weintraub M, Sundaresan PR, Schuster B, Ginsberg G, Madan M, Balder A, Stein EC, Byrne L. Long-term weight control study. II (weeks 34 to 104). An open-label study of continuous fenfluramine plus phentermine versus targeted intermittent medication as adjuncts to behavior modification, caloric restriction, and exercise. *Clin Pharmacol Ther.* 1992;**51**(5):595–601.

15. Smith SR, Garvey WT, Greenway FL, Zhou S, Fain R, Pilson R, Fujioka K, Aronne LJ. Coadministration of lorcaserin and phentermine for weight management: A 12-week, randomized, pilot safety study. *Obesity (Silver Spring).* 2017;**25**(5):857–865.

16. Bohula EA, Wiviott SD, McGuire DK, Inzucchi SE, Kuder J, Im K, Fanola CL, Qamar A, Brown C, Budaj A, Garcia-Castillo A, Gupta M, Leiter LA, Weissman NJ, White HD, Patel T, Francis B, Miao W, Perdomo C, Dhadda S, Bonaca MP, Ruff CT, Keech AC, Smith SR, Sabatine MS, Scirica BM, for the CAMELLIA–TIMI 61 Steering Committee and Investigators. Cardiovascular safety of lorcaserin in overweight or obese patients. *N Engl J Med.* 2018;**379**(12):1107–1117.

17. Bohula EA, Scirica BM, Inzucchi SE, McGuire DK, Keech AC, Smith SR, Kanevsky E, Murphy SA, Leiter LA, Dwyer JP, Corbalan R, Hamm C, Kaplan L, Nicolau JC, Ophuis TO, Ray KK, Ruda M, Spinar J, Patel T, Miao W, Perdomo C, Francis B, Dhadda S, Bonaca MP, Ruff CT, Sabatine MS, Wiviott SD, for the CAMELLIA-TIMI 61 Steering Committee Investigators. Effect of lorcaserin on prevention and remission of type 2 diabetes in overweight and obese patients (CAMELLIA-TIMI 61): A randomised, placebo-controlled trial. *Lancet.* 2018;**392**(10161): 2269–2279.

18. Khera R, Murad MH, Chandar AK, Dulai PS, Wang Z, Prokop LJ, Loomba R, Camilleri M, Singh S. Association of pharmacological treatments for obesity with weight loss and adverse events: A systematic review and meta-analysis. *JAMA.* 2016;**315**(22):2424–2434.

19. Nissen SE, Wolski KE, Prcela L, Wadden T, Buse JB, Bakris G, Perez A, Smith SR. Effect of naltrexone-bupropion on major adverse cardiovascular events in overweight and obese patients with cardiovascular risk factors: A randomized clinical trial. *JAMA.* 2016;**315**(10):990–1004.

20. Burcelin R, Gourdy P. Harnessing glucagon-like peptide-1 receptor agonists for the pharmacological treatment of overweight and obesity. *Obes Rev.* 2017;**18**(1):86–98.

21. Astrup A, Rössner S, Van Gaal L, Rissanen A, Niskanen L, Al Hakim M, Madsen J, Rasmussen MF, Lean ME, for the NN8022-1807 Study Group. Effects of liraglutide in the treatment of obesity: A randomised, double-blind, placebo-controlled study. *Lancet.* 2009;**374**(9701): 1606–1616.

22. Armstrong MJ, Gaunt P, Aithal GP, Barton D, Hull D, Parker R, Hazlehurst JM, Guo K, Abouda G, Aldersley MA, Stocken D, Gough SC, Tomlinson JW, Brown RM, Hübscher SG, Newsome PN, for the LEAN Trial Team. Liraglutide safety and efficacy in patients with non-alcoholic steatohepatitis (LEAN): A multicentre, double-blind, randomised, placebo-controlled phase 2 study. *Lancet.* 2016;**387**(10019): 679–690.

23. Marso SP, Daniels GH, Brown-Frandsen K, Kristensen P, Mann JF, Nauck MA, Nissen SE, Pocock S, Poulter NR, Ravn LS, Steinberg WM, Stockner M, Zinman B, Bergenstal RM, Buse JB, for the LEADER Steering Committee; LEADER Trial Investigators. Liraglutide and cardiovascular outcomes in type 2 diabetes. *N Engl J Med.* 2016; **375**(4):311–322.

24. le Roux CW, Astrup A, Fujioka K, Greenway F, Lau DCW, Van Gaal L, Ortiz RV, Wilding JPH, Skjøth TV, Manning LS, Pi-Sunyer X, for the SCALE Obesity Prediabetes NN8022-1839 Study Group. 3 years of liraglutide versus placebo for type 2 diabetes risk reduction and weight management in individuals with prediabetes: A randomised, double-blind trial. *Lancet.* 2017;**389**(10077):1399–1409.

25. Kumar RB, Aronne LJ. Efficacy comparison of medications approved for chronic weight management. *Obesity (Silver Spring).* 2015; **23**(Suppl 1):S4–S7.

26. Yanovski SZ, Yanovski JA. Long-term drug treatment for obesity: A systematic and clinical review. *JAMA.* 2014;**311**(1):74–86.

27. Ruban A, Uthayakumar A, Ashrafian H, Teare JP. Endoscopic interventions in the treatment of obesity and diabetes. *Dig Dis Sci.* 2018; **63**(7):1694–1705.

28. Sullivan S, Stein R, Jonnalagadda S, Mullady D, Edmundowicz S. Aspiration therapy leads to weight loss in obese subjects: A pilot study. *Gastroenterology.* 2013;**145**(6):1245-1252.e1-5.

29. Thompson CC, Abu Dayyeh BK, Kushner R, Sullivan S, Schorr AB, Amaro A, Apovian CM, Fullum T, Zarrinpar A, Jensen MD, Stein AC, Edmundowicz S, Kahaleh M, Ryou M, Bohning JM, Ginsberg G, Huang C, Tran DD, Glaser JP, Martin JA, Jaffe DL, Farraye FA, Ho SB, Kumar N, Harakal D, Young M, Thomas CE, Shukla AP, Ryan MB, Haas M, Goldsmith H, McCrea J, Aronne LJ. Percutaneous gastrostomy device for the treatment of class II and class III obesity: Results of a randomized controlled trial. *Am J Gastroenterol.* 2017;**112**(3): 447–457.

30. Mechanick JI, Youdim A, Jones DB, Timothy Garvey W, Hurley DL, Molly McMahon M, Heinberg LJ, Kushner R, Adams TD, Shikora S, Dixon JB, Brethauer S. Clinical practice guidelines for the perioperative nutritional, metabolic, and nonsurgical support of the bariatric surgery patient--2013 update: Cosponsored by American Association of Clinical Endocrinologists, the Obesity Society, and American Society for Metabolic & Bariatric Surgery. *Surg Obes Relat Dis.* 2013;**9**(2):159–191.

31. Jensen MD, Ryan DH, Apovian CM, Ard JD, Comuzzie AG, Donato KA, Hu FB, Hubbard VS, Jakicic JM, Kushner RF, Loria CM, Millen BE, Nonas CA, Pi-Sunyer FX, Stevens J, Stevens VJ, Wadden TA, Wolfe BM, Yanovski SZ, Jordan HS, Kendall KA, Lux LJ, Mentor-Marcel R, Morgan LC, Trisolini MG, Wnek J, Anderson JL, Halperin JL, Albert NM, Bozkurt B, Brindis RG, Curtis LH, DeMets D, Hochman JS, Kovacs RJ, Ohman EM, Pressler SJ, Sellke FW, Shen WK, Smith SC, Jr, Tomaselli GF, for the American College of Cardiology/American Heart Association Task Force on Practice Guidelines; Obesity Society. 2013 AHA/ ACC/TOS guideline for the management of overweight and obesity in adults: A report of the American College of Cardiology/American Heart Association Task Force on Practice Guidelines and The Obesity Society [published correction appears in Circulation. 2014; 129(25 Suppl 2):S139-S140]. *Circulation.* 2014;**129**(25 Suppl 2): S102–S138.

32. Sakran N, Sherf-Dagan S, Blumenfeld O, Romano-Zelekha O, Raziel A, Keren D, Raz I, Hershko D, Gralnek IM, Shohat T, Goitein D. Incidence and risk factors for mortality following bariatric surgery: A nationwide registry study [correction appears in *Obes Surg.* doi: 10.1007/s11695-018-3274-0]. *Obes Surg.* 2018;**28**(9):2661–2669.

33. Inaba CS, Koh CY, Sujatha-Bhaskar S, Silva JP, Chen Y, Nguyen DV, Nguyen NT. One-year mortality after contemporary laparoscopic bariatric surgery: An analysis of the bariatric outcomes longitudinal database. *J Am Coll Surg.* 2018;**226**(6):1166–1174.

34. Mulla CM, Middelbeek RJW, Patti ME. Mechanisms of weight loss and improved metabolism following bariatric surgery. *Ann N Y Acad Sci.* 2018;**1411**(1):53–64.

35. Arterburn D, Wellman R, Emiliano A, Smith SR, Odegaard AO, Murali S, Williams N, Coleman KJ, Courcoulas A, Coley RY, Anau J, Pardee R, Toh S, Janning C, Cook A, Sturtevant J, Horgan C, McTigue KM, for the PCORnet Bariatric Study Collaborative. Comparative effectiveness and safety of bariatric procedures for weight loss: A PCORnet cohort study. *Ann Intern Med.* 2018;**169**(11):741–750.

36. Salminen P, Helmiö M, Ovaska J, Juuti A, Leivonen M, Peromaa-Haavisto P, Hurme S, Soinio M, Nuutila P, Victorzon M. Effect of laparoscopic sleeve gastrectomy vs laparoscopic Roux-en-Y gastric bypass on weight loss at 5 years among patients with morbid obesity: The SLEEVEPASS randomized clinical trial. *JAMA.* 2018;**319**(3):241–254.

37. Schauer PR, Bhatt DL, Kirwan JP, Wolski K, Aminian A, Brethauer SA, Navaneethan SD, Singh RP, Pothier CE, Nissen SE, Kashyap SR, for the STAMPEDE Investigators. Bariatric surgery versus intensive medical therapy for diabetes: 5-Year outcomes. *N Engl J Med.* 2017;**376**(7):641–651.

38. Arterburn DE, Olsen MK, Smith VA, Livingston EH, Van Scoyoc L, Yancy WS, Jr, Eid G, Weidenbacher H, Maciejewski ML. Association between bariatric surgery and long-term survival. *JAMA.* 2015;**313**(1):62–70.

39. Courcoulas AP, Yanovski SZ, Bonds D, Eggerman TL, Horlick M, Staten MA, Arterburn DE. Long-term outcomes of bariatric surgery: A National Institutes of Health symposium. *JAMA Surg.* 2014;**149**(12):1323–1329.

40. Courcoulas AP, King WC, Belle SH, Berk P, Flum DR, Garcia L, Gourash W, Horlick M, Mitchell JE, Pomp A, Pories WJ, Purnell JQ, Singh A, Spaniolas K, Thirlby R, Wolfe BM, Yanovski SZ. Seven-year weight trajectories and health outcomes in the Longitudinal Assessment of Bariatric Surgery (LABS) study. *JAMA Surg.* 2018;**153**(5):427–434.

41. King WC, Chen JY, Mitchell JE, Kalarchian MA, Steffen KJ, Engel SG, Courcoulas AP, Pories WJ, Yanovski SZ. Prevalence of alcohol use disorders before and after bariatric surgery. *JAMA.* 2012;**307**(23):2516–2525.

42. Neovius M, Bruze G, Jacobson P, Sjöholm K, Johansson K, Granath F, Sundström J, Näslund I, Marcus C, Ottosson J, Peltonen M, Carlsson LMS. Risk of suicide and non-fatal self-harm after bariatric surgery: Results from two matched cohort studies. *Lancet Diabetes Endocrinol.* 2018;**6**(3):197–207.

43. Salehi M, Vella A, McLaughlin T, Patti ME. Hypoglycemia after gastric bypass surgery: Current concepts and controversies. *J Clin Endocrinol Metab.* 2018;**103**(8):2815–2826.

44. Garvey WT, Mechanick JI, Brett EM, Garber AJ, Hurley DL, Jastreboff AM, Nadolsky K, Pessah-Pollack R, Plodkowski R, for the Reviewers of the AACE/ACE Obesity Clinical Practice Guidelines. American Association of Clinical Endocrinologists and American College of Endocrinology comprehensive clinical practice guidelines for medical care of patients with obesity. *Endocr Pract.* 2016;**22**(Suppl 3):1–203.

45. Ard JD, Cook M, Rushing J, Frain A, Beavers K, Miller G, Miller ME, Nicklas B. Impact on weight and physical function of intensive medical weight loss in older adults with stage II and III obesity. *Obesity (Silver Spring).* 2016;**24**(9):1861–1866.

46. Flum DR, Belle SH, King WC, Wahed AS, Berk P, Chapman W, Pories W, Courcoulas A, McCloskey C, Mitchell J, Patterson E, Pomp A, Staten MA, Yanovski SZ, Thirlby R, Wolfe B, for the Longitudinal Assessment of Bariatric Surgery (LABS) Consortium. Perioperative safety in the longitudinal assessment of bariatric surgery. *N Engl J Med.* 2009;**361**(5):445–454.

47. Adams TD, Davidson LE, Litwin SE, Kim J, Kolotkin RL, Nanjee MN, Gutierrez JM, Frogley SJ, Ibele AR, Brinton EA, Hopkins PN, McKinlay R, Simper SC, Hunt SC. Weight and metabolic outcomes 12 years after gastric bypass. *N Engl J Med.* 2017;**377**(12):1143–1155.

Calories, Composition, Ketones, or Clock: What Is Most Important for Dietary Management of Type 2 Diabetes and Obesity

M52
Presented, March 23–26, 2019

William Donahoo, MD. Division of Endocrinology, Diabetes & Metabolism, University of Florida, Gainesville, Florida 32610, E-mail: troy.donahoo@medicine.ufl.edu

SIGNIFICANCE OF THE CLINICAL PROBLEM

Hippocrates is often misquoted as having said, "let food be thy medicine and medicine be thy food." Although the importance of food was well described in the *Hippocratic Corpus* from the 5th century BC, the texts did not state that medicine and food were not interchangeable. In 1746, James Lind carried out the "first controlled trial in clinical nutrition" when he treated 12 sailors with scurvy with one of six treatments (n = 2 per group), including two oranges and a lemon in one group. It took Lind until 1753 to publish these findings and it was not until 1795 that the British Navy adopted treating sailors with lemon (and later, lime) juice, based on the dramatic results of an experiment with only two participants. Upton Sinclair published in 1911 *The Fasting Cure*, which was probably the first collection of "patient reported outcomes" with the use of therapeutic fasting. Over the last century, a PubMed search reveals there are >4500 human clinical trials with key words "diet therapy" and "obesity" and >3600 human clinical trials with key words "diabetes" and "diet therapy." With the interest in the relationship between diet and health dating back millennia, the first nutrition clinical trials dating back almost 300 years, published reports on the benefits of one nutritional intervention (fasting) from over 100 years ago, and thousands of papers in the literature evaluating diet therapy's effects on obesity and diabetes in human clinical trials, why are there still so many questions regarding the best diet for weight loss and diabetes management?

How we have, and continue to do dietary research is part of the problem. In 2013, Dr. Ioannidis published an editorial entitled "Implausible results in human nutrition research: definitive solutions won't come from another million observational papers or small randomized trials" (1). The very poor track record of observational studies compared with randomized controlled trial (RCT) results is the first reason why. Since much of the research has related to single nutrients, dramatically positive results were often seen when a deficiency was corrected, but rarely (if ever) have micronutrients or vitamins been shown to be beneficial with excess supplementation. We continue to hold the belief that we will find magical curative results from the right food, as we have misquoted Hippocrates, and as was seen when vitamins were discovered and miraculously cured deadly deficiency-related diseases like scurvy. With few genuinely positive results from >9000 published human clinical dietary trials, it is exceedingly unlikely we will ever find a magic food or macronutrient beneficial for everyone. This can become a futile situation for the provider with a patient in the exam room when counseling on dietary therapy of diabetes and attempting to use the traditional prescriptive medical management. However, the lack of a definitive single answer is actually very freeing for the provider engaging in shared-decision clinical management.

BARRIERS TO OPTIMAL PRACTICE
- Lack of definitive evidence-based dietary guidelines
- Lack of long-term patient adherence to medical nutrition therapy
- Lack of insurance/reimbursement for medical nutrition therapy counseling

LEARNING OBJECTIVES
As a result of participating in this session, learners should be able to
- Identify the limitations of nutrition research in obesity and diabetes management
- Compare and contrast the risks and benefits of caloric restriction versus macronutrient alteration in the management of weight loss and diabetes
- Evaluate the risks and benefits of ketosis obtained through fasting (standard or new alternative methods) or extreme carbohydrate restriction in the management of weight loss and diabetes

STRATEGIES FOR DIAGNOSIS, THERAPY, AND/OR MANAGEMENT

Prior to the availability of insulin therapy, the diet for a person with (type 1) diabetes was nearly without any carbohydrate. Since the 1920s the optimal carbohydrate versus fat content in the diet for a patient with diabetes has been debated, and it shifted dramatically in the 1960s and 70s from more fat based to more carbohydrate based. The pendulum shifted so far over that the American Diabetes Association's Nutrition and Dietary Recommendations in 1971 stated "There no longer appears to be a need to restrict disproportionally the intake of carbohydrates in the diet of most diabetic patients. Increase of dietary carbohydrate, even to extremes, without increase of total calories..." (2). However, with the questions raised about the validity of Ancel Key's Seven Countries study (which correlated lower fat intake with less cardiovascular disease) and with the continued growth of the diabetes and obesity epidemics, many have called into question the low-fat paradigm. Diet Intervention Examining the Factors Interacting With Treatment Success (DIETFITS) is the best study to date to evaluate the effect of low-fat (LF) versus low-carbohydrate (LC) diet in overweight adults with varying levels of insulin resistance (3). In this 12-month study of >600 randomized participants, 481 or 79% completed the trial. The LC group was eating 45% fat and 30% carbohydrate at the end, whereas the LF group was eating 29% fat and 48% carbohydrate. This study found no differences in weight loss nor was there any interaction between diet and level of insulin resistance or between diet and a genotype predicting better response (3). A recent systematic review also found no difference in glucose control between LF and LC diets in people with type 2 diabetes mellitus (T2DM) (4). There is emerging evidence that an LC diet (~20% carbohydrate and 60% fat) over a relatively short period of time (20 weeks) might increase energy expenditure by ~200 kcal/d compared with an LF diet (20% fat and 60% carbohydrate) (5). Unfortunately, the practical clinical applicability of this diet is unknown, especially over the long-term (5). The question of long-term feasibility and efficacy of any dietary intervention is highly relevant, of course, and must be considered carefully. For example, the Atkins™ diet was hyped after several studies showed it to be superior for weight loss at 6 months, but then enthusiasm dissipated when benefits were found to be attenuated at 1 year or longer. In addition, the effects of low carbohydrate intake, or any dietary intervention, may depend heavily on the context of other macronutrients. For example, a recent cohort study and meta-analysis suggested that a lower-carbohydrate diet might reduce total mortality but only when the carbohydrates are substituted with plant-based protein and fat and not with animal-based protein and fat (6). In addition, although this last cohort study and meta-analysis could easily lead to the conclusion that plant-based diets are indeed "the best," this analysis was based on observational (albeit prospective) studies and not on RCTs, and thus must be viewed with caution.

Finally, there are several RCTs in T2DM showing that vegetarian/plant-based diets can benefit several surrogate outcomes, such as glycemic control, lipids, body weight, blood pressure, and quality of life (7, 8). However, long-term adherence to plant-based diets is extremely difficult for the majority of the population, and it has yet to be determined how to implement such a diet. In addition, it is not yet known which patients will respond best to this type of a prescription.

"The Science of Obesity Management: An Endocrine Society Scientific Statement" (9) validates a variety of options (see table 3 from this reference; Table 1). With respect to macronutrient composition, a lower carbohydrate diet such as the Dietary Approaches to Stop Hypertension (DASH) diet is favored, in part due to the meta-analysis by Hall and Guo (10).

Ketosis, whether through fasting/severe caloric restriction or through very low carbohydrate intake, has become popular recently. In part this is due to emerging findings suggesting health benefits beyond weight loss, including decreasing appetite, decreased sympathetic nervous system activation, and neuroprotection, which may be due to epigenetic changes and/or other mechanisms (11). Ketogenic diets based on very low carbohydrate intake have been shown to be safe and modestly more effective for weight loss and improved glycemic control when compared with moderate-carbohydrate diets over 4 to 12 months in participants with T2DM (12, 13). A recent online survey of people with T1DM suggests that following a very-low-carbohydrate diet (mean intake 36 ± 15 g/d) resulted in very good glycemic control (HbA$_{1c}$, 5.7 ± 0.7) (14). Surprisingly, there were rare diabetes-related hospitalizations for either diabetic ketoacidosis (1.2%) or hypoglycemia (0.6%) (14). These data must be interpreted with extreme caution given that they are self-reported, and there was selection bias in subject recruitment, but they do provide preliminary evidence for possible short-term beneficial effects of very-low-carbohydrate diets in T1DM. Long-term ketogenic diets have been used for many years in children with intractable seizure disorders. Although not a fair comparison with people with diabetes and obesity, many severe side effects have been reported in long-term observational studies of ketogenic diets, including hyperuricemia and nephrolithiasis, hyperlipidemia, increased liver function enzymes, electrolyte abnormalities, pancreatitis, sepsis, cardiomyopathy, lipoid pneumonia, and death (up to 3% in some reviews).

Prolonged fasting has a range of severe side effects similar to those of a ketogenic diet from very low carbohydrate intake. These include edema, motor neuropathy, urate nephropathy, abnormal liver function tests, decreased bone density, Wernicke encephalopathy, renal failure, cardiac arrhythmias, and death from lactic acidosis. This is why prolonged fasting was abandoned many decades ago by the medical profession in favor of protein-sparing modified fasting and other very-low-calorie diets. Recently, alternative forms of fasting that might have similar benefits to prolonged fasting, but with improved safety, have emerged:

- Intermittent fasting (fasting for 12 hours or longer)
  - True alternate-day fasting (fasting one full day, alternating with a day of ad lib eating)
  - Time-restricted feeding (restricting food intake to a small time window of 2 to 12 hours a day)
  - Periodic fasting (fasting 1 to 2 nonconsecutive days per week and eating ad lib the other 5 to 6 days per week)
- Modified fasting (consuming 25% or less of baseline calories on modified fasting days and ad lib on nonfasting days)
  - Alternate-day modified fasting (eating <25% of energy needs every other day, alternating with ad lib feeding)
  - Periodic modified fasting (eating <25% of energy needs 1 to 2 days per week, *e.g.*, the 5:2 diet)
- Fasting-mimicking diet (5-day cycles of low-calorie, low-carbohydrate diets to generate ketosis occurring once a month)

Table 1.   A Comparison of Various Diet Programs and Eating Plans to a Typical American Diet

Type of Diet	Example	General Dietary Characteristic	Comments	AHA/ACC/TOS Evaluation and Others
Typical American diet		Carbohydrate: 50%	Low in fruits and vegetables, dairy, and whole gains	
		Protein: 75%	High in saturated fat and unrefined carbohydrates	
		Fat 35%		
		Average of 2200 kcal/d		
Balanced-nutrient moderate-calorie approach	DASH Diet or diet based on MyPyramid food guide commercial diet plans such as: Diet Center, Jenny Craig®, Nutrisystem®, Physician's Weight Loss Shapedown Pediatric Program, Weight Watchers®, Setpoint, Sonomo, Volumetrics	Carbohydrate: 55%–60%	Based on set pattern of selections from food lists using regular grocery store food or prepackaged food supplemented by fresh food items	Meta-analysis showing DASH approach better than control or healthy diets (weight mean difference 0.87–7.5 kg)
		Protein: 15%–20%	Low in saturated fat and ample in fruits, vegetables, and fiber	
		Fat: 20%–30%	Recommended reasonable weight-loss goal of as 20 pounds/wk	
		Usually 1200–1800 kcal/d	Prepackeged plans may limit food choice	
			Most recommend exercise plan	
			Many encouraged deitary record keeping	
			Some offer weight-maintenance plans/support	
Low- and very-low-fat, high-carbohydrate approach	Ornish Diet (Eat More, Weightless) Pritikin Diet, T-factor Diet, Choose to Lose Diet, Fit or Fat Diet	Carbohydrate: 65%	Long-term compliance with some plans may be difficult because of low level of fat	Same weight loss at 6 months comparing 30% fat to >40% strength of evidence moderate
		Protein: 10%–20%	Diet can be low in calcium	
		Fat: <10%–19%	Some plans restrict healthful foods (seafood LF dairy, poultry)	
		Limited intake of animal protein, nuts, seeds, other fats	Some encourage exercise and stress management techniques	
Low energy density	Volumetrics Diet	Carbohydrate: 55%	Four food categories:	More weight loss at 6 months with low energy-dense diet, strength of evidence RCT
		Protein: 10%–25%	(1) Very-low-density nonstarchy fruits and vegetables, nonfat milk, broth-based soups	
		Fat: 20%–35%	(2) Low-density starchy fruits/ vegetables, grains, breakfast cereal, LF meats, and mixed dishes	
		Focus on fruits, vegetables, and soups	(3) Medium-density meat, cheese, pizza, fries, dressings, bread, and such	
			(4) High-density desserts, nuts, butter, oils	
			Focus on categories 1 and 2, some from 3, minimum from 4	
Portion controlled	Use of meal replacements, both liquid and solid meals			Weight loss at 1 year in Look AHEAD trial related to frequency of consuming portion-control meals

(Table Continues)

Table 1. A Comparison of Various Diet Programs and Eating Plans to a Typical American Diet (Continued)

Type of Diet	Example	General Dietary Characteristic	Comments	AHA/ACC/TOS Evaluation and Others
Mediterranean-style diets		Carbohydrate: 35%–40%	Eat primarily plant-based foods (fruits, vegetable, whole grains, legumes, and nuts)	
		Protein: 12%–20%	Healthy oils instead of saturated fats	
		Fat: 40%–50%	Limit red meat to a few times a month	
		Approximately 25%–30% of energy from monounsaturated fat	Eat fish and poultry at least twice a week	
			Red wine in moderation for individuals who choose to drink alcohol	
			Be active and enjoy meals with family and friends	
LC, high-protein, high-fat approach	Atkins™ New Diet Revolution, Protein Power Diet, Stillman Diet (The Doctor's Quick Weight Loss Diet), Carbohydrate Addict's Diet, Scarsdale Diet	Carbohydrate: <20%	Promotes quick weight loss (much is water loss rather than fat loss)	Some weight loss at 6 months comparing <30 g/d vs. 55% carbohydrate and 15% protein or 40% carbohydrate and 30% protein
		Protein: 25%–40%	Ketosis causes loss of appetite	Strength of evidence low
		Fat: >55%–65%	Can be too high in saturated fat	
		Strictly limits carbohydrates to <100–125 g/d	Low in carbohydrates, vitamins, minerals, and fiber	
			Not practical for long-term because of rigid diet or restricted food choices	
Higher-protein, moderate-carbohydrate, moderate-fat approach	The Zone® Diet, Sugar Busters Diet, South Beach Diet	Carbohydrate: 40%–50%	Diet rigid and difficult to maintain	Same weight loss at 6 months comparing 25% to 30% vs. 15% protein; strength of evidence high
		Protein: 25%–40%	Enough carbohydrates to avoid ketosis	
		Fat: 30%–40%	Low in carbohydrates, can be low in vitamins and minerals	
Glycemic load	The Glycemic-load Diet Rob Thompson	Carbohydrate: 40%–>55%	Focus on low-glycemic-load foods	Same weight loss at 6 months comparing high vs. low glycemic load; strength of evidence low
		Protein: 15%–30%		
		Fat: 30%		
Low-sugar or nonsugar-sweetened beverages	Not really a diet but just a call to reduce sugar-sweetened beverage intake as a preventive strategy	No recommendation other than to reduce/remove sugar-sweetened beverages from your overall diet plan	Meta-analyses show that consumption of sugar-sweetened beverages is related to risk of obesity, T2DM, and heart disease	Weight loss less in adolescents comparing artificial vs. sugar-sweetened drinks; strength of evidence RCT comparing artificially sweetened vs. sugar-sweetened beverages
Novelty diets	Immune Power Diet, Rotation Diet, Cabbage Soup Diet, Beverly Hills Diet, Dr. Phil Diet	Most promote certain foods, or combinations of foods, or nutrients as having allegedly magical qualities	No scientific basis for recommendations	

Reproduced with permission from Bray GA, Heisel WE, Afshin A, et al. The science of obesity management: An Endocrine Society Scientific Statement. *Endocrine Reviews* 2018; 39:9–132.

Abbreviations: ACC, American College of Cardiology; AHA, American Heart Association; TOS, The Obesity Society.

Several recent studies have demonstrated the safety and benefits of alternate-day fasting, alternate-day modified fasting, and fasting-mimicking diet on body weight and other cardiovascular risk factors (15–17). A recent study showed that periodic modified fasting (500 to 600 kcal on two non-consecutive days per week) resulted in similar weight loss and improvements in glycemic control as a 1200 to 1500 kcal/d restriction over 12 months in participants with T2DM (18). Finally, a case series showed that with intermittent fasting/time-restricted feeding, three men with T2DM were able to come off almost all diabetes medications (one continued to use canagliflozin) and achieve very good glycemic control (19). It should be noted that few of these studies actually measured ketosis; thus the seeming lack of benefit with some studies might be due to inadequate reduction of carbohydrate intake.

MAIN CONCLUSIONS

Although we have improved in our performance of nutrition research in diabetes and obesity management, this remains a very difficult area of study due to limitations in accurately tracking provided diets in free-living settings, the unknown reasons for dramatic individual variation in response, and often-unrecognized bias among researchers. Given continued conflicting data with respect to calorie restriction versus altered macronutrient composition, we have made little, if any, progress over the past decade. One large remaining challenge is to find a hypocaloric diet to which the patient can best adhere. Emerging data are showing potential benefits of ketosis by alternative types of fasting; however, few studies have measured the degree of ketosis achieved, if any, and valid concerns remain about the long-term safety of sustained or intermittent ketosis.

CASES

Case 1

Dr. S is a 50-year-old physiology professor who comes to see you after being diagnosed with diabetes (HbA$_{1c}$ 6.9%) and hypertriglyceridemia (triglyceride 300 mg/dL). His body mass index is 38 kg/m^2. He has reviewed "Endocrine Daily Briefing" to determine what will be the best diet for him. He brings in 15 postings on this topic, but they differ in their conclusions and so he remains confused. He does not want to do anything drastic like "keto" right now. Your best advice is that he eat:

A. A diet with as much "healthy" fat and as little carbohydrate as tolerable
B. A diet with as much "healthy" carbohydrate and as little fat as possible
C. A plant-based diet
D. The DASH diet with a modest caloric deficit

Case 2

Dr. S returns for follow-up after working through several diets with only modest success. His HbA$_{1c}$ is now 8.2% (on no

diabetes medications) and his body mass index is now 41 kg/m^2, but his lipids are well controlled on a statin. He says "diets don't work" and he now wants to do something more drastic like "keto" or fasting. He again reviewed "Endocrine Daily Briefing" to determine what will be the best diet for him. Your best advice is now that he:

A. Start a reduced-carbohydrate, ketogenic diet, which is safe for long-term use
B. Work on eating three meals a day with at least 30 g of carbohydrate per meal and a bedtime snack
C. Start a modified fasting regimen with close follow-up
D. Avoid anything that might result in ketosis

DISCUSSION OF CASES and ANSWERS

Case 1

Answers A and B are incorrect as it was shown in the DIETFITS study (3) that neither higher-fat nor higher-carbohydrate diets were superior when compared head to head. Although a plant-based diet (answer C) has evidence to support the use (7, 8), long-term adherence is low; thus, this is less than optimal for most patients. Answer D is the most correct and is based on the Endocrine Society's recent Scientific Statement (9).

Case 2

Although short-term studies have shown safety and efficacy of ketogenic diets (nutritional ketosis) in people with T2DM (12, 13) and self-reported data suggest the same for T1DM (14), long-term studies are lacking and there is concern for the long-term safety of true ketogenic diets (assuming the validity of data from ketogenic diets in people with seizure disorders). Thus, answers A and D are incorrect. Answer B is incorrect as the patient clearly stated he did not want that advice. Answer C is the best choice and is based on the study by Carter et al. (18).

References

1. Ioannidis JP. Implausible results in human nutrition research. *BMJ.* 2013;**347**:f6698.
2. Principles of nutrition and dietary recommendations for patients with diabetes mellitus: 1971. *Diabetes.* 1971;**20**(9):633–634.
3. Gardner CD, Trepanowski JF, Del Gobbo LC, Hauser ME, Rigdon J, Ioannidis JPA, Desai M, King AC. Effect of low-fat vs low-carbohydrate diet on 12-month weight loss in overweight adults and the association with genotype pattern or insulin secretion: the DIETFITS randomized clinical trial. *JAMA.* 2018;**319**(7):667–679.
4. Van Zuuren EJ, Fedorowicz Z, Kuijpers T, Pijl H. Effects of low-carbohydrate compared with low-fat diet interventions on metabolic control in people with type 2 diabetes: a systematic review including GRADE assessments. *AJCN.* 2018;**108**(2):300–331
5. Ebbeling CB, Feldman HA, Klein GL, Wong JMW, Bielak L, Steltz SK, Luoto PK, Wolfe RR, Wong WW, Ludwig DS. Effects of a low carbohydrate diet on energy expenditure during weight loss maintenance: randomized trial. *BMJ.* 2018;**363**:k4583.
6. Seidelmann SB, Claggett B, Cheng S, Henglin M, Shah A, Steffen LM, Folsom AR, Rimm EB, Willett WC, Solomon SD. Dietary carbohydrate intake and mortality: a prospective cohort study and meta-analysis. *Lancet Public Health.* 2018;**3**(9):e419–e428.
7. Viguilouk E, Kendall CWC, Kahleova H, Rahelic D, Salas-Salvado J, Choo VL, Mejia SB, Stewart SE, Leiter LA, Jenkins DJA, Sievenpiper JL.

Effect of vegetarian dietary patterns on cardiometabolic risk factors in diabetes: a systematic review and meta-analysis of randomized controlled trials [published online ahead of print 13 June 2018]. *Clin Nutr.* doi:10.1016/j.clnu.2018.05.032.

8. Toumpanakis A, Turnbull T, Alba-Barba I. Effectiveness of plant-based diets in promoting well-being in the management of type 2 diabetes: a systematic review [published online ahead of print 30 October 2018]. *BMJ Open Diabetes Res Care.* doi:10.1136/bmjdrc-2018-000534.

9. Bray GA, Heisel WE, Afshin A, Jensen MD, Dietz WH, Long M, Kushner RF, Daniels SR, Wadden TA, Tsai AG, Hu FB, Jakicic JM, Ryan DH, Wolfe BM, Inge TH. The science of obesity management: an Endocrine Society scientific statement. *Endocr Rev.* 2018;**39**(2):79–132.

10. Hall KD, Guo J. Obesity energetics: body weight regulation and the effects of diet composition. *Gastroenterology.* 2017;**152**(7):1718.e3–1727.e3.

11. Anton SD, Moehl K, Donahoo WT, Marosi K, Lee SA, Mainous AG III, Leeuwenburgh C, Mattson MP. Flipping the metabolic switch: understanding and applying the health benefits of fasting. *Obesity (Silver Spring).* 2018;**26**(2):254–268.

12. Goday A, Bellido D, Sajoux I, Crujeiras AB, Burguera B, García-Luna PP, Oleaga A, Moreno B, Casanueva FF. Short-term safety, tolerability and efficacy of a very low-calorie-ketogenic diet interventional weight loss program versus hypocaloric diet in patients with type 2 diabetes mellitus. *Nutr Diabetes.* 2016;**6**(9):e230.

13. Saslow LR, Daubenmier JJ, Moskowitz JT, Kim S, Murphy EJ, Phinney SD, Ploutz-Snyder R, Goldman V, Cox RM, Mason AE, Moran P, Hecht FM. Twelve-month outcomes of a randomized trial of a moderate-carbohydrate versus very low-carbohydrate diet in overweight adults with type 2 diabetes mellitus or prediabetes. *Nutr Diabetes.* 2017;**7**(12):304.

14. Lennerz BS, Barton A, Bernstein RK, Dikeman RD, Diulus C, Hallberg S, Rhodes ET, Ebbeling CB, Westman EC, Yancy WS, Jr, Ludwig DS. Management of type 1 diabetes with a very low-carbohydrate diet. *Pediatrics.* 2018;**141**(6):e20173349.

15. Catenacci VA, Pan Z, Ostendorf D, Brannon S, Gozansky WS, Mattson MP, Martin B, MacLean PS, Melanson EL, Troy Donahoo W. A randomized pilot study comparing zero-calorie alternate-day fasting to daily caloric restriction in adults with obesity. *Obesity (Silver Spring).* 2016;**24**(9):1874–1883.

16. Trepanowski JF, Kroeger CM, Barnosky A, Klempel MC, Bhutani S, Hoddy KK, Gabel K, Freels S, Rigdon J, Rood J, Ravussin E, Varady KA. Effect of alternate-day fasting on weight loss, weight maintenance, and cardioprotection among metabolically healthy obese adults: a randomized clinical trial. *JAMA Intern Med.* 2017;**177**(7):930–938.

17. Wei M, Brandhorst S, Shelehchi M, Mirzaei H, Cheng CW, Budniak J, Groshen S, Mack WJ, Guen E, Di Base S, Cohen P, Morgan TE, Dorff T, Hong K, Michalsen A, Laviano A, Longo VD. Fasting-mimicking diet and markers/risk factors for aging, diabetes, cancer, and cardiovascular disease. *Sci Transl Med.* 2017;**9**(377):eaai8700.

18. Carter S, Clifton PM, Keogh JB. Effect of intermittent compared with continuous energy restricted diet on glycemic control in patients with type 2 diabetes. *JAMA Netw Open.* 2018;**1**(3):e180756.

19. Furmli S, Elmasry R, Ramos M, Fung J. Therapeutic use of intermittent fasting for people with type 2 diabetes as an alternative to insulin. *BMJ Case Rep.* 2018;pii:bcr-2017-221854.

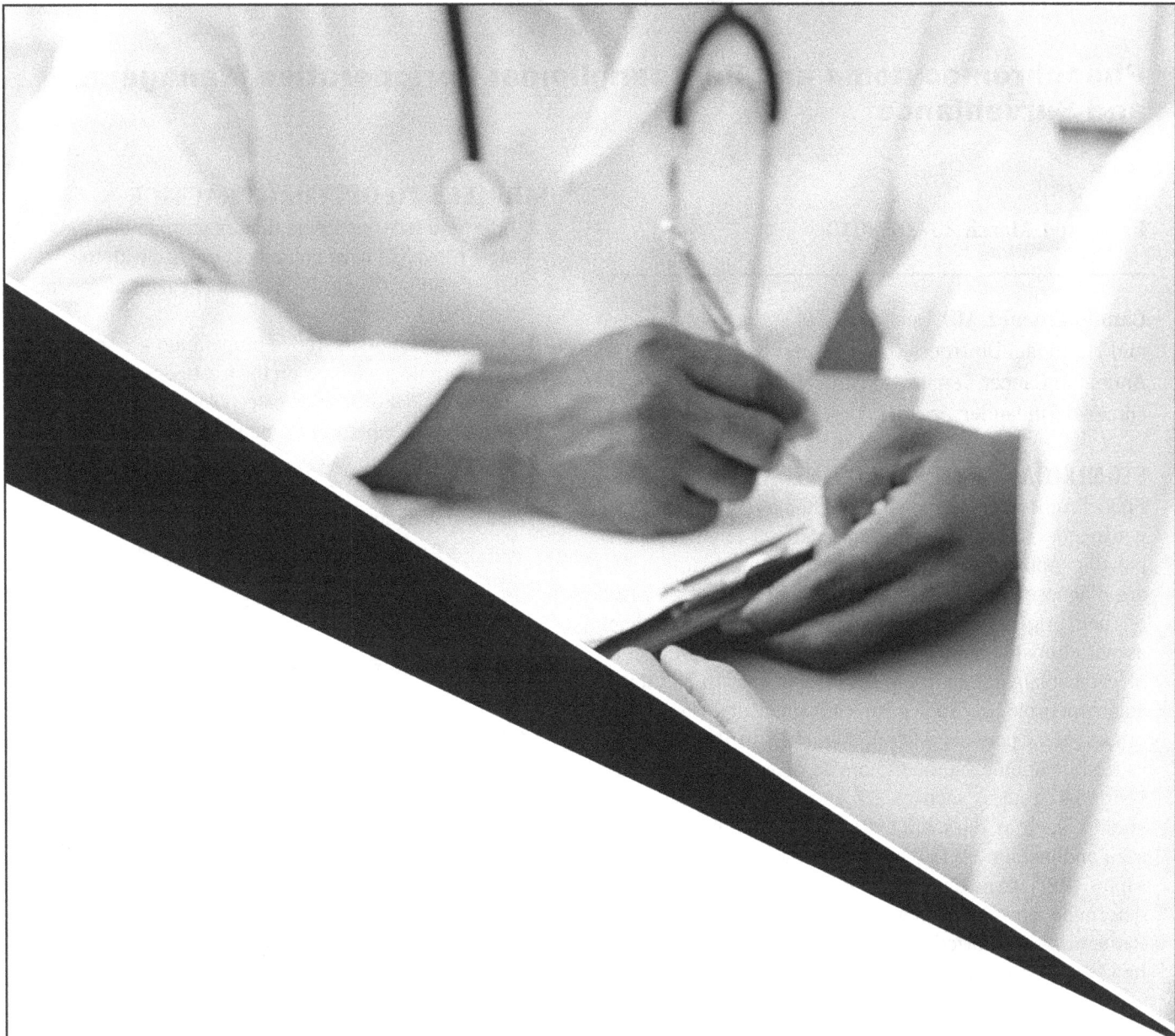

ADRENAL

Pheochromocytoma and Paraganglioma: Perioperative Management and Surveillance

M02
Presented, March 23–26, 2019

Camilo Jimenez, MD. Department of Endocrine Neoplasia and Hormonal Disorders, The University of Texas, MD Anderson Cancer Center, Houston, Texas 77004, E-mail: cjimenez@mdanderson.org

SIGNIFICANCE OF THE CLINICAL PROBLEM

Pheochromocytomas and paragangliomas (PHPGs) are rare neuroendocrine tumors that are derived from the paraganglia. Approximately 1000 new patients with PHPGs are diagnosed every year in the United States. As a result of their origin, PHPGs may secrete catecholamines, such as noradrenaline and/or adrenaline. Excessive production of catecholamines may predispose patients to cardiovascular, neurologic, and gastrointestinal disease, among others. Most patients with PHPGs (83% to 85%) have localized or nonmetastatic tumors as demonstrated by conventional studies, such as CT and MRI. Complementary studies, such as the meta-iodine-benzyl guanidine (MIBG) scan and gallium 68 DOTATATE positron emission tomography (PET) scan, may provide valuable information to determine how patients with PHPGs should be treated. Patients with localized PHPGs may be cured with surgery; however, surgery could be a challenging procedure. Several aspects related to surgery may predispose patients to acute complications and mortality. Preoperative preparation with α- and β-blockers and other medications, isotonic fluids, and adequate salt intake may prevent perioperative complications (1).

Approximately 30% to 40% of patients with PHPGS have a hereditary predisposition. Most mutations that predispose patients to PHPGs have been identified over the last two decades. Some mutations are quite rare, the penetrance of some mutations is low, and the long-term experience with these patients and their families is still insufficient to determine how to clearly observe most patients with hereditary disease (1). Patients with malignant PHPGs (15% to 17%) represent the biggest challenge in clinical practice (2). Currently, the definition of malignancy relies on the presence of metastases. Most patients with metastatic PHPGs have advanced disease and are not curable with surgery. Systemic therapies are rather palliative than curative (3, 4). Fifty percent of patients with malignant disease have metachronous metastases. Clinical predictors of malignancy and survivorship have led to the development of the first PHPG TNM staging system (5).

BARRIERS TO OPTIMAL PRACTICE

- PHPG are rare endocrine tumors (orphan disease).
- Most providers have limited experience with the identification, diagnosis, and management of patients with PHPG.
- Guidelines on preoperative preparation are scant.
- There are no guidelines on the treatment of emergencies related to PHPG, such as catecholamine crisis, hypertensive emergency, and severe constipation.
- There are no histologic, molecular, genetic, or biochemical markers that could help to differentiate benign from malignant tumors.
- There are no guidelines on the diagnosis and treatment of patients with metastatic disease.
- Therapies for patients with metastatic disease are limited.

LEARNING OBJECTIVES

As a result of participating in this session, learners should be able to:

- Prevent complications related to hormonal excess in patients undergoing surgical resection of PHPGs
- Identify clinical predictors of metastases
- Provide a clear plan of care and follow-up for patients PHPGs

STRATEGIES FOR DIAGNOSIS, THERAPY, AND/OR MANAGEMENT

Preoperative Management

Surgery, fortunately, is an effective approach by which to treat and cure patients with localized PHPGs; however, surgery may be associated with complications as a result of the excessive tumor secretion of catecholamines. Several aspects at the time of surgery may predispose patients to a catecholamine crisis (1). Mechanical intubation, tumor palpation, and peritoneal insufflation during laparoscopic procedures may induce an excessive release of catecholamines. Medications used during surgery, such as opiates, antiemetics (metoclopramide), muscle relaxants, tranquilizers (droperidol), and sympathomimetics, may also precipitate a catecholamine crisis. Atropine and vagolytics may prevent protective responses to the catecholamine excess (6).

Historical observations have clearly demonstrated that patients who are not prepared with α- and β-blockers before surgery are at high risk of cardiovascular complications. A classical study on surgical outcomes noted that up to 70% of patients with PHPG who did not receive treatment with α-blockers before surgery had cardiovascular complications, whereas only 3% of pretreated patients with α-blockers experienced complications (7). Cardiovascular complications include hypertensive emergencies, angina, heart attacks, arrhythmias, congestive heart failure, pulmonary edema, renal failure, intestinal ischemia, and hypertensive retinopathy.

α-Blockers

α-Blockers have been used to lower and stabilize blood pressure in patients with PHPGs in preparation for surgery. α-Blockers will prevent catecholamine toxicity on the arterioles and arteries of the coronary, pulmonary, brain, ocular, and splanchnic vascular bed. α-Blockers are classified in two different categories on the basis of their interactions with the α-1 and α-2 receptors. Selective α-blockers interact exclusively with α-1 receptors. Selective α-blockers include such medications as prazosin, terazosin, and doxazosin. Nonselective α-blockers interact with both α-1 and α-2 receptors. The only nonselective α-blocker used in clinical practice is phenoxybenzamine. Selective α-blockers establish ionic bonds with the α-1 receptor. Subsequently, their half-lives are short. The half-life of prazosin is only 3 hours and that of terazosin and doxazosin is 24 hours. Conversely, phenoxybenzamine establishes covalent bonds with α-receptors. Subsequently, its half-life is longer. The half-life of phenoxybenzamine is approximately 10 days. Hypotension is the main adverse effect associated with α-blockers. In preparation for surgery, hypotension, in reality, is a desired adverse effect. In fact, adequate α-blockage occurs when the patient develops orthostatic hypotension with reflex tachycardia. Once the patient develops orthostatic hypotension, he or she may start treatment with β-blockers. The patient should continue treatment with α- and β-blockers until the day of surgery. However, it is important to remember that once the PHPG is removed, patients may exhibit persistent hypotension during the postoperative period. The duration of this adverse effect may be long in patients who are treated with phenoxybenzamine. Patients with postoperative hypotension need IV isotonic fluids, mainly normal saline or ringer lactate, to re-establish normal blood pressure while waiting for the actions of the α-blocker to vanish. Occasionally, in cases of severe hypotension, transient use of vasopressors is indicated (8, 9).

β-Blockers

β-Blockers are important medications to provide to patients with PHPGs in preparation for surgery. β-Blockers interact with the B1 receptors located in the heart. β-Blockers have beneficial negative inotropic and chronotropic effects. By decreasing cardiac muscle contractibility and heart rate, β-blockers decrease cardiac oxygen consumption, which prevents angina, heart attacks, heart failure, and arrhythmias. Treatment with β-blockers should be initiated once adequate α-blockage has been instituted. β-Blockers must be started at the time that the patient has orthostatism and reflex tachycardia, which indicate that adequate α-blockage has been achieved. β-Blockers should not be initiated before the α-blockers. Use of β-blockers before α-blockage

may cause a rebound hypertension as a result of skeletal muscle vascular bed contraction. Like α-blockers, β-blockers could be selective and nonselective. Propranolol is a nonselective β-blocker that antagonizes the interaction of catecholamines with β-1 and β-2 receptors. Metoprolol, atenolol, and nadolol are selective β-1 receptor blockers. Both nonselective and selective β-blockers protect patients with PHPGs from cardiac events. Labetalol and carvedilol are medications that block α- and β-receptors. For clinical purposes, in the context of PHPG disease, labetalol and carvedilol are β-blockers and should therefore be used once α-blockage has been achieved (1). Labetalol and carvedilol interact mainly on β-receptors. For instance, the potency of labetalol on β-receptors compared with α-receptors is 7 to 1. It is also important to remember that propranolol, metoprolol, or atenolol are more effective medications to prevent arrhythmias than carvedilol.

Calcium Channel Blockers, Angiotensin-Converting Enzyme Inhibitors, and Angiotensin Receptor Blockers

Calcium channel blockers, angiotensin-converting enzyme inhibitors, and angiotensin receptor blockers are useful medications with which to treat patients with PHPG in preparation for surgery. These medications could be prescribed in different situations and could be useful to prepare patients with a mild catecholamine surge (e.g., small tumors identified by radiographic screening in patients with hereditary predisposition) or those who are unable to tolerate α-blockers. These medications can also supplement α- and β-blockers when hypertension is still difficult to control. These agents may also supplement α- and β-blockers to prevent their toxicity when high doses to control blood pressure are needed. The latter two situations are mainly observed in patients with large nonmetastatic PHPGs or in those with metastatic PHPGs (10). Although patients with metastatic disease are not usually curable with surgery, these patients may benefit from resection of the primary tumor, and preoperative preparation with α- and β-blockers and other antihypertensive medications is frequently needed. Resection of the primary tumor in the context of metastatic disease is associated with lower catecholamine secretion and easier to control hypertension. In addition, surgery is associated with improvement of overall survival and, perhaps, better responses to systemic therapy (11).

Inhibitors of Catecholamine Secretion

α-Metyrosine inhibits tyrosine hydroxylase. Tyrosine hydroxylase is the regulatory enzyme of the catecholamine synthesis pathway. α-Metyrosine lowers the secretion of adrenaline and/or noradrenaline, which makes it easier to control the patient's hypertension. A recent retrospective study suggested that patients who were treated with α-metyrosine, together with α- and β-blockers had a significantly lower rate of cardiovascular complications compared with patients treated with only α- and β-blockers (12). Use of α-metyrosine in clinical practice, however, is not straightforward. Effective doses of α-metyrosine are usually higher than 2500 mg/d. Adverse effects associated with α-metyrosine are proportional to the dose. Adverse effects could be overwhelming and include anxiety, fatigue, and diarrhea, and patients frequently discontinue treatment. Furthermore, α-metyrosine is expensive. The price of this medication in the United States is approximately USD $2000 per prescription despite being an old medication. In addition, it is not available in most pharmacies and hospitals in the United States, nor in most countries around the world. Therefore, treatment mainly relies on the medications previously described (13).

Maintenance of Volemia

It is important to remember that excessive secretion of catecholamines in patients with PHPG may predispose them to water consumption and insensitive water loss. Despite hypertension, patients are frequently hypovolemic; therefore, patients should be encouraged to follow a diet with normal salt content and good hydration. In preparation for surgery, patients should receive normal saline at the time of admission and during and immediately after the procedure. It is recommended to avoid the use of diuretics unless the patient has fluid congestion (*i.e.*, pulmonary edema and/or cardiac failure) (1).

Surveillance

Thirty to 40% of patients with PHPG have a genetic predisposition for disease. Follow-up of patients with multiple endocrine neoplasia type 2 (MEN2), von Hippel-Lindau (VHL), and neurofibromatosis type 1 (NF1) seems straightforward. Approximately 50% of patients with MEN2 and 40% of those with VHL would develop PHPGs. Less than 10% of patients with NF1 would develop PHPGs. Patients with MEN2 develop PHs. These tumors secrete noradrenaline and adrenaline and are rarely metastatic. Most patients with VHL develop PHs (90%); some patients may develop PGs (10%). Most VHL PGs are subdiaphragmatic and are rarely metastatic (10%). VHL PHPGs secrete only noradrenaline. Most patients with MEN2 and VHL who develop PHPGs are young adults; however, the earliest PHPGs have been described during adolescence. PHPG screening for patients with MEN2 and VHL should then start at adolescence. Screening tests should include periodic measurement of plasma or 24-hour urinary fractionated metanephrines and MRIs of the abdomen (in patients with MEN2) or abdomen and pelvis (in patients with VHL). Most patients with NF1 will not develop PHPGs. It is important to recognize that up to 50% of patients with NF1 with hypertension may have a PHPG (14). For patients with paraganglioma syndromes and carriers of less common mutations, such as TMEM127, MAX, and others, long-term follow-up with periodic biochemical and radiographic studies is guarantee; however, the characteristics of their follow-up are still to be determined (1).

Currently, there are no histologic, molecular, genetic, or biochemical markers that help to differentiate benign from malignant disease. Subsequently, the definition of malignancy relies on the presence of metastases. Because of this issue, the World Health Organization has recommended classifying PHPGs as metastatic and nonmetastatic (15). There are some clinical predictors of metastatic potential. Location of the primary tumor [extra-adrenal (abdominal, pelvic, or thoracic) *vs.* adrenal], primary tumor size > 5 cm, and the presence of germline mutations of the mitochondrial enzymatic complex 2 or succinate dehydrogenase subunit B gene are recognized predictors of aggressiveness (2). Patients with any of these characteristics need long-term follow-up (16). Clinical experience suggests that patients with PHPGs with clinical predictors need long-term follow-up. In fact, metastases have been described up to 40 years after the initial diagnosis and removal of the primary tumor (2). Follow-up evaluations should include clinical assessments with a particular focus on symptoms that are suggestive of catecholamine excess and tumor burden. Biochemical testing with periodic plasma metanephrines and MRI is recommended. MRI is preferable to CT scan as MRI is not associated with radiation exposure. As the experience with these patients is still limited, it is up to the clinician to consider other testing periodically (*i.e.*, bone scan) to assess the presence of disease (16, 17). Screening with nuclear medicine studies, such as MIBG, fluorodeoxyglucose (FDG)-, and DOTATATE PET scans, has been suggested (16); however, such aspects as their price, limited sensitivity (MIBG scan is not able to identify tumors that do not express the catecholamine transporter), and long-term radiation exposure, especially with PET modalities, limit the use of these imaging modalities. Benefits related to screening are several. Screening testing allows for the identification of early recurrences or localized metastases that could be treated with surgery. Screening may identify advanced but no massive disease that could respond better to systemic chemotherapy or high specific-activity MIBG. High specific activity is the first and only therapy approved by the US Food and Drug Administration for the treatment of patients with metastatic/unresectable PHPGs (18).

MAIN CONCLUSIONS

PHPGs are challenging endocrine tumors. Surgery is the main therapy for most patients. Patients should be prepared with α- and β-blockers and sometimes with other interventions before surgery. These interventions will guarantee good clinical outcomes. Patients with genetic predisposition and/or clinical predictors of metastases need long-term follow-up.

CASE 1

An 18-year-old man presents to the emergency room with sudden abdominal pain. A CT scan shows a 3.1-cm right adrenal nodule. Plasma normetanephrines are 2300 ng/mL (normal, <400 ng/mL). Blood pressure is 120/60 mm Hg and heart rate is 60 beats/min. The patient is diagnosed with a pheochromocytoma and is a candidate for surgery. In preparation for surgery, you would recommend:

A. Treatment with phenoxybenzamine and proceed with surgery

B. Treatment with doxazosin followed by propranolol once the patient is orthostatic

C. Treatment with labetalol only as this medication offers α- and β-blockage

D. No additional treatment is needed as his blood pressure and pulse are normal

E. Treatment with prazosin followed by metoprolol and a diet with salt restriction

Answer: B

CASE 2

A 33-year-old man presents to the clinic with hypertension. The patient has normal body mass index and an athletic complexion. His blood pressure is 140/90 mm Hg and pulse is 80 beats/min. The patient indicates that his tolerance to exercise has declined over the last 3 months. Plasma metanephrines are 3500 ng/mL (normal, <400 ng/mL). CT scan shows a 3.2-cm retroperitoneal mass. FDG-PET scan confirms CT findings. Gene testing is normal. The patient undergoes surgery. The pathology report indicates that the tumor resection was complete (R0) and Ki-67 is <1%. The patient is asymptomatic and has normal blood pressure 6 months after surgery. Plasma metanephrines are normal. What do you recommend next?

A. The tumor was small and benign. The patient is cured. No follow-up is needed.

B. The tumor was not associated with metastases. Subsequently, no additional follow-up is required.

C. The tumor is sporadic and resection was complete. No follow-up is needed.

D. The patient needs long-term follow-up, despite the fact that the tumor is sporadic.

Answer: D

References

1. Lenders JW, Duh QY, Eisenhofer G, Gimenez-Roqueplo AP, Grebe SK, Murad MH, Naruse M, Pacak K, Young WF, Jr, Endocrine S, for the Endocrine Society. Pheochromocytoma and paraganglioma: An Endocrine Society clinical practice guideline. *J Clin Endocrinol Metab.* 2014;**99**(6):1915–1942.
2. Ayala-Ramirez M, Feng L, Johnson MM, Ejaz S, Habra MA, Rich T, Busaidy N, Cote GJ, Perrier N, Phan A, Patel S, Waguespack S, Jimenez C. Clinical risk factors for malignancy and overall survival in patients with pheochromocytomas and sympathetic paragangliomas: Primary tumor size and primary tumor location as prognostic indicators. *J Clin Endocrinol Metab.* 2011;**96**(3):717–725.
3. Jimenez P, Tatsui C, Jessop A, Thosani S, Jimenez C. Treatment for malignant pheochromocytomas and paragangliomas: 5 years of progress. *Curr Oncol Rep.* 2017;**19**(12):83.
4. Hamidi O, Young WF, Jr, Gruber L, Smestad J, Yan Q, Ponce OJ, Prokop L, Murad MH, Bancos I. Outcomes of patients with metastatic
5. Roman-Gonzalez A, Jimenez C. Malignant pheochromocytoma-paraganglioma: Pathogenesis, TNM staging, and current clinical trials. *Curr Opin Endocrinol Diabetes Obes.* 2017;**24**(3):174–183.
6. Eisenhofer G, Rivers G, Rosas AL, Quezado Z, Manger WM, Pacak K. Adverse drug reactions in patients with phaeochromocytoma: Incidence, prevention and management. *Drug Saf.* 2007;**30**(11):1031–1062.
7. Goldstein RE, O'Neill JA, Jr., Holcomb GW, 3rd, Morgan WM, 3rd, Neblett WW, 3rd, Oates JA, Brown N, Nadeau J, Smith B, Page DL, Abumrad NN, Scott HW, Jr. Clinical experience over 48 years with pheochromocytoma. *Ann Surg.* 1999;**229**(6):755-764; discussion 764-756.
8. Gu YW, Poste J, Kunal M, Schwarcz M, Weiss I. Cardiovascular manifestations of pheochromocytoma. *Cardiol Rev.* 2017;**25**(5):215–222.
9. Malec K, Miśkiewicz P, Witkowska A, Krajewska E, Toutounchi S, Gałązka Z, Piotrowski M, Kącka A, Bednarczuk T, Ambroziak U. Comparison of phenoxybenzamine and doxazosin in perioperative management of patients with pheochromocytoma. *Kardiol Pol.* 2017;**75**(11):1192–1198.
10. Plouin PF, Fitzgerald P, Rich T, Ayala-Ramirez M, Perrier ND, Baudin E, Jimenez C. Metastatic pheochromocytoma and paraganglioma: Focus on therapeutics. *Horm Metab Res.* 2012;**44**(5):390–399.
11. Roman-Gonzalez A, Zhou S, Ayala-Ramirez M, Shen C, Waguespack SG, Habra MA, Karam JA, Perrier N, Wood CG, Jimenez C. Impact of surgical resection of the primary tumor on overall survival in patients with metastatic pheochromocytoma or sympathetic paraganglioma. *Ann Surg.* 2018;**268**(1):172–178.
12. Wachtel H, Kennedy EH, Zaheer S, Bartlett EK, Fishbein L, Roses RE, Fraker DL, Cohen DL. Preoperative metyrosine improves cardiovascular outcomes for patients undergoing surgery for pheochromocytoma and paraganglioma. *Ann Surg Oncol.* 2015;**22**(Suppl 3) S646–S654.
13. Butz JJ, Weingarten TN, Cavalcante AN, Bancos I, Young WF, Jr, McKenzie TJ, Schroeder DR, Martin DP, Sprung J. Perioperative hemodynamics and outcomes of patients on metyrosine undergoing resection of pheochromocytoma or paraganglioma. *Int J Surg.* 2017;**46**:1–6.
14. Jiménez C, Cote G, Arnold A, Gagel RF. Review: Should patients with apparently sporadic pheochromocytomas or paragangliomas be screened for hereditary syndromes? *J Clin Endocrinol Metab.* 2006;**91**(8):2851–2858.
15. Lam AK. Update on adrenal tumours in 2017 World Health Organization (WHO) of endocrine tumours. *Endocr Pathol.* 2017;**28**(3):213–227.
16. Plouin PF, Amar L, Dekkers OM, Fassnacht M, Gimenez-Roqueplo AP, Lenders JW, Lussey-Lepoutre C, Steichen O, Guideline Working G, for the Guideline Working Group. European Society of Endocrinology Clinical Practice Guideline for long-term follow-up of patients operated on for a phaeochromocytoma or a paraganglioma. *Eur J Endocrinol.* 2016;**174**(5):G1–G10.
17. Jimenez C, Rohren E, Habra MA, Rich T, Jimenez P, Ayala-Ramirez M, Baudin E. Current and future treatments for malignant pheochromocytoma and sympathetic paraganglioma. *Curr Oncol Rep.* 2013;**15**(4):356–371.
18. Pryma DA, Chin BB, Noto RB, Dillon JS, Perkins S, Solnes L, Kostakoglu L, Serafini AN, Pampaloni MH, Jensen J, Armor T, Lin T, White T, Stambler N, Apfel S, DiPippo V, Mahmood S, Wong V, Jimenez C. Efficacy and safety of high-specific-activity I-131 MIBG therapy in patients with advanced pheochromocytoma or paraganglioma [published online ahead of print 5 October 2018]. *J Nucl Med.* doi:10.2967/jnumed.118.217463.

Pheochromocytoma and Paraganglioma: New Imaging Modalities and Management of Advanced Disease

M02
Presented, March 23–26, 2019

Daniel A. Pryma, MD. Perelman School of Medicine, University of Pennsylvania, Philadelphia, Pennsylvania 19104, E-mail: dpryma@pennmedicine.upenn.edu

SIGNIFICANCE OF THE CLINICAL PROBLEM

Pheochromocytoma (pheo) and paraganglioma (para) are related rare diseases originating from the adrenal medulla or autonomic paraganglia, respectively. Although pheo arises from sympathetic/catecholaminergic cells, para can be either sympathetic (usually arising in the abdomen or pelvis) or parasympathetic (generally arising in the neck and sometimes the chest). Sympathetic pheo and para often secrete high levels of catecholamines, resulting in cardiovascular presentations including malignant hypertension, arrhythmia, and stroke. However, it is important to note that ~50% of sympathetic pheos and paras do not have catecholaminergic symptoms. Parasympathetic para is rarely functioning. Most sympathetic and a vast majority of parasympathetic pheos and paras are benign, but they can be locally aggressive and recurrent. The definition of malignancy has been challenging; therefore, in recent World Health Organization guidelines, pheo and para have been defined only as metastatic or not metastatic. In most patients, metastatic disease has a relatively indolent behavior, and patients can have stable disease for many years. Furthermore, metastatic disease can present decades after curative-intent resection of presumed benign disease. Advanced disease can be challenging to identify with anatomic imaging; therefore, functional imaging tests play an important role in pheo/para. Until recently, there were no US Food and Drug Administration (FDA)–approved treatments for patients with advanced disease.

BARRIERS TO OPTIMAL PRACTICE

- Pheo and para are rare diseases, and a majority are benign.
- Advanced disease can present years or decades after curative-intent treatment of presumed benign disease.
- Recognition of the importance of genetic predispositions to pheo or para is increasing; in some genetic syndromes, management of pheo or para is complicated by other neoplasms.
- Primary tumors can arise in a myriad of sites and can have associated hormonal symptoms. Biochemical aberrations and/or hormonal symptoms do not reliably predict the primary site.

- Even in the setting of indolent, small-volume disease, hormonal effects can be fatal or life threatening.
- Few prospective data are available to inform management of advanced disease; prospective clinical trials are challenging, given the rarity and relatively long survival of patients with advanced pheo or para.

LEARNING OBJECTIVES

- Understand the optimal imaging workup of patients with benign or metastatic pheo or para
- Appreciate treatment options for advanced disease and identify patients in whom systemic therapy is indicated
- Understand the expected outcomes of systemic therapy

STRATEGIES FOR IMAGING AND THERAPY
Screening

There are emerging, although as yet incomplete, data suggesting a potential role for imaging screening with rapid whole-body MRI for germ line mutation carriers predisposed to pheo or para. MRI is attractive because it has relatively high sensitivity for detection of pheo and para independent of their many possible sites of origin, and it exposes the patient to no ionizing radiation. However, the appropriate age at first screening and interval for screening remain uncertain. A multicenter trial would be required to optimally answer these questions.

Preoperative Imaging

A majority of pheos and paras are benign and, as such, require only local anatomic imaging in most cases. Although functional imaging is not routinely indicated, there should be a low threshold to imaging patients at risk for multifocal or metastatic disease. For example, patients with catecholaminergic symptoms and bilateral adrenal nodules may benefit from iodine-123 (I-123) metaiodobenzylguanidine (MIBG; also known as iobenguane) imaging, as would patients with an identified primary and germ line mutation conveying an elevated risk of metastatic or multiple primary disease, such as *SDHB* mutation. Patients with head and neck para may be referred for functional imaging when anatomic findings reveal suspicious or equivocal nodal or osseous lesions. For example, osseous metastasis from para can be easily confused with atypical hemangioma on MRI. Although MIBG imaging is the mainstay of functional imaging of sympathetic pheo and para, indium-111 (In-111) pentetreotide imaging has higher sensitivity and specificity for head and neck para, which is usually of parasympathetic origin. Furthermore, In-111 pentetreotide imaging has been largely replaced by gallium-68 (Ga-68) DOTATATE positron emission tomography (PET)/CT, which has higher sensitivity, lower radiation dose to the patient, and much shorter overall imaging time. Early studies have shown a high sensitivity of DOTATATE PET/CT in SDHB-related pheo and para, but data are limited in other types of pheo/para; therefore, MIBG imaging remains the standard for the time being. Of note, MIBG analogs for PET/CT imaging labeled with either I-124 or fluorine-18 are being evaluated but are not yet available for clinical use. There is almost no role for fluorodeoxyglucose (FDG) PET/CT in pheo or para, especially at initial presentation, because a majority of patients, even those with widespread advanced disease, have low FDG uptake.

Postsurgical Imaging

There is no clear role for surveillance imaging in the routine postsurgical setting after resection of presumed benign disease. However, because patients can present with advanced disease years or decades later, it is critically important to not lose patients to follow-up and to have a low threshold for symptom- or biomarker-prompted imaging. In most cases, the initial imaging test should be directed anatomic imaging of the surgical site. In patients with known or suspected metastatic disease, functional imaging plays a primary role. The mainstays of functional imaging are akin to those for preoperative imaging: Ga-68 DOTATATE PET/CT in head and neck para and I-123 MIBG in other types of pheo and para, noting early clinical evidence for an emerging role for Ga-68 DOTATATE PET/CT broadly in pheo and para. FDG PET/CT is rarely indicated in pheo or para; its appropriate use is largely limited to characterization of seemingly aggressive disease. Rarely patients have highly aggressive disease that is highly FDG avid, and those patients are likely to require a more aggressive conventional cytotoxic therapeutic approach.

Treatment Options in Advanced Disease
Local Disease

Surgery remains the mainstay therapy for local disease, whether primary or recurrent. However, local disease may be unresectable because of local invasion or adjacency to nerves or vessels. In these cases, external-beam radiotherapy plays a significant role. Patients in whom external beam is contraindicated can occasionally benefit from systemic therapy in the setting of local disease only. More frequently, local disease is accompanied by a smaller burden of distant disease in which case systemic therapy can be favored. Of note, anecdotal evidence suggests that external-beam radiotherapy for bulky local disease can be safely combined with systemic therapy for metastatic disease. This strategy may be helpful because local disease is thought to likely represent a reservoir for metastasis. It is important to note that after external-beam radiotherapy for pheo or para, even at curative-intent doses, disease often remains positive on functional imaging tests, although long-term follow-up shows no progression even over the course of many years and in the presence of progression of

nonirradiated sites. Therefore, positive functional imaging within the radiotherapy field alone is not an indication for further treatment.

Distant Disease

When metastatic, pheo and para have a predilection for nodal and osseous disease, with hepatic and pulmonary metastases also frequent but less common. Median overall survival of patients with metastatic pheo or para disease has been reported to be ~5 years, but long-term retrospective series have shown that survival for decades is not uncommon. Therefore, presence of metastatic disease alone is not an indication for systemic therapy. The mainstay of treatment focuses on hormonal control, largely with α blockade. Systemic therapy should be reserved for patients with clear progression of disease or those with hormonal symptoms that are severe and cannot be adequately controlled. The only currently FDA-approved therapy for advanced pheo or para is high specific-activity I-131 MIBG; this should be the first consideration for treatment of patients in whom systemic therapy is indicated. Therefore, patients with advanced pheo or para who may require imminent systemic therapy should undergo I-123 MIBG scan to assess for MIBG-positive disease. Of note, even patients with parasympathetic paragangliomas often have MIBG avidity and could be amenable to MIBG therapy. Those with macroscopic, anatomic metastatic disease with no significant MIBG uptake are not good candidates for MIBG therapy. Other treatment options for metastatic disease may include palliative surgery and/or external-beam radiotherapy, chemotherapy, or other targeted agents. The traditional chemotherapy regimen described in advanced pheo and para is the three-drug combination of cyclophosphamide, vincristine, and dacarbazine (CVD), but there is some more recent anecdotal evidence supporting use of capecitabine and temozolomide. There have been small series testing targeted agents, mostly tyrosine kinase inhibitors, with some evidence of activity. However, many of these have been limited in pheo and para, because they can exacerbate baseline severe disease-related hypertension. Finally, given the emerging evidence of positive Ga-68 DOTATATE PET/CT in pheo and para, there has been interest in targeting the somatostatin receptor with both unlabeled somatostatin analogs as well as with radioactive somatostatin analogs [currently only lutetium-177 (Lu-177) DOTATATE is FDA approved in the United States for gastroenteropancreatic neuroendocrine tumors].

Outcomes of Therapy

Controlled clinical trials with survival end points are incredibly difficult in pheo and para, given the rarity of the diseases coupled with highly variable clinical behaviors. Therefore, trials have generally focused on anatomic, biomarker, or symptomatic improvement as surrogate markers of efficacy. Furthermore, because these are generally relatively indolent cancers, anatomic responses can be slow and subtle. Disease stabilization, pain control, and symptom relief are common, seen in >80% of patients treated with MIBG. However, there are no clear data showing a survival advantage from systemic therapy for pheo and para, and it is unlikely that such data will ever be feasibly collected.

MAIN CONCLUSIONS

Pheo and para make up a heterogeneous group of neoplasms that are largely benign but can be locally aggressive and/or metastatic, with behaviors ranging from highly aggressive to extremely indolent. Metastatic disease in a majority of patients has a relatively indolent course. Systemic therapy is indicated for advanced disease with meaningful progression and/or uncontrolled symptoms. High specific-activity I-131 MIBG is now FDA approved as systemic therapy for advanced pheo and para; other systemic treatments are also available, with varying levels of evidence to support their use.

CASES

Case 1

A 68-year-old patient with long-standing, poorly controlled hypertension and history of myocardial infarction and stroke presents for evaluation of suspected osseous metastasis because of multifocal bone pain, with marrow-based lesions seen on hip MRI. The patient has a remote history of right adrenalectomy 18 years previously for pheochromocytoma. What is the most appropriate next step?

A. Fine-needle aspiration
B. CT chest/abdomen/pelvis
C. I-123 MIBG scan
D. FDG PET/CT
Answer: C

Case 2

A 43-year-old patient was recently diagnosed with widely metastatic para to lymph nodes and bones on both I-123 MIBG and Ga-68 DOTATATE imaging. The patient is asymptomatic, and biochemical testing reveals a nonfunctioning cancer. What is the most appropriate next step?

A. Active surveillance
B. I-131 MIBG therapy
C. Lu-177 DOTATATE therapy
D. CVD chemotherapy
E. Somatostatin analog therapy
Answer: A

Recommended Reading

Breen W, Bancos I, Young WF Jr, Bible KC, Laack NN, Foote RL, Hallemeier CL. External beam radiation therapy for advanced/unresectable malignant paraganglioma and pheochromocytoma. *Adv Radiat Oncol.* 2017;**3**(1):25–29.

Carrasquillo JA, Pandit-Taskar N, Chen CC. I-131 metaiodobenzylguanidine therapy of pheochromocytoma and paraganglioma. *Semin Nucl Med.* 2016;**46**(3):203–214.

Fishbein L. Pheochromocytoma and paraganglioma: genetics, diagnosis, and treatment. *Hematol Oncol Clin North Am.* 2016;**30**(1):135–150.

Fishbein L, Ben-Maimon S, Keefe S, Cengel K, Pryma DA, Loaiza-Bonilla A, Fraker DL, Nathanson KL, Cohen DL. *SDHB* mutation carriers with malignant pheochromocytoma respond better to CVD. *Endocr Relat Cancer.* 2017;**24**(8):L51–L55.

Fishbein L, Bonner L, Torigian DA, Nathanson KL, Cohen DL, Pryma D, Cengel KA. External beam radiation therapy (EBRT) for patients with malignant pheochromocytoma and non-head and -neck paraganglioma: combination with 131I-MIBG. *Horm Metab Res.* 2012;**44**(5):405–410.

Han S, Suh CH, Woo S, Kim YJ, Lee JJ. Performance of (68)Ga-DOTA-conjugated somatostatin receptor targeting peptide PET in detection of pheochromocytoma and paraganglioma: a systematic review and meta-analysis [published online ahead of print 20 July 2018]. *J Nucl Med.* doi:10.2967/jnumed.118.211706.

Huang H, Abraham J, Hung E, Averbuch S, Merino M, Steinberg SM, Pacak K, Fojo T. Treatment of malignant pheochromocytoma/paraganglioma with cyclophosphamide, vincristine, and dacarbazine: recommendation from a 22-year follow-up of 18 patients. *Cancer.* 2008;**113**(8):2020–2028.

Jing H, Li F, Wang L, Wang Z, Li W, Huo L, Zhang J. Comparison of the 68Ga-DOTATATA PET/CT, FDG PET/CT, and MIBG SPECT/CT in the evaluation of suspected primary pheochromocytomas and paragangliomas. *Clin Nucl Med.* 2017;**42**(7):525–529.

Kroiss AS, Uprimny C, Pichler R, Gasser RW, Virgolini IJ. A rare case of a ¹²³I-MIBG SPECT/CT positive, but ⁶⁸Ga-DOTA-TOC PET/CT negative pheochromocytoma of the bladder. *Rev Esp Med Nucl Imagen Mol.* 2018;**37**(5):315–317.

Lam AK. Update on adrenal tumours in 2017 World Health Organization (WHO) of endocrine tumours. *Endocr Pathol.* 2017;**28**(3):213–227.

Maignan A, Guerin C, Julliard V, Paladino NC, Kim E, Roche P, Castinetti F, Essamet W, Mancini J, Imperiale A, Clifton-Bligh R, Romanet P, Barlier A, Pacak K, Sebag F, Taïeb D. Implications of SDHB genetic testing in patients with sporadic pheochromocytoma. *Langenbecks Arch Surg.* 2017;**402**(5):787–798.

Nastos K, Cheung VTF, Toumpanakis C, Navalkissoor S, Quigley AM, Caplin M, Khoo B. Peptide receptor radionuclide treatment and (131)I-MIBG in the management of patients with metastatic/progressive phaeochromocytomas and paragangliomas. *J Surg Oncol.* 2017;**115**(4):425–434.

Niemeijer ND, Alblas G, van Hulsteijn LT, Dekkers OM, Corssmit EP. Chemotherapy with cyclophosphamide, vincristine and dacarbazine for malignant paraganglioma and pheochromocytoma: systematic review and meta-analysis. *Clin Endocrinol (Oxf).* 2014;**81**(5):642–651.

Nomura K, Kimura H, Shimizu S, Kodama H, Okamoto T, Obara T, Takano K. Survival of patients with metastatic malignant pheochromocytoma and efficacy of combined cyclophosphamide, vincristine, and dacarbazine chemotherapy. *J Clin Endocrinol Metab.* 2009;**94**(8):2850–2856.

Noto RB, Pryma DA, Jensen J, Lin T, Stambler N, Strack T, Wong V, Goldsmith SJ. Phase 1 study of high-specific-activity I-131 MIBG for metastatic and/or recurrent pheochromocytoma or paraganglioma. *J Clin Endocrinol Metab.* 2018;**103**(1):213–220.

Pandit-Taskar N, Zanzonico P, Staton KD, Carrasquillo JA, Reidy-Lagunes D, Lyashchenko S, Burnazi E, Zhang H, Lewis JS, Blasberg R, Larson SM, Weber WA, Modak S. Biodistribution and dosimetry of ¹⁸F-meta-fluorobenzylguanidine: a first-in-human PET/CT imaging study of patients with neuroendocrine malignancies. *J Nucl Med.* 2018;**59**(1):147–153.

Pryma DA, Chin BB, Noto RB, Dillon JS, Perkins S, Solnes L, Kostakoglu L, Serafini AN, Pampaloni MH, Jensen J, Armor T, Lin T, White T, Stambler N, Apfel S, DiPippo V, Mahmood S, Wong V, Jimenez C. Efficacy and safety of high-specific-activity I-131 MIBG therapy in patients with advanced pheochromocytoma or paraganglioma [published online ahead of print 5 October 2018]. *J Nucl Med.* doi:10.2967/jnumed.118.217463.

Tanabe A, Naruse M, Nomura K, Tsuiki M, Tsumagari A, Ichihara A. Combination chemotherapy with cyclophosphamide, vincristine, and dacarbazine in patients with malignant pheochromocytoma and paraganglioma. *Horm Cancer.* 2013;**4**(2):103–110.

Vogel J, Atanacio AS, Prodanov T, Turkbey BI, Adams K, Martucci V, Camphausen K, Fojo AT, Pacak K, Kaushal A. External beam radiation therapy in treatment of malignant pheochromocytoma and paraganglioma. *Front Oncol.* 2014;**4**:166.

Yamaguchi A, Hanaoka H, Higuchi T, Tsushima Y. Radiolabeled (4-fluoro-3-Iodobenzyl) guanidine improves imaging and targeted radionuclide therapy of norepinephrine transporter-expressing tumors. *J Nucl Med.* 2018;**59**(5):815–821.

Ten Rules of Adrenal Insufficiency

M14
Presented, March 23–26, 2019

James W. Findling, MD. Medical College of Wisconsin, Milwaukee, Wisconsin 53051, E-mail: james.findling@ froedtert.com

SIGNIFICANCE OF THE CLINICAL PROBLEM AND BARRIERS TO OPTIMAL PRACTICE

Hypocortisolemia is a commonly recognized finding that is usually due to the administration of exogenous glucocorticoids or opioids. Some of these patients develop adrenal insufficiency (AI), and there are no guidelines on how to best manage them. Secondary AI may also be due to hypothalamic-pituitary disorders, and assessment of the integrity of pituitary-adrenal function may be challenging. Primary adrenal failure is much less common. Although clinical recognition may be difficult for primary care providers, the biochemical diagnosis is simple. Treatment of all forms of AI include glucocorticoid administration (hydrocortisone preferably) with lots of emphasis on sick day/stress management strategies. Despite our best efforts, adrenal crisis is a common problem and a significant cause of death in patients with AI.

LEARNING OBJECTIVES
Ten Rules of Adrenal Insufficiency
- Adrenal fatigue does not exist, but "adrenal" supplements all contain T_3 and many contain biologically active glucocorticoids.
- AI should be excluded in all patients with hyponatremia.
- New specific cortisol assays (*e.g.,* liquid chromatography–tandem mass spectrometry) will yield a lower threshold peak cortisol response to stimulation with cosyntropin [~14 to 15 μg/dL (400 nmol/L)].
- The cosyntropin test is an imperfect test and clinical parameters must be known for its proper interpretation; there is no difference between high- and low-dose cosyntropin testing.
- Plasma adrenocorticotropic hormone (ACTH) should not be used as a barometer of the adequacy of glucocorticoid therapy.
- Drugs that impact steroid binding proteins (estrogens) or glucocorticoid metabolic clearance (inhibitors of CYP3A4) must be taken into account when assessing hypothalamic-pituitary-adrenal axis function.
- The most common cause of hypocortisolemia in the United States is exogenous glucocorticoid administration (millions of patients daily) and chronic opioid use. Protracted therapy of either may cause secondary AI.

- Glucocorticoid therapy is needed in patients with AI, and hydrocortisone is the therapy of choice. Replacement dosing should take into consideration the patient's weight, endogenous cortisol production, and, most importantly, general well-being.
- Adrenal insufficiency is a potentially life-threatening problem, and all patients need clear, repetitive teaching regarding sick day/stress dose management: every patient, every visit.
- All patients with AI/hypocortisolemia should be evaluated and managed by an endocrinologist.

Some of these rules would be considered low evidence (possibly no evidence) by the epidemiologists who perform meta-analysis that dictates endocrine guidelines. Many are based on my personal clinical experience. I change the Rules frequently, and, not surprisingly, some clinicians do not follow them.

CASE SUBJECTS
Case 1
A 34-year-old woman with a history of radiotherapy for an optic glioma in 1999 presents in 2003 with secondary amenorrhea and hyperprolactinemia. Treatment with cabergoline normalizes prolactin but she has persistent amenorrhea with low gonadotropins. Oral contraceptives are initiated. In 2004, she has papillary thyroid cancer (s/p surgery/ radioactive iodine) and remains in remission on levothyroxine. In 2009, she complains of fatigue and myalgias; she has no appetite change and her weight is stable. She is taking the following medications: drospirenone/ethinyl estradiol, cabergoline, and levothyroxine. The results of the physical exam are as follows: blood pressure 98/70 mm Hg, pulse 66 beats/min, body mass index 24 kg/m^2, clinically euthyroid, and normal examination. The laboratory results are as follows: Na 134 mEq/L, K 3.9 mEq/L, Cl 100 mEq/L, CO_2 25 mEq/L, blood urea nitrogen 9 mg/dL, creatinine 0.7 mg/dL, glucose 86 mg/dL, thyrotropin 0.09, and free T_4 1.2 ng/dL (SI unit: 15.5 pmol/L). In light of her pituitary hypogonadism, you consider pituitary hypoadrenalism.

Which of the following studies would you obtain?
A. Pituitary MRI
B. Morning cortisol, ACTH, dehydroepiandrosterone sufate (DHEAS)
C. Metyrapone stimulation
D. Insulin-induced hypoglycemia
E. Cosyntropin stimulation test

Patients with AI often present with vague, nonspecific complaints such as fatigue, malaise, and myalgias. The majority of patients with significant cortisol deficiency will have a decreased appetite and weight loss, but this woman does not have any change in her appetite or weight. Nonetheless, this woman has well-established radiotherapy-induced pituitary hypofunction, and she is at a high risk for the development of secondary AI. In addition, she has mild hyponatremia. Hyponatremia is the most common biochemical abnormality in patients with cortisol deficiency, including both primary AI (PAI) and secondary AI. Cortisol exerts negative feedback on vasopressin secretion, and, therefore, hypocortisolemia may cause impaired free water clearance. Anyone with unexplained hyponatremia should have assessment of adrenocortical function.

Securing a morning measurement of serum cortisol, plasma ACTH, and serum DHEAS is a very reasonable place to start when disorders of pituitary-adrenal function are suspected. Obviously, the pituitary-adrenal axis is dynamic with a well-known diurnal rhythm. If the patient has an unusual sleep-wake cycle, this may obfuscate this approach. Consistently subnormal morning serum cortisol levels <4 μg/dL (120 nmol/L) are consistent with AI; however, it must be remembered that hypocortisolemia is not always associated with AI. In fact, the most common cause of low cortisol levels in the United States is exogenous corticosteroid administration (topical, oral, inhaled, and injected). Of course, these patients have excessive glucocorticoid exposure and do not benefit from giving them more. Moreover, serum cortisol levels >14 μg/dL exclude the diagnosis of AI, and no further testing is needed. Needless to say, there are many patients who fall between 4 and 14 μg/dL so that additional testing is often required.

Plasma ACTH measurements, obtained in a reliable method, help to distinguish primary from secondary adrenal failure. All patients with PAI have elevations of plasma ACTH, whereas patients with secondary AI have subnormal or normal levels.

Of course, DHEAS reflects adrenal androgen secretion, and it is the most abundant circulating steroid. It often provides important clues for the diagnosis of adrenal dysfunction. Most importantly, DHEAS is almost always <85 μg/dL in patients with AI, and levels above this would be uncommon in patients with clinically significant adrenal hypofunction. It should, of course, be remembered that adrenal androgen secretion declines with age so there are age-adjusted normal levels. Patients who have had a protracted course of exogenous steroid therapy for any reason may often have low DHEAS levels for many years.

The morning laboratory studies show the following: cortisol 10.8 μg/dL (292 nmol/L), ACTH 15 pg/mL (3.3 pmol/L), and DHEAS 66 μg/dL (1848 nmol/L).

What would you do next?
A. Pituitary MRI
B. Insulin-induced hypoglycemia
C. Metyrapone stimulation test
D. Low-dose cosyntropin stimulation test
E. High-dose cosyntropin stimulation test

This woman appears to have a normal morning cortisol concentration; however, she is on oral contraceptives (OC),

which cause significant increases in corticosteroid binding globulin (CBG), the hepatic-derived major binding protein for cortisol. Women receiving oral estrogen therapy usually have morning cortisol levels >18 to 20 μg/dL. The level in this woman is considerably lower than expected. The DHEAS level is within the normal range, but it is <85 μg/dL. Because DHEA has little binding to CBG, OC do not affect its concentration. The plasma ACTH level is not helpful in this case.

Insulin-induced hypoglycemia is considered by pituitary experts to be the "gold standard" for the diagnosis of secondary AI. Unfortunately, this test induces torture for the patient and the person responsible for executing the test. In the United States, it is often done in academic medical centers where an endocrinology fellow usually provides supervision of this time-consuming and anxiety-provoking exercise. In my opinion, it is rarely needed. In the past 35 years, since I left my fellowship, I have only done it in two patients.

Metyrapone stimulation testing (not readily available in the United States) was actually introduced in the late 1950s. Metyrapone, an 11-β-hydroxylase inhibitor, is administered orally, usually on a weight-based dose of 30 mg/kg at 11:00 PM, with measurement of 11-deoxycortisol and cortisol the following morning. An increase of 11-deoxycortisol of >7 μg/dL (200 nmol/L) is considered normal. This test can be dangerous in patients with clinically significant AI, and hospitalization may be needed in some patients, decreasing its clinical utility.

In the United States, this woman would have a cosyntropin stimulation test. For many years, there has been controversy about the potential advantages of administering a low-dose (1 μg) ACTH stimulation test compared with the conventional high-dose (250 μg) test. Most studies have shown that there is no difference in the diagnostic outcomes of the studies, and this is not surprising. After a 1-μg dose of ACTH, the plasma ACTH concentration exceeds 1000 pg/mL. After the 250-μg dose, plasma ACTH exceeds 100,000 pg/mL. The adrenal cortex never sees concentrations of this magnitude. In fact, a plasma ACTH concentration >100 pg/mL induces maximum adrenal production of cortisol, and the dose-response curve is pretty flat after that. This is why the cosyntropin stimulation study is superfluous in patients with PAI; when you give cosyntropin to a patient with an elevated plasma ACTH due to PAI, there will be very little further increase in cortisol.

A cosyntropin (250 μg) test is performed in 2009 (basal and +30 min): cortisol 12.8 μg/dL (350 nmol/L) and 23.3 μg/dL (640 nmol/L).

What would you recommend next?
A. Repeat test with 60-minute post-ACTH sample
B. Insulin-induced hypoglycemia
C. Reassure the patient she has normal hypothalamic-pituitary-adrenal axis function
D. Secure "free" cortisol levels
E. Discontinue birth control pills for 1 week and repeat test

The normal peak cortisol level after ACTH varies considerably now depending on the specificity of the cortisol assay. New specific cortisol assays (liquid chromatography–tandem mass spectrometry and monoclonal antibody assays) yield a normal peak cortisol of 14 to 15 μg/dL (400 nmol/L) compared with the older methods where the normal peak response is 18 μg/dL. You must know what cortisol assay your laboratory uses. In the United States, many clinical hospital laboratories change their assay methodology without informing the clinicians. Although some studies have demonstrated occasional discordance between a 30- and 60-minute post-ACTH cortisol level, I usually secure only a 30-minute sample. My rationale is simple: if the adrenal cortex sees an ACTH concentration of 100,000 pg/mL and cannot generate a cortisol level >14 to 15 μg/dL in 30 minutes, additional glucocorticoid support needs to be considered.

Of course, this patient is receiving OC that confound the interpretation of this test. The peak post-ACTH cortisol level in women taking OC varies from 570 to 780 nmol/L (20 to 28 μg/dL). Discontinuation of OC certainly may help to eliminate the confounding factor of increased CBG, but the time frame is much longer than 1 week. Usually it takes at least 3 months for the estrogen-induced increases in CBG to completely return to baseline. This test is very hard to interpret in this patient; your index of suspicion is high, so assessment of the free cortisol concentration should be helpful.

A cosyntropin (250 μg) test is performed in 2009 (basal and +30 min): cortisol 12.8 μg/dL (350 nmol/L) and 23.3 μg/dL (640 nmol/L); salivary cortisol 0.1 μg/dL (3.3 nmol/L) and 0.3 μg/dL (8.4 nmol/L). The total peak cortisol response to ACTH (cosyntropin) is normal, but the basal "free" cortisol, as reflected by salivary cortisol and the peak free cortisol response, is subnormal. These findings suggest that this woman has early secondary AI. Normative ranges for free cortisol (saliva or serum) are not well established in some assays; however, the normal late-night salivary cortisol is <3.5 nmol/L in most assays, so it seems logical that an early morning level should be higher.

A cosyntropin (250 μg) test is performed in 2017 six months after discontinuing OC (basal and +30 min): cortisol 2.3 μg/dL (63 nmol/L) and 8.9 μg/dL (245 nmol/L).

What therapy would you recommend in 2009? In 2017?
A. Prednisone 5 mg in the morning and 2.5 mg in the afternoon
B. Stress dosing 20 to 30 mg daily in divided doses with parenterally available steroid
C. Hydrocortisone 5 to 10 mg in the morning with stress dose management
D. Continuous subcutaneous hydrocortisone infusion
E. Refer the patient to a European center for Plenadrin

In the United States, the preferred treatment of AI is hydrocortisone. In some countries, hydrocortisone is not available and prednisolone may be used. Physiologic replacement of glucocorticoids is challenging, and therapy needs to be individualized depending on the patient's basal cortisol production and weight. The majority of patients, like this woman, with secondary AI rarely require more than 10 to 15 mg daily. In contrast, patients with PAI with negligible cortisol production may need more. Since studies have clearly shown that hydrocortisone metabolic clearance is most affected by body weight, heavier patients will require larger doses. Although thrice daily dosing has been shown to more closely mimic physiologic cortisol secretion throughout the day, this is a bit impractical and unacceptable in many patients. Obviously, the first early morning dose should be the highest with a smaller dose in the early afternoon and sometimes early evening. Physiologic prednisone replacement is very difficult, but 7.5 mg daily is too much in almost anyone. Since prednisone needs to be converted in the liver to prednisolone to create a biologically active glucocorticoid, the Endocrine Society guidelines recommend prednisolone 3 to 5 mg daily for replacement treatment. Some patients feel fine, even with a fairly low morning cortisol, and may not feel better with supplemental morning hydrocortisone (this woman did not from 2009 to 2017); however, stress dosing is always crucial in these patients (see case 3).

Since the quality of life is often impaired in patients with chronic AI, other glucocorticoid preparations and different administration vehicles have been reported. Continuous subcutaneous hydrocortisone administration has been reported to improve the quality of life in patients with congenital adrenal hyperplasia, with better reductions in 17-hydroxyprogesterone and probably less glucocorticoid exposure. Although there is no question that this would most likely provide our AI patients with much more physiologic cortisol profiles than oral dosing, this technique is currently being used in only investigational settings. In Europe, a once-daily, modified-release hydrocortisone preparation is available. In a much-heralded, single-blinded, randomized control trial, this formulation (Plenadrin) reduced body weight, normalized the immune cell profile, reduced recurrent infections, and improved quality of life compared with a group of patients on "conventional" glucocorticoid replacement treatment two to three times daily. Of course, it is possible that a simple dose reduction scheme in the "conventional" group may have done the same thing. Nonetheless, new time-released glucocorticoid preparations may provide patients with a more physiologic glucocorticoid profile and improved sense of well-being. Currently, none of these preparations are being studied or are available in the United States.

Case 2

A 22-year-old man, accompanied by his mother, is referred for suspected adrenal fatigue. He has been more lethargic and irritable, but there has been no change in his weight. Six months ago, he was seen by an "integrative health professional" and after a salivary cortisol day curve (see below), he was started on three different "adrenal support" compounds and DHEA 50 mg daily (sold in the office for cash). The patient's mother wanted an endocrinology evaluation since her son had not improved.

You secure the following laboratory studies in the morning of your visit: cortisol 1.4 µg/dL, ACTH 8 pg/mL, and DHEAS 462 µg/dL. Peak cortisol after cosyntropin stimulation is 11 µg/dL and pituitary MRI is normal.

Which of the following is most likely responsible for his low cortisol?
 A. Adrenal fatigue
 B. Adrenal supplements
 C. Isolated ACTH deficiency
 D. Surreptitious opioid use
 E. DHEA therapy

Adrenal fatigue is a nonexistent clinical entity without any pathophysiologic foundation. This unfortunate fantasy has been perpetrated by naturopathic physicians for several years with the concept of downregulation of adrenal function related to chronic physical or psychologic stress factors. Nothing could be further from the truth: patients with posttraumatic stress disorder and chronic fatigue syndrome and patients dying from AIDS (circa late 1980s) maintain normal basal and stress-induced cortisol secretion. There is also no evidence that glucocorticoid therapy provides any sustained benefit in these conditions.

Isolated ACTH deficiency and pituitary hypoadrenalism was once a very rare clinical disorder; however, the commonly used immune checkpoint inhibitors are often complicated by autoimmune-mediated hypophysitis, which may result in isolated ACTH deficiency. DHEA therapy resulted in a robust level in this young man, but DHEA does not bind to the glucocorticoid receptor and has no impact on ACTH secretion.

Many adrenal "supplements" are available on the internet and, as in this case, may be sold by naturopaths directly to their patients. Recently, it has been discovered that all of these supplements contain T_3 and many contain potent glucocorticoids such as budesonide...so it is possible that the adrenal supplements may have exerted some glucocorticoid negative feedback in this young man.

Two weeks after his visit, his mother called my office to tell us that she found buprenorphine in his dresser drawer. Opioid-induced suppression of the pituitary-adrenal axis is an underappreciated phenomenon that is mediated by CRH suppression (tertiary AI). In light of the widespread use of narcotics in the United States, it is a common cause of hypocortisolemia. The suppression of adrenal function is, however, short-lived and superimposed significant stress presumably overcomes this suppression. To date, there are no reports of adrenal crisis related to opioid use. Nonetheless, ~5% to 10% of patients on chronic opioid treatment have been shown to have a low morning cortisol and blunted peak cortisol response to stimulation with ACTH (cosyntropin).

There are no evidence-based recommendations for the management of these patients. I personally offer glucocorticoid replacement only in patients who have clear symptomatic hypoadrenalism (anorexia with weight loss, hypotension, etc). Withdrawal of opioids results in prompt resurrection of pituitary-adrenal function. This young man failed any follow-up care.

Case 3

A 57-year-old woman is seen for her annual follow-up visit for evaluation and management of PAI after bilateral adrenalectomy 12 years earlier for Cushing disease. She offers no new complaints, and a pituitary MRI done 6 months ago showed no evidence of any pituitary lesions. She has never experienced an adrenal crisis.

She takes hydrocortisone 15 mg in the morning and 5 mg in the early afternoon (although she acknowledges that she often misses this dose), fludrocortisone 100 µg daily, pravastatin 20 mg daily, and amlodipine 5 mg daily. She has injectable hydrocortisone at home.

The results of the physical exam are as follows: blood pressure 142/84, pulse 78 beats/min, height 66.7 inches (169 cm), and weight 246 pounds (112 kg), and normal examination; she is well pigmented in sun-exposed areas. The laboratory results are as follows: normal electrolyte composition, ACTH 503 pg/mL, and plasma renin activity 3.7 ng/mL per hour.

Which of the following would you recommend for this woman?
 A. Increase her hydrocortisone to 25 mg in morning and 15 mg in afternoon
 B. Add dexamethasone 0.5 mg at bedtime
 C. Change her steroid replacement to prednisolone 3 mg in morning and 2 mg in afternoon
 D. Increase her fludrocortisone to 150 µg/daily
 E. Review sick day management

This woman is doing well and her glucocorticoid replacement dose is reasonable. There is no reason to increase her hydrocortisone doses or switch her to a synthetic steroid. Dexamethasone use is strongly discouraged for the treatment of AI. Elevations of ACTH are usually present in patients with PAI and, of course, much higher in patients with a residual corticotroph adenoma; however, the absence of a pituitary imaging abnormality excludes Nelson syndrome or the corticotroph tumor progression syndrome. Plasma ACTH usually exceeds 1000 pg/mL with corticotroph tumor progression. Accordingly, plasma ACTH measurements should not be measured to gauge glucocorticoid replacement in PAI. Nonetheless, I occasionally measure ACTH since low levels (*i.e.*, <25 to 30 pg/mL) may suggest excessive glucocorticoid exposure in PAI. A normal plasma renin activity and electrolyte composition support adequate mineralocorticoid therapy, and an increase is not justified particularly in light of her hypertension.

Two weeks after this visit, I received a call at 6:30 AM from the medical examiner's office. Her husband found her dead in bed. The day before, she had a gastrointestinal illness with nausea, vomiting, and diarrhea. Her husband was sure that she had not used the injectable hydrocortisone and possibly had not even increased her dose of hydrocortisone.

Adrenal crisis is a common problem in patients with AI, and 8% of patients with AI will experience an adrenal crisis each year. This occurs even in patients who have been educated about sick day/stress steroid management. Unfortunately, 0.5% of patients with AI die each year of this preventable situation. Management of adrenal crisis should be reviewed at every visit. I recommend a 3 × 3 rule: triple the steroid dose for 3 days or until the patient has recovered from their illness. If gastrointestinal problems are prominent, the patient should use parenteral hydrocortisone (100 mg) and be seen in a health care facility. Subcutaneous hydrocortisone has been shown to achieve more than adequate cortisol levels and is usually easier for the patients to administer. In Europe, rectal and vaginal hydrocortisone suppositories are also available, but neither may provide adequate levels of cortisol during a crisis.

Recommended Reading

Akturk HK, Chindris AM, Hines JM, Singh RJ, Bernet VJ. Over-the-counter "adrenal support" supplements contain thyroid and steroid-based adrenal hormones. *Mayo Clin Proc.* 2018;**93**(3):284–290.

Al-Aridi R, Abdelmannan D, Arafah BM. Biochemical diagnosis of adrenal insufficiency: the added value of dehydroepiandrosterone sulfate measurements. *Endocr Pract.* 2011;**17**(2):261–270.

Bancos I, Erickson D, Bryant S, Hines J, Nippoldt TB, Natt N, Singh R. Performance of free versus total cortisol following cosyntropin stimulation testing in an outpatient setting. *Endocr Pract.* 2015;**21**(12): 1353–1363.

Bornstein SR, Allolio B, Arlt W, Barthel A, Don-Wauchope A, Hammer GD, Husebye ES, Merke DP, Murad MH, Stratakis CA, Torpy DJ. Diagnosis and treatment of primary adrenal insufficiency: an Endocrine Society Clinical Practice Guideline. *J Clin Endocrinol Metab.* 2016;**101**(2): 364–389.

Gibb FW, Stewart A, Walker BR, Strachan MWJ. Adrenal insufficiency in patients on long-term opioid analgesia. *Clin Endocrinol (Oxf).* 2016; **85**(6):831–835.

Hahner S, Spinnler C, Fassnacht M, Burger-Stritt S, Lang K, Milovanovic D, Beuschlein F, Willenberg HS, Quinkler M, Allolio B. High incidence of adrenal crisis in educated patients with chronic adrenal insufficiency: a prospective study. *J Clin Endocrinol Metab.* 2015;**100**(2):407–416.

He X, Findling JW, Auchus RJ, Levine A, ed. Diagnosis and management of adrenal insufficiency. In: *Adrenal Disorders: Physiology, Pathophysiology and Treatment.* Philadelphia, PA: Springer; 2017:199–215.

Isidori AM, Venneri MA, Graziadio C, Simeoli C, Fiore D, Hasenmajer V, Sbardella E, Gianfrilli D, Pozza C, Pasqualetti P, Morrone S, Santoni A, Naro F, Colao A, Pivonello R, Lenzi A. Effect of once-daily, modified-release hydrocortisone versus standard glucocorticoid therapy on metabolism and innate immunity in patients with adrenal insufficiency (DREAM): a single-blind, randomised controlled trial. *Lancet Diabetes Endocrinol.* 2018;**6**(3):173–185.

Mah PM, Jenkins RC, Rostami-Hodjegan A, Newell-Price J, Doane A, Ibbotson V, Tucker GT, Ross RJ. Weight-related dosing, timing and monitoring hydrocortisone replacement therapy in patients with adrenal insufficiency. *Clin Endocrinol (Oxf).* 2004;**61**(3):367–375.

Mayenknecht J, Diederich S, Bähr V, Plöckinger U, Oelkers W. Comparison of low and high dose corticotropin stimulation tests in patients with pituitary disease. *J Clin Endocrinol Metab.* 1998;**83**(5):1558–1562.

Ospina NS, Al Nofal A, Bancos I, Javed A, Benkhadra K, Kapoor E, Lteif AN, Natt N, Murad MH. ACTH stimulation tests for the diagnosis of adrenal insufficiency: systemic review and meta-analysis. *J Clin Endocrinol Metab.* 2016;**101**(2):427–434.

Raff H, Brock S, Findling JW. Cosyntropin-stimulated salivary cortisol in hospitalized patients with hypoproteinemia. *Endocrine.* 2008;**34**(1-3): 68–74.

Ueland GA, Methlie P, Øksnes M, Thordarson HB, Sagen J, Kellmann R, Mellgren G, Ræder M, Dahlqvist P, Dahl SR, Thorsby PM, Løvås K, Husebye ES. The short cosyntropin test revisited: new normal reference range using LC-MS/MS. *J Clin Endocrinol Metab.* 2018;**103**(4): 1696–1703.

Adrenal Incidentalomas: Medical and Surgical Aspects

M24
Presented, March 23–26, 2019

Sheila Fraser, MB ChB, MD, FRCS. Leeds Teaching Hospitals NHS Trust and University of Leeds, Leeds LS9 7TF, United Kingdom, E-mail: sheila.fraser7@nhs.net

Paul Stewart, MB ChB, MD, FRCP, FMedSci. Leeds Teaching Hospitals NHS Trust and University of Leeds, Leeds LS2 9NL, United Kingdom, E-mail: p.m.stewart@leeds.ac.uk

SIGNIFICANCE OF THE CLINICAL PROBLEM

The widespread use of abdominal CT/MRI has resulted in a new and common diagnosis for the clinical endocrinologist—the management of patients with adrenal incidentalomas (AIs). Defined as an adrenal mass discovered incidentally in the workup or treatment of clinical conditions not related to suspicion of adrenal disease, incidentalomas cover a spectrum of underlying adrenal pathologies with a common pathway of discovery.

Because of the risk of malignancy, they raise uncertainty, confusion, and concern in doctors and patients alike and consume substantial resources. We will define the scale of the problem and discuss diagnostic challenges as they relate to hormone hypersecretion and the ascertainment of benign vs malignant. The natural history and the suggested follow-up and treatment of patients based on published clinical guidelines will be addressed; such guidelines perhaps overinflate the real risk of malignancy, and a more risk-averse approach to management is now required. One particular area of debate is the term "subclinical" Cushing syndrome reported in up to 15% of all cases, where the overarching issue is the determination of "autonomous cortisol secretion" and ascribing its role in age-related phenotypes, such as obesity/diabetes, hypertension, low bone mineral density (BMD), and cognitive decline. Here our diagnostic tests and tissue markers of cortisol excess are far from ideal.

The management of patients in Leeds (England's third largest city) is coordinated through a multidisciplinary team comprising clinical endocrinologists, endocrine specialist nurses, radiologists, and dedicated endocrine surgeons.

BARRIERS TO OPTIMAL PRACTICE

- Awareness of the diagnosis and its prevalence
- Risk stratification of care pathways in excluding a diagnosis of adrenocortical cancer
- Accuracy of diagnostic tests and awareness of the impact of false-positive and false-negative results
- The need to refer to specialist centers working within multidisciplinary teams

LEARNING OBJECTIVES

As a result of participating in this session, learners should be able to

- Appreciate the prevalence of adrenal incidentaloma as a common finding in clinical practice and its link to an aging population
- Be aware of the differential diagnosis
- Embark on a pathway of care patients in guiding patients to address two key questions: (a) is this benign or malignant and (b) is it secreting hormones or is it nonfunctional
- Be aware of the pitfalls in making the above conclusions and in ascribing patients symptoms and signs to the adrenal lesion
- Appreciate the need to work in large multidisciplinary teams for effective patient management

CASE 1

Geraldine is a 52-year-old housewife who presented via her general practitioner to the emergency room with acute abdominal pain at another hospital. She had a 5-year history of hypertension controlled on a calcium channel blocker. Details are vague, but cholelithiasis was suspected, and for reasons that are unclear, Geraldine had a CT scan of the abdomen. The CT scan revealed no cause for the abdominal pain but did show a left-sided 2.5-cm adrenal mass (arrow in Fig. 1). Geraldine was referred to our endocrine team having been told that she had an adrenal tumor.

Geraldine was puzzled and confused, because she had been admitted with one diagnosis, for which no cause was identified, and then, was given another. She was worried that she had cancer. She had performed an Internet search and noted a connection between adrenal tumors and blood pressure. She wanted to know the answer to three questions.

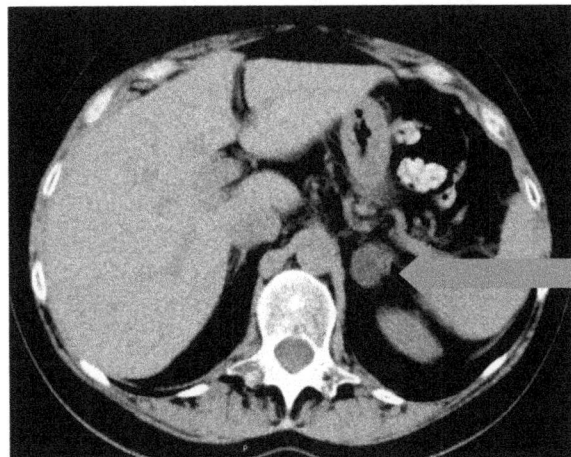

Figure 1. Case 1: CT scan.

1. What could this be?
2. Do I have cancer? Benign or malignant?
3. Is there a link with my blood pressure or any other risks?

Prevalence and Pathology

As predicted from historical postmortem data, AIs are common and largely a "disease" of aging; <1% of the population below 40 years of age will have an AI, but this prevalence rate rises to 7% by the age of 70 years of age, potentially rendering AI one of the most common endocrine conditions in current clinical practice.

In total, 80% to 85% of all AIs are benign endocrine-inactive adenomas. Up to 10% are metastatic lesions, 2% are adrenocortical carcinomas (ACCs), 2% are aldosterone secreting adenomas, 5% to 7% are pheochromocytomas, and 5% to 10% are cortisol secreting adenomas. Rarely, other lesions, such as myelolipomas, ganglioneuromas, and cysts, are reported. Metastatic lesions are obviously more common in patients with a history of underlying malignancy (commonly lung, renal, breast, or melanoma), but even in this subgroup, 25% of identified lesions are not metastatic and require endocrine workup.

Management

Two key questions must be addressed in every case. First, is the AI benign or malignant, and second, is it secretory or nonsecretory?

Malignant/Benign?

The presenting diagnostic test is usually a nonenhanced CT scan. CT (unlike MRI) has high spatial resolution that allows for assessment of tissue density through quantification of X-ray absorption of tissues measured as Hounsfield units (HUs; where zero equates to a radiodensity of water). HU of <10 invariably indicates a lipid-rich benign adrenal adenoma, but up to 30% of "benign" adenomas will have an HU score of >10, overlapping with malignant lesions and pheochromocytoma. Nonhomogeneous masses with irregular margins, younger age (<40 years old), and >4 cm in diameter are additional pointers toward malignancy; indeed, the ACC risk is <0.1% in lesions that are <4 cm, but this rises to 20% in lesions that are >4 cm. Contrast-enhanced washout CT is another aid to differential diagnosis in cases of uncertainty; generally, AIs enhance rapidly after contrast, but benign adenomas also show rapid washout compared with delayed washout in ACCs. Nuclear imaging with agents, such as ^{18}F-fluorodeoxyglucose–positron emission tomography, is reserved for patients with a history of underlying malignancy.

Geraldine's adrenal lesion was well circumscribed with an HU score of −4 and a size of 2.5 cm. We could be confident in reassuring her that this lesion was benign.

Secretory/Nonsecretory?

In excluding hormone secretion, every patient should have a clinical examination specifically recording blood pressure and assessing any discriminatory features for Cushing syndrome, Conn, or pheochromocytoma. All patients should have plasma free metanephrines or urinary fractionated metanephrines measured to exclude pheochromocytoma. We perform resting random plasma aldosterone/renin ratios only on patients with underlying hypertension and/or unexplained hypokalemia. Sex hormones are measured in patients suspected of having ACC. The greatest challenge arises in excluding a diagnosis of autonomous cortisol secretion. The optimal test is a 1-mg overnight dexamethasone suppression test measuring 9:00 AM plasma cortisol the following morning. A value of <50 nmol/L (<1.8 μg/dL) effectively excludes autonomous secretion, but values in excess of this are challenging. No diagnostic test has 100% sensitivity or specificity. Even with a cutoff of 140 nmol/L (5 μg/dL), specificity is only 95%; 5% of the "normal" population by definition will fail this test, and ascribing age-related comorbidities to borderline normal/high levels of cortisol secretion remains challenging. With little evidence base and no consistent reported relationship at such low levels between cortisol secretion and metabolic traits, our advice has been to adopt a personalized approach. Higher concentrations of cortisol, evidence of autonomy on other testing (ACTH), determination of BMD/fracture, glucose tolerance and other discriminatory markers of Cushing syndrome, and patient consent might all be pointers for unilateral adrenalectomy. However, comorbidities in all patients should be treated rigorously with medical therapies; with this in place, we adopt a conservative approach to surgical intervention at this moment in time. Finally, bilateral AI lesions are common, and they should be investigated such as for unilateral AI but with the addition of measurement of 17-OH progesterone and a short synachten test to exclude congenital adrenal hyperplasia and adrenal insufficiency.

Geraldine's endocrine tests were undertaken as above, and they showed normal plasma free metanephrine concentrations and a plasma cortisol value of 48 nmol/L after a 1-mg overnight dexamethasone suppression test. Because of her hypertension, her random plasma aldosterone/renin ratio was measured, and this too showed values within the normal reference range.

The diagnosis is a nonfunctioning benign AI.

An exciting development is the possible utility of an individual steroid metabolite "fingerprint" measuring a panel of adrenal steroids and their precursors in urine. It is hoped that such a test will help to confirm or refute a diagnosis of ACC and help define adrenocortical hormone hypersecretion.

Follow-Up

Patients with an adrenal mass of <4 cm and no other indication of malignancy or hormone hypersecretion can be discharged without follow-up imaging or repeat endocrine testing.

In patients with an indeterminant adrenal lesion not progressing to surgery (see below), we repeat the adrenal scan at 6 months. An increase in size of the lesion (indicative 20%

increase) would be an indication for surgery. If the lesion is unchanged, we would undertake a scan in 12 months and discharge if unchanged.

Which Patients for Surgery?

Patients are referred for surgery after discussion at the adrenal multidisciplinary team meeting. The decision for surgery is made on an individualized basis, but it is usually indicated for functional masses, masses suspicious for ACC, and indeterminate nodules on imaging, especially if the nodules have increased in size.

More complex situations include bilateral adrenal masses and patients with multiple comorbidities, particularly in the setting of autonomous cortisol secretion but not overt Cushing syndrome.

CASE 2

Laura is an 82-year-old retired nurse with a recent diagnosis of esophageal cancer. A staging CT scan before a course of potentially curative chemoradiotherapy revealed a well-circumscribed homogenous 2-cm adrenal left adrenal lesion (arrow) with HU = 8 (Fig. 2).

Laura has a 5-year history of type 2 diabetes mellitus and generalized obesity (body mass index = 32 kg/m²). Blood pressure is mildly elevated (168/98 mm Hg), but a normal bone mineral density was documented on dual-energy x-ray absorptiometry scanning.

Endocrine investigations revealed normal plasma free metanephrines and a normal plasma aldosterone/renin ratio, but plasma cortisol was elevated on two occasions after an overnight 1-mg dexamethasone suppression test (162 and 178 nmol/L).

Laura understands that she has a cancer diagnosis and is worried that the adrenal lesion might signify spread of her esophageal cancer.

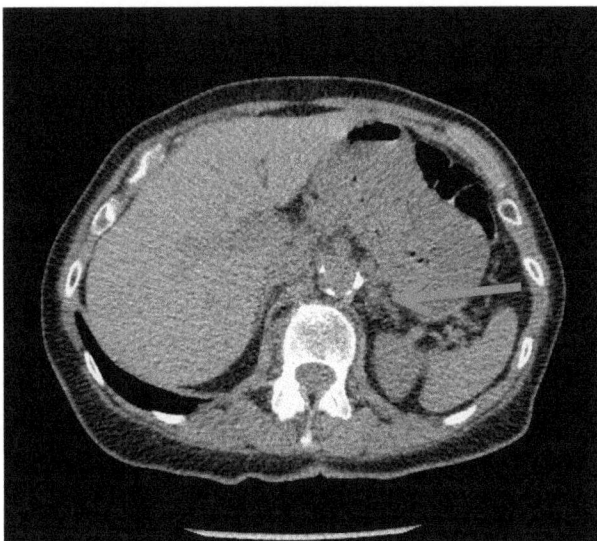

Figure 2. Case 2: CT scan.

Laura had a positron emission tomography-CT scan before her esophageal cancer therapy that showed uptake in the esophagus but no evidence of metastatic disease and no uptake in the adrenal lesion. This together with HU = 8 indicated that this was a benign adenoma, and she was reassured accordingly.

Is the adrenal lesion functioning? Does she have autonomous cortisol secretion? Should she undergo adrenalectomy?

In patients with multiple comorbidities and autonomous cortisol secretion, the decision to operate is not always straightforward. These patients have increased risks of peri- and postoperative morbidity, and it can be difficult to predict the long-term effect of an adrenalectomy on their medical comorbidities.

In addition, an overnight dexamethasone suppression test is not always easy to interpret. Several medications, including antiepileptics, can enhance hepatic dexamethasone metabolism. False-positive results are also seen in patients with "physiological hypercortisolism," such as obesity, diabetes, depression, chronic illness, alcohol abuse, and hemodialysis.

Although Laura has type 2 diabetes, she had no other clinical signs of Cushing syndrome. She was very anxious about the treatment of her esophageal cancer and did not feel that she could tolerate surgery for this. Therefore, she was not willing to consider the possibility of an adrenalectomy, especially when she felt that there were no definite long-term health benefits and that the prognosis of her esophageal cancer was not yet known.

Bilateral adrenal masses should be investigated the same way as a unilateral lesion, with each adrenal nodule assessed separately on imaging and functional testing undertaken. Although most bilateral masses are benign adenomas, there is also a chance of different coexisting conditions. We use various imaging modalities, including adrenal venous sampling, norcholesterol adrenal scintigraphy scans, and iodine-123 meta-iodobenzylguanidine, to differentiate which adrenal gland should be removed.

Synchronous bilateral adrenalectomies are rare, but they are the recommended treatment of bilateral pheochromocytomas (often hereditary) and overt Cushing syndrome. A bilateral adrenalectomy leaves the patient with the need for lifelong corticosteroid replacement treatment, and therefore, the benefit of surgery must be balanced against continued medical management of the underlying condition.

Laparoscopic surgery is now considered routine for an adrenalectomy. Laparoscopic surgery can be undertaken via the transperitoneal or retroperitoneal approach. We use the retroperitoneal approach as standard in Leeds, which has been shown to have the shortest length of stay and operating time. Open adrenal surgery is still advised if there is a risk of adrenal cortical cancer, especially if the mass is >6 cm and there is any suspicion of local invasion. Laparoscopic surgery can be considered in smaller cancers with no evidence of extra-adrenal spread. We would consider an adrenalectomy in a patient with an adrenal metastasis if there were no other sites of disease, as a curative procedure, or occasionally, for a definitive diagnosis.

Postoperatively, patients are started on adrenal replacement therapy (hydrocortisone with or without fludrocortisone) after a bilateral adrenalectomy. If there is a diagnosis of Cushing syndrome preoperatively due to an adenoma or autonomous cortisol secretion, patients are usually started on hydrocortisone in consultation with the endocrine team due to the risk of contralateral adrenal suppression.

Recommended Reading

Alemanno G, Bergamini C, Prosperi P, Valeri A. Adrenalectomy: indications and options for treatment [published correction appears in *Updates Surg.* 2017;69(4):555]. *Updates Surg.* 2017;**69**(2):119–125.

Arlt W, Biehl M, Taylor AE, Hahner S, Libé R, Hughes BA, Schneider P, Smith DJ, Stiekema H, Krone N, Porfiri E, Opocher G, Bertherat J, Mantero F, Allolio B, Terzolo M, Nightingale P, Shackleton CH, Bertagna X, Fassnacht M, Stewart PM. Urine steroid metabolomics as a biomarker tool for detecting malignancy in adrenal tumors. *J Clin Endocrinol Metab.* 2011;**96**(12):3775–3784.

Bourdeau I, El Ghorayeb N, Gagnon N, Lacroix A. MANAGEMENT OF ENDOCRINE DISEASE: differential diagnosis, investigation and therapy of bilateral adrenal incidentalomas. *Eur J Endocrinol.* 2018;**179**(2): R57–R67.

Fassnacht M, Arlt W, Bancos I, Dralle H, Newell-Price J, Sahdev A, Tabarin A, Terzolo M, Tsagarakis S, Dekkers OM. Management of adrenal incidentalomas: European Society of Endocrinology Clinical Practice Guideline in collaboration with the European Network for the Study of Adrenal Tumors. *Eur J Endocrinol.* 2016;**175**(2): G1–G34.

Heger P, Probst P, Hüttner FJ, Gooßen K, Proctor T, Müller-Stich BP, Strobel O, Büchler MW, Diener MK. Evaluation of open and minimally invasive adrenalectomy: a systematic review and network meta-analysis. *World J Surg.* 2017;**41**(11):2746–2757.

Maccora D, Walls GV, Sadler GP, Mihai R. Bilateral adrenalectomy: a review of 10 years' experience. *Ann R Coll Surg Engl.* 2017;**99**(2):119–122.

Palazzo F, Dickinson A, Phillips B, Sahdev A, Bliss R, Rasheed A, Krukowski Z, Newell-Price J. Adrenal surgery in England: better outcomes in high-volume practices. *Clin Endocrinol (Oxf).* 2016;**85**(1):17–20.

Stewart PM. Is subclinical Cushing's syndrome an entity or a statistical fallout from diagnostic testing? Consensus surrounding the diagnosis is required before optimal treatment can be defined. *J Clin Endocrinol Metab.* 2010;**95**(6):2618–2620.

Neuroendocrine Tumors of Gut and Pancreas

M53
Presented, March 23–26, 2019

Wouter W. de Herder, MD, PhD. Department of Internal Medicine, Sector of Endocrinology, Erasmus MC, 3062 EC, Rotterdam, The Netherlands, E-mail: w.w.deherder@erasmusmc.nl

SIGNIFICANCE OF THE CLINICAL PROBLEM
- The reported incidence of gastroenteropancreatic neuroendocrine tumors (GEP-NENs) ranges from 1.4 to 7.0 per 100,000 persons and is rising.
- NENs of the gastrointestinal tract were formerly known as carcinoids.
- Pancreatic NEN types:
  - Insulinoma
  - Gastrinoma
  - VIPoma (VIP, vasoactive intestinal polypeptide)
  - Glucagonoma
  - Somatostatinoma
  - Nonsyndromic/nonfunctioning pancreatic NEN

BARRIERS TO OPTIMAL PRACTICE
- Orphan diseases; however, the incidence of GEP-NENs is rapidly increasing
- Variable clinical manifestations
- Variable clinical courses
- Symptom control vs tumor control
- Multidisciplinary diagnostic and therapeutic approaches

POTENTIAL ROLE OF THE ENDOCRINOLOGIST
- Rare functioning tumor syndromes
- Duodenal NEN in the spectrum of multiple endocrine neoplasia type 1. Pancreatic NENs are generally sporadic, but can be multiple and a component of familial syndromes, including multiple endocrine neoplasia type 1, von Hippel-Lindau disease, or neurofibromatosis type 1.
- Medical therapy and management of hormonal and peptide hypersecretion
- Receptor-mediated therapies

LEARNING OBJECTIVES
As a result of participating in this session, learners should be able to:
- Recognize the clinical relevant endocrine features of GEP-NENs
- Optimal diagnose functioning = syndromic GEP-NENs

As a result of participating in this session, learners will attain knowledge on:
- Diagnostic strategies in GEP-NENs
- Treatment modalities for symptom control and tumor control in patients with GEP-NENs

DIGESTIVE NENs
Digestive NENs (Carcinoid Tumors), Nonfunctioning
- Mainly diagnosed either incidentally or by local mass effects

Digestive NENs (Carcinoid Tumors) and the Carcinoid Syndrome
Typical carcinoid syndrome usually has the following clinical manifestations:
- Cutaneous flushing, secretory diarrhea, right-sided heart failure caused by tricuspid and pulmonic valve fibrosis and endocardial fibrosis (carcinoid heart disease), abdominal pain, and pellagra
  - Carcinoid crisis is an extreme, life-threatening manifestation of the carcinoid syndrome. It occurs as a consequence of the massive release of vasoactive peptides into the circulation following anesthesia, interventional procedures, or administration of certain medications. Main features are: hypotension, rarely hypertension, tachycardia, bronchial wheezing, and central nervous system dysfunction.
  - Carcinoids in the distal jejunum and ileum can be associated with extensive mesenteric fibrosis (desmoplastic reaction) associated with a mesenterial lymph node metastasis resulting in abdominal pain, venous congestion of the bowel, and arterial insufficiency leading to life-threatening bowel ischemia

PANCREATIC NENs (PNENs)
PNENs, Nonfunctioning
- Mainly diagnosed either incidentally or by local mass effects

Insulinomas
- Mostly benign, small-sized tumors
- Characterized by insulin hypersecretion and resulting hypoglycemia features

Gastrinomas
- Duodenum and pancreas
- Hypergastrinemia causes acid hypersecretion with esophagitis, peptic ulcerations in the upper gastrointestinal tract, and diarrhea

Glucagonomas
- Large tumors
- Weight loss, diabetes mellitus, cheilosis, diarrhea, and necrolytic migratory erythema

VIPomas
- Rare; usually large and metastatic
- Very severe secretory diarrhea and metabolic derangements (hypovolemia, hypokalemia, hypomagnesemia, hypophosphatemia, hypochlorhydria, and acidosis)

Somatostatinomas
- Extremely rare

BIOCHEMICAL AND TISSUE MARKERS
- All GEP-NENs
- Plasma: Chromogranin A
- Carcinoid syndrome:
  - Urine (plasma): Breakdown product of serotonin (5-hydroxindolacetic acid. Plasma serotonin.
  - PNENs
  - Plasma: Insulin, C-peptide, proinsulin, gastrin, VIP, somatostatin, glucagon, and pancreatic polypeptide can be measured in plasma on indication.
- On indication, further specific diagnostic tests can be performed:
  - 72-hour fast for the diagnosis of insulinoma
  - Secretin test for the diagnosis of gastrinoma

LOCALIZING STUDIES
Assessment of the location and extent of GEP-NENs is essential for management, including:
- Determination of when surgery should be performed, as well as the extent of surgery
- Timing/aggressiveness of antitumor treatment
- Possible role of surgery in advanced disease
- Monitoring and diagnosis of recurrent disease
- Monitoring of progression

Imaging modalities include the following:
- Endoscopic ultrasound in patients with PNENs (preferred diagnostic technique)
- Positron emission tomography (PET) using ^{68}Ga-DOTATOC or ^{68}Ga-DOTATATE (^{111}In-pentetreotide scintigraphy with single-photon emission computed tomography imaging [somatostatin receptor scintigraphy] is becoming redundant)
- Three-phase computed tomography (CT)
- Magnetic resonance imaging
- Transabdominal ultrasound
- ^{18}F-fluorodeoxyglucose PET in poorly differentiated NEN or neuroendocrine carcinoma (NEC). May have an additional role in well-differentiated NEN.
- Scintigraphy with single-photon emission computed tomography imaging using ^{111}In-DOTA-exendin-4 or ^{68}Ga-DOTA-exendin-4 PET/CT in patients with insulinoma

TUMOR STAGING AND GRADING
- 2017 World Health Organization classification:
  - Neuroendocrine tumor, NET G1
  - Neuroendocrine tumor, NET G2
  - Neuroendocrine tumor, NET G3
  - Neuroendocrine carcinoma, NEC G3 (small-cell type/large-cell type)
  - Mixed neuroendocrine–nonneuroendocrine neoplasias
- World Health Organization/National Comprehensive Cancer Network/European Neuroendocrine Tumor Society grading and staging (TNM) systems

THERAPY
I. Controlling tumor growth
II. Inhibition of the secretion of bioactive agents with consequent symptom amelioration

1. Surgical Therapy
- Surgery is essential in many phases of the management of GEP-NENs
- In most patients with limited disease, it remains the primary method of obtaining a cure
- In advanced disease, cytoreductive surgery is used for palliation, symptom reduction in patients with functional tumors, and improved survival
- Even in unresectable metastatic carcinoid tumors, there is a role for surgery to prevent symptoms of obstruction and to reduce the possibility of obstruction

Procedures for treatment of liver metastases include the following:
- Metastasectomy
- Partial hepatectomy
- Radiofrequency ablation, microwave ablation, and cryoablation
- High-intensity focused ultrasound
- Laser
- Brachytherapy
- Irreversible electroporation
- Bland embolization and chemoembolization (transarterial chemoembolization; only performed in the presence of a patent portal vein)
- Radioembolization (selective internal radiation therapy) using Y^{90} microspheres
- Liver transplantation (only performed when extrahepatic tumors can be ruled out)

2. Medical Therapy
- Biotherapy: somatostatin analogs (*e.g.*, octreotide, lanreotide):
  - Effective in controlling tumor-related symptoms as well as reducing tumor secretion
  - Delay disease progression (progression-free survival/time to progression)

- Well-tolerated, safe drugs with minor side effects
- Telotristat etiprate for the control of secretory diarrhea in patients with carcinoid syndrome not controlled by treatment with somatostatin analogs
- Chemotherapy and targeted therapy
- Everolimus in patients with G1 or G2 GEP-NENs
- Sunitinib in patients with G1 or G2 PNENs
- Etoposide plus cisplatin as first-line treatment of G3 GEP-NEC
- Streptozotocin plus fluorouracil plus doxorubicin in patients with PNENs
- Temozolomide with or without capecitabine in patients with PNENs
- Experimental studies

3. Peptide Receptor Radionuclide Therapy
- ^{177}Lu-DOTATATE in patients with G1 or G2 GEP-NENs

4. Miscellaneous
- ^{131}I-meta-iodobenzylguanidine in patients with G1 or G2 GEP-NENs

CONCLUSIONS: AREAS DISCUSSED
- Improvements in the diagnosis of GEP-NENs and their associated syndromes
- Identification of prognostic markers
- Improvements in tumor localization
- Improvements in control of hormonal/hormone-related symptoms and syndromes
- Improvements in control of tumor growth

CASE 1

A 44-year-old woman was referred because of hypoglycemic symptoms. For 2.5 years, she had been complaining of attacks of tremors, vision blurriness, loss of attention, and headaches. There was no excessive perspiration, hunger, or loss of consciousness. She had fewer complaints when she ate frequent meals. Her weight is 77 kg; it has gradually increased over a period of 3 years, with a gain of 1 to 2 kg/y. Using a portable glucose sensor, her physician has measured very low blood glucose levels during an attack.

Additional investigations included:
- 72-hour fast: Glucose 1.4 mmol/L (25 mg/dL), insulin 3.0 mU/L after a 60.5-hour fast. Hypoglycemic symptoms were reported by the patient (the test was stopped, the patient was allowed to eat, and hypoglycemic symptoms disappeared).
- Toxicology testing of urine was negative for sulfonylurea derivatives.

Questions
1. Do the findings support the diagnosis of insulinoma?
2. Which imaging procedures would you request?
3. Which therapeutic procedure(s) would you prefer?

Answers
1. Yes
2. Ultrasonography of the abdomen, CT or magnetic resonance imaging of the pancreas, endoscopic ultrasound of the pancreas (most sensitive)
3. Enucleation or larger resections for a small localized (benign) insulinoma. Targeted therapies for metastatic insulinomas.

CASE 2

A 61-year-old man was referred to a urologist for prostate hyperplasia. Subsequent imaging with CT revealed pathological lesions in the pancreas and liver. There were no bone lesions. He complained of involuntary weight loss, fatigue, and polyuria. His Eastern Cooperative Oncology Group/World Health Organization/Zubrod performance status was 1.

An inoperable, well-differentiated (grade 1) NET in the pancreatic body with multilobar liver metastases was diagnosed.

Additional investigations revealed the following:
- Serum calcium levels were elevated
- Serum phosphate levels were reduced
- Serum creatinine levels were within the reference range
- Plasma parathyroid hormone concentrations were undetectable
- Serum levels of chromogranin A were elevated
- ^{68}Ga-DOTATATE PET/CT showed a scan-positive lesion in the pancreas and multiple liver lesions. There was no pathologic uptake in the bones.

Questions
1. Are the findings in line with the diagnosis of a parathyroid hormone–related protein–producing pancreatic neuroendocrine tumor?
2. Which additional investigations would you request?
3. Which therapeutic procedure(s) would you prefer?

Answers
1. Yes
2. Parathyroid hormone–related protein measurements in the blood
3. Isotonic saline, somatostatin analogs, peptide receptor radionuclide therapy

Recommended Reading

Brabander T, van der Zwan WA, Teunissen JJM, Kam BLR, Feelders RA, de Herder WW, van Eijck CHJ, Franssen GJH, Krenning EP, Kwekkeboom DJ. Long-term efficacy, survival, and safety of [^{177}Lu-DOTA^0,Tyr^3]octreotate in patients with gastroenteropancreatic and bronchial neuroendocrine tumors. *Clin Cancer Res.* 2017;**23**(16):4617–4624.

Garcia-Carbonero R, Rinke A, Valle JW, Fazio N, Caplin M, Gorbounova V, O Connor J, Eriksson B, Sorbye H, Kulke M, Chen J, Falkerby J, Costa F, de Herder W, Lombard-Bohas C, Pavel M; Antibes Consensus Conference participants. ENETS Consensus Guidelines for the Standards of Care in

Neuroendocrine Neoplasms. Systemic Therapy 2: Chemotherapy. *Neuroendocrinology*. 2017;**105**(3):281–294.

Hicks RJ, Kwekkeboom DJ, Krenning E, Bodei L, Grozinsky-Glasberg S, Arnold R, Borbath I, Cwikla J, Toumpanakis C, Kaltsas G, Davies P, Hörsch D, Tiensuu Janson E, Ramage J; Antibes Consensus Conference participants. ENETS Consensus Guidelines for the Standards of Care in Neuroendocrine Neoplasia: Peptide Receptor Radionuclide Therapy with Radiolabeled Somatostatin Analogues. *Neuroendocrinology*. 2017;**105**(3):295–309.

Hofland J, Feelders RA, Brabander T, Franssen GJH, de Herder WW. Recent developments in the diagnosis and therapy of well-differentiated neuroendocrine tumours. *Neth J Med*. 2018;**76**(3): 100–108.

Kaltsas G, Caplin M, Davies P, Ferone D, Garcia-Carbonero R, Grozinsky-Glasberg S, Hörsch D, Tiensuu Janson E, Kianmanesh R, Kos-Kudla B, Pavel M, Rinke A, Falconi M, de Herder WW; Antibes Consensus Conference participants. ENETS Consensus Guidelines for the Standards of Care in Neuroendocrine Tumors: Pre- and Peri-operative Therapy in Patients with Neuroendocrine Tumors. *Neuroendocrinology*. 2017;**105**(3):245–254.

Knigge U, Capdevila J, Bartsch DK, Baudin E, Falkerby J, Kianmanesh R, Kos-Kudla B, Niederle B, Nieveen van Dijkum E, O'Toole D, Pascher A, Reed N, Sundin A, Vullierme MP; Antibes Consensus Conference Participants; Antibes Consensus Conference participants. ENETS Consensus Recommendations for the Standards of Care in Neuroendocrine Neoplasms: Follow-Up and Documentation. *Neuroendocrinology*. 2017;**105**(3):310–319.

Oberg K, Couvelard A, Delle Fave G, Gross D, Grossman A, Jensen RT, Pape UF, Perren A, Rindi G, Ruszniewski P, Scoazec JY, Welin S, Wiedenmann B, Ferone D; Antibes Consensus Conference participants. ENETS Consensus Guidelines for Standard of Care in Neuroendocrine Tumours: Biochemical Markers. *Neuroendocrinology*. 2017;**105**(3):201–211.

O'Toole D, Grossman A, Gross D, Delle Fave G, Barkmanova J, O'Connor J, Pape UF, Plöckinger U; Mallorca Consensus Conference participants; European Neuroendocrine Tumor Society. ENETS Consensus Guidelines for the Standards of Care in Neuroendocrine Tumors: Biochemical Markers. *Neuroendocrinology*. 2009;**90**(2):194–202.

Partelli S, Bartsch DK, Capdevila J, Chen J, Knigge U, Niederle B, Nieveen van Dijkum EJM, Pape UF, Pascher A, Ramage J, Reed N, Ruszniewski P, Scoazec JY, Toumpanakis C, Kianmanesh R, Falconi M; Antibes Consensus Conference participants. ENETS Consensus Guidelines for Standard of Care in Neuroendocrine Tumours: Surgery for Small Intestinal and Pancreatic Neuroendocrine Tumours. *Neuroendocrinology*. 2017;**105**(3):255–265.

Pavel M, Valle JW, Eriksson B, Rinke A, Caplin M, Chen J, Costa F, Falkerby J, Fazio N, Gorbounova V, de Herder W, Kulke M, Lombard-Bohas C, O'Connor J, Sorbye H, Garcia-Carbonero R; Antibes Consensus Conference Participants; Antibes Consensus Conference participants. ENETS Consensus Guidelines for the Standards of Care in Neuroendocrine Neoplasms: Systemic Therapy - Biotherapy and Novel Targeted Agents. *Neuroendocrinology*. 2017;**105**(3):266–280.

Perren A, Couvelard A, Scoazec JY, Costa F, Borbath I, Delle Fave G, Gorbounova V, Gross D, Grossma A, Jense RT, Kulke M, Oeberg K, Rindi G, Sorbye H, Welin S; Antibes Consensus Conference participants. ENETS Consensus Guidelines for the Standards of Care in Neuroendocrine Tumors: Pathology: Diagnosis and Prognostic Stratification. *Neuroendocrinology*. 2017;**105**(3):196–200.

Sundin A, Arnold R, Baudin E, Cwikla JB, Eriksson B, Fanti S, Fazio N, Giammarile F, Hicks RJ, Kjaer A, Krenning E, Kwekkeboom D, Lombard-Bohas C, O'Connor JM, O'Toole D, Rockall A, Wiedenmann B, Valle JW, Vullierme MP; Antibes Consensus Conference participants. ENETS Consensus Guidelines for the Standards of Care in Neuroendocrine Tumors: Radiological, Nuclear Medicine & Hybrid Imaging. *Neuroendocrinology*. 2017;**105**(3):212–244.

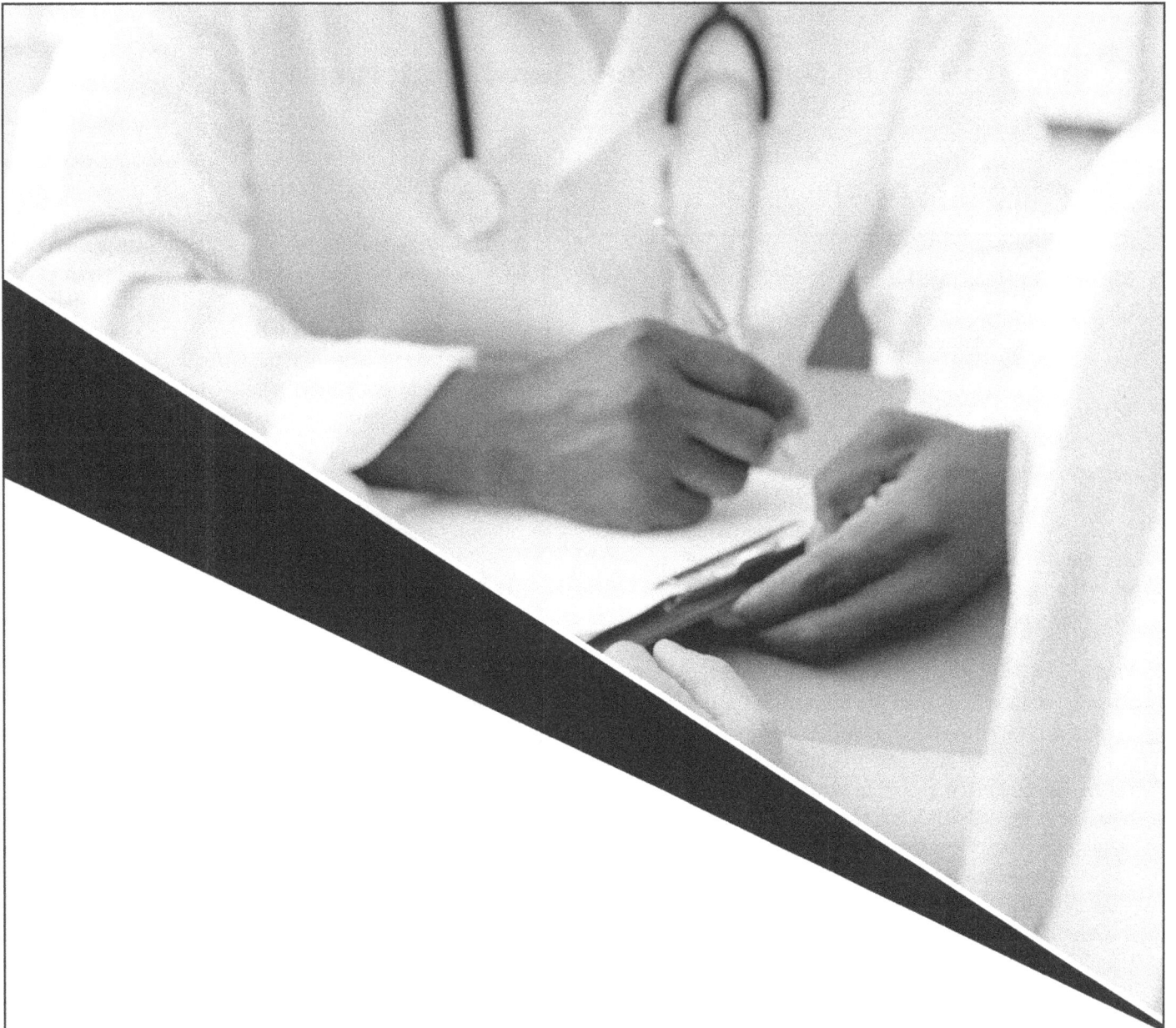

BONE AND MINERAL METABOLISM

From "T to Z": The Basics of Bone Density Interpretation

M03
Presented, March 23–26, 2019

Micol S. Rothman, MD. University of Colorado School of Medicine, Aurora, Colorado 80045, E-mail: micol. rothman@ucdenver.edu

SIGNIFICANCE OF THE CLINICAL PROBLEM

Bone mineral density (BMD) testing using dual-energy X-ray absorptiometry (DXA) has been a part of clinical practice since the 1980s. It remains the gold standard for measuring bone density at the spine and hip. BMD is the bone mineral content in grams per two-dimensional projected area of bone, reported as grams per square centimeter. In 1994, the World Health Organization defined osteoporosis on the basis of BMD testing by DXA and T-score defined as follows: (patient's BMD − young normal mean)/SD of young normal. In postmenopausal women and men older than age 50 years, a T-score of −1.0 or greater is considered normal BMD, less than −1.0 to −2.5 is defined as low bone mass or osteopenia, and less than or equal to −2.5 is considered to be osteoporosis (1). Osteoporosis can also be diagnosed after a low-trauma fracture (fall from a standing height). In younger patients, Z-score is used to compare patients' BMD with others of their age. A Z-score of less than −2.0 indicates an abnormal bone mineral density for age (1, 2).

Osteoporosis is a common bone disease. Fractures affect morbidity and mortality and cost the health care system billions of dollars each year. There are more than 2 million fractures in the United States each year, and the risk of having a broken bone after age 50 years is one in two for women and one in four for men. Twenty percent of women will die in the first year after hip fracture, and 60% of patients never regain their prefracture level of independence. Osteoporosis in men is often underdiagnosed and undertreated, but a man is more likely to die after a hip fracture than a woman (3).

Although DXA is still the most widely used clinical tool with which to screen for osteoporosis, it has limitations. Additional tools can be used to evaluate fracture risk, as many patients who experience a fracture have bone density scores in the osteopenic or even normal range. Thus, DXA in combination with FRAX (fracture risk assessment tool; https://www.shef.ac.uk/FRAX/) is used as a fracture prediction tool for untreated patients with a diagnosis of osteopenia. FRAX takes into account BMD-independent risks for fracture, including age, glucocorticoid treatment, current tobacco use, parental history of hip fracture, rheumatoid arthritis and alcohol use of more than three times per day. FRAX can also be used to calculate fracture risk when BMD is not available. Other risk prediction tools include the Garvan calculator, which also incorporates falls, and the osteoporosis self-assessment tool, which looks at body weight and age alone.

Additional imaging techniques and/or measurements of bone quality can be used in patient care in addition to DXA. Trabecular bone score (TBS), a gray-level textural measurement, is now being used in both research and clinical practice (4). TBS can take lumbar spine data from standard DXA testing to noninvasively asses bone microarchitecture. It projects a three-dimensional structure onto a two-dimensional plane and uses gray-level variation in images of the lumbar spine to calculate a score. This score has been shown to predict fracture in primary osteoporosis, as well as several forms of secondary osteoporosis. Dedicated vertebral imaging *via* vertebral fracture assessment with DXA or with plain X-ray films of the spine can also be useful, particularly in adults with osteopenia and additional risk factors for osteoporosis where the finding of a silent fracture would change recommendations for pharmacologic therapy. Other modalities, such as quantitative CT, can measure volumetric BMD at the spine and hip. Although high-resolution peripheral quantitative CT is thought to be a good measure of bone quality as a result of cost and radiation exposure, it is generally used for research only at this time. Bone biopsies provide the most direct information about bone microarchitecture and bone turnover, but are invasive procedures.

BARRIERS TO OPTIMAL PRACTICE

Although BMD testing is widely used, measurements are frequently not reported in concordance with International Society of Clinical Densitometry (ISCD) guidelines. Many clinicians are not familiar with how to interpret DXA images in the face of artifacts and other limitations. In addition, use of T-scores *vs.* Z-scores is often misunderstood. ISCD suggests that even when multiple sites are measured, such as hips and spine, still only the lowest site T-score should be used for a diagnosis (1). That is, one should not report "The hip has osteoporosis but the spine shows osteopenia." Furthermore, many DXA centers do not have a measurement of least significant change (LSC), which can make it difficult to interpret change in BMD over time.

There are also ongoing controversies about the frequency of DXA for screening and monitoring. Guidelines from national societies provide conflicting advice about when to screen and how often to repeat DXA (5). Medicare coverage for screening in some groups differs from that which the ISCD and National Osteoporosis Foundation recommend. Many women who are eligible for screening DXA still do not receive it. In a study of Medicare beneficiaries from 2002 to 2008, 48% of women had no testing performed at all. Less than 4% received four or more DXA studies, and, thus, undertesting may be more of a problem than overtesting (6).

LEARNING OBJECTIVES

As a result of participating in this session, learners should be able to:

- Interpret BMD testing for men and women of all ages
- Use DXA to help guide secondary work-up of low BMD or bone loss
- Be familiar with the guidelines—and controversies—regarding DXA screening and follow-up intervals
- Be familiar with the unknowns of the use of DXA in the transgender population
- Use TBS

STRATEGIES FOR DIAGNOSIS, THERAPY, OR MANAGEMENT

The National Osteoporosis Foundation (NOF) Clinician's Guide for 2014 recommends osteoporosis screening for all women older than age 65 years and men older than age 70 years. The guide also advises screening for post-menopausal women and men older than age 50 years with other risk factors. In addition, a DXA is suggested after a fracture to define the extent of low BMD. NOF also suggests that DXA be performed at facilities that use accepted quality assurance measures. The US Preventive Services Task Force recommends bone density screening for all women older than age 65 years (grade B) and women younger than age 65 years whose 10-year risk of fracture as calculated by FRAX is greater than a 65-year-old white woman without risk factors (9.3%; grade B) (7). Use of additional vertebral imaging for those with low BMD is also suggested in the following groups: women older than age 70 and men older than age 80 with T-scores less than −1.0, women age 65 to 69 and men 70 to 79 years with T-scores less than −1.5, and men and women older than age 50 years with adult low-trauma fractures, height loss, and glucocorticoid treatment (3). NOF advises follow-up testing for those on treatment in 1 to 2 years and every 2 years thereafter, but note that certain clinical situations may warrant more- or less-frequent follow-up.

LSC and precision should be calculated by each technician at a bone density facility. Here, technicians can measure a patient multiple times (15 patients × 3 or 30 patients × 2) to determine their precision and, thus, what change in BMD can be interpreted as a true change. There is a formula on the ISCD Web site (http://www.ISCD.org) where patients' data can be entered and the precision for each technician can then be calculated. LSC is reported as grams per square centimeter for hip and spine. T-scores are not used because they can change with alterations in the database reference population. If a patient's change in BMD does not exceed the LSC, it is not considered a significant change; however, even if changes do exceed the LSC, this does not mean they are clinically significant. A loss of 1% to 2% per year can be observed with normal aging, and BMD testing performed at long intervals

may demonstrate loss that exceeds the LSC but is not considered pathologic.

In the setting of a low T-score—or low Z-score in a young patient—a work-up to rule out secondary causes is advised. This includes looking for common causes of low BMD (renal disease, liver disease, vitamin D deficiency, hyperthyroidism, hyperparathyroidism, hypogonadism, or hypercalciuria) as well as less-common causes as clinical suspicion dictates (Cushing's syndrome, multiple myeloma, celiac disease, mastocytosis, or osteogenesis imperfecta).

MAIN CONCLUSIONS

BMD should be interpreted using T-scores for men older than age 50 years and postmenopausal women. Younger groups should have Z-scores reported.

Low Z-scores at any age many indicate the need for a secondary work-up of low bone density.

BMD testing should be repeated at a time interval when a change is likely to be significant and/or lead to a treatment change. This may vary by patient factors, treatments used, and other clinical indicators. For those patients who are at highest risk, that interval may be 1 to 2 years. For those at lower risk, it can be longer.

TBS is a new tool that can help predict fracture risk in many groups. It may be of particular use in populations in whom BMD has not historically been low.

CASES

Case 1

A 65-year-old woman with no risk factors for osteoporosis undergoes a screening DXA (image shown) that shows am L1-L4 T-score of 0.8 and right femoral neck T-score of −1.2.

Which of the following is appropriate to put on the DXA report?

A. This is a screening study for a 65-year-old woman with no reported risk factors for osteoporosis.
B. This patient has normal bone density at the lumbar spine and osteopenia at the right hip.
C. This patient's BMD test does not need to be repeated.
D. There has been significant bone loss in this patient.

Case 1 Discussion
Answer: A

ISCD guidelines specifically note that osteoporosis is a systemic disease and that one unifying diagnosis should be given—not osteopenia at one site and normal at another (1). Therefore, answer B is incorrect. Answer D is incorrect as we do not know in a screening study whether bone loss has occurred. As to answer C, the issue of monitoring intervals for bone density is controversial. In 2012, Gourlay *et al.* (8) investigated the use of screening DXA for osteoporosis. They examined a subgroup of women from the Study on Osteo-porotic Fractures and assessed the time it took women with normal BMD or osteopenia to transition to osteoporosis. This time varied with changes in age, estrogen use, and body mass index. Less than 5% of women with mild osteopenia, which would be the patient in this case, made the transition to osteoporosis during the 15-year period. A more recent study from this group suggests that a single DXA may predict fracture risk for up to 25 years, although the authors note that additional risk factor data, including follow-up BMD, may optimize risk prediction further (9). None of the evidence would support retesting this patient in 1 year, and she is unlikely to have loss that would indicate a need for pharmacologic therapy, but we cannot say at this time that her DXA should never be repeated. Patient history and risk factors can help to determine the interval. ISCD does suggest that all DXA reports include the following as a minimum: patient demographics, machine manufacture and model, skeletal sites scanned, and BMD in grams per square centimeter, as well as T-score and/or Z-score where appropriate, World Health Organization criteria for diagnosis, recommendations for the timing of the next study, risk factors with a statement about fracture risk, and a statement that medical evaluation for causes of low BMD may be indicated.

We will use this case vignette to discuss the guidelines for what should be included on a DXA report as well as controversies surrounding testing intervals.

Case 2

A postmenopausal woman undergoes BMD testing on several occasions (DXA slide shown here). You are concerned that, although the hip BMD is stable, there has been a large decrease in BMD in the spine in a rapid time frame.

What step would you take next?
A. Change her oral bisphosphonate to an alternative therapy
B. Add estrogen to her current regimen to increase her spine BMD
C. Order makers of bone turnover to assess for increased osteoclast activity
D. View the images yourself, particularly the spine

Case 2 Discussion
Answer: D
Looking at images for accuracy is a key part of bone density interpretation. Before taking costly steps, such as ordering blood or urine tests, or changing to alternative therapies, it is important to view the images. Thus, answers A, B, and C are incorrect. As shown here, when the 2016 spine outline was redrawn to match 2015, the changes were no longer significant.

This case highlights the need to view images. Other examples of imaging issues and artifacts will be shown.

Case 3

A 23-year-old woman with a history of an eating disorder is seen for amenorrhea. She has not had menses in 7 months. She has experienced prior but not recent fractures. Recent studies from her primary care physician show a vitamin D level of 35 ng/mL. She brings a bone density with her as shown in PowerPoint slides.

Which of the following do you suggest?
A. Begin teriparatide
B. Further assess the amenorrhea and think about a bone mineral apparent density calculation.
C. Add 50,000 IU of vitamin D once per week
D. Begin alendronate on the basis of her low T-score

Case 3 Discussion
Answer: B
This case addresses the larger issue of how to approach low BMD in younger patients. Oftentimes, young patients with low BMD have not reached peak bone mass and their bone density should be interpreted with caution. Use of T-scores in men younger than age 50 years and premenopausal women is not appropriate, and in young patients who are not fracturing we try to avoid pharmacologic therapy (10). Answer D, therefore, is incorrect. In addition, teriparatide is contraindicated in young patients (answer A), as there can still be concerns for open epiphyses until age 25. With a vitamin D level of 35 ng/mL, additional supplementation is unlikely to help her bone health; thus, answer C is incorrect. Patients with eating disorders in adolescence may have delayed bone age and it is important to keep this in mind when thinking about DXA Z-scores. In addition, growing patients or those who are of smaller stature will have smaller bones. Fracture risk can be overestimated in patients with short stature. A calculation can be performed to estimate bone mineral apparent density and provide more of a volumetric BMD. The term was coined in 1992 and a University of Washington Web site provides a calculator (https://courses.washington.edu/bonephys/opBMAD.html) (11). Additional questioning about the amenorrhea and laboratory work-up would be appropriate.

We will use this case vignette to talk about the use of T- and Z-scores in young people and when pharmacologic intervention should be considered.

Case 4

A 24-year-old transgender man has been on testosterone for 2 years and is exploring options for ongoing bleeding, including the use of leuprolide and aromatase inhibitors. A DXA is obtained.

With what reference population should the DXA be interpreted?
A. Male reference range, as he has been on testosterone
B. Female reference range, as that was the predominant sex steroid during puberty accrual of bone
C. The answer is unknown at this time, especially in people who are still attaining peak bone mass.

Case 4 Discussion
Answer: C

There are no data to guide us in this area yet. Most researchers use the sex assigned at birth when interpreting DXA, as many patients did reach peak bone mass under the influence of natal sex steroids. However, it remains unclear, and this may change with more patients undergoing pubertal blockade with GnRH agonists and transitioning earlier in life (12). Our current practice is to request additional interpretation, which does not entail an additional visit for the patient, when bone density results are unexpected or would require intervention and then discuss both results with the patient.

We will use this case vignette to talk about the unknowns in the interpretation of bone density and osteoporosis screening in the transgender population.

Case 5

A postmenopausal woman with diabetes has a humeral fracture. She has an HbA_{1c} of 7.2 and takes metformin, pioglitazone, and canagliflozin. You decide to obtain a TBS.

Which of the following is true?

A. TBS requires additional images and radiation exposure for the patient.

B. TBS can be used in combination with FRAX to stratify fracture risk.

C. High TBS indicates poor bone architecture.

D. ISCD advised that TBS should be used to monitor response to bisphosphonate treatment in people with diabetes.

Case 5 Discussion
Answer: B

TBS is a gray-level textural measurement that uses images already obtained by two-dimensional images (4, 13, 14). Answer A is incorrect. A high score is indicative of better microarchitecture; therefore, answer C is incorrect. A lower score indicates poor bone architecture. TBS has been shown to be an independent predictor of fracture risk. FRAX scores can now be adjusted with the inclusion of TBS on the FRAX Web site (answer B is correct).

TBS may be of particular help in populations in whom DXA may seem to be falsely reassuring (patients with diabetes or those who are on long-term glucocorticoids). A study of women in Manitoba with diabetes demonstrated that lumbar spine TBS predicted fracture independent of BMD (15). Although some studies suggest that TBS increases with osteoporosis therapy at this time, ISCD and other group do not yet recommend that TBS be used for monitoring of therapy; therefore, answer D is incorrect.

This case will serve as a discussion point for talking about the uses and limitations of TBS and the populations in whom it has been studied.

References

1. The International Society for Clinical Densitometry. 2015 ISCD official positions. Available at: https://www.iscd.org/official-positions/. Accessed 8 January 2019.
2. Lewiecki EM. Bone density measurement and assessment of fracture risk. *Clin Obstet Gynecol.* 2013;**56**(4):667–676.
3. Cosman F, de Beur SJ, LeBoff MS, Lewiecki EM, Tanner B, Randall S, Lindsay R. Clinician's Guide to Prevention and Treatment of Osteoporosis [published correction appears in Osteoporos Int. 2015;26(7):2045]. *Osteoporos Int.* 2014;**25**(10):2359–2381.
4. Silva BC, Leslie WD, Resch H, Lamy O, Lesnyak O, Binkley N, McCloskey EV, Kanis JA, Bilezikian JP. Trabecular bone score: A noninvasive analytical method based upon the DXA image. *J Bone Miner Res.* 2014;**29**(3):518–530.
5. Rothman MS, Lewiecki EM, Miller PD. Bone density testing is the best way to monitor osteoporosis treatment. *Am J Med.* 2017;**130**(10):1133–1134.
6. King AB, Fiorentino DM. Medicare payment cuts for osteoporosis testing reduced use despite tests' benefit in reducing fractures. *Health Aff (Millwood).* 2011;**30**(12):2362–2370.
7. Golob AL, Laya MB. Osteoporosis: Screening, prevention, and management. *Med Clin North Am.* 2015;**99**(3):587–606.
8. Gourlay ML, Fine JP, Preisser JS, May RC, Li C, Lui LY, Ransohoff DF, Cauley JA, Ensrud KE, for the Study of Osteoporotic Fractures Research Group. Bone-density testing interval and transition to osteoporosis in older women. *N Engl J Med.* 2012;**366**(3):225–233.
9. Black DM, Cauley JA, Wagman R, Ensrud K, Fink HA, Hillier TA, Lui LY, Cummings SR, Schousboe JT, Napoli N. The ability of a single BMD and fracture history assessment to predict fracture over 25 years in postmenopausal women: The study of osteoporotic fractures *J Bone Miner Res.* 2018;**33**(3):389–395.
10. Abraham A, Cohen A, Shane E. Premenopausal bone health: Osteoporosis in premenopausal women. *Clin Obstet Gynecol.* 2013;**56**(4):722–729.
11. Carter DR, Bouxsein ML, Marcus R. New approaches for interpreting projected bone densitometry data. *J Bone Miner Res.* 1992;**7**(2):137–145.
12. Hembree WC, Cohen-Kettenis PT, Gooren L, Hannema SE, Meyer WJ, Murad MH, Rosenthal SM, Safer JD, Tangpricha V, T'Sjoen GG. Endocrine treatment of gender-dysphoric/gender-incongruent persons: An Endocrine Society clinical practice guideline. *J Clin Endocrinol Metab.* 2017;**102**(11):3869–3903.
13. Martineau P, Silva BC, Leslie WD. Utility of trabecular bone score in the evaluation of osteoporosis. *Curr Opin Endocrinol Diabetes Obes.* 2017;**24**(6):402–410.
14. Shevroja E, Lamy O, Kohlmeier L, Koromani F, Rivadeneira F, Hans D. Use of trabecular bone score (TBS) as a complimentary approach to dual-energy X-ray absortiometry (DXA) for fracture risk assessment in clinical practice *J Clin Densitom.* 2017;**20**(3):334–345.
15. Leslie WD, Aubry-Rozier B, Lamy O, Hans D, for the Manitoba Bone Density Program. TBS (trabecular bone score) and diabetes-related fracture risk. *J Clin Endocrinol Metab.* 2013;**98**(2):602–609.

Hypercalcemia of Malignancy

M04
Presented, March 23–26, 2019

Azeez Farooki, MD. Division of Endocrinology, Memorial Sloan Kettering Cancer Center, New York, New York 10065, E-mail: farookia@mskcc.org

SIGNIFICANCE OF THE CLINICAL PROBLEM

Hypercalcemia in patients with malignancy is a common clinical scenario, occurring in 20% to 30% of patients with advanced cancer (1). This condition can occur in patients with both solid and hematologic malignancies, the most common being breast cancer, lung cancer, multiple myeloma, and renal cell carcinoma. Hypercalcemia of malignancy may be recurrent and/or refractory requiring inpatient hospitalizations, thereby severely impairing quality of life and contributing to increased health care costs.

Endocrinologists' possess an in-depth knowledge of the workup of hypercalcemia. For example, primary hyperparathyroidism can coexist with hypercalcemia of malignancy and may not be detected by treating oncologists. Endocrinologists also have extensive expertise in bone and mineral metabolism, antiresorptive drug action, and adverse effects. Thus, they can and should play a key role in helping to comanage this condition along with oncologists. Hypercalcemia of malignancy can occur via various mechanisms (2), and endocrinologists should appreciate these mechanisms to best guide treatment of this debilitating condition.

BARRIERS TO OPTIMAL PRACTICE

- There is a paucity of literature and interventional trials on management of refractory hypercalcemia in patients with malignancy.
- There is underappreciation of a mechanism-driven approach to treat hypercalcemia of malignancy.

LEARNING OBJECTIVES

As a result of participating in this session, learners should be able to

- Appreciate the various mechanisms by which hypercalcemia of malignancy is caused
- Understand and implement mechanism-based treatments for hypercalcemia germane to endocrinologists

CASE 1

A 41-year-old woman was referred to the endocrinology clinic for refractory hypercalcemia. She had a history of breast cancer initially diagnosed in 2009 with pathological examination consistent with invasive ductal carcinoma (BRACA1+ ER+ PR− Her2/neu−). She underwent bilateral mastectomy and received multiple lines of chemotherapies. Her course was complicated by biopsy-proven liver metastasis and bone metastases. At the time of presentation, she was enrolled in an investigational protocol with cyclophosphamide and a poly (ADP-ribose) polymerase inhibitor and had suffered from hypercalcemia for 6 months despite receiving multiple courses of IV fluid hydration, monthly denosumab (120 mg), and two doses of IV zoledronic acid (4 mg) within a 6-month time period. Approximately 2.5 weeks before endocrine consultation, her peak corrected calcium was equal to 13.9 mg/dL [8.5 to 10.5 mg/dL; international system unit (SI): 3.48 mmol/L (2.13 to 2.63 mmol/L)] in the setting of normal renal function and volume status. The patient, however, was also taking calcium carbonate 600 mg once daily for bone health, which was discontinued a few days before endocrinology evaluation.

On initial evaluation, elevations in calcium equal to 11.6 mg/dL [8.5 to 10.5 mg/dL; SI: 2.90 mmol/L (2.13 to 2.63 mmol/L)] and $1,25(OH)_2D$ level at 327 pg/mL [18 to 72 pg/mL; SI: 850.2 pmol/L (46.8 to 187.2 pmol/L)] were noted (Table 1, case 1). Calcium levels were often above 12.0 mg/dL (SI: 3 mmol/L). Her $1,25(OH)_2D$ levels had been increasing steadily from 177 pg/mL (SI: 460.2 pmol/L) 1 month earlier and 248 pg/mL (SI: 644.8 pmol/L) 10 days earlier. Phosphorus was low at 1.4 mg/dL [2.5 to 4.2 mg/dL; SI: 0.45 mmol/L (0.81 to 1.36 mmol/L)]. The patient had normal angiotensin-converting enzyme at 58 U/L [9 to 67 U/L; SI: 0.97 μkat/L (0.15 to 1.12 μkat/L)], suppressed PTH at 11.2 pg/mL [12 to 88 pg/mL; SI: 11.2 ng/L (12 to 88 ng/L)], a 25(OH)D level at 19 ng/dL [30 to 100 ng/dL; SI: 47.42 nmol/L (74.88 to 249.60 nmol/L)], "low" urine N-telopeptide at 12 nmol bone collagen equivalents (BCE) per millimole creatinine (3 to 63 nmol BCE per millimole creatinine), and normal bone-specific alkaline phosphatase at 19.9 U/L [14.2 to 42.7 U/L; SI: 0.33 μkat/L (0.24 to 0.71 μkat/L)]. Of note, the patient also had slightly elevated PTH-related peptide (PTHrp) at 28 pg/mL [14 to 27 pg/mL; SI: 28 ng/L (14 to 27 ng/L)], which had increased from 18 pg/mL (SI: 18 ng/L) 1 month earlier. Phosphorus levels remained <2 mg/dL [2.5 to 4.2 mg/dL; SI: 0.65 mmol/L (0.81 to 1.36 mmol/L)] despite repletion; fractional excretion of phosphate was calculated at 33%, indicating phosphaturesis. Fibroblast growth factor 23 level was normal. The patient declined collection of a 24-hour urine for calcium. She had a repeat whole-body positron emission tomography/CT scan, which revealed diffuse osseous metastases (right sacrum and throughout the axial and appendicular skeleton). There was no evidence of granulomatous disease on imaging.

Questions for Discussion

1. What mechanisms were responsible for hypercalcemia in this patient with metastatic breast cancer?

Table 1. Baseline Laboratory Workup for Patients

Unit System	Laboratory Tests										
	Ca	**P**	**PTH**	**PTHrp**	**1,25(OH)$_2$D**	**25(OH)D**	**ACE**	**BSAP**	**CTX**	**Urine NTX**	**24 Urine Ca**
Normal range (CU)	8.5–10.5	2.5–4.2	12–88	14–27	18–72	30–100	9–67	14.2–42.7	40–465	3–63	50–150
Normal range (SI)	2.13–2.63	0.81–1.36	12–88	14–27	46.8–187.2	74.88–249.60	0.15–1.12	0.24–0.71	40–465	3–63	1.25–3.75
Case 1 (CU)	11.6 mg/dL	1.4 mg/dL	11.2 pg/mL	28 pg/mL	327 pg/mL	19 ng/dL	58 U/L	19.9 U/L	—	12 BCE	—
Case 1 (SI)	2.90 mmol/L	0.45 mmol/L	11.2 ng/L	28 ng/L	850.2 pmol/L	47.42 nmol/L	0.97 μkat/L	0.33 μkat/L	—	12 BCE	—
Case 2 (CU)	12.0 mg/dL	1.5 mg/dL	<4.0 pg/mL	132 pg/mL	234 pg/mL	14 ng/dL	34 U/L	8.3 U/L	67 pg/mL	— BCE	60 mg/24 h
Case 2 (SI)	3.0 mmol/L	0.48 mmol/L	11.2 ng/L	132 ng/L	608.4 pmol/L	34.94 nmol/L	0.57 μkat/L	0.14 μkat/L	67 ng/L	— BCE	1.50 mmol/d

Abbreviations: ACE, angiotensin-converting enzyme; BCE, bone collagen equivalents; BSAP, bone-specific alkaline phosphatase; Ca, calcium; CTX, C-telopeptide; CU, conventional unit; NTX, N-telopeptide; P, phosphorous; PTHrp, PTH-related peptide; SI, international system unit; 24 urine Ca, 24-hour urine calcium.

2. Should the patient's 25-hydroxyvitamin D level be repleted?
3. What other management strategies might be used?

Given the elevated 1,25(OH)$_2$D levels from presumed increased 1-α-hydroxylase activity related to breast cancer, prednisone 40 mg daily was started. After 5 days of prednisone 40 mg daily, repeat calcium normalized from 11.6 mg/dL (SI: 2.9 mmol/L) to 10.3 mg/dL (SI: 2.58 mmol/L), at which time prednisone taper was started. After the patient reached a prednisone dose of 15 mg daily after 5 weeks, repeat calcium level was slightly increased again to 11.1 mg/dL [8.5 to 10.5 mg/dL; SI: 2.78 mmol/L (2.13 to 2.63 mmol/L)]. The patient's repeat 1,25(OH)$_2$D level remained elevated but stable at 306 pg/mL [18 to 72 pg/mL; SI: 795.6 pmol/L (46.8 to 187.2 pmol/L)]. The patient transferred her oncology care outside the institution; anticancer therapy was changed, serum calcium remained mildly elevated between 10 and 11 mg/dL (SI: 2.50 to 2.75 mmol/L), and phosphate requirement improved.

Discussion With Strategies for Diagnosis and Management

This patient likely had hypercalcemia of malignancy due to

1. Extrarenal production of calcitriol from tumor-associated macrophages and/or PTHrp stimulation
2. Increased bone resorption; this resulted from osteolysis mediated by "local" cytokines stimulating bone resorption in the context of metastatic bone disease or osteolysis mediated by systemically measured PTHrp
3. Increased distal tubular calcium reabsorption and proximal tubular–mediated phosphaturia (due to PTHrp)

Workup for hypercalcemia in patients with malignancy should start by excluding PTH-dependent hypercalcemia. In this patient's case, PTH was suppressed, and it is unlikely that it was contributing to the hypercalcemia. The rest of the workup should include phosphorus, PTHrp, 25-hydroxyvitamin D, and 1,25 dihydroxyvitamin D levels. Other causes of PTH-independent hypercalcemia, such as granulomatous disease not related to cancer diagnosis, vitamin A toxicity, hyperthyroidism, and milk alkali syndrome, should be excluded.

This patient had marked elevation in calcitriol, which Memorial Sloan–Kettering data suggest may be associated with refractory hypercalcemia in patients with solid tumor (3). Although this patient's calcitriol level was clearly inappropriately elevated, it is important to note that a "high normal" calcitriol level in the face of PTH-independent hypercalcemia is also inappropriate. PTHrp is thought to only weakly stimulate calcitriol production and was minimally elevated. Thus, this case suggests a source of calcitriol, such as tumor-associated macrophages, which have been described in lymphoma (4). Increased intestinal calcium absorption induced by high serum calcitriol concentrations is probably the main mechanism of hypercalcemia, although elevations in calcitriol have also been shown to increase bone resorption and possibly, inhibit bone mineralization (5), which also probably contributes.

This patient also had hypophosphatemia. Patients with calcitriol-mediated hypercalcemia do not typically have hypophosphatemia, and therefore, PTHrp was probably the mechanism of hypophosphatemia (via inhibition of proximal tubular phosphate transport).

Treatment

Given the multiple mechanisms contributing to hypercalcemia and the fact that this patient was refractory to standard antiresorptive therapies given at approved oncologic doses (monthly zoledronic acid and denosumab), a multipronged treatment approach makes sense.

First, to reduce calcitriol production in a manner analogous to therapy of granulomatous diseases causing hypercalcemia, steroid therapy can be started at a dose of 10 to 30 mg/d of prednisone. As second-line therapy for those unable to take steroids, a general inhibitor of P450 enzymes, such as ketoconazole, should also decrease calcitriol production via inhibition of 1-α-hydroxylase. Gastrointestinal absorption of calcium is markedly increased due to elevated calcitriol levels. Such patients should be advised to avoid both calcium and vitamin D supplements; hypocalcemia resulting from antiresorptive therapy is not a concern in the context of refractory hypercalcemia. Furthermore, some patients with cancer receive highly calcium-fortified supplements, such as Ensure—these should be avoided, and low-calcium nutritional supplements should be advised. A low-calcium diet is also prudent. However, relevant dietary calcium restriction should also be accompanied by a low-oxalate diet to lower the risk for calcium oxalate kidney stones.

Second, to address the increased bone resorption due to metastatic bone disease and PTHrp, denosumab was continued at 120 mg subcutaneously monthly. It is important to note that weekly denosumab at 120 mg may be given in the setting of hypercalcemia refractory to monthly IV bisphosphonates and may offer better calcium lowering (6), such as would be expected with the increased dosing schedule and the slightly higher antiresorptive potency of denosumab. Given that refractory hypercalcemia is an acute situation compromising quality of life and that many such patients have a limited life expectancy, concern for long-term adverse effects (*e.g.*, osteonecrosis of the jaw or atypical femur fracture) with more intensive dosing schedules should not drive treatment decisions.

Third, addressing the PTHrp-driven hypophosphatemia may also ameliorate the hypercalcemia. Before the advent of bisphosphonates, IV and/or oral phosphate was shown to improve hypercalcemia of malignancy (7, 8). Calcium phosphate is thought to complex in the blood and be eliminated via the reticuloendothelial system. Furthermore, some patients with PTHrp-driven hypercalcemia have dangerously low phosphorus levels, and these patients should be treated regardless of the severity of the hypercalcemia.

CASE 2

A 52-year-old woman was referred for refractory hypercalcemia. She had a history of clear cell carcinoma of the ovary. The patient underwent resection and received multiple chemotherapies and immunotherapy, which were followed by a recurrence. On initial presentation, the patient's hypercalcemia was refractory to zoledronic acid 4 mg for two doses followed by denosumab 120 mg dosed weekly for three doses, with calcium in the 12 to 13 mg/dL (SI: 3.0 to 3.25 mmol/L) range.

On initial evaluation, calcium was consistently elevated to 12 mg/dL or higher [8.5 to 10.5 mg/dL; SI: 3 mmol/L (2.13 to 2.63 mmol/L)] (Table 1, case 2). Phosphorus was low at 1.5 mg/dL [2.5 to 4.2 mg/dL; SI: 0.48 mmol/L (0.81 to 1.36 mmol/L)]. The patient had normal angiotensin-converting enzyme at 34 U/L [9 to 67 U/L; SI: 0.57 μkat/L (0.15 to 1.12 μkat/L)], suppressed PTH < 4.0 pg/mL [12 to 88 pg/mL; SI: <4 ng/L (12 to 88 ng/L)], low 25(OH)D level at 14 ng/dL [30 to 100 ng/dL; SI: 34.94 nmol/L (74.88 to 249.6 nmol/L)], elevated 1,25(OH)$_2$D level at 234 pg/mL [18 to 72 pg/mL; SI: 608.4 pmol/L (46.8 to 187.2 pmol/L)], suppressed serum C-telopeptide at 67 pg/mL [40 to 465 pg/mL; SI: 67 (40 to 465 ng/L)], and normal bone-specific alkaline phosphatase at 8.3 U/L [premenopausal range < 14.3 U/L; SI: 0.14 μkat/L (premenopausal range < 0.24 μkat/L)]. The patient also had a markedly elevated PTHrp at 132 pg/mL [14 to 27 pg/mL; SI: 132 ng/L (14 to 27 ng/L)]. Her 24-hour urine levels for calcium, sodium, and phosphorus were 60 mg/24 h (SI: 1.5 mmol/d), 328 mEq/24 h (SI: 328 mmol/d), and 1360 mg/24 h (SI: 43.93 mmol/d), respectively. On imaging, there was no evidence of osseous metastases or granulomatous disease.

Questions for Discussion

1. What mechanisms were responsible for hypercalcemia?
2. Should the patient's 25-hydroxyvitamin D level be repleted?
3. What other management strategies might be used?

This patient had intermittent gastrointestinal bleeding related to her tumor, and thus, prednisone therapy could not be attempted to reduce calcitriol levels. Similar to case 1, this patient was advised to avoid both dietary calcium (especially calcium-fortified foods, such as Ensure) and vitamin D. The deficient vitamin D level should not be treated, because there could be accelerated conversion to 1,25 dihydroxyvitamin D, exacerbating the hypercalcemia. Ketoconazole therapy was attempted as an alternative strategy to reduce both 1-α-hydroxylase activity and calcitriol levels (9, 10); however, the patient's liver function tests were elevated, and ketoconazole seemed to be poorly tolerated.

The patient had suppressed levels of bone turnover markers as would be expected after denosumab 120 mg.

Another management strategy would be trying to overcome PTHrp-mediated renal calcium retention via intermittent furosemide IV (along with vigorous normal saline hydration) and/or oral furosemide, the latter on a daily basis. Furosemide should be administered in the setting of vigorous hydration and adequate volume status, which is problematic for some patients who are hypercalcemic to achieve via oral hydration due to nausea.

Discussion With Strategies for Diagnosis and Management

This patient likely had hypercalcemia of malignancy due to

1. Ectopic production of calcitriol from tumor-associated macrophages and/or PTHrp stimulation

2. Increased bone resorption (due to markedly elevated PTHrp levels)
3. Increased distal tubular calcium reabsorption and proximal tubular–mediated phosphaturia (due to PTHrp)

Treatment

Like the first case, there are multiple mechanisms contributing to hypercalcemia in this case. Because this patient was refractory to standard antiresorptive therapies given at approved oncologic doses (monthly zoledronic acid and denosumab), a multipronged treatment approach was necessary.

First, because this patient was not a good candidate for prednisone use to reduce calcitriol production, ketoconazole, a general inhibitor of P450 enzymes, was attempted (9, 10), which the patient was unable to tolerate at the necessary doses. Of note, ketoconazole at a high dose may cause hypogonadism, hypoadrenalism, hepatotoxicity, and adverse effects (*e.g.*, headache, sedation, nausea, and vomiting).

Second, to address the increased bone resorption due to PTHrp, denosumab was continued at 120 mg subcutaneously monthly. It is important to note that weekly denosumab 120 mg may be given in the setting of hypercalcemia refractory to monthly IV bisphosphonates and may offer better calcium lowering (6), such as would be expected with the increased dosing schedule and the slightly higher antiresorptive potency of denosumab. Given that refractory hypercalcemia is an acute situation compromising quality of life and that many such patients have a limited life expectancy, concern for long-term adverse effects (*e.g.*, osteonecrosis of the jaw or atypical femur fracture) with more intensive dosing schedules should not drive treatment decisions.

Third, addressing the PTHrp-driven increase in distal tubular calcium reabsorption featured very prominently in this case. The patient's low 24-hour urine calcium value in the setting of hypercalcemia was most certainly driven by PTHrp. She was given weekly hydration with 2 to 3 L normal saline in addition to IV furosemide 40 mg. This strategy succeeded in temporarily reducing the calcium level, but there was a rapid rise in serum calcium over the next few days. The patient was given furosemide to take at home daily along with vigorous hydration with 1 L of normal saline self-administered via gravity through her port (4 hours for 1 L).

Of note, PTHrp is not thought to stimulate calcitriol production to the same extent as the PTH (11). Ectopic calcitriol production in solid tumors has rarely been described (12). Thus, the etiology of this patient's marked calcitriol elevation is unclear.

Treatment of hypophosphatemia was also started in an attempt to ameliorate the hypercalcemia. Before the advent of bisphosphonates, IV and/or oral phosphate was shown to improve hypercalcemia of malignancy (7, 8). Calcium phosphate is thought to complex in the blood and be eliminated via the reticuloendothelial system. Furthermore, some such patients with PTHrp-driven hypercalcemia have dangerously low phosphorus levels, which should be treated regardless of the severity of the hypercalcemia.

Ultimately, through the above measures and a change in anticancer therapy, this patient's calcium normalized.

MAIN CONCLUSIONS

Hypercalcemia of malignancy may be refractory to standard measures, such as Food and Drug Administration–approved oncologic doses of zoledronic acid and denosumab, greatly impairing quality of life via the symptoms of hypercalcemia and repeated inpatient admissions. Multiple mechanisms may contribute to hypercalcemia in this context, and therapy should be directed toward the various mechanistic drivers present in a given patient as clinically feasible. Elevations in bone resorption, increased calcitriol production, PTHrp-driven renal calcium retention, and hypophosphatemia may all contribute to hypercalcemia of malignancy. Calcitriol levels should be checked, because elevation may occur in patients with solid tumors (in addition to the well-described elevations that may occur in lymphoma and granulomatous diseases). If elevated calcitriol is detected, vitamin D supplements and calcium-fortified foods should be avoided. Additionally, corticosteroid therapy may be attempted. PTHrp elevations may cause renal calcium retention, and theoretically, they may be responsive to frequent IV fluids along with furosemide to induce calciuresis. Finally, it is also logical to diagnose and treat substantial hypophosphatemia with the aim of improving hypercalcemia.

References

1. Stewart AF. Clinical practice. Hypercalcemia associated with cancer. *N Engl J Med.* 2005;**352**(4):373–379.
2. Clines GA, Guise TA. Hypercalcaemia of malignancy and basic research on mechanisms responsible for osteolytic and osteoblastic metastasis to bone. *Endocr Relat Cancer.* 2005;**12**(3):549–583.
3. Chukir T, Liu Y, Farooki A. Retrospective evaluation of solid tumor patients with PTH-independent hypercalcemia and their response to bisphosphonates or denosumab. In: Proceedings of the ASBMR; September 8–9, 2017; Denver, CO. Abstract FR0003.
4. Hewison M, Kantorovich V, Liker HR, Van Herle AJ, Cohan P, Zehnder D, Adams JS. Vitamin D-mediated hypercalcemia in lymphoma: evidence for hormone production by tumor-adjacent macrophages. *J Bone Miner Res.* 2003;**18**(3):579–582.
5. Lieben L, Masuyama R, Torrekens S, Van Looveren R, Schrooten J, Baatsen P, Lafage-Proust MH, Dresselaers T, Feng JQ, Bonewald LF, Meyer MB, Pike JW, Bouillon R, Carmeliet G. Normocalcemia is maintained in mice under conditions of calcium malabsorption by vitamin D-induced inhibition of bone mineralization. *J Clin Invest.* 2012;**122**(5):1803–1815.
6. Hu MI, Glezerman I, Leboulleux S, Insogna K, Gucalp R, Misiorowski W, Yu B, Ying W, Jain RK. Denosumab for patients with persistent or relapsed hypercalcemia of malignancy despite recent bisphosphonate treatment. *J Natl Cancer Inst.* 2013;**105**(18):1417–1420.
7. Goldsmith RS, Ingbar SH. Inorganic phosphate treatment of hypercalcemia of diverse etiologies. *N Engl J Med.* 1966;**274**(1):1–7.
8. Thalassinos N, Joplin GF. Phosphate treatment of hypercalcaemia due to carcinoma. *BMJ.* 1968;**4**(5622):14–19.

9. Conron M, Beynon HL. Ketoconazole for the treatment of refractory hypercalcemic sarcoidosis. *Sarcoidosis Vasc Diffuse Lung Dis.* 2000; **17**(3):277–280.

10. Adams JS, Sharma OP, Diz MM, Endres DB. Ketoconazole decreases the serum 1,25-dihydroxyvitamin D and calcium concentration in sarcoidosis-associated hypercalcemia. *J Clin Endocrinol Metab.* 1990; **70**(4):1090–1095.

11. Schilling T, Pecherstorfer M, Blind E, Leidig G, Ziegler R, Raue F. Parathyroid hormone-related protein (PTHrP) does not regulate 1,25-dihydroxyvitamin D serum levels in hypercalcemia of malignancy. *J Clin Endocrinol Metab.* 1993;**76**(3):801–803.

12. Kallas M, Green F, Hewison M, White C, Kline G. Rare causes of calcitriol-mediated hypercalcemia: a case report and literature review. *J Clin Endocrinol Metab.* 2010;**95**(7):3111–3117.

Challenges in Treatment of Patients With Hypoparathyroidism

M15
Presented, March 23–26, 2019

Michael Mannstadt, MD. Endocrine Unit, Massachusetts General Hospital, Boston, Massachusetts 02114, E-mail: mannstadt@mgh.harvard.edu

SIGNIFICANCE OF THE CLINICAL PROBLEM

Hypoparathyroidism affects ~80,000 people in the United States (1). It most commonly occurs after the parathyroid glands are inadvertently removed or damaged during neck surgery. The hallmarks of hypoparathyroidism are hypocalcemia and inappropriately low PTH concentrations. Standard therapy consists of oral calcium and active vitamin D (calcitriol or α-calcidol); however, this approach increases serum calcium levels without replacing the regulatory actions of PTH. Without parathyroid regulation of serum and urine calcium concentrations, patients can develop long-term complications (2, 3), including renal disease and reduced quality of life (4–6). Although replacement therapy with recombinant PTH has been approved for treatment of patients with hypoparathyroidism and is an enrichment of current treatment options, daily injections do not fully replicate the normal endocrine response.

Complications of standard therapy and poor biochemical control present a unique challenge for clinicians. A full understanding of these challenges is needed to improve quality of life and long-term outcomes for patients.

BARRIERS TO OPTIMAL PRACTICE

- The need to measure 24-hour urinary calcium excretion is not well appreciated.
- Measuring blood calcium regularly and at different times during the day presents a technical challenge.
- Many clinicians lack extensive experience with PTH replacement therapy.

LEARNING OBJECTIVES

As a result of participating in this session, learners should be able to

- Summarize the complications of hypoparathyroidism
- Identify the principles of treatment of hypoparathyroidism with calcium and active vitamin D
- Discuss treatment of hypoparathyroidism with PTH and PTH analogs

STRATEGIES FOR MANAGEMENT

The broad goals of therapy of hypoparathyroidism are

- Control symptoms of hypocalcemia
- Minimize long-term complications

The 2016 summary statement provides more details on the goals of treatment (7):

- Prevent signs and symptoms of hypocalcemia
- Maintain low-normal serum calcium concentrations
- Maintain calcium-phosphate product <55 mg^2/dL^2 (4.4 mmol^2/L^2)
- Avoid hypercalciuria
- Avoid hypercalcemia
- Avoid renal and other extraskeletal calcifications

Renal Complications

PTH interacts with receptors in the renal tubule to promote calcium reabsorption. In the absence of PTH, high urinary calcium excretion is of particular concern. Hypercalciuria is a risk factor for developing kidney stones, nephrocalcinosis, and chronic renal insufficiency, which are some of the most dreaded long-term complications of hypoparathyroidism and its treatment. One retrospective chart review of 120 patients from a tertiary-care hospital system found that 38% of patients had at least one 24-hour urine calcium measurement of >300 mg/24 h (2). Of those who had imaging of the kidney, 31% had renal calcifications. Rates of chronic kidney disease stage 3 or higher were 2- to 17-fold greater than age-appropriate norms. In a multivariate analysis, the age of the patient, duration of hypoparathyroidism, and time spent at calcium levels >9.5 mg/dL were associated with renal impairment. In a large Danish study of 688 patients with postsurgical hypoparathyroidism, renal complications were 3.7-fold higher compared with a control group of 2064 age- and sex-matched controls (3).

Shockingly, about half of the 120 patients in the above study did not have a record of 24-hour urinary calcium measurement. High serum calcium concentrations are known to lead to a higher filtered load of calcium and higher urinary calcium excretion. Lowering serum calcium is one of the most effective ways to decrease urinary calcium excretion. Thus, the risk for renal complications drives the need to target as low a serum calcium concentration as can be tolerated by the patient.

Strategies to lower urinary calcium include

- Lowering serum calcium as tolerated (see above)
- Avoiding high peak serum calcium values by more evenly spreading supplements throughout the day
- Using thiazides in combination with low salt diet (8)
- Consider treatment with recombinant human PTH(1-84) [rhPTH(1-84)] (9)

MAIN CONCLUSIONS

In summary, patients with chronic hypoparathyroidism who are on conventional therapy with calcium and vitamin D have a substantial rate of complications. Strategies to reduce urinary calcium include the use of thiazides, avoiding elevated peak calcium levels, and lowering the target serum calcium level if tolerated by the patient. Treatment with PTH is an emerging modality, and more experience and data are needed to identify the best target patient group for this replacement therapy.

CASES

Case 1

A 63-year-old woman with postsurgical hypoparathyroidism (duration 10 years) has muscle twitching and cramps when she goes on a strenuous hike. She takes 500 mg of elemental calcium (as calcium carbonate) three times a day, calcitriol 0.25 μg twice daily, and levothyroxine 137 μg daily. Her laboratory results are as follows: serum calcium 8.0 to 8.6 mg/dL, serum phosphate 4.0 to 5.0 mg/dL, 25OHD 11 ng/mL, and 24-hour urinary calcium 330 mg/d (normal, <250 mg/d).

How can you improve her management?

A. Decrease oral calcium and calcitriol

B. Increase calcitriol and add thiazide

C. Add thiazide and give vitamin D 2000 units daily

D. All of the above

Discussion

Answer C: Add Thiazide and Give Vitamin D 2000 Units Daily

This patient has hypercalciuria, a risk factor for developing renal complications. A renal ultrasound might be indicated to check for calcifications. In addition to encouraging adequate fluid intake and examining her urinary stone risk profile further, efforts should focus on reducing her urinary calcium. Thiazides are used to reduce urinary calcium. They are effective in combination with a low-salt diet. Serum potassium and sodium should be checked after starting a thiazide. The Institute of Medicine recommends a vitamin D level of at least 20 ng/mL, and vitamin D supplements should be started.

Case 2

A 39-year-old woman with autoimmune polyglandular syndrome type 1 (APS-1) (also known as autoimmune polyendocrinopathy-candidiasis-ectodermal dystrophy or APECED) and hypoparathyroidism is maintained on calcium citrate 315 mg two tablets three times a day and calcitriol 0.5 μg twice daily. She has periods of hypocalcemia for several days and adds extra calcium and sometimes calcitriol. This is followed by hypercalcemia that can last for weeks. She was not able to tolerate thiazides. Her laboratory results are as follows: serum calcium 6.8 to 11.0 mg/dL, serum phosphate 3.9 to 5.5 mg/dL, 24-hour urinary calcium 180 to 430 mg/d (normal, <250 mg/d), and estimated glomerular filtration rate >60 mL/min per 1.73 m².

To improve management, you would

A. Switch from calcium citrate to calcium carbonate

B. Decrease calcitriol and add a thiazide

C. Start rhPTH(1-84) and down-titrate calcitriol and calcium

D. Switch from calcitriol to high-dose ergocalciferol

Discussion

Answer C: Start rhPTH(1-84)

rhPTH(1-84) is approved in the United States as an adjunct to calcium and vitamin D to control hypocalcemia in patients with hypoparathyroidism. Per Food and Drug Administration label, it is recommended "only for patients who cannot be well controlled on calcium supplements and active forms of vitamin D alone." As more experience with this new drug is obtained, the indication for its use and the interpretation of "[not] well controlled" is evolving. A U.S. consensus paper suggests the following selection criteria for rhPTH(1-84) therapy: inadequate control of serum calcium, high doses of calcium/activated vitamin D, hypercalciuria and renal complications, hyperphosphatemia and high calcium-phosphate product, gastrointestinal malabsorption, and reduced quality of life (10). European guidelines recommend against the routine use of replacement therapy with PTH or PTH analogs (11).

The patient in this vignette likely has problems with gastrointestinal absorption, perhaps due to her APS-1. These periods of hypocalcemia (perhaps when her absorption is low) followed by hypercalcemia (when her absorption is improved) lead to insufficient control of her serum calcium levels. Treatment with PTH(1-84) (answer C) has the advantage of bypassing gastrointestinal absorption problems and may result in better blood calcium control. High-dose nonactivated vitamin D (answer D) was previously the mainstay for the treatment of hypoparathyroidism, but it is now rarely used given the availability of active vitamin D.

References

1. Clarke BL, Brown EM, Collins MT, Jüppner H, Lakatos P, Levine MA, Mannstadt MM, Bilezikian JP, Romanischen AF, Thakker RV. Epidemiology and diagnosis of hypoparathyroidism. *J Clin Endocrinol Metab.* 2016;**101**(6):2284–2299.

2. Mitchell DM, Regan S, Cooley MR, Lauter KB, Vrla MC, Becker CB, Burnett-Bowie SA, Mannstadt M. Long-term follow-up of patients with hypoparathyroidism. *J Clin Endocrinol Metab.* 2012;**97**(12):4507–4514.

3. Underbjerg L, Sikjaer T, Mosekilde L, Rejnmark L. Cardiovascular and renal complications to postsurgical hypoparathyroidism: a Danish nationwide controlled historic follow-up study. *J Bone Miner Res.* 2013;**28**(11):2277–2285.

4. Sikjaer T, Rolighed L, Hess A, Fuglsang-Frederiksen A, Mosekilde L, Rejnmark L. Effects of PTH(1-84) therapy on muscle function and quality of life in hypoparathyroidism: results from a randomized controlled trial. *Osteoporos Int.* 2014;**25**(6):1717–1726.

5. Cho NL, Moalem J, Chen L, Lubitz CC, Moore FD, Jr, Ruan DT. Surgeons and patients disagree on the potential consequences from hypoparathyroidism. *Endocr Pract.* 2014;**20**(5):427–446.

6. Cusano NE, Rubin MR, McMahon DJ, Irani D, Tulley A, Sliney J, Jr, Bilezikian JP. The effect of PTH(1-84) on quality of life in hypoparathyroidism. *J Clin Endocrinol Metab.* 2013;**98**(6):2356–2361.

7. Bilezikian JP, Brandi ML, Cusano NE, Mannstadt M, Rejnmark L, Rizzoli R, Rubin MR, Winer KK, Liberman UA, Potts JT, Jr. Management of

hypoparathyroidism: present and future. *J Clin Endocrinol Metab.* 2016;**101**(6):2313–2324.

8. Brickman AS, Coburn JW, Koppel MH, Peacock M, Massry SG. The effect of hydrochlorothiazide administration on serum and urinary calcium in normal, hypoparathyroid and hyperparathyroid subjects. Studies on mechanisms. *Isr J Med Sci.* 1971;**7**(3):518–519.

9. Mannstadt M, Clarke BL, Vokes T, Brandi ML, Ranganath L, Fraser WD, Lakatos P, Bajnok L, Garceau R, Mosekilde L, Lagast H, Shoback D, Bilezikian JP. Efficacy and safety of recombinant human parathyroid hormone (1-84) in hypoparathyroidism (REPLACE): a double-blind, placebo-controlled, randomised, phase 3 study [published correction appears in Lancet Diabetes Endocrinol. 2014;2(1):e3]. *Lancet Diabetes Endocrinol.* 2013;**1**(4):275–283.

10. Brandi ML, Bilezikian JP, Shoback D, Bouillon R, Clarke BL, Thakker RV, Khan AA, Potts JT, Jr. Management of hypoparathyroidism: summary statement and guidelines. *J Clin Endocrinol Metab.* 2016; **101**(6):2273–2283.

11. Bollerslev J, Rejnmark L, Marcocci C, Shoback DM, Sitges-Serra A, van Biesen W, Dekkers OM; European Society of Endocrinology. European Society of Endocrinology Clinical Guideline: treatment of chronic hypoparathyroidism in adults. *Eur J Endocrinol.* 2015;**173**(2): G1–G20.

Vertebral Fracture Assessment: How to Find Vertebral Fractures and What to Do When You Find Them

M16
Presented, March 23–26, 2019

Tamara Vokes, MD. Section of Endocrinology, University of Chicago, Chicago, Illinois 60637, E-mail: tvokes@uchicago.edu

Nelson Watts, MD, FACP, MACE. Mercy Health Osteoporosis and Bone Health Services, Cincinnati, Ohio 45236, E-mail: nelson.watts@hotmail.com

IMPORTANCE OF VERTEBRAL FRACTURES

Vertebral fractures are the most common osteoporotic fractures (1). They are important to detect because they are associated with increased morbidity (2, 3) and mortality (4, 5) and because they are strongly predictive of future vertebral and other fractures, including hip fractures (6–8). Some years ago, vertebral fractures were often considered an unavoidable consequence of aging. Today, however, when we know that vertebral fractures are a result of osteoporosis rather than aging *per se* and when we have very effective therapies for preventing vertebral fractures, it is imperative to increase the awareness of the importance of vertebral fractures and develop effective clinical pathways for their detection (9).

CHALLENGES IN DIAGNOSING VERTEBRAL FRACTURES

Vertebral Fractures Are Often Not Clinically Apparent

In some cases, they are truly not symptomatic, but more often, their symptoms, most commonly back pain, are nonspecific and attributed to other causes. Although vertebral fractures are clinically recognized in fewer than one-third of those who have them on imaging (10), patients with vertebral fractures have more back pain and impaired activities of daily living (11).

Vertebral Fractures Require Imaging for Diagnosis

However, imaging is usually not performed when evaluating patients for osteoporosis and assessing fracture risk. Furthermore, even when imaging (performed for other purposes such as chest x-ray) is available, vertebral fractures are not reported, and even if they are mentioned in the report, patients are not evaluated or treated for osteoporosis (12, 13). Appreciation of this unmet need has led to the development of technology for imaging the spine for detection of vertebral fracture on dual-energy x-ray absorptiometry (DXA), now known as vertebral fracture assessment (VFA) (14). Because VFA is usually performed together with bone mineral density (BMD) and interpreted by clinicians who are interested in osteoporosis, it can be integrated with the results of bone density and clinical risk factors (15).

Radiographic Diagnosis of Vertebral Fractures Is Not Straightforward

In contrast to fractures of long bones, which are generally associated with a defined traumatic injury and clear findings of bone discontinuity on imaging, vertebral fractures are often not a result of a discrete event but rather may develop gradually with a progressive loss of height of the vertebral bodies (Fig. 1) (16).

Consequently, the degree of height reduction that is defined as fracture is somewhat arbitrary and has been the main reason for lack of consensus regarding the precise definition of what is normal and what is a fractured vertebra. The additional problem in assessing vertebral fractures is that vertebrae can be deformed (*i.e.*, have alterations in size and shape that are not fractures). Therefore, although every fracture is also a vertebral deformity, not every deformity is a fracture, and differentiating fractures from nonfracture deformities can be difficult. Therefore, many investigators have proposed methods for evaluating, grading, and reporting vertebral fractures. Broadly, these methods can be grouped into morphologic (qualitative visual assessment, where a trained professional, usually a radiologist, determines that the shape of the vertebra is consistent with a fracture) and morphometric (where points are placed in the vertebral endplates by a trained person or by software, and dimensions of the vertebrae are compared with normal). A commonly used hybrid of the two is the Genant semiquantitative (GSQ) tool (17), where the appearance of the vertebra is compared with a chart (Fig. 2) to assign a grade and type of deformity (wedge, concave, or crush).

This method has been criticized because of the fact that mild (grade 1) deformities are not always due to a fracture but may be caused by normal variation in vertebral shape or degenerative remodeling. Jiang *et al.* (18) proposed a different approach, where diagnosis of fracture requires that the endplate is discontinuous (*i.e.*, broken) and that the endplate abnormality is not due to other causes (*e.g.*, Schmorl's nodes). This algorithm-based method (ABQ), however, does not provide the grade or severity of fracture, and it has been shown that the risk of future fracture is higher with greater severity and greater number of fractures (19). Although consensus still does not exist on which method should be used for assessing vertebral fracture, there is perhaps more clarity in the field because of three recent population studies that compared the GSQ method with a modification of the ABQ method (20–22). In these three studies, a modified ABQ method, which included assessment of grade (severity) in addition to the presence of broken endplate, performed best in terms of being associated with lower bone density and higher risk for future fractures. On the basis of these data, it seems that the GSQ method is useful for more severe fractures, but for mild (grade 1) fractures, presence of endplate defect required by the ABQ method is a reasonable

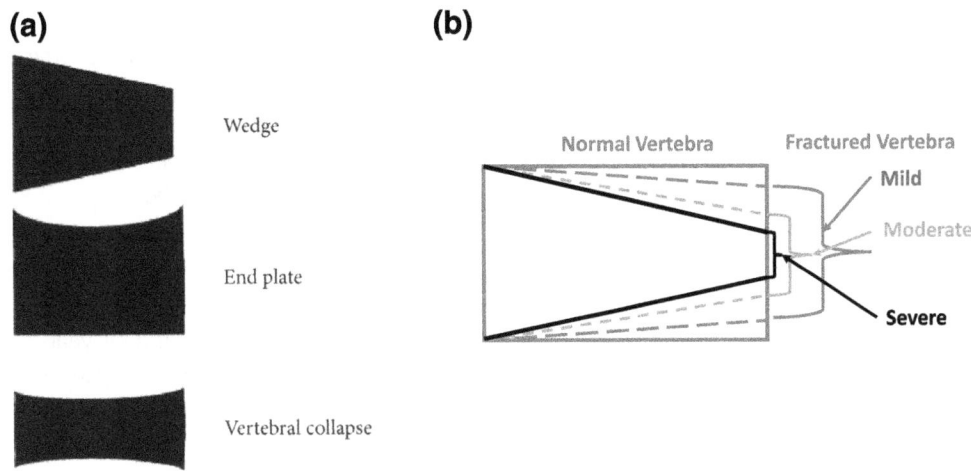

Figure 1. The transition from normal vertebra to progressive degree of fracture may be gradual. (a) Reproduced under a Creative Commons CC BY 3.0 license from Tosi P. Diagnosis and treatment of bone disease in multiple myeloma: spotlight on spinal involvement. *Scientifica*. 2013; article ID 104546.

approach to avoid overdiagnosing and aggressively treating patients who do not have high fracture risk.

INDICATIONS FOR PERFORMING VERTEBRAL IMAGING

Both the International Society for Clinical Densitometry (ISCD) and National Osteoporosis Foundation (NOF) have put forward recommendations for performing vertebral imaging when evaluating a patient for osteoporosis (23, 24). NOF also notes that presence of vertebral fracture, unless due to trauma or a pathologic process such as malignancy, is diagnostic of osteoporosis and is an indication for pharmacologic therapy for osteoporosis. For many, if not most, osteoporosis specialists, finding vertebral fractures often leads to a more aggressive therapeutic approach and at least a consideration of anabolic therapy.

According to ISCD, VFA or other vertebral imaging is indicated when T-score is < −1.0 and one or more of the following is present: age ≥70 years in women and age ≥80 years in men, historical height loss >4 cm (>1.5 in), self-reported but undocumented prior vertebral fracture, and glucocorticoid therapy equivalent to ≥5 mg of prednisone or equivalent per day for ≥3 days.

NOF indications for vertebral imaging are as follows: age ≥65 years in women and age ≥70 years in men, if T-score is ≤ −1.5; age ≥70 years in women and age ≥80 years in men, regardless of T-score; postmenopausal women and men age ≥50 years with a low trauma fracture; and postmenopausal women and men age 50 to 69 years with historical height loss of ≥1.5 in, prospective height loss of ≥1.5 in, or recent or ongoing long-term glucocorticoid treatment.

However, finding a vertebral fracture on VFA or spine x-ray does not mean that the fracture is recent and that the therapy

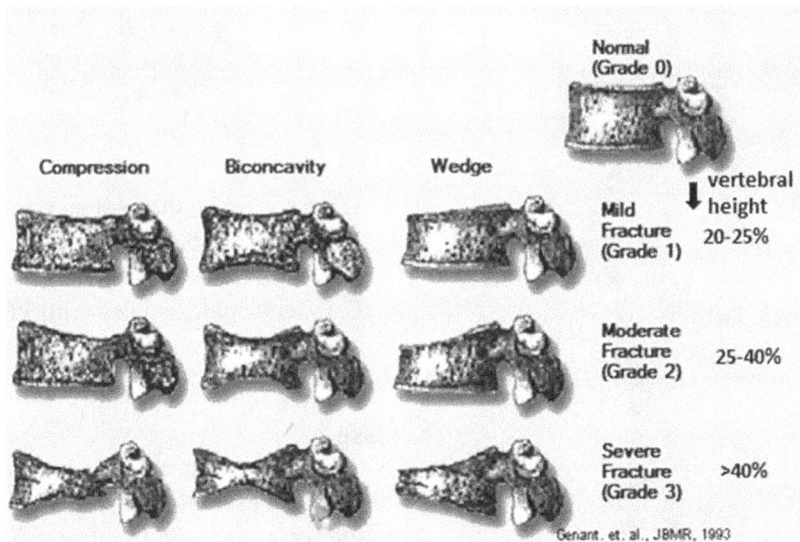

Figure 2. GSQ chart. The examiner compares the vertebrae with the images on the chart to assign the type and grade of fracture. Reproduced with permission from Genant HK, Wu CY, van Kuijk C, Nevitt MC. Vertebral fracture assessment using a semiquantitative technique. *J Bone Miner Res.* 1993;8(9):1137–1148.

needs to be altered accordingly. Evaluation of prior imaging [chest radiographs or computed tomography (CT) or MRI examination] can help determine the acuteness and clinical implications of the fracture. Similarly, there are situations where a fracture found on VFA or spine radiograph may warrant further imaging with CT, MRI, or radionucleotide bone scan. Examples include finding lesions in the vertebrae that cannot be clearly attributed to benign causes (*e.g.*, sclerotic or lytic changes), vertebral deformities in patients with known malignancy, unidentifiable vertebrae between T7 and L4, and similar. In cases where it is not clear whether the fracture is new (*i.e.*, no prior images), MRI or radionucleotide bone scan can be useful.

Case 1

A 75-year-old white woman presents for management of osteoporosis. Two years earlier, she had been diagnosed with osteoporosis on bone density test but did not want to take medication. Instead, she began jogging 1 mile daily and lifting weights. Nine months before coming to the osteoporosis clinic, she had presented to the emergency room with back pain; 2 days earlier, she had done some back stretches with a 90-lb weight burden; a day later, she had helped her husband carry a file cabinet drawer. The next day, she woke up in great pain, was unable to get out of bed, and presented to the emergency room. Lumbar spine radiograph showed no fractures, and she was given analgesics. At our evaluation, she no longer has back pain and is still resistant to taking medication. Repeat bone density shows a T-score of −2.1 at the lumbar spine and −2.6 at the femoral neck, with no significant change from prior examination. On further questioning, the

VFA and reverse VFA May 2016

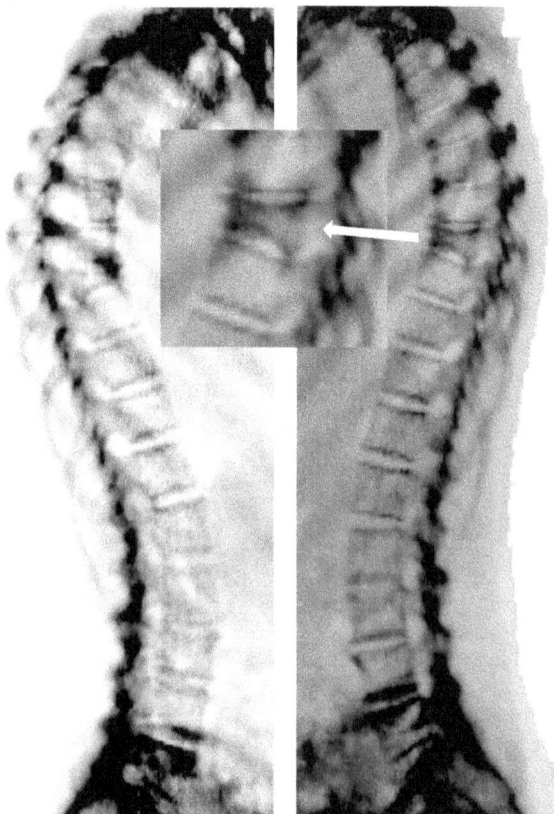

patient reports that her back pain was midthoracic and not lumbar. VFA shows a severe (grade 3) fracture at T8.

Next steps should include:
A. Treatment with bisphosphonate
B. Treatment with an anabolic agent
C. Vertebroplasty or kyphoplasty
D. Continued observation and reassurance

Case 2

DXA results are presented for a 74-year-old man with chronic obstructive pulmonary disease. He uses inhaled steroids chronically and needs occasional steroid tapers (two to three times per year).

	Area (cm²)	BMD (g)	T-Score
L1	12.71	7.61	−3.7
L2	13.99	12/16	−2.0
L3	15.9	11.37	−3.6
L4	18.87	12.77	−4.0
Total	60.72	43.91	−3.3

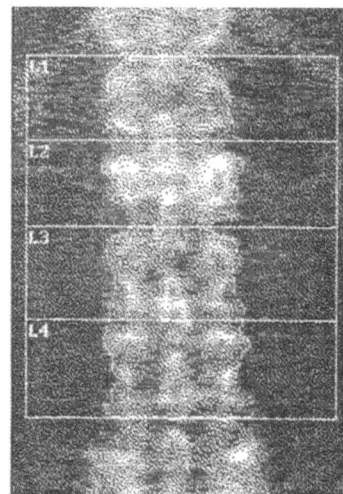

What should be the next step in managing this patient?
A. Nuclear medicine bone scan
B. MRI of the lumbar spine
C. Lateral spine imaging with VFA or radiography
D. Refer for kyphoplasty or vertebroplasty

Case 3

A 36-year-old woman with no known health problems is seen for an executive physical. Lateral chest x-ray shows a grade 3 compression fracture of T8. She has no back pain, cannot recall any trauma, and has no apparent height loss. DXA shows a Z-score of −1.1 at the spine and −0.9 at the left femoral neck.

Next steps should include:

A. Workup for malignancy
B. Treatment with an anabolic agent
C. Vertebroplasty or kyphoplasty
D. Review of prior imaging

Case 4

An 81-year-old white woman presents in March 2018 after sustaining spontaneous vertebral fractures. She had been diagnosed with osteoporosis in 2009, with a T-score of −2.6 at the lumbar spine and −2.7 at the femoral neck. Her main risk factor was taking suppressive doses of levothyroxine for remote history of thyroid cancer. She was using the Juvent platform as well as vitamin D3 at 5000 IU/d and calcium at 1000 mg. By 2011, her BMD had decreased (T-score of −3.3 at the lumbar spine and −3 at the femoral neck), and treatment with 60 mg of denosumab every 6 months was started. She had no fracture despite being in a motor vehicle accident in 2012. By 2016, her BMD had increased by 14.2% at the lumbar spine and 11.4% at the total hip. She reports several falls but no fractures. In January 2018, she failed to come for an injection of denosumab. Three months later, she has developed severe back pain without any trauma and is found to have multiple compression fractures.

What should be the next step in managing this patient?
A. Start alendronate or zoledronic acid
B. Start teriparatide or abaloparatide
C. Resume denosumab
D. Refer for kyphoplasty or vertebroplasty

AUGMENTATION OF VERTEBRAL FRACTURES WITH BONE CEMENT (VERTEBROPLASTY AND KYPHOPLASTY)

Percutaneous injection of bone cement was introduced in 1987 (25) for stabilization of vertebral fractures resulting from metastatic malignancy and hemangiomas. It was later extended to treatment of vertebral fractures in patients with osteoporosis (25), with the primary goal of pain relief. Use of a balloon before cement injection (kyphoplasty) added the potential for restoring lost vertebral height (26). Even as new modifications are being explored [*e.g.*, vertebral body stenting, OsseoFix (ATEC Spine, Carlsbad, CA), and SpineJack (Stryker, Kalamazoo, MI)] (27), the true value of vertebral augmentation remains unclear.

Proper evaluation in clinical trials is challenging because of procedure-related and patient variables.

Efficacy goals of vertebral augmentation	Safety goals of vertebral augmentation
• Relief of pain • Restore vertebral height • Restore/maintain spinal contours • Improve overall mobility and function • Reduce mortality	• Avoid/minimize cement leakage • Prevent further loss of vertebral height • Minimize risk of fracture of adjacent vertebrae • Minimize risk of fracture of other vertebrae

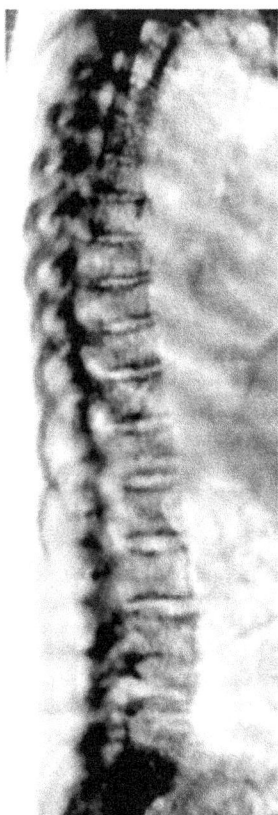

VFA 2013

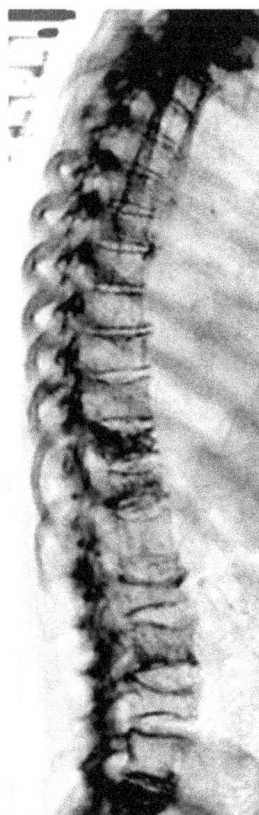

VFA 2018

Procedural Variables	Patient Variables
• Operator/learning curve • Bilateral or unilateral • Direct injection or balloon • Cement composition • Cement viscosity • Cement volume	• Time from fracture to intervention • Magnitude of compression • Intravertebral cleft/mobility • Disruption of cortex • Degree of kyphosis • Amount of height restoration • Multilevel/sandwich

Several studies of vertebroplasty for pain relief have been positive, but enthusiasm for vertebroplasty was diminished (28), although not extinguished (29, 30), after publication of sham-controlled trials that failed to show a difference in postprocedure pain (31, 32); interest in vertebroplasty is unlikely to fade, even in the face of a third negative trial (33). Some comparative studies have suggested that kyphoplasty may provide greater pain relief compared with vertebroplasty (34), but the difference in outcome may not justify the difference in cost (35). Restoration of vertebral height is not a given but is more likely with kyphoplasty; however, later further compression of the treated vertebra or fractures of adjacent or distant vertebrae may offset the height restoration of the treated vertebra (36, 37).

Criteria for patient selection include pain that is unusually severe or prolonged. The choice of vertebroplasty or kyphoplasty may depend on extent of compression (≤30% for vertebroplasty, >30% compression for kyphoplasty); however, in large part because of the heterogeneity of both procedures and patients, there are no proven standards (38, 39).

Patients with vertebral fractures are at high risk for future fractures. Often, postprocedure, they are not evaluated further or offered treatment to reduce future fracture risk. In one study, orthopedists were more likely than neurosurgeons or interventional radiologists to refer patients for osteoporosis management (40). Interestingly, use of vertebral augmentation for fractures resulting from discontinuing denosumab does not seem to be a good strategy, because it has been associated with development of additional fractures (41).

References

1. Johnell O, Kanis JA. An estimate of the worldwide prevalence and disability associated with osteoporotic fractures. *Osteoporos Int.* 2006;**17**(12):1726–1733.
2. Ström O, Borgstrom F, Zethraeus N, Johnell O, Lidgren L, Ponzer S, Svensson O, Abdon P, Ornstein E, Ceder L, Thorngren KG, Sernbo I, Jonsson B. Long-term cost and effect on quality of life of osteoporosis-related fractures in Sweden. *Acta Orthop.* 2008;**79**(2):269–280.
3. Burger H, Van Daele PL, Grashuis K, Hofman A, Grobbee DE, Schütte HE, Birkenhäger JC, Pols HA. Vertebral deformities and functional impairment in men and women. *J Bone Miner Res.* 1997;**12**(1):152–157.
4. Kado DM, Browner WS, Palermo L, Nevitt MC, Genant HK, Cummings SR; Study of Osteoporotic Fractures Research Group. Vertebral fractures and mortality in older women: a prospective study. *Arch Intern Med.* 1999;**159**(11):1215–1220.
5. Kanis JA, Oden A, Johnell O, De Laet C, Jonsson B. Excess mortality after hospitalisation for vertebral fracture. *Osteoporos Int.* 2004;**15**(2):108–112.
6. Black DM, Arden NK, Palermo L, Pearson J, Cummings SR; Study of Osteoporotic Fractures Research Group. Prevalent vertebral deformities predict hip fractures and new vertebral deformities but not wrist fractures. *J Bone Miner Res.* 1999;**14**(5):821–828.
7. Johnell O, Kanis JA, Odén A, Sernbo I, Redlund-Johnell I, Petterson C, De Laet C, Jönsson B. Fracture risk following an osteoporotic fracture. *Osteoporos Int.* 2004;**15**(3):175–179.
8. Lindsay R, Silverman SL, Cooper C, Hanley DA, Barton I, Broy SB, Licata A, Benhamou L, Geusens P, Flowers K, Stracke H, Seeman E. Risk of new vertebral fracture in the year following a fracture. *JAMA.* 2001;**285**(3):320–323.
9. Kendler DL, Bauer DC, Davison KS, Dian L, Hanley DA, Harris ST, McClung MR, Miller PD, Schousboe JT, Yuen CK, Lewiecki EM. Vertebral fractures: clinical importance and management. *Am J Med.* 2016;**129**(2):221.e1–221.e10.
10. Fink HA, Milavetz DL, Palermo L, Nevitt MC, Cauley JA, Genant HK, Black DM, Ensrud KE; Fracture Intervention Trial Research Group. What proportion of incident radiographic vertebral deformities is clinically diagnosed and vice versa? *J Bone Miner Res.* 2005;**20**(7):1216–1222.
11. Nevitt MC, Ettinger B, Black DM, Stone K, Jamal SA, Ensrud K, Segal M, Genant HK, Cummings SR. The association of radiographically detected vertebral fractures with back pain and function: a prospective study. *Ann Intern Med.* 1998;**128**(10):793–800.
12. Delmas PD, van de Langerijt L, Watts NB, Eastell R, Genant H, Grauer A, Cahall DL; IMPACT Study Group. Underdiagnosis of vertebral fractures is a worldwide problem: the IMPACT study. *J Bone Miner Res.* 2005;**20**(4):557–563.
13. Gehlbach SH, Bigelow C, Heimisdottir M, May S, Walker M, Kirkwood JR. Recognition of vertebral fracture in a clinical setting. *Osteoporos Int.* 2000;**11**(7):577–582.
14. Lewiecki EM, Laster AJ. Clinical review: clinical applications of vertebral fracture assessment by dual-energy x-ray absorptiometry. *J Clin Endocrinol Metab.* 2006;**91**(11):4215–4222.
15. Siris ES, Genant HK, Laster AJ, Chen P, Misurski DA, Krege JH. Enhanced prediction of fracture risk combining vertebral fracture status and BMD. *Osteoporos Int.* 2007;**18**(6):761–770.
16. Szulc P. Vertebral fracture: diagnostic difficulties of a major medical problem. *J Bone Miner Res.* 2018;**33**(4):553–559.
17. Genant HK, Wu CY, van Kuijk C, Nevitt MC. Vertebral fracture assessment using a semiquantitative technique. *J Bone Miner Res.* 1993;**8**(9):1137–1148.
18. Jiang G, Eastell R, Barrington NA, Ferrar L. Comparison of methods for the visual identification of prevalent vertebral fracture in osteoporosis. *Osteoporos Int.* 2004;**15**(11):887–896.
19. Delmas PD, Genant HK, Crans GG, Stock JL, Wong M, Siris E, Adachi JD. Severity of prevalent vertebral fractures and the risk of subsequent vertebral and nonvertebral fractures: results from the MORE trial. *Bone.* 2003;**33**(4):522–532.
20. Deng M, Zeng XJ, He LC, Leung JCS, Kwok AWL, Griffith JF, Kwok T, Leung PC, Wang YXJ. Osteoporotic vertebral fracture prevalence in elderly Chinese men and women: a comparison of endplate/cortex fracture-based and morphometrical deformity-based methods [published online ahead of print 2 December 2017]. *J Clin Densitom.* doi:10.1016/j.jocd.2017.11.004.
21. Lentle BC, Berger C, Probyn L, Brown JP, Langsetmo L, Fine B, Lian K, Shergill AK, Trollip J, Jackson S, Leslie WD, Prior JC, Kaiser SM, Hanley DA, Adachi JD, Towheed T, Davison KS, Cheung AM, Goltzman D; CaMos Research Group. Comparative analysis of the radiology of osteoporotic vertebral fractures in women and men: cross-sectional and longitudinal observations from the Canadian Multicentre Osteoporosis Study (CaMos). *J Bone Miner Res.* 2018;**33**(4):569–579.
22. Oei L, Koromani F, Breda SJ, Schousboe JT, Clark EM, van Meurs JB, Ikram MA, Waarsing JH, van Rooij FJ, Zillikens MC, Krestin GP, Oei EH, Rivadeneira F. Osteoporotic vertebral fracture prevalence varies widely between qualitative and quantitative radiological assessment

methods: the Rotterdam study. *J Bone Miner Res.* 2018;**33**(4): 560–568.

23. Cosman F, de Beur SJ, LeBoff MS, Lewiecki EM, Tanner B, Randall S, Lindsay R; National Osteoporosis Foundation. Clinician's guide to prevention and treatment of osteoporosis. *Osteoporos Int.* 2014; **25**(10):2359–2381.

24. Rosen HN, Vokes TJ, Malabanan AO, Deal CL, Alele JD, Olenginski TP, Schousboe JT. The official positions of the International Society for Clinical Densitometry: vertebral fracture assessment. *J Clin Densitom.* 2013;**16**(4):482–488.

25. Galibert P, Deramond H, Rosat P, Le Gars D. Preliminary note on the treatment of vertebral angioma by percutaneous acrylic verte-broplasty [in French]. *Neurochirurgie.* 1987;**33**(2):166–168.

26. Belkoff SM, Mathis JM, Fenton DC, Scribner RM, Reiley ME, Talmadge K. An ex vivo biomechanical evaluation of an inflatable bone tamp used in the treatment of compression fracture. *Spine.* 2001;**26**(2):151–156.

27. Vanni D, Galzio R, Kazakova A, Pantalone A, Grillea G, Bartolo M, Salini V, Magliani V. Third-generation percutaneous vertebral augmentation systems. *J Spine Surg.* 2016;**2**(1):13–20.

28. Laratta JL, Shillingford JN, Lombardi JM, Mueller JD, Reddy H, Saifi C, Fischer CR, Ludwig SC, Lenke LG, Lehman RA. Utilization of verte-broplasty and kyphoplasty procedures throughout the United States over a recent decade: an analysis of the Nationwide Inpatient Sample. *J Spine Surg.* 2017;**3**(3):364–370.

29. Chandra RV, Maingard J, Asadi H, Slater LA, Mazwi TL, Marcia S, Barr J, Hirsch JA. Vertebroplasty and kyphoplasty for osteoporotic ver-tebral fractures: what are the latest data? *AJNR Am J Neuroradiol.* 2018;**39**(5):798–806.

30. Davies E. No more vetebroplasty for acute vertebral compression fractures? *BMJ.* 2018;**361**:k1756.

31. Kallmes DF, Comstock BA, Heagerty PJ, Turner JA, Wilson DJ, Di-amond TH, Edwards R, Gray LA, Stout L, Owen S, Hollingworth W, Ghdoke B, Annesley-Williams DJ, Ralston SH, Jarvik JG. A randomized trial of vertebroplasty for osteoporotic spinal fractures. *N Engl J Med.* 2009;**361**(6):569–579.

32. Buchbinder R, Osborne RH, Ebeling PR, Wark JD, Mitchell P, Wriedt C, Graves S, Staples MP, Murphy B. A randomized trial of vertebroplasty for painful osteoporotic vertebral fractures. *N Engl J Med.* 2009; **361**(6):557–568.

33. Firanescu CE, de Vries J, Lodder P, Venmans A, Schoemaker MC, Smeet AJ, Donga E, Juttmann JR, Klazen CAH, Elgersma OEH, Jansen FH, Tielbeek AV, Boukrab I, Schonenberg K, van Rooij WJJ, Hirsch JA, Lohle PNM. Vertebroplasty versus sham procedure for painful acute osteoporotic vertebral compression fractures (VERTOS IV): rando-mised sham controlled clinical trial. *BMJ.* 2018;**361**:k1551.

34. Robinson Y, Olerud C. Vertebroplasty and kyphoplasty--a systematic review of cement augmentation techniques for osteoporotic vertebral compression fractures compared to standard medical therapy. *Maturitas.* 2012;**72**(1):42–49.

35. Omidi-Kashani F, Samini F, Hasankhani EG, Kachooei AR, Toosi KZ, Golhasani-Keshtan F. Does percutaneous kyphoplasty have better functional outcome than vertebroplasty in single level osteoporotic compression fractures? A comparative prospective study. *J Osteoporos.* 2013;**2013**:690329.

36. Li YX, Guo DQ, Zhang SC, Liang D, Yuan K, Mo GY, Li DX, Guo HZ, Tang Y, Luo PJ. Risk factor analysis for re-collapse of cemented vertebrae after percutaneous vertebroplasty (PVP) or percutaneous kypho-plasty (PKP). *Int Orthop.* 2018;**42**(9):2131–2139.

37. Jacobson RE, Palea O, Granville M. Progression of vertebral com-pression fractures after previous vertebral augmentation: technical reasons for recurrent fractures in a previously treated vertebra. *Cureus.* 2017;**9**(10):e1776.

38. Luthman S, Widén J, Borgström F. Appropriateness criteria for treatment of osteoporotic vertebral compression fractures. *Osteo-poros Int.* 2018;**29**(4):793–804.

39. Sahota O, Ong T, Salem K. Vertebral fragility fractures (VFF)--who, when and how to operate. *Injury.* 2018;**49**(8):1430–1435.

40. Daffner SD, Karnes JM, Watkins CM. Surgeon specialty influences referral rate for osteoporosis management following vertebral com-pression fractures. *Global Spine J.* 2016;**6**(6):524–528.

41. Anastasilakis AD, Polyzos SA, Makras P, Aubry-Rozier B, Kaouri S, Lamy O. Clinical features of 24 patients with rebound-associated vertebral fractures after denosumab discontinuation: systematic review and additional cases. *J Bone Miner Res.* 2017;**32**(6):1291–1296.

Kidney Stones: Diagnosis, Management, and Prevention

M25
Presented, March 23–26, 2019

Naim Maalouf, MD. Charles and Jane Pak Center for Mineral Metabolism and Clinical Research, Department of Internal Medicine, Division of Mineral Metabolism, University of Texas, Southwestern Medical Center, Dallas, Texas 75390-8885, E-mail: naim.maalouf@utsouthwestern.edu

SIGNIFICANCE OF THE CLINICAL PROBLEM

Urinary stone disease is an important medical and public health problem in the United States. Urinary stones lead to considerable pain, absenteeism, diminished quality of life, and at times to urinary tract infection, chronic kidney disease, and even end-stage renal disease. In the United States, the prevalence of urinary stones has doubled in the last 20 years, currently affecting 1 in 11 persons. Urinary stones recur at a high rate (>50% at 10 years), particularly in patients with family history of stones and in stone formers with obesity, diabetes, or other metabolic risk factors.

In view of the substantial morbidity and cost associated with urinary stones, a medical evaluation to identify abnormalities responsible for stone formation has been advocated to guide therapy to reduce the risk of stone recurrence. The evaluation of stone formers generally comprises an extensive medical history and laboratory studies (including stone composition analysis and serum and urinary chemistries) to assess for any underlying systemic disorders, detect environmental and metabolic processes contributing to stone disease, and guide initial and follow-up dietary and pharmacological therapy.

BARRIERS TO OPTIMAL PRACTICE

Although the costs of metabolic evaluation and medical treatment of remediable causes can be substantial in stone formers, this cost is balanced by the reductions in stone-related events and medical encounters. This is particularly the case for recurrent stone formers, in whom conservative therapy (*i.e.*, dietary advice without metabolic testing) is unsatisfactory because of a high recurrence rate. Still, the vast majority of kidney stone formers do not undergo evaluation to detect the cause of their stone disease. This is in part related to the perceived complexity of such an evaluation by treating physicians, who frequently do not think that they are competent to conduct testing for stone risk assessment.

LEARNING OBJECTIVES

As a result of participating in this session, learners should be able to:
- Identify major risk factors for commonly encountered kidney stones
- Become familiar with the recommended evaluation of first-time and recurrent stone formers
- Assess the impact of lifestyle and pharmacological interventions on the risk of stone recurrence
- Recognize diabetes and obesity as risk factors for uric acid kidney stones

STRATEGIES FOR DIAGNOSIS, THERAPY, AND/OR MANAGEMENT
Overview

Urinary stones result from the formation of solid concretions consisting of both protein and crystalline materials in the lumen of the urinary tract. Nephrolithiasis is not a true diagnosis in the sense that urinary stones can form because of a wide range of underlying diseases. Clinicians can unveil the underlying pathophysiology and cause of stone formation in a substantial proportion of patients, which can guide therapy to prevent stone recurrence.

Pathogenesis and Risk Factors for Urinary Stones

The pathogenesis of urinary stone disease is complex and multifactorial. It involves a combination of acquired factors and inherited conditions. The process of stone formation is thought to begin by formation of a crystal nidus in a super-saturated urinary environment, with subsequent transformation of this nidus into a stone through crystal growth and aggregation.

Urinary stones are generally classified by composition, with calcium-containing (calcareous) stones [including calcium oxalate (approximately 70% of all stones analyzed) and calcium phosphate (15%) stones] and noncalcareous stones [uric acid (10%), struvite (infection stones), cystine, and others].

Major abnormalities and potential etiologies for the most commonly encountered stone types are listed in Table 1.

Evaluation of Stone Former
History

Evaluation of a patient with urinary stones requires the identification of factors contributing to stone formation. Historical factors to be reviewed include age at onset and rate of stone formation, a detailed medical history, medication use, and family and dietary history. Onset of stone disease at an earlier age and a family history of stones can suggest an underlying inherited condition. History assessment should include the identification of medical conditions associated with metabolic abnormalities that lead to urinary stones (*e.g.*, primary hyperparathyroidism, granulomatous disorders, inflammatory bowel disease, chronic diarrhea, recurrent urinary tract infections, gout, and others). Medications associated with urinary stone formation may be identified and discontinued. These include drugs that are poorly soluble in the urinary environment (*e.g.*, triamterene, sulfonamides, indinavir, and others), or drugs

Table 1. Metabolic Abnormalities in Commonly Encountered Kidney Stones

Metabolic Abnormality	Potential Etiologies	Stone Type		
		Calcium Oxalate	Calcium Phosphate	Uric Acid
Low urine volume	Low fluid intake, diarrhea, or excessive sweating	X	X	X
High urine calcium	Hypercalcemia, high protein or salt intake, medication, idiopathic	X	X	
Low urine citrate	States of acidosis (RTA, drugs, diarrhea, high protein intake)	X	X	
High urine oxalate	Primary (genetic) or secondary (enteric or high dietary sources)	X		
High urine uric acid	Excessive purine intake or purine production	X		X
High urine pH	Distal renal tubular acidosis, infection, medications		X	
Low urine pH	GI alkali loss, excessive dietary protein intake, or idiopathic			X

Abbreviation: RTA, renal tubular acidosis.

that lead to metabolic stones (*e.g.*, calcium, vitamin D, or vitamin C supplements; furosemide; and carbonic anhydrase inhibitors).

Collecting a dietary history should elicit risk factors for low urine volume (*e.g.*, low fluid intake, excessive perspiration and/or intestinal loss). Although high dietary calcium was previously thought to predispose to stone formation, several large observational epidemiologic studies have found a lower incidence of urinary stones in individuals with a higher dietary calcium intake. This probably occurs through the complexation of intestinal luminal oxalate by dietary calcium, ultimately reducing urinary oxalate excretion. High salt and high protein consumption also significantly increases stone formation by enhancing urinary calcium excretion. High animal protein consumption also results in dietary acid and purine loads that lower urine pH and citrate, and raise urinary uric acid.

Laboratory Testing
If a sample is available, stone analysis is essential to guiding diagnosis and therapy. Blood tests should include assessment of renal function, serum electrolytes (hypokalemia and metabolic acidosis are observed with chronic diarrhea and/or renal tubular acidosis), serum uric acid, and serum calcium (hypercalcemia can lead to identification of primary hyperparathyroidism or granulomatous disorders). A urinalysis can identify hematuria, crystalluria, and/or urinary tract infection. In the assessment of recurrent stone formers, the evaluation of urine chemistries on a 24-hour urine collection is recommended. Included parameters, reference ranges, and interpretations are listed in Table 2.

Management
Lifestyle Modification
Fluid intake is an effective, low risk, and inexpensive intervention for the secondary prevention of urinary stones. In a

randomized trial of adult stone formers, fluid intake that resulted in a urine output greater than 2 L/d decreased stone recurrence by 55% and increased the time to recurrence by more than 1 year. In another randomized trial, a diet low in sodium and animal protein content also lowered stone recurrence rate in patients with calcium stones. A diet rich in fruits and vegetables is generally recommended to most stone formers to raise urine pH and enhance citrate excretion.

Medications
In hypercalciuric calcium nephrolithiasis, thiazide diuretics plus potassium citrate are used to lower calcium excretion and prevent stone recurrence. Normocalciuric stone formers are frequently prescribed potassium citrate alone because the resulting rise in urinary citrate inhibits the crystallization of calcium oxalate and calcium phosphate. In hyperuricosuric calcium stone formers without hypercalciuria, allopurinol has been shown to reduce stone recurrence rate versus placebo.

Uric acid stones, which are more common in obese and/or diabetic stone formers, are primarily caused by overly acidic urine (*i.e.*, low urine pH), whereas hyperuricosuria is a less common risk factor. Alkali therapy (most frequently in the form of potassium citrate) to raise urine pH is therefore the mainstay of uric acid stones, whereas hypo-uricosuric agents (such as allopurinol or febuxostat) are less commonly used.

MAIN CONCLUSIONS
The evaluation of kidney stone formers generally comprises an extensive medical history and laboratory studies to assess for processes contributing to stone disease and to guide initial and follow-up therapy. The most commonly encountered stone types (calcium oxalate and calcium phosphate stones) share common metabolic risk factors (*e.g.*, hypercalciuria, hypocitraturia), but

Table 2. Interpretation and Management of 24-hour Urinary Parameters in Kidney Stone Formers

24-Hour Urine Parameter	Reference Range	Interpretation	Risk Modification
Creatinine	♀: 15–20 mg/kg/d; ♂: 20–25 mg/kg/d	Used to verify adequacy of 24-h urine collection	N/A
Volume	>2.0–2.5 L/d	Determines urine saturation	Increase fluid intake
pH	5.7–6.3	pH altered by acid-base status, buffers, diet, medications	Potassium citrate raises urine pH[a]
Calcium	♀: <250 mg/d; ♂: <300 mg/d	Hypercalciuria may be environmental or metabolic	Low salt, low protein diet,[a] thiazide,[a] and potassium citrate[a]
Oxalate	<45 mg/d	Hyperoxaluria may be genetic or environmental	Restriction of oxalate-containing foods
Citrate	>320 mg/d	Inhibitor of calcium stones	Potassium citrate,[a] sodium bicarbonate raise urine citrate
Uric acid	<700 mg/d	Marker of purine intake	Allopurinol[a]; reduce purine intake
Phosphorus	<1100 mg/d	Marker of protein intake	Reduce protein intake
Sodium	<200 mEq/d	Marker of salt intake	Reduce salt intake
Sulfate	<40 mEq/d	Marker of protein intake	Reduce protein intake

Abbreviation: N/A, not applicable.

[a] Interventions shown to reduce stone recurrence rate in long-term randomized clinical trials.

also exhibit other unique pathophysiological abnormalities. Uric acid stones, which are more common in obese and/or diabetic stone formers, are primarily caused by overly acidic urine (*i.e.*, low urine pH). Lifestyle modifications that have been shown to reduce recurrent nephrolithiasis include an increase in fluid intake and a reduction in salt and animal protein intake. Pharmacological agents that have been shown to reduce stone recurrence include thiazide diuretics, allopurinol, and potassium citrate.

CASES
Case 1
Which of the Following Increases the Risk of Urinary Stones?

A. A high intake of calcium from dietary sources and a high intake of calcium from supplements

B. A low intake of calcium from dietary sources and a high intake of calcium from supplements

C. A high intake of calcium from dietary sources and a low intake of calcium from supplements

D. A low intake of calcium from dietary sources and a low intake of calcium from supplements

Case 2
Which of the Following Measures Has Been Shown to Reduce the Recurrence of Calcium Stones in Randomized, Placebo-Controlled, Clinical Trials?

A. Thiazide diuretics

B. Potassium citrate

C. Allopurinol

D. A and B only

E. A, B, and C

Case 3
Which of the Following Statements Is True Regarding Uric Acid Stones?

A. Allopurinol is the primary therapy because it corrects hyperuricemia, the most commonly encountered metabolic abnormality.

B. Allopurinol is the primary therapy because it corrects hyperuricosuria, the most commonly encountered metabolic abnormality.

C. Potassium citrate is the primary therapy because it corrects hypocitraturia, the most commonly encountered metabolic abnormality.

D. Potassium citrate is the primary therapy because it corrects low urine pH, the most commonly encountered metabolic abnormality.

DISCUSSION OF CASES AND ANSWERS
Case 1
Correct answer: B

Several large observational epidemiologic studies (Nurses' Health Study I and II, Health Professionals Follow-Up Study, and Women's Health Initiative Observational Study) have found a lower incidence of urinary stones in individuals with a higher dietary calcium intake. This probably occurs through the complexation of intestinal luminal oxalate by dietary calcium, thereby reducing urinary oxalate excretion and urinary stone formation. Contrary to dietary calcium, the use of calcium and vitamin D supplements results in an increased risk of nephrolithiasis.

Case 2
Correct Answer: E
In controlled clinical trials conducted in patients with calcium stones, recurrent stone formation was reduced by:
- Thiazide diuretics (in six clinical trials comparing thiazides with placebo or control)
- Citrate therapy (in the form of potassium citrate, potassium-magnesium citrate, or sodium-potassium citrate, in four clinical trials)
- Allopurinol (in calcium stone formers with hyperuricosuria in four clinical trials)

Case 3
Correct Answer: D
The single most important pathogenic factor in uric acid stone disease is overly acidic urine. Low urine pH (<5.5, the pKa for uric acid) promotes the protonation of urate to insoluble uric acid. Potassium citrate treatment creates a urinary environment less conducive to uric acid by increasing urine pH and reducing the amount of undissociated uric acid, resulting in dissolution of uric acid stones. Although allopurinol can reduce serum and urine uric acid concentration, these parameters are minor contributors to the pathogenesis of uric acid stone formation.

Recommended Reading
Lotan Y, Cadeddu JA, Roerhborn CG, Pak CY, Pearle MS. Article 1. Cost-effectiveness of medical management strategies for nephrolithiasis. *J Urol.* 2004;**172**(6 Pt 1):2275–2281.

Maalouf N. Approach to the adult kidney stone former. *Clin Rev Bone Miner Metab.* 2012;**10**(1):38–49.

Pearle MS, Goldfarb DS, Assimos DG, Curhan G, Denu-Ciocca CJ, Matlaga BR, Monga M, Penniston KL, Preminger GM, Turk TM, White JR; American Urological Association. Medical Management of Kidney Stones: AUA Guideline. *J Urol.* 2014;**192**(2):316–324.

Sakhaee K, Maalouf NM, Sinnott B. Article I. Clinical review. Kidney stones 2012: pathogenesis, diagnosis, and management. *J Clin Endocrinol Metab.* 2012;**97**(6):1847–1860.

Song L, Maalouf NM. 24-hour urine calcium in the evaluation and management of nephrolithiasis. *JAMA.* 2017;**318**(5):474–475.

Metabolic Bone Disease in Patients With Renal Insufficiency/Failure

M35
Presented, March 23–26, 2019

Peter R. Ebeling, MD. Department of Medicine, School of Clinical Sciences, Faculty of Medicine, Nursing and Health Sciences, Monash University, Clayton, Victoria 3168, Australia, E-mail: peter.ebeling@monash.edu.

Jasna Aleksova, MD. Department of Medicine, School of Clinical Sciences, Faculty of Medicine, Nursing and Health Sciences, Monash University, Clayton, Victoria 3168, Australia, E-mail: jasna.aleksova@hudson.org.au.

SIGNIFICANCE OF THE CLINICAL PROBLEM

Chronic kidney disease (CKD) is one of the most common medical problems in the United States, affecting 20 million Americans. A majority of patients have stage 1, 2, or 3 CKD with estimated glomerular filtration rates (eGFRs) of $\geq$90 mL/min plus kidney damage, 60 to 89 mL/min plus kidney damage, and 30 to 59 mL/min, respectively (1). However, 300,000 Americans had stage 4 CKD (eGFR, 15 to 29 mL/min) and 452,957 had stage 5 CKD (eGFR, <15 mL/min) or were on dialysis in 2003 (2). CKD is associated with excess morbidity and mortality and increased health care costs. CKD metabolic bone disorder (MBD) occurs in stage 4 and 5 CKD and is characterized by bone (renal osteodystrophy), soft tissue (calcifications), and mineral (phosphate, calcium, fibroblast growth factor-23, calcitriol, sclerostin, and Dikkopf-1) abnormalities. However, the pathologic end points of CKD-MBD are increased cardiovascular risk, mortality, and fractures.

Hip fracture incidence increases with age in the general population, but is increased at every age for patients with stage 3b, 4, and 5 CKD. Mortality after any fracture is also increased in patients with CKD and is highest in patients with stage 5 CKD. Total annual costs of treating fractures associated with stage 5 CKD are $100 million and $500 million for nondialysis CKD.

BARRIERS TO OPTIMAL PRACTICE

Physicians are unsure whether conventional antiosteoporosis drugs are either appropriate or effective in patients with CKD. In particular, there is a reluctance to measure bone mineral density (BMD) using dual-energy absorptiometry (DXA) as there is concern that it may not be as predictive of fractures in patients with CKD as in the general population. There is also a reluctance to use antiresorptive drugs as patients may have low turnover renal osteodystrophy so that treatment could theoretically worsen skeletal fragility.

LEARNING OBJECTIVES

As a result of participating in this session, learners should be able to:
- Understand the epidemiology of CKD and fractures
- Distinguish between the CKD-related bone disorders that comprise renal osteodystrophy
- Take a case-based approach, including fracture risk assessment, bone disease diagnostic strategies, and treatment with bisphosphonates, denosumab, and teriparatide.

BONE DISEASE IN CKD (RENAL OSTEODYSTROPHY)

The TMV classification system exists for CKD and is based on bone turnover, mineralization, and volume, and each can be low/absent, normal, or high. The combination of each component can be used to classify the disease—for example, in adynamic bone disease, turnover is low, mineralization is normal, and volume is low, whereas in hyperparathyroidism, turnover is high, mineralization is normal, and volume is low. In contrast, in osteomalacia, turnover is low, mineralization is low, and volume is normal (3).

CKD-MBD GUIDELINES

Previous Kidney Disease: Improving Global Outcomes (KDIGO) guidelines from 2009 suggest a cutoff for parathyroid hormone (PTH), above which high turnover renal osteodystrophy would be treated with the calcimimetic drug, cinacalcet, and the active form of vitamin D. However, new 2017 KDIGO guidelines state that the optimal PTH level is not known. Instead, there should be a renewed focus on an assessment of both fracture risk and bone turnover in the individual patient with CKD. In patients with high turnover bone disease, an antiresorptive drug with or without vitamin D should be used, whereas in patients with low turnover bone disease, an anabolic drug with or without vitamin D should be used.

2017 KDIGO CKD-MBD GUIDELINE UPDATE

Per the 2017 KDIGO CKD-MBD update (4), in patients with CKD G3a to G5D with evidence of CKD-MBD
- And/or risk factors for osteoporosis, BMD testing to assess fracture risk is suggested if results will affect treatment decisions (Fig. 1)
- It is reasonable to perform a bone biopsy if knowledge of the type of renal osteodystrophy will affect treatment decisions.
- Optimal PTH level is not known.
- Vitamin D_3 supplements should be provided in patients with stage 3 CKD to correct vitamin D deficiency.
- Reserve the use of calcitriol or vitamin D analogs for patients with stage 4 and 5 CKD with severe and progressive hyperparathyroidism.

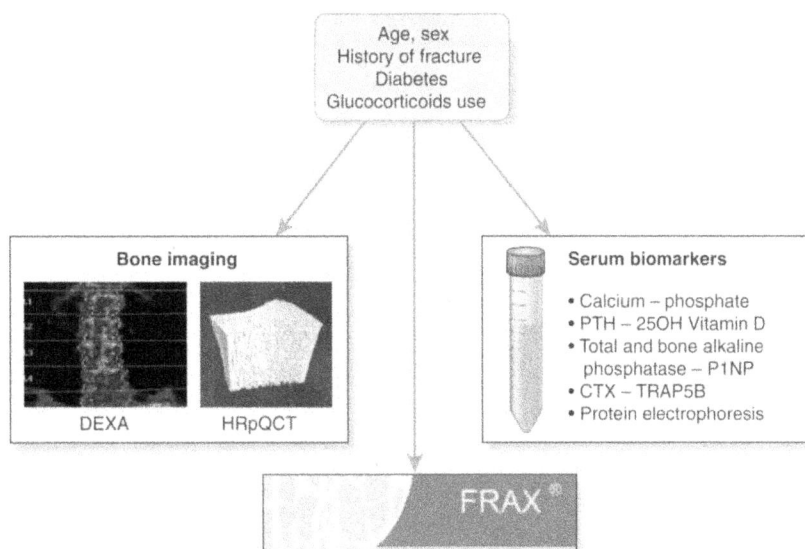

Figure 1. Assessing bone in CKD-MBD. Reproduced under a Creative Commons BY-NC-ND 4.0 license from Pimentel A, Urena-Torres P, Zillikens C, et al. Fractures in patients with CKD—diagnosis, treatment, and prevention: a review by members of the European Calcified Tissue Society and the European Renal Association of Nephrology Dialysis and Transplantation. *Kidney Int.* 2017;92(6):1343–1355.

- Antifracture efficacy for any osteoporosis therapy in severe (stage 4 and 5) CKD is lacking.

CKD-MBD: REVIEW FROM EUROPEAN CALCIFIED TISSUE SOCIETY AND EUROPEAN RENAL ASSOCIATION OF NEPHROLOGY DIALYSIS AND TRANSPLANTATION

This alternative guideline (5) suggests that there is still value in measuring PTH to differentiate between high and low turnover states in renal osteodystrophy. The aim of both guidelines is to recommend treatment of renal osteodystrophy on the basis of whether bone turnover is likely to be high or low. The combination of PTH levels with the bone formation marker, bone-specific alkaline phosphatase (BSAP), which is not affected by renal function, remains the best noninvasive way to divide patients into high or low bone turnover. However, in cases with either low PTH or low or intermediate levels of BSAP, bone biopsy may be required to exclude causes of low turnover renal osteodystrophy (adynamic bone disease and osteomalacia) (Fig. 2).

NOVEL RESEARCH INTO BONE HEALTH IN PATIENTS WITH CKD-MBD
Gonadal Hormones in CKD-MBD

In the general population without CKD, the effect of hypogonadism on skeletal outcomes is well recognized and is associated with lower BMD and increased fracture rates in both men and women (6–8), whereas hormone replacement therapy increases BMD and reduces fracture risk (9–11).

Disturbances in gonadal hormones are also frequent in patients with CKD, reported in up to 50% of men with stage 3 to 5 CKD (12, 13), increasing to up to 75% of men undergoing dialysis (14–16). In these patients, low total testosterone levels likely result from a combination of primary testicular failure and secondary hypothalamic–pituitary dysfunction (17). Similarly, in premenopausal women with CKD, menstrual irregularities are common, with approximately 50% of women with stage 5 CKD experiencing amenorrhea and low estrogen levels. Few regain menses after the commencement of dialysis once amenorrhoeic (17). Recently, increased sex hormone binding globulin levels have also been associated with nonvertebral fractures in men receiving dialysis, which suggests an important role for free testosterone in bone health (18). Although the KDIGO workgroup recognizes the potential effects of altered gonadal hormones on bone quality in patients with CKD-MBD (19), the contribution of gonadal hormone disturbances on the pathogenesis of renal osteodystrophy, or the benefits of hormone-replacement therapy on bone outcomes in CKD-MBD, remains uncertain (4, 20) and is an area that requires future research.

Novel Bone Imaging Techniques
Given the limited ability of areal BMD by DXA to capture the complex and varied microarchitectural changes in CKD-MBD, as well as the large proportion of patients with CKD-MBD who fracture with normal BMD, newer imaging techniques are under investigation for their utility in fracture prediction.
- Trabecular bone score (TBS) is a novel gray-level imaging tool obtained from lumbar spine DXA images (Fig. 3). It provides surrogate information on trabecular

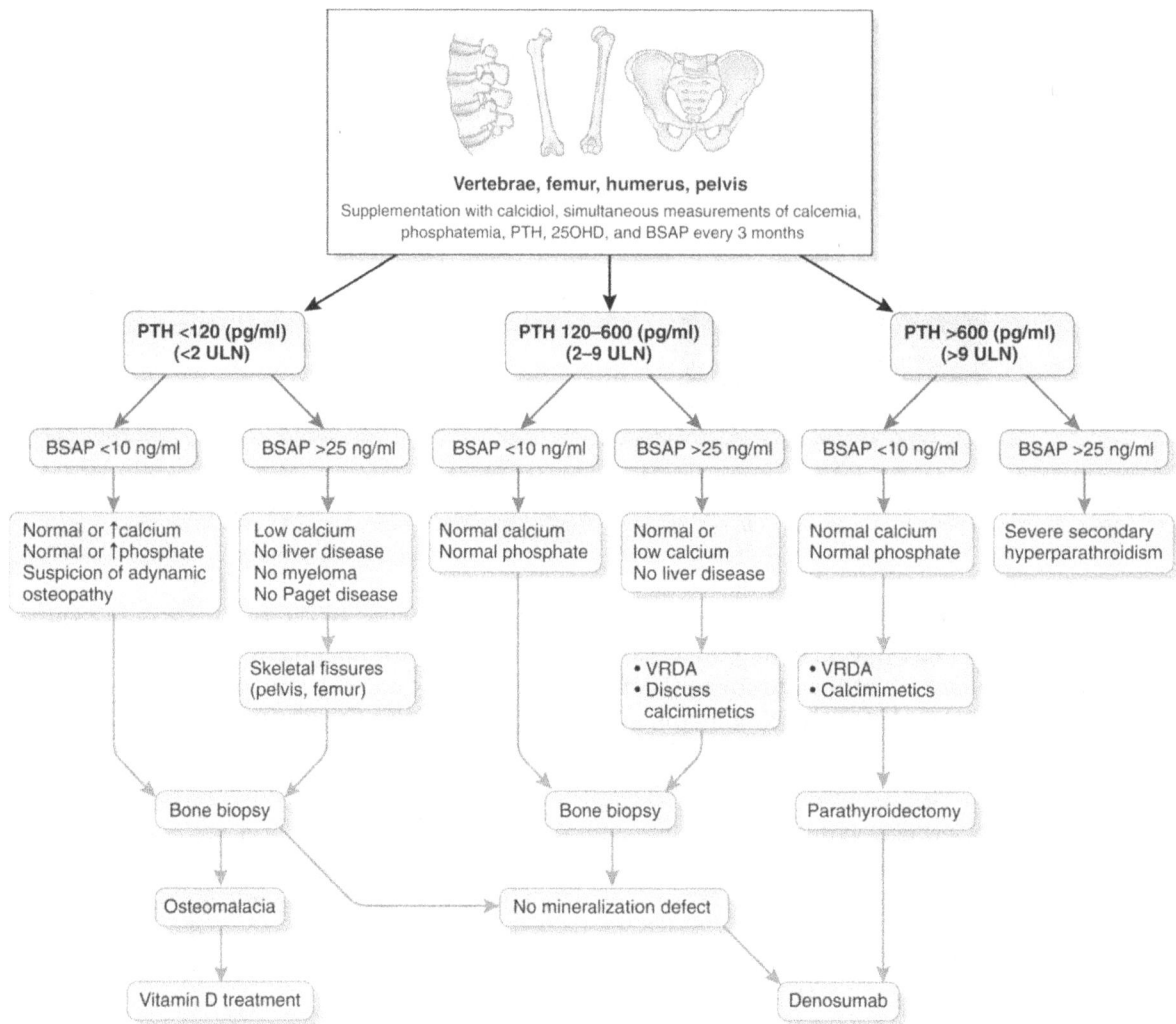

Figure 2. Treatment algorithm in patients with CKD-MBD according to bone turnover.

microarchitectural integrity not captured by BMD (21). Studies have shown that patients receiving dialysis have lower TBS (22, 23), which indicates deterioration of trabecular bone, and one study has demonstrated lower TBS to be associated with nonvertebral fractures (24).

• High-resolution peripheral quantitative CT provides noninvasive three-dimensional images of bone microarchitecture with a resolution to approximately 62 μm. Its use has greatly improved our understanding of microarchitectural abnormalities in patients with CKD-MBD, showing predominantly rapid and early cortical deterioration (25). It has also shown promise in its ability to delineate fracture risk, but the cost, availability, and expertise required for data acquisition and interpretation limits its clinical application (25, 26).

SUMMARY AND CONCLUSION
CKD-MBD: Differentiate and Manage Accordingly
• Almost all healthy adults have an age-related decline in renal function.

• Fracture risk and fracture-related complications and costs are higher in patients with CKD.
• DXA T-score helps to classify fracture risk in patients with CKD, but has limitations.
• The combination of PTH and bone turnover markers, particularly BSAP, predict bone loss and help guide treatment.
• Bone biopsies are needed when turnover and/or osteomalacia cannot be diagnosed noninvasively.
• An individual and tailored approach to managing bone disease is needed in patients with CKD.

CASES
Case 1
A 63-year-old postmenopausal white woman with stage 3 CKD is referred for clinical vertebral fracture (L4/L5). Her prior medical history includes hypertension and remote tobacco use. Medications include lisinopril 10 mg once per day. DXA T-scores Fracture Risk Assessment Tool (FRAX) are as follows: lumbar spine, -1.5 major osteoporotic fracture: 11%; total hip, -1.3 hip: 1.9%; femoral neck, -2.2; and 1/3 radius: 0.1.

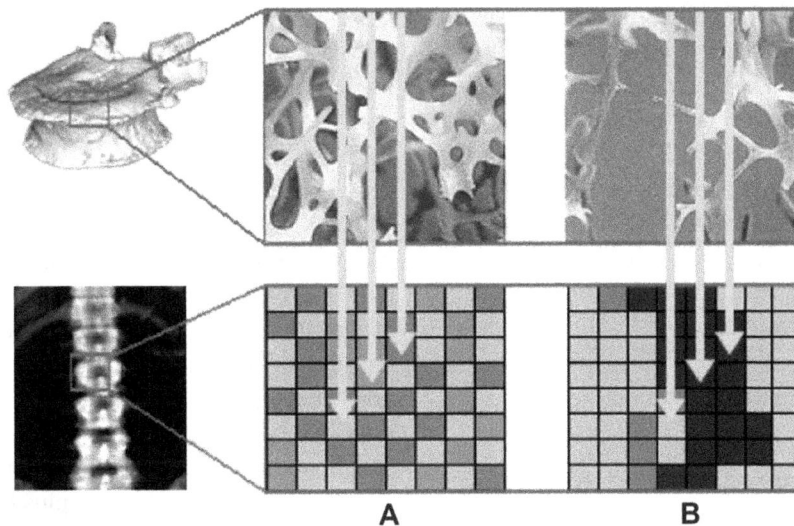

Figure 3. Derivation of the TBS. Reproduced with permission from Hans D, Barthe N, Boutroy S, et al. Correlations between trabecular bone score, measured using anteroposterior dual-energy x-ray absorptiometry acquisition, and 3-dimensional parameters of of bone microarchitecture: an experimental study on human cadaver vertebrae. *J Clin Densitom.* **2011;14:302–312.**

1. What is the patient's diagnosis on the basis of the KDIGO TMV system?
2. Should we measure bone turnover in this patient and, if so, how should it be measured?
3. What treatment would be best for this patient?

Case 2

A 43-year-old female is referred for low bone density on a knee plain film (osteonecrosis of the knee), refractory hyperparathyroidism, and end-stage renal disease (hereditary renal retinal syndrome). Patient underwent hemodialysis (HD) from 1978 to 2003 and received a successful kidney transplantation from a deceased donor from 2003 to 2007. In 2007, she experienced graft failure as a result of BK virus. From 2007 to present, she has received hemodialysis.

The patients' history includes the following: blind; HD-related neuropathy (walks with unsteady gait); normal menstruation; no tobacco, alcohol, or drugs; and a family history of renal disease (a sister with end-stage renal disease).

Patient has a dialysis prescription of Kt/v > 1.2 and 2.5 mEq calcium bath (standard). Patient's medications include prednisone 2.5 to 5 mg since transplantation failure, phenobarbital for seizures, sevelamer 800 mg three times per day with meals, paricalcitol 9 μg IV on HD days, and cinacalcet 30 mg once every day for 2 months before her visit and the dose was increased recently to 60 mg once every day (PTH > 400 pg/mL). Patient has never taken a bisphosphonate.

Spine X-rays reveal no fractures. DXA T-scores are as follows: spine, −0.5 (aortic calcification and end-plate osteosclerosis); total hip, −1.5; femoral neck, −2.0; 1/3 radius, −3.4 (90% cortical bone); and ultradistal radius, −1.7 (80% trabecular bone).

Laboratory test results include the following: calcium, 8.4 mg/dL (reference, 8.6 to 10.2 mg/dL); phosphorus, 5.6 mg/dL (reference, 2.5 to 4.5 mg/dL); PTH, 545 pg/mL (reference, 10 to 65 pg/mL); 25-hydroxyvitamin D (25-OHD), 20 ng/mL (reference, 20 to 100 ng/mL); bone alkaline phosphatase, 32 U/L (reference, 4.5 to 16.9 U/L); and C-terminal telopeptide (CTX), 4159 pg/mL (reference, 40 to 465 pg/mL).

1. What is the patient's diagnosis on the basis of the KDIGO TMV system?
2. Why is there a larger deficit in cortical bone than trabecular bone?
3. Should we measure bone turnover in this patient and, if so, how should it be measured?
4. What treatment would be best for this patient?

DISCUSSION
Case 1

In this patient with severe osteoporosis, both BMD and FRAX demonstrate poor sensitivity. In addition, CKD and osteoporosis are coprevalent with just less than 10% of women with an eGFR of <60 mL/min having osteoporosis and 21.3% of women age 70 to 79 years with osteoporosis having an eGFR of <35 mL/min (27, 28).

2017 KDIGO CKD-MBD recommendations are as follows: In patients with stages 3a to 5D CKD with evidence of CKD-MBD and/or risk factors for osteoporosis, we suggest BMD testing to assess fracture risk if results will affect treatment decisions (4).

Limitations of DXA in Patients With CKD

- DXA does not assess microarchitecture or bone strength.
- DXA does not assess turnover, mineralization, or the type of renal osteodystrophy.
- You cannot base treatment decisions on the DXA results.

Noninvasive tests, such as PTH and BSAP, can be used to differentiate between low and nonlow turnover renal osteodystrophy, as well as high and nonhigh turnover renal osteodystrophy, with cutoffs for each being available with areas under the curve ranging from 0.70 to 0.76 (29–32).

Bone biopsy is required to guide treatment decisions when
- The type of renal osteodystrophy is not clear
  ○ Low turnover or adynamic bone disease
  ○ Osteomalacia
- There are unexplained fractures
  ○ Normal BMD
  ○ No evidence of hyperparathyroidism
  ○ GFR < 45 mL/min

In this case the bone biopsy demonstrated the following:
- Turnover
  ○ Low–normal bone formation rate
  ○ Rare osteoclasts and osteoblasts
- Mineralization
  ○ No defect
- Volume
  ○ Cortical thinning (25)
  ○ Endosteal trabecularization
  ○ Normal trabecular microarchitecture

On the basis of a secondary analysis of the Fracture Prevention Trial with teriparatide, which contained low numbers of patients with CKD, regardless of whether eGFR was less than or greater than 80 mL/min, recombinant human PTH (1–33) increased lumbar spine and femoral neck BMD and reduced vertebral and nonvertebral fractures (33). The patient was treated with teriparatide as bone formation was low–normal (Fig. 4). In the Fracture Prevention Trial, teriparatide treatment was associated with increased serum calcium in all patients and uric acid in patients with CKD; however, no nephrolithiasis, gout, symptomatic hypercalcemia, or acute renal failure were seen in patients receiving teriparatide.

Repeat DXA 6 months later demonstrated a 3% increase in lumbar spine BMD, a 5% increase in femoral neck BMD, and a 4% increase in 1/3 radius BMD.

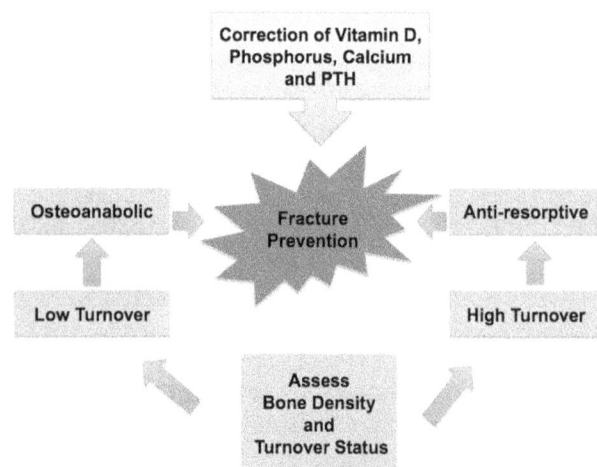

Figure 4. Approach to treatment in CKD-MBD.

Repeat bone biopsy showed increased cortical width, a mild decrease in cancellous bone, and an increase in bone formation rate in the low–normal range.

Case 2

This patient has severe secondary hyperparathyroidism causing cortical osteoporosis. In this situation, the combination of total hip BMD and BSAP is the best at predicting fracture risk (34). Her fracture risk is high given the degree of elevation of BSAP and her increased propensity to falls because of her blindness and peripheral neuropathy. The goal of treatment is to reduce her PTH levels to reduce bone remodeling, increase BMD, and reduce fracture risk. Treatment should include the following: increase sevelamer 1600 mg three times per day plus 800 mg with snacks (goal is phosphorus < 4.5 mg/dL); maintain <2.5 mEq/L calcium bath; vitamin D_3 repletion: goal is 30 to 40 ng/mL; change phenobarbital to lamictal to reduce adverse effects on vitamin D and bone; paricalcitol: adjust as needed, but avoid hypercalcemia; and cinacalcet: increase dose to 60 mg two times per day, but there is limited evidence from the EVOLVE trial—in which fractures were reduced from 13.2% to 12.2% over 5 years compared with placebo (secondary study outcome) —that this would reduce fracture risk (35).

One year later, laboratory results were as follows: PTH, 413 pg/mL (reference, 10 to 65 pg/mL); 25-OHD, 18 ng/mL (reference, 20 to 100 ng/mL); total ALP, 95 U/L (reference, 33 to 115 U/L); and CTX, 1216 pg/mL (reference, 40 to 465 pg/mL).

Repeat DXA T-scores (% change) were as follows: spine, −1.0 (−5.6%*); total hip, −1.7 (−3.2%*); femoral neck, −2.0; and 1/3 radius, −3.6 (−1.9%*).

Medical treatment has been ineffective at preventing bone loss or reducing PTH levels adequately. The best treatment would be parathyroidectomy. In patients with stage 5D CKD matched for age, sex, race, HD duration, and vitamin D dose, parathyroidectomy reduced hip fractures by 32% and any fractures by 31% over 10 years of follow-up. Parathyroid imaging in this patient revealed a mildly enlarged right upper parathyroid gland (87 mg) and slightly enlarged left lower parathyroid gland (67 mg) (36); however, the patient refused parathyroid surgery, so the dose of cinacalcet was increased to 90 mg two times per day.

A deceased donor kidney transplantation was then performed. Post-transplant immunosuppression regimen consisted of prednisone 5 mg once per day, tacrolimus 3 mg two times per day, mycophenolate 750 mg once every 12 hours, IV Ig × 6 weeks, and cholecalciferol 1000 IU daily.

Post-transplant test results included the following: creatinine, 1.4 (eGFR > 45 mL/min), phosphorus, 3.6 mg/dL (reference, 2.5 to 4.5 mg/dL); calcium, 9.0 mg/dL (reference, 8.6 to 10.2 mg/dL); albumin, 4.0 g/dL; PTH, 267 pg/mL (reference, 10 to 65 pg/mL); 25-OHD, 35 ng/mL (reference, 20 to 100 ng/mL); BSAP, 24.2 U/L (reference, 14.2 to 42.7 U/L); and CTX, 1222 pg/mL (reference, 40 to 465 pg/mL).

Post-transplant DXA T-scores (% change) included the following: spine, −1.3 (−3.5%*); total hip, −2.1 (−7.3%*); femoral neck, −2.0; and 1/3 radius, −4.1 (−6.4%*).

Continuing post-transplant hyperparathyroidism will increase the risk of fracture if PTH levels are >130 pg/mL.

Treatment Options
- Do nothing (masterly inactivity)
- Vitamin D analog
- Cinacalcet
- Parathyroidectomy
- Antiresorptive
- Anabolic agent teriparatide

Antiresorptive agents (37–40) are the best treatment option, combined with continuing medical management of hyperparathyroidism with cinacalcet, as the patient was still refusing parathyroidectomy.

Both risedronate and denosumab have been shown to reduce vertebral fractures in patients with mild CKD (stage 2 to 4 CKD for risedronate and stage 2 to 3 CKD for denosumab). Data on nonvertebral fracture reduction are lacking. Regardless of renal function, the incidence of adverse events (nonrenal/renal) were similar (serum creatinine, calcium, and phosphorous) in risedronate- and placebo-treated groups. Iliac crest biopsies from risedronate-treated patients with stage 3 or 4 CKD demonstrated a 68% decrease in mineralizing surface and a 54% decrease in activation frequency, but no evidence of adynamic bone disease.

Denosumab should be cautiously used in patients with stage 4 CKD, as cases of hypocalcemia have been reported, despite normal serum calcium and vitamin D levels. Its use should probably be avoided in patients with stage 5D CKD.

After 2 years of treatment with risedronate and cinacalcet, laboratory results were as follows: creatinine, 1.25 (eGFR, 46 mL/min); phosphorus, 4.2 mg/dL (reference, 2.5 to 4.5 mg/dL); calcium, 8.8 mg/dL (reference, 8.6 to 10.2 mg/dL); albumin, 4.3 g/dL; PTH, 132 pg/mL (down from 168 pg/mL; reference, 10 to 65 pg/mL); 25-OHD, 48 ng/mL (reference, 20 to 100 ng/mL); BSAP, 10.1 U/L (reference, 4.5 to 16.9 U/L); and CTX, 743 pg/mL (down from 1222 pg/mL; reference, 40 to 465 pg/mL).

DXA T-scores (% change) were as follows: spine, −0.8 (+5.5*%); total hip, −1.7 (+5.5%*); femoral neck, −1.8; and 1/3 radius, −3.5 (+8.0%*).

References

1. Coresh J, Byrd-Holt D, Astor BC, Briggs JP, Eggers PW, Lacher DA, Hostetter TH. Chronic kidney disease awareness, prevalence, and trends among U.S. adults, 1999 to 2000. *J Am Soc Nephrol.* 2005; **16**(1):180–188.
2. United States Renal Data System. 2005 annual data report. Available at: https://www.usrds.org/atlas05.aspx. Accessed 10 January 2018.
3. Cesini J, Cheriet S, Breuil V, Lafage-Proust MH. Osteoporosis: Chronic kidney disease in rheumatology practice. *Joint Bone Spine.* 2012; **79**(Suppl 2):S104–S109.
4. Ketteler M, Block GA, Evenepoel P, Fukagawa M, Herzog CA, McCann L, Moe SM, Shroff R, Tonelli MA, Toussaint ND, Vervloet MG, Leonard MB. Executive summary of the 2017 KDIGO Chronic Kidney Disease-Mineral and Bone Disorder (CKD-MBD) Guideline Update: What's changed and why it matters [published correction appears in Kidney Int. 2017;92(6):1558]. *Kidney Int.* 2017;**92**(1): 26–36.
5. Pimentel A, Ureña-Torres P, Zillikens MC, Bover J, Cohen-Solal M. Fractures in patients with CKD-diagnosis, treatment, and prevention: A review by members of the European Calcified Tissue Society and the European Renal Association of Nephrology Dialysis and Transplantation. *Kidney Int.* 2017;**92**(6):1343–1355.
6. Fink HA, Ewing SK, Ensrud KE, Barrett-Connor E, Taylor BC, Cauley JA, Orwoll ES. Association of testosterone and estradiol deficiency with osteoporosis and rapid bone loss in older men. *J Clin Endocrinol Metab.* 2006;**91**(10):3908–3915.
7. Zhu L, Jiang X, Sun Y, Shu W. Effect of hormone therapy on the risk of bone fractures: A systematic review and meta-analysis of randomized controlled trials. *Menopause.* 2016;**23**(4):461–470.
8. ESHRE Capri Workshop Group. Bone fractures after menopause. *Hum Reprod Update.* 2010;**16**(6):761–773.
9. Crofton PM, Evans N, Bath LE, Warner P, Whitehead TJ, Critchley HO, Kelnar CJ, Wallace WH. Physiological versus standard sex steroid replacement in young women with premature ovarian failure: Effects on bone mass acquisition and turnover. *Clin Endocrinol (Oxf).* 2010; **73**(6):707–714.
10. Finkelstein JS, Lee H, Leder BZ, Burnett-Bowie SA, Goldstein DW, Hahn CW, Hirsch SC, Linker A, Perros N, Servais AB, Taylor AP, Webb ML, Youngner JM, Yu EW. Gonadal steroid-dependent effects on bone turnover and bone mineral density in men. *J Clin Invest.* 2016;**126**(3): 1114-1125.
11. Cauley JA, Danielson ME, Jammy GR, Bauer DC, Jackson R, Wactawski-Wende J, Chlebowski RT, Ensrud KE, Boudreau R. Sex steroid hormones and fracture in a multiethnic cohort of women: The Women's Health Initiative Study (WHI). *J Clin Endocrinol Metab.* 2017;**102**(5): 1538-1547.
12. Albaaj F, Sivalingham M, Haynes P, McKinnon G, Foley RN, Waldek S, O'Donoghue DJ, Kalra PA. Prevalence of hypogonadism in male patients with renal failure. *Postgrad Med J.* 2006;**82**(972):693-696.
13. Khurana KK, Navaneethan SD, Arrigain S, Schold JD, Nally JV, Shoskes DA. Serum testosterone levels and mortality in men with CKD stages 3-4. *Am J Kidney Dis.* 2014;**64**(3):367-374.
14. Carrero JJ, Qureshi AR, Nakashima A, Arver S, Parini P, Lindholm B, Bárány P, Heimbürger O, Stenvinkel P. Prevalence and clinical implications of testosterone deficiency in men with end-stage renal disease. *Nephrol Dial Transplant.* 2011;**26**(1):184–190.
15. Gungor O, Kircelli F, Carrero JJ, Asci G, Toz H, Tatar E, Hur E, Sever MS, Arinsoy T, Ok E. Endogenous testosterone and mortality in male hemodialysis patients: Is it the result of aging? *Clin J Am Soc Nephrol.* 2010;**5**(11):2018-2023.
16. Yilmaz MI, Sonmez A, Qureshi AR, Saglam M, Stenvinkel P, Yaman H, Eyileten T, Caglar K, Oguz Y, Taslipinar A, Vural A, Gok M, Unal HU, Yenicesu M, Carrero JJ. Endogenous testosterone, endothelial dysfunction, and cardiovascular events in men with nondialysis chronic kidney disease. *Clin J Am Soc Nephrol.* 2011;**6**(7):1617-1625.
17. Handelsman DJ. Hypothalamic-pituitary gonadal dysfunction in renal failure, dialysis and renal transplantation. *Endocr Rev.* 1985;**6**(2): 151–182.
18. Aleksova J, Wong P, McLachlan R, Choy KW, Ebeling PR, Milat F, Elder GJ. Sex hormone-binding globulin is a biomarker associated with nonvertebral fracture in men on dialysis therapy. *Kidney Int.* 2018; **94**(2):372–380.
19. Ketteler M, Elder GJ, Evenepoel P, Ix JH, Jamal SA, Lafage-Proust MH, Shroff R, Thadhani RI, Tonelli MA, Kasiske BL, Wheeler DC, Leonard MB. Revisiting KDIGO clinical practice guideline on chronic kidney disease-mineral and bone disorder: a commentary from a Kidney Disease: Improving Global Outcomes controversies conference. *Kidney Int.* 2015;**87**(3):502–528.
20. Aleksova J, Rodriguez AJ, McLachlan R, Kerr P, Milat F, Ebeling PR. Gonadal hormones in the pathogenesis and treatment of bone health

in patients with chronic kidney disease: A systematic review and meta-analysis. *Curr Osteoporos Rep.* 2018;**16**(6):674–692.

21. Silva BC, Leslie WD, Resch H, Lamy O, Lesnyak O, Binkley N, McCloskey EV, Kanis JA, Bilezikian JP. Trabecular bone score: A noninvasive analytical method based upon the DXA image. *J Bone Miner Res.* 2014;**29**(3):518–530.

22. Brunerová L, Ronová P, Verešová J, Beranová P, Potoèková J, Kasalický P, Rychlík I. Osteoporosis and impaired trabecular bone score in hemodialysis patients. *Kidney Blood Press Res.* 2016;**41**(3): 345–354.

23. Yavropoulou MP, Vaios V, Pikilidou M, Chryssogonidis I, Sachinidou M, Tournis S, Makris K, Kotsa K, Daniilidis M, Haritanti A, Liakopoulos V. Bone quality assessment as measured by trabecular bone score in patients with end-stage renal disease on dialysis. *J Clin Densitom.* 2017;**20**(4):490–497.

24. Aleksova J, Kurniawan S, Elder GJ. The trabecular bone score is associated with bone mineral density, markers of bone turnover and prevalent fracture in patients with end stage kidney disease. *Osteoporos Int.* 2018;**29**(6):1447–1455.

25. Nickolas TL, Stein EM, Dworakowski E, Nishiyama KK, Komandah-Kosseh M, Zhang CA, McMahon DJ, Liu XS, Boutroy S, Cremers S, Shane E. Rapid cortical bone loss in patients with chronic kidney disease. *J Bone Miner Res.* 2013;**28**(8):1811–1820.

26. Nickolas TL, Stein E, Cohen A, Thomas V, Staron RB, McMahon DJ, Leonard MB, Shane E. Bone mass and microarchitecture in CKD patients with fracture. *J Am Soc Nephrol.* 2010;**21**(8):1371–1380.

27. Nickolas TL, McMahon DJ, Shane E. Relationship between moderate to severe kidney disease and hip fracture in the United States. *J Am Soc Nephrol.* 2006;**17**(11):3223–3232.

28. Klawansky S, Komaroff E, Cavanaugh PF, Jr, Mitchell DY, Gordon MJ, Connelly JE, Ross SD. Relationship between age, renal function and bone mineral density in the US population. *Osteoporos Int.* 2003; **14**(7):570–576.

29. Yenchek RH, Ix JH, Shlipak MG, Bauer DC, Rianon NJ, Kritchevsky SB, Harris TB, Newman AB, Cauley JA, Fried LF, for the Health, Aging, and Body Composition Study. Bone mineral density and fracture risk in older individuals with CKD. *Clin J Am Soc Nephrol.* 2012;**7**(7): 1130–1136.

30. Bervoets ARJ, Spasovski GB, Behets GJ, Dams G, Polenakovic MH, Zafirovska K, Van Hoof VO, De Broe ME, D'Haese PC. Useful biochemical markers for diagnosing renal osteodystrophy in predialysis end-stage renal failure patients. *Am J Kidney Dis.* 2003;**41**(5): 997–1007.

31. Sprague SM, Bellorin-Font E, Jorgetti V, Carvalho AB, Malluche HH, Ferreira A, D'Haese PC, Drüeke TB, Du H, Manley T, Rojas E, Moe SM. Diagnostic accuracy of bone turnover markers and bone histology in patients with CKD treated by dialysis. *Am J Kidney Dis.* 2016;**67**(4): 559–566.

32. Malluche HH, Mawad HW, Monier-Faugere MC. Renal osteodystrophy in the first decade of the new millennium: Analysis of 630 bone biopsies in black and white patients. *J Bone Miner Res.* 2011;**26**(6): 1368–1376.

33. Miller PD, Schwartz EN, Chen P, Misurski DA, Krege JH. Teriparatide in postmenopausal women with osteoporosis and mild or moderate renal impairment. *Osteoporos Int.* 2007;**18**(1):59–68.

34. Iimori S, Mori Y, Akita W, Kuyama T, Takada S, Asai T, Kuwahara M, Sasaki S, Tsukamoto Y. Diagnostic usefulness of bone mineral density and biochemical markers of bone turnover in predicting fracture in CKD stage 5D patients: A single-center cohort study. *Nephrol Dial Transplant.* 2012;**27**(1):345–351.

35. Moe SM, Abdalla S, Chertow GM, Parfrey PS, Block GA, Correa-Rotter R, Floege J, Herzog CA, London GM, Mahaffey KW, Wheeler DC, Dehmel B, Goodman WG, Drüeke TB, for the Evaluation of Cinacalcet HCl Therapy to Lower Cardiovascular Events (EVOLVE) Trial Investigators. Effects of cinacalcet on fracture events in patients receiving hemodialysis: The EVOLVE trial. *J Am Soc Nephrol.* 2015; **26**(6):1466–1475.

36. Rudser KD, de Boer IH, Dooley A, Young B, Kestenbaum B. Fracture risk after parathyroidectomy among chronic hemodialysis patients. *J Am Soc Nephrol.* 2007;**18**(8):2401–2407.

37. Miller PD, Roux C, Boonen S, Barton IP, Dunlap LE, Burgio DE. Safety and efficacy of risedronate in patients with age-related reduced renal function as estimated by the Cockcroft and Gault method: A pooled analysis of nine clinical trials. *J Bone Miner Res.* 2005;**20**(12): 2105–2115.

38. Jamal SA, Bauer DC, Ensrud KE, Cauley JA, Hochberg M, Ishani A, Cummings SR. Alendronate treatment in women with normal to severely impaired renal function: An analysis of the fracture intervention trial. *J Bone Miner Res.* 2007;**22**(4):503–508.

39. Jamal SA, Ljunggren O, Stehman-Breen C, Cummings SR, McClung MR, Goemaere S, Ebeling PR, Franek E, Yang YC, Egbuna OI, Boonen S, Miller PD. Effects of denosumab on fracture and bone mineral density by level of kidney function. *J Bone Miner Res.* 2011;**26**(8): 1829–1835.

40. Broadwell A, Ebeling PR, Franek E, Goemaere S, Wagman RB, Yin X, Yue S, Miller PD. Safety and efficacy of denosumab among subjects with mild-to-moderate chronic kidney disease (CKD) in the "Fracture REduction Evaluation of Denosumab in Osteoporosis every 6 Months" extension study [abstract]. *Arthritis Rheumatol.* 2017;**69**(Suppl 10): Abstract 1889.

Osteoporosis: Sequential Therapy, Treatment Failure, and Drug Holiday

M41
Presented, March 23–26, 2019

Dolores Shoback, MD. University of California, San Francisco, San Francisco, California 94158; and San Francisco Veterans Affairs Medical Center, San Francisco, California 94158, E-mail: dolores.shoback@ucsf.edu

Kelly Wentworth, MD. University of California, San Francisco, San Francisco, California 94158, E-mail: kelly.wentworth@ucsf.edu

SIGNIFICANCE OF THE CLINICAL PROBLEM

Osteoporosis is a common medical condition and a major public health concern, particularly as the population ages. Osteoporosis leads to debilitating fractures of the hip, spine, and other sites, causing substantial morbidity and mortality. Approximately 40% of women and one fifth of men over the age of 50 years will sustain a fragility fracture in their remaining lifetimes (1). We now have strong, randomized, placebo-controlled clinical trials that support the use of bisphosphonates, a receptor activator of nuclear factor κ-B ligand inhibitor, and parathyroid hormone (1–33) [PTH (1–33)] and a PTH-related protein analog in the treatment of men and women with osteoporosis, with the overall goal of reducing fracture risk and maintaining quality of life.

Although most practitioners are comfortable with implementing initial treatment strategies for osteoporosis, decisions about how long to treat patients, when to consider a drug holiday, and when to implement sequential therapy for refractory disease are considerably more challenging. During this session, we will review the recommended approach toward patients in whom current treatment has failed or who might benefit from switching to an alternative agent. We also will provide a data-driven approach to using sequential therapy in patients with severe osteoporosis or in those who are at high risk of fracture. Finally, we will provide an approach to help to determine which patients might be candidates for a drug holiday, how to monitor them during the holiday, and when to consider reinitiating pharmacotherapy.

BARRIERS TO OPTIMAL PRACTICE

- Lack of consensus about what constitutes treatment failure and when to consider switching to a different pharmacologic agent
- Difficulty in identifying patients who might benefit from a drug holiday vs those who are at high risk of fracture and should remain on pharmacotherapy
- Lack of clear guidelines on how to monitor patients during a drug holiday, how long to continue the drug holiday, and when to reinitiate pharmacotherapy

LEARNING OBJECTIVES

As a result of participating in this session, learners should be able to:

- Apply an evidence-based approach to sequential therapy in patients with osteoporosis
- Identify patients who might be at risk for treatment failure
- Identify patients who might benefit from escalation in pharmacotherapy
- Identify appropriate candidates for a drug holiday and develop a careful monitoring plan

MANAGEMENT STRATEGIES

Initial Therapy

Oral bisphosphonates are the initial recommended pharmacotherapy for most patients with osteoporosis on the basis of randomized controlled clinical trials that have demonstrated a reduction in vertebral, nonvertebral, and hip fractures with these treatments (2). For patients who cannot tolerate an oral bisphosphonate (esophageal disorders, inability to remain upright for 30 minutes after taking the medication) or who have underlying malabsorptive conditions (Roux-en-Y gastric bypass surgery, untreated celiac disease), an intravenous (IV) bisphosphonate may be given (3).

In patients with severe osteoporosis (defined as a T-score of < −3.5 at any site or a history of fragility fracture and a T-score of < −2.5 at any site), it is reasonable to consider an anabolic agent (teriparatide, abaloparatide) as initial therapy (4, 5). In the Fracture Prevention Trial, postmenopausal women who were treated with teriparatide (20 μg) for approximately 21 months had an increase in bone mineral density (BMD) (9% at lumbar spine, 3% at femoral neck) and a reduction in both vertebral and nonvertebral fractures (5% vs 14% and 3% vs 6%, respectively) compared with placebo (4). Similarly, in the ACTIVE trial, patients who were randomized to receive abaloparatide (80 μg) for 18 months had an increase in BMD at all sites and a decrease in vertebral fractures (0.5% vs 4.22% vs 0.84%) compared with placebo and teriparatide, respectively, and a decrease in nonvertebral fractures (2.7% vs 4.7%) compared with placebo (5). The results of these studies show that treatment with an anabolic agent for 2 years results in a substantial increase in BMD and a decrease in vertebral and nonvertebral fractures.

Sequential Therapy

Clinical trial data have shown that BMD begins to steadily decline after completion of anabolic therapy. This decline in

BMD can be mitigated by initiating an antiresorptive agent after treatment with an anabolic agent. In the PaTH trial, women who were treated for 1 year with PTH followed by 1 year of alendronate had an additional 6% increase in BMD compared with those who received 1 year of PTH followed by 1 year of placebo (6). Similarly, the EUROFORS trial evaluated the use of 1 year of teriparatide followed by raloxifene vs placebo and noted a 7.8% vs 3.8%, respectively, increase in lumbar spine BMD from baseline at 24 months (7). The DATA-Switch trial showed that 2 years of teriparatide followed by 2 years of denosumab leads to a sustained increase in BMD (8.6% at the lumbar spine, 5.6% at the femoral neck, and 4.7% at the total hip) compared with baseline (8). There are no available data at this time to assess definitively whether ongoing fracture risk is reduced in these patients. Preliminary data from the ongoing ACTIVExtend trial showed similar findings (9). In this study, patients received 18 months of abaloparatide or placebo followed by alendronate. After 6 months of treatment with alendronate, BMD improved at all sites, and the number of new vertebral and nonvertebral fractures was lower in the abaloparatide-alendronate group than in the placebo-alendronate group (0.55% vs 4.4%) (9). The results from these clinical trials support the use of an antiresorptive agent or raloxifene after 2 years of anabolic therapy.

Combination Therapy

Several trials have explored whether administering a PTH peptide concomitantly with another agent (bisphosphonate, denosumab, raloxifene, or estrogen) results in cumulative gains in BMD and additional fracture risk reduction. When PTH was given along with alendronate, no additional increase in BMD was noted compared with PTH alone (10–12). In one study, patients in the PTH-alone group had twice the increase in volumetric trabecular bone density compared with those receiving combination therapy (12). Of note, we have no data evaluating the effect of combination therapy on fracture rates. At this time, there does not seem to be any additional benefit to combination therapy with teriparatide and bisphosphonates. Similar findings were noted using combination therapy with teriparatide and raloxifene or estrogen (7, 13, 14). The DATA Extension Study evaluated the combination of teriparatide and denosumab therapy (15). In this study, patients who received 1 year of teriparatide and denosumab had a significantly higher increase in BMD than with either drug alone. This effect persisted at 2 years on this therapy. However, after the 2-year time point, the increase in BMD was the same among all groups. This study did not assess fracture outcomes. Because the differences did not persist after 2 years and costs of treatment are higher with two agents, we do not currently recommend combined treatment with teriparatide and denosumab (15).

One remaining question is whether initiating treatment with an antiresorptive medication before starting an anabolic agent has any effect on the response to anabolic therapy. In the DATA-Switch trial, women who received pretreatment with 1 year of denosumab followed by teriparatide had a lower overall BMD response than those treated with teriparatide first followed by denosumab (8). As such, when possible, we recommend using teriparatide followed by denosumab and avoiding the sequence of denosumab followed by teriparatide (8). In contrast, no data suggest that treatment with a bisphosphonate before an anabolic agent attenuates the effect on BMD or fracture risk reduction.

Treatment Failure

The primary goal in osteoporosis treatment is to reduce the risk of developing a fragility fracture at the hip, spine, and other skeletal sites. Response to therapy typically is monitored by obtaining a duel-energy x-ray absorptiometry (DXA) scan 1 to 2 years after therapy is initiated. If the BMD remains stable as defined by not exceeding the least significant change (LSC) or increases above the LSC, these are considered to be expected treatment responses. The situation becomes more complex if the BMD decreases (exceeding the LSC) or if the patient develops a fracture during therapy. Both of these scenarios should prompt additional evaluation, and consideration should be given to changing therapies. There are no clear consensus guidelines about when treatment has failed in a patient; therefore, the course of action for each patient must be individualized. The International Osteoporosis Foundation and National Osteoporosis Foundation have published guidelines on what constitutes treatment failure that are heavily based on expert opinion. They define treatment failure as follows (16):

1. Two or more incident fragility fractures
2. One incident fracture and elevated serum β-C-telopeptide (CTX) or P1NP at baseline with no substantial reduction during treatment, a substantial decrease in BMD, or both
3. Both no substantial decrease in β-CTX or P1NP and a substantial decrease in BMD

For patients in whom the BMD decreases by greater than or equal to the LSC on DXA scan, we recommend evaluating for medication adherence as well as for any factors that might contribute to decreased gastrointestinal absorption, particularly if a patient is taking an oral bisphosphonate. If adherence or malabsorption are the primary issues, then consideration should be given to switching to parenteral therapy with an IV bisphosphonate. These recommendations are predicated on the idea that BMD correlates with fracture risk.

In a patient with osteoporosis who sustains two fragility fractures while on at least 1 year of therapy, consideration should be given to switching to an anabolic agent, such as teriparatide or abaloparatide. This therapy then can be followed by an antiresorptive agent such as a bisphosphonate or denosumab. We now have solid data to support the use of sequential medications in osteoporosis, when clinically indicated, as discussed above.

Clinicians should be aware of risk factors that might lead to a poor response to treatment. These include ongoing or untreated secondary causes of osteoporosis, inadequate calcium or vitamin D intake, and history of osteoporotic fracture. Additional risk factors for fracture risk include glucocorticoid use, frequent falls, and weight loss (17).

When to Consider a Drug Holiday

The FLEX and HORIZON extension trials demonstrated that long-term bisphosphonate use (10 years of alendronate or 6 years of zoledronic acid) is associated with an ongoing decrease in vertebral fracture rates (18, 19). Subgroup analyses have shown that the greatest benefit is gained in high-risk patients, as defined by age >70 years, femoral neck T-score < −2.5, history of major osteoporotic fracture before therapy, or fracture during therapy. In these patients, the benefit of continuing therapy for an additional 5 years (alendronate) or 3 years (zoledronic acid) likely outweighs the potential risks (1). In lower-risk patients, however, the increased risks associated with prolonged bisphosphonate therapy, particularly the risk of developing an atypical femoral fracture, may outweigh the benefits of continuing therapy. Thus, it is reasonable to consider a drug holiday for these lower-risk patients.

The American Society of Bone and Mineral Research Task Force has developed clear, evidence-based guidelines for when to continue long-term bisphosphonate therapy vs when to consider a drug holiday (1). These recommendations are heavily based on the results from the FLEX and HORIZON extension trials described above (Fig. 1). We agree with these guidelines and recommend that patients with osteoporosis who have received a total of 3 to 5 years of oral bisphosphonate therapy or 3 years of IV bisphosphonate therapy and are at low risk for future fractures [age <70 years, have no history of fracture, have not experienced a fracture while on therapy, and have stable or improved BMD at the femoral neck (T-score > −2.5)] be considered for a drug holiday. Conversely, bisphosphonate treatment should be extended to a total of 10 years (for oral bisphosphonates) or 6 years (for IV bisphosphonates) if a patient is at high risk of future fragility fracture, as defined above. Note that these guidelines are based on studies in postmenopausal women, and whether they are applicable to men with osteoporosis and patients with glucocorticoid-induced osteoporosis remains unknown.

No consensus exists on the appropriate length of a drug holiday or what factors should prompt reinitiation of pharmacotherapy. The American Association of Clinical Endocrinologists guidelines recommend following serial DXA scans and bone turnover markers (BTMs) and reinitiating therapy either when the BMD declines beyond the LSC or when the BTMs return to pretreatment baseline (20). The American Society of Bone and Mineral Research Task Force also recommends monitoring during a drug holiday, but the optimal frequency of DXA and BTM measurements is not clearly defined, particularly because BTM and DXA measurements at 1 year posttreatment did not accurately predict future fracture risk during the FLEX trial (18, 21). The ASBMR recommendations to resume therapy once the T-score falls below −2.5 or

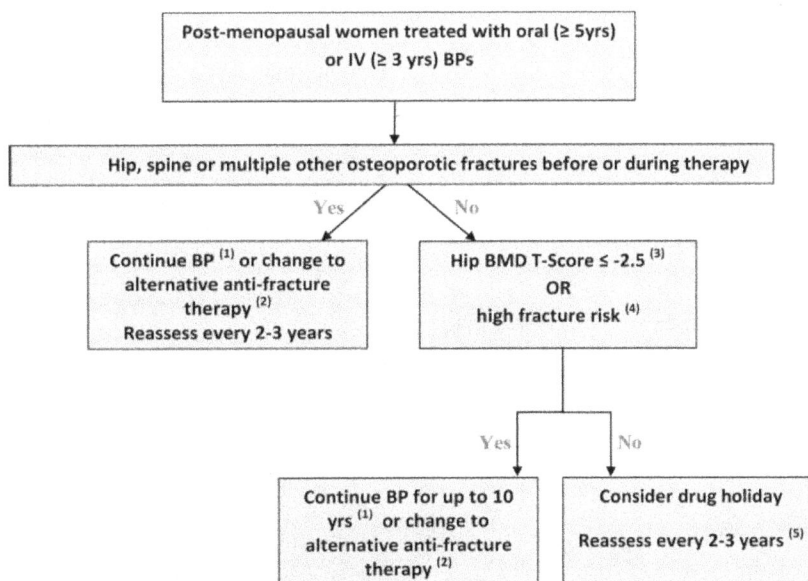

Figure 1. Algorithm for the management of postmenopausal women on long-term bisphosphonate (BP) therapy. Reproduced with permission from Adler RA, Fuleihan GE-H, Bauer DC, et al. Managing osteoporosis in patients on long-term bisphosphonate treatment: Report of a task force of the American Society for Bone and Mineral Research. *J Bone Miner Res.* 2016;31(1):16–35.

when the fracture risk has increased come primarily from expert opinion. All groups recommend close monitoring of calcium and vitamin D intake to ensure that patients receive at least 1200 mg/d of elemental calcium and maintain vitamin D levels >30 ng/mL.

At the start of the drug holiday, we recommend obtaining a DXA scan and BTM measurement to confirm that bone turnover currently is suppressed. We then encourage adequate calcium and vitamin D repletion for the duration of the drug holiday. We recommend assessing the patient annually for new fractures and repeating DXA and BTM measurements at 2 years. If the patient continues to meet criteria for a drug holiday, this can be continued with the same monitoring strategy. If the patient's BMD declines or a new fracture occurs, this is an indication to resume therapy.

DISCUSSION OF CASES AND ANSWERS
Case 1: Treatment Failure
A 66-year-old white woman is referred to the clinic for evaluation of possible treatment failure and lack of response to osteoporosis medications. In 2004, at age 56 years, she underwent menopause with hot flashes and cessation of menses and did not take any hormonal therapy. Her first DXA scan was done at that time, and she was diagnosed with osteoporosis [lumbar spine BMD, 0.593 g/cm^2 (T-score, −4.1); total hip BMD, 0.618 g/cm^2 (T-score, −2.7); femoral neck BMD, 0.514 g/cm^2 (T-score, −3.0)].

Medical and Surgical History
1. Hypothyroidism since age 40 years treated with levothyroxine 0.100 mg/d
2. Mild stable anemia with negative colonoscopy
3. Mild stable asthma and receipt of inhaled corticosteroids for 3 to 4 years (10 years prior) but not using recently
4. Xanthogranulomatous pyelonephritis status post–right nephrectomy
5. Cesarean sections in 1977 and 1979

Family History
The patient believes that her mother had osteoporosis because her height decreased over time, but she never had a DXA scan, and there is no history of fractures in the patient's mother, father, or grandparents. There is a history of cardiovascular disease leading to death in family members, breast cancer in mother, and Alzheimer disease in other family members.

Social History
The patient is a former smoker (less than one pack per day for approximately 7 years; quit in 1972); she drinks approximately one glass of wine three times a week. She exercises three times a week. Her diet includes at least two dairy servings per day.

Treatment Course
The patient was initiated on weekly risedronate (35 mg) in 2005 and was told to take calcium supplements and 1000 IU vitamin D3, which she did, in addition to continuing her levothyroxine replacement and daily montelukast. In 2008, raloxifene was added to the regimen because of a minimal response in BMD and a family history of breast cancer. In 2010, repeat DXA showed stable BMD, and both medications were continued. In 2012, she sustained a right-sided comminuted radial fracture after a ground-level fall, which required surgical repair. In 2014, both risedronate and raloxifene were stopped because of declining BMD and no consistent response to treatment. At that time, the patient was referred to our institution for further consultation. Her treatment course is summarized in Table 1.

Review of Systems
The patient had no dermatologic, ophthalmic, pulmonary, cardiovascular, gastrointestinal, neurologic, psychiatric, rheumatologic, or urologic complaints. There was no weight loss, height loss, or back pain.

Medications in 2014
The patient took calcium supplements, vitamin D3 1000 IU/d, montelukast 10 mg, and levothyroxine 0.1 mg/d.

Physical Examination
The patient was a well-developed, well-nourished–appearing woman in no distress. She was 5 ft tall and weighed 100.9 lb. Her pulse was 56 beats/min and blood pressure, 102/55 mm Hg. There was no rash or skin lesions and no bone deformities or back pain. The remainder of the examination was within normal limits. We next conducted a secondary evaluation for osteoporosis.

Laboratory Evaluation in 2014
The patient's chemistry panel findings were as follows: sodium, 134 mmol/L; potassium, 4.1 mmol/L; chloride, 100 mmol/L; carbon dioxide, 28 mmol/L; blood urea nitrogen, 16 mg/dL; chromium, 0.8 μg/L; calcium, 9.6 mg/dL; total protein, 7.3 g/dL; albumin, 4.3 g/dL; glucose, 89 mg/dL; alkaline phosphatase, 48 U/L (30 to 115 U/L); aspartate aminotransferase, 32 U/L; alanine aminotransferase, 27 U/L; uric acid, 5.7 mg/dL; PTH, 45 pg/mL (normal range, 12 to 65 pg/mL); and 25-hydroxy (25-OH) vitamin D, 44 ng/mL (normal range, 20 to 100 ng/mL).

Her 24-hour urine findings were 84.6 mg/24 h calcium, volume 1968 mL, and 742 mg/24 h creatinine. The patient's complete blood count (CBC) findings were hemoglobin, 10.8 g/dL (mean corpuscular volume, 85 μm^3) with normal white blood cell and differential and platelet counts. Her iron study findings were as follows: iron 32 (initial measurement),

Table 1.   Case 1 Treatment Course

Date (Patient's Age)[a]	LS BMD (g/cm²) (T-Score)	Total Hip BMD (g/cm²) (T-Score)	Femoral Neck BMD (g/cm²) (T-Score)	Actions/Events
11/2004 (56 years)	0.593 (−4.1)	0.618 (−2.7)	0.514 (−3.0)	
2005				Started weekly risedronate
5/2006 (58 years)	0.595 (−4.1)	0.624 (−2.6)	0.509 (−3.1)	
9/2007 (59 years)	0.613 (−3.9)	0.655 (−2.4)	0.515 (−3.0)	
Change in BMD (2004–2007), %	+3.4	+6	No change	
2008				Raloxifene daily added
9/2010 (62 years)	0.602 (−4.0)	0.621 (−2.6)	0.511 (−3.0)	BMD considered stable, both medications continued
2012				Ground-level fall after tripping, right radial fracture, repaired surgically
4/2012 (64 years)	0.573 (−4.3)	0.598 (−2.8)	0.540 (−2.8)	Medications continued
5/2014 (66 years)	0.570 (−4.3)	0.554 (−3.2)	0.510 (−3.1)	
Change in BMD (2010–2014), %	−5.3	−10.6	No change	
2014				Both risedronate (7–8 years treatment) and raloxifene (6 years treatment) stopped

Abbreviation: LS, lumbar spine.
[a] At another facility.

41 (repeated measurement) μg/dL (normal range, 29 to 189 μg/dL); saturation, 11% (10% to 47%); transferrin, 269 mg/dL (182 to 360 mg/dL); ferritin, 7 μg/L (10 to 291 μg/L); sedimentation rate, 43.7 mm/h; serum protein electrophoresis (SPEP), normal with no M spike; thyrotropin (TSH), 4.2 mIU/L, free T_4, 1.42 ng/dL, total T_3, 91.3 ng/dL; antitissue transglutaminase, >100 CU (strongly positive, positive >30 CU).

November 2014 Thoracolumbar Spine X-Ray (Anteroposterior and Lateral)
The patient had moderately severe osteopenia throughout the thoracic and lumbar spine without substantial compression fracture. Disc spaces are well preserved. Alignment was satisfactory with a minimal upper thoracic curve to the right at the T5 to T6 level.

Endoscopy and Colonoscopy
The patient's endoscopy and colonoscopy showed gastritis as well as mucosal atrophy in the duodenum consistent with celiac disease. The pathology report showed severe mucosal atrophy.

Management
A gluten-free diet and iron supplements were initiated along with daily teriparatide therapy in 2015 (Table 2). Bowel habits remained the same, with one or two formed stools per day, her lifelong pattern. Over the next 2 years, antitissue transglutaminase antibody titers normalized, iron studies improved to normal, levels of ferritin and hemoglobin improved, and urinary calcium levels increased to 170 mg/24 h. 25-OH vitamin D levels remained in the range of 40 to 45 ng/mL.

1. What is a sufficient workup for secondary etiologies for osteoporosis in postmenopausal women, premenopausal women, and men with low BMD?

In patients in whom a secondary cause of osteoporosis is suspected, a thorough evaluation includes a complete metabolic panel, PTH, calcium, phosphorus, 25-OH vitamin D, CBC with differential, thyroid hormone levels, SPEP/urinary protein electrophoresis, iron and ferritin, gonadal status, glucocorticoid use or Cushing syndrome, and malabsorptive diseases such as celiac disease (22–26).

2. What is a treatment failure?

There is no clearly defined answer for what constitutes treatment failure. The International Osteoporosis Foundation and National Osteoporosis Foundation suggest that a substantial decline in BMD after 2 years on a therapy or sustaining two fractures while on therapy is consistent with treatment failure, as reviewed above. When a patient fails to respond to therapy as anticipated, this should prompt a thorough evaluation for possible secondary causes of osteoporosis.

3. How does malabsorption affect the response to treatment of osteoporosis?

Table 2. Case 1 Management

Date (Patient's Age)[a]	LS BMD (g/cm²) (T-Score)	Total Hip BMD (g/cm²) (T-Score)	Femoral Neck BMD (g/cm²) (T-Score)	Actions/Events
1/2015				Teriparatide started
11/2015 (67 years)	0.658 (−3.5)	0.636 (−2.5)	0.518 (−3.0)	10 months on teriparatide
11/2016 (68 years)	0.679 (−3.3)	0.636 (−2.5)	0.522 (−2.9)	
1/2017				Teriparatide stopped after 24 months, denosumab started
2/2018 (70 years)	0.761 (−2.6)	0.685 (−2.1)	0.547 (−2.7)	Denosumab continued every 6 months
Change in BMD (2015–2018), %	+7.3	+7.7	+5.6	
Nadir T-score to present T-score	−4.3 to −2.6	−3.2 to −2.1	−3.1 to −2.7	

Abbreviation: LS, lumbar spine.

[a] At the University of California, San Francisco, DXA laboratory.

Diseases that result in malabsorption affect both calcium and vitamin D absorption from the intestine as well as some of the oral medications like bisphosphonates. This can substantially affect the response to treatment.

4. Do treatments for osteoporosis work in patients who have secondary etiologies for low bone mass or fractures?

Treatments for osteoporosis work in some patients who have secondary etiologies for low bone mass, including glucocorticoid-induced osteoporosis or hypogonadal-induced osteoporosis. However, responses depend on the etiology for the bone loss.

Case 2: Sequential/Combination Therapy

A 58-year-old white woman was referred after a hospital admission for the management of osteoporosis and fracture. One week before the office visit, she was admitted to University of California, San Francisco, Medical Center for evaluation and management of intractable back pain. The patient relates that she was on her way to work in the morning and noted acute severe lumbar back pain and heard a "pop." She rated the initial pain as 10 out of 10, radiating into both legs. She missed 3 days of work and presented to the emergency department with intractable pain and an inability to care for herself. She denied saddle anesthesia, numbness, and bowel or bladder incontinence or weakness. An x-ray done in the emergency department showed a moderate compression fracture of L1 of indeterminate age.

Medical History

The patient experienced menarche at age 12 years, had one full-term pregnancy, lactated 1 to 2 months, and began menopause with hot flushes at age 50 to 51 years. She had no history of eating disorders, amenorrhea, or corticosteroid or medroxyprogesterone acetate injection use. After menopause, she took no estrogen therapy.

At age 54 years, while cleaning her house, the patient tripped over a table and hit her rib cage. She did not present for x-rays, but she had several weeks of rib pain and wondered whether she fractured a rib. At her annual examination, her gynecologist ordered a DXA scan [L2 to L4 BMD, 0.717 g/cm² (T-score, –3.3); total hip BMD, 0.754 g/cm² (T-score, –1.5); femoral neck BMD, 0.583 g/cm² (T-score, 2.4)].

Fracture Risk Assessment Scores

The patient's fracture risk assessment scores showed a 10-year major osteoporotic fracture risk of 5.5% and a 10-year hip fracture risk of 0.6%. On the basis of these scores, calcium and vitamin D3 supplements and weight-bearing exercise were recommended.

Medications

The patient's medications included 1000 mg calcium, 1000 IU vitamin D3, nasal spray calcitonin 200 IU/d (started in the hospital), cyclobenzaprine 10 mg/d, and acetaminophen 1000 mg three times daily.

Family History

The patient had a family history of osteoporosis in her mother and father (both treated) and breast cancer in her mother. She is a nonsmoker and drinks one glass of wine 5 d/wk. She has minimal dairy intake and exercises infrequently.

Physical Examination (in Clinic)

The patient was 5 ft, 7 in (170.2 cm), tall and weighed 136 lb (61.8 kg). She was noted to be in pain, wearing brace, and unable to sit still during the interview.

Table 3. Case 2 DXA Findings

Age at DXA Scan	L2–L4 (g/cm^2) (T-Score)	Total Hip (g/cm^2) (T-Score)	Femoral Neck (g/cm^2) (T-Score)
54 years	0.717 (−3.3)	0.754 (−1.5)	0.583 (−2.4)
58 years	0.683 (−3.6)	0.737 (−1.7)	0.551 (−2.7)
Change, %	−4.7	−2.3	−5.5

Her spine was diffusely tender with guarding. The patient was unable to lean forward without pain or lie flat. No Cushing stigmata, no blue sclerae, no long bone pain or deformity was present. She was neurologically intact to motor and sensory testing but had a slow gait.

Imaging Review (From the Hospitalization)

Thoracic and lumbar spine x-rays showed an L1 compression fracture (50% to 60% height loss) with mild osseous retropulsion and a T7 compression fracture (~40% height loss); both were age indeterminate.

Spine CT

A CT scan of the patient's spine showed acute an L1 compression fracture (50% height loss) with a 1-cm bony retropulsion; no lytic or sclerotic bone lesions were otherwise noted.

Spine MRI (T2 Weighted, Fat Suppressed)

The patient had a posterior-superior endplate L1 fracture with retropulsion and mild canal narrowing at this level but no abnormal cord signal, cord compression, or epidural hematoma. High signal intensity on MRI suggested an acute or subacute fracture.

1. What would be your evaluation at this time?

We recommend performing the following laboratory and imaging studies. The patient's chemistry panel, CBC, SPEP, urinary protein electrophoresis, quantitative immunoglobulin levels, liver and thyroid function tests, antitissue transglutaminase, intact PTH, and 25-OH vitamin D were all normal. Her DXA findings at ages 54 and 58 years are shown in Table 3.

2. Now that you know that the patient is actively losing bone mass and has two vertebral compression fractures (one moderate, one severe), what therapy would you consider? What important adjunctive treatment should be included?

The decision at this time is whether the patient would benefit from antiresorptive therapy, anabolic therapy, or a combination of both. As reviewed above, combination therapy regimens that have been reported include: estrogen plus PTH (13, 27), alendronate plus PTH (12), and PTH plus denosumab (15). Sequential regimens reported include PTH followed by denosumab or denosumab followed by PTH (8) and abaloparatide followed by alendronate (9). Given the advantageous combination of PTH followed by denosumab, we decided to treat this patient with teriparatide for 2 years with the plan to follow this with denosumab.

3. What course would you take after initiating anabolic therapy with teriparatide? For how long would you treat this patient? Are there any precautions that you would warn this patient about regarding timeliness and compliance with future treatments?

Anabolic therapy should be followed by an antiresorptive agent, such as a bisphosphonate or denosumab. Lack of adherence to the antiresorptive agent will lead to a subsequent decline in BMD compared with strict adherence. Denosumab in particular has a rapid on-off effect, with a return to the baseline BMD within 12 to 18 months after treatment is stopped (28). It is, therefore, strongly recommended that patients treated with denosumab not miss doses and receive doses of this medication exactly on schedule to avoid rebound increases in bone turnover; rapid loss of BMD; and the small, but real possibility of experiencing rebound vertebral fractures in the setting of discontinuing this therapy (29–33). Table 4 summarizes the patient's DXA findings over 4 years.

Follow-up therapy was with denosumab (60 mg every 6 months). No further fractures have occurred.

Case 3: Drug Holiday

A 64-year-old woman presents for assessment of skeletal status. Her history includes normal age of menarche at 12 years with two full-term pregnancies. She had regular menstrual cycles until age 52 to 53 years when she went through menopause. She took no hormone therapy. At age 55 years, she sustained a fall in her garage and had a severe tibial fracture that required repeated casting and nonweight bearing for ~6 months. Her internist obtained a DXA scan and referred her to the clinic for evaluation.

Table 4. Case 2 Summary of DXA Findings Over 4 Years

Age at DXA Scan	L2–L4 (g/cm^2) (T-Score)	Total Hip (g/cm^2) (T-Score)	Femoral Neck (g/cm^2) (T-Score)
54 years	0.717 (−3.3)	0.754 (−1.5)	0.583 (−2.4)
58 years	0.683 (−3.6)	0.737 (−1.7)	0.551 (−2.7)
60 years	0.793 (−2.6)	0.761 (−1.5)	0.585 (−2.4)
Change in 2-year teriparatide, %	+16.1	+3.3	+6.2

Medical History

1. Chronic lymphocytic leukemia with minimal lymph-adenopathy, no infections, organomegaly, or cytopenias; with routine follow-up, no indications for treatment (stage 0 to 1)
2. Multinodular goiter, euthyroid, with two biopsy specimens negative for malignant cells
3. Esophagitis and chronic reflux
4. Scoliosis since teenage years, progressively worsening
5. Hypertension

Family History

The patient has a family history for cardiovascular disease, diabetes, and hypertension but no history for fractures and osteoporosis.

Social History

The patient is a nonsmoker, rarely consumes alcohol, exercises infrequently, and consumes dairy daily.

Medications

The patients takes ranitidine, omeprazole, calcium carbonate 500 mg, vitamin D3 3000 IU/d, trazodone, escitalopram, gabapentin, and valsartan.

Physical Examination

The patient's physical examination was positive for moderate scoliosis, multinodular goiter, and minimal cervical lymph-adenopathy but otherwise was normal.

Laboratory Studies (2018)

The patient had a normal CBC (white blood cell count, 12,700/μL with 8,070/μL lymphocytes) and normal liver function tests; chemistry panel findings; and calcium, albumin, and PTH levels. Her 25-OH vitamin D level was 48 ng/mL, and free T_4 and TSH were normal.

Management

On the basis of the patient's DXA scan in 2010, the initial plan was to treat her with 3 years of IV bisphosphonate. She received her last dose of IV zoledronic acid in 2012 and has been on drug holiday since 2013 (now at 4 years in 2018). She is now 10 years since onset of menopause at her current age of 64 years. The patient has not had any new fractures. Her spinal BMD has declined from the peak response to first course of treatment by –9%, with a more-modest change at the femoral neck. Her bone resorption marker serum CTX has risen to near the premenopausal upper limit of normal. The patient's orthopedic surgeon has noted that her scoliosis may require surgery at some point and that his general preference for spine healing is to avoid bisphosphonate. The patient's treatment course is summarized in Table 5.

1. How do you interpret the BMD changes and the changes in serum CTX?

The serum CTX was initially appropriately suppressed while treated with bisphosphonate but has now risen to the upper limit of normal for a premenopausal woman. The patient's BMD at the total hip is stable but has decreased by greater than the LSC in the spine.

Table 5.   Case 3 Treatment Course Summary

Year (Patient's Age)	LS (L1, L2) (g/cm²) (T-Score)	Total Hip (g/cm²) (T-Score)	Femoral Neck (g/cm²) (T-Score)	Serum CTX (40–465 pg/mL)	Actions/Events
2007 (52–53 years)					Menopause
2009 (55 years)					Slowly healing tibial fracture
2010 (56 years)	0.680 (−3.0)	0.809 (−1.1)	0.656 (−1.7)	283, 299	5 mg zoledronic acid given after fracture healed
2011 (57 years)				70	5 mg zoledronic acid
2012 (58 years)				99	5 mg zoledronic acid
2013 (59 years)	0.766 (−1.9)	0.812 (−1.1)	0.671 (−1.6)	202	Drug holiday starts
Change (2010–2013), %	+12.6	Not different	Not different		
2015 (60 years)	0.727 (−2.3)	0.811 (−1.1)	0.680 (−1.5)	286	Drug holiday continued
2017 (62 years)	0.697 (−2.6)	0.807 (−1.1)	0.650 (−1.7)	435	Drug holiday continued
Change (2013–2017), %	−9.0	Not different	−3.1		
2018					Drug holiday continued

Abbreviation: LS, lumbar spine.

2. Would you continue the drug holiday? When do you resume treatment? What factors do you consider? What monitoring plan do you use?

A patient should be assessed for any new fractures annually at a clinic visit, and DXA and BTM measurements should be performed every 2 years, although evidence-based guidelines are lacking for setting these intervals. When considering whether to continue the drug holiday, we recommend initiating treatment when either a fracture has occurred, the BMD decrement exceeds the LSC, or the BTMs exceed the upper limit of normal. In this patient, consideration should be given to resuming therapy with an antiresorptive agent.

References

1. Adler RA, El-Hajj Fuleihan G, Bauer DC, Camacho PM, Clarke BL, Clines GA, Compston JE, Drake MT, Edwards BJ, Favus MJ, Greenspan SL, McKinney R, Jr, Pignolo RJ, Sellmeyer DE. Managing osteoporosis in patients on long-term bisphosphonate treatment: report of a task force of the American Society for Bone and Mineral Research. *J Bone Miner Res.* 2016;**31**(1):16–35.
2. Cummings SR, Black DM, Thompson DE, Applegate WB, Barrett-Connor E, Musliner TA, Palermo L, Prineas R, Rubin SM, Scott JC, Vogt T, Wallace R, Yates AJ, LaCroix AZ. Effect of alendronate on risk of fracture in women with low bone density but without vertebral fractures: results from the Fracture Intervention Trial. *JAMA.* 1998;**280**(24):2077–2082.
3. Eastell R, Lang T, Boonen S, Cummings S, Delmas PD, Cauley JA, Horowitz Z, Kerzberg E, Bianchi G, Kendler D, Leung P, Man Z, Mesenbrink P, Eriksen EF, Black DM; HORIZON Pivotal Fracture Trial. Effect of once-yearly zoledronic acid on the spine and hip as measured by quantitative computed tomography: results of the HORIZON Pivotal Fracture Trial. *Osteoporos Int.* 2010;**21**(7):1277–1285.
4. Neer RM, Arnaud CD, Zanchetta JR, Prince R, Gaich GA, Reginster JY, Hodsman AB, Eriksen EF, Ish-Shalom S, Genant HK, Wang O, Mitlak BH. Effect of parathyroid hormone (1-34) on fractures and bone mineral density in postmenopausal women with osteoporosis. *N Engl J Med.* 2001;**344**(19):1434–1441.
5. Miller PD, Hattersley G, Riis BJ, Williams GC, Lau E, Russo LA, Alexandersen P, Zerbini CA, Hu MY, Harris AG, Fitzpatrick LA, Cosman F, Christiansen C; ACTIVE Study Investigators. Effect of abaloparatide vs placebo on new vertebral fractures in postmenopausal women with osteoporosis: a randomized clinical trial. *JAMA.* 2016;**316**(7):722–733.
6. Black DM, Bilezikian JP, Ensrud KE, Greenspan SL, Palermo L, Hue T, Lang TF, McGowan JA, Rosen CJ; PaTH Study Investigators. One year of alendronate after one year of parathyroid hormone (1-84) for osteoporosis. *N Engl J Med.* 2005;**353**(6):555–565.
7. Eastell R, Nickelsen T, Marin F, Barker C, Hadji P, Farrerons J, Audran M, Boonen S, Brixen K, Gomes JM, Obermayer-Pietsch B, Avramidis A, Sigurdsson G, Glüer CC. Sequential treatment of severe postmenopausal osteoporosis after teriparatide: final results of the randomized, controlled European Study of Forsteo (EUROFORS). *J Bone Miner Res.* 2009;**24**(4):726–736.
8. Leder BZ, Tsai JN, Uihlein AV, Wallace PM, Lee H, Neer RM, Burnett-Bowie SA. Denosumab and teriparatide transitions in postmenopausal osteoporosis (the DATA-Switch study): extension of a randomised controlled trial. *Lancet.* 2015;**386**(9999):1147–1155.
9. Cosman F, Miller PD, Williams GC, Hattersley G, Hu MY, Valter I, Fitzpatrick LA, Riis BJ, Christiansen C, Bilezikian JP, Black D. Eighteen months of treatment with subcutaneous abaloparatide followed by 6 months of treatment with alendronate in postmenopausal women with osteoporosis: results of the ACTIVExtend Trial. *Mayo Clin Proc.* 2017;**92**(2):200–210.
10. Finkelstein JS, Hayes A, Hunzelman JL, Wyland JJ, Lee H, Neer RM. The effects of parathyroid hormone, alendronate, or both in men with osteoporosis. *N Engl J Med.* 2003;**349**(13):1216–1226.
11. Finkelstein JS, Leder BZ, Burnett SM, Wyland JJ, Lee H, de la Paz AV, Gibson K, Neer RM. Effects of teriparatide, alendronate, or both on bone turnover in osteoporotic men. *J Clin Endocrinol Metab.* 2006;**91**(8):2882–2887.
12. Black DM, Greenspan SL, Ensrud KE, Palermo L, McGowan JA, Lang TF, Garnero P, Bouxsein ML, Bilezikian JP, Rosen CJ; PaTH Study Investigators. The effects of parathyroid hormone and alendronate alone or in combination in postmenopausal osteoporosis. *N Engl J Med.* 2003;**349**(13):1207–1215.
13. Ste-Marie LG, Schwartz SL, Hossain A, Desaiah D, Gaich GA. Effect of teriparatide [rhPTH(1-34)] on BMD when given to postmenopausal women receiving hormone replacement therapy. *J Bone Miner Res.* 2006;**21**(2):283–291.
14. Cosman F, Nieves J, Woelfert L, Formica C, Gordon S, Shen V, Lindsay R. Parathyroid hormone added to established hormone therapy: effects on vertebral fracture and maintenance of bone mass after parathyroid hormone withdrawal. *J Bone Miner Res.* 2001;**16**(5):925–931.
15. Leder BZ, Tsai JN, Uihlein AV, Burnett-Bowie SA, Zhu Y, Foley K, Lee H, Neer RM. Two years of denosumab and teriparatide administration in postmenopausal women with osteoporosis (the DATA Extension Study): a randomized controlled trial. *J Clin Endocrinol Metab.* 2014;**99**(5):1694–1700.
16. Diez-Perez A, Adachi JD, Agnusdei D, Bilezikian JP, Compston JE, Cummings SR, Eastell R, Eriksen EF, Gonzalez-Macias J, Liberman UA, Wahl DA, Seeman E, Kanis JA, Cooper C; IOF CSA Inadequate Responders Working Group. Treatment failure in osteoporosis. *Osteoporos Int.* 2012;**23**(12):2769–2774.
17. Diez-Pérez A, Adachi JD, Adami S, Anderson FA, Jr, Boonen S, Chapurlat R, Compston JE, Cooper C, Gehlbach SH, Greenspan SL, Hooven FH, LaCroix AZ, Nieves JW, Netelenbos JC, Pfeilschifter J, Rossini M, Roux C, Saag KG, Silverman S, Siris ES, Wyman A, Rushton-Smith SK, Watts NB; Global Longitudinal Study of Osteoporosis in Women (GLOW) Investigators. Risk factors for treatment failure with antiosteoporosis medication: the global longitudinal study of osteoporosis in women (GLOW). *J Bone Miner Res.* 2014;**29**(1):260–267.
18. Black DM, Schwartz AV, Ensrud KE, Cauley JA, Levis S, Quandt SA, Satterfield S, Wallace RB, Bauer DC, Palermo L, Wehren LE, Lombardi A, Santora AC, Cummings SR; FLEX Research Group. Effects of continuing or stopping alendronate after 5 years of treatment: the Fracture Intervention Trial Long-term Extension (FLEX): a randomized trial. *JAMA.* 2006;**296**(24):2927–2938.
19. Black DM, Reid IR, Boonen S, Bucci-Rechtweg C, Cauley JA, Cosman F, Cummings SR, Hue TF, Lippuner K, Lakatos P, Leung PC, Man Z, Martinez RL, Tan M, Ruzycky ME, Su G, Eastell R. The effect of 3 versus 6 years of zoledronic acid treatment of osteoporosis: a randomized extension to the HORIZON-Pivotal Fracture Trial (PFT). *J Bone Miner Res.* 2012;**27**(2):243–254.
20. Watts NB, Bilezikian JP, Camacho PM, Greenspan SL, Harris ST, Hodgson SF, Kleerekoper M, Luckey MM, McClung MR, Pollack RP, Petak SM; AACE Osteoporosis Task Force. American Association of Clinical Endocrinologists Medical Guidelines for Clinical Practice for the diagnosis and treatment of postmenopausal osteoporosis. *Endocr Pract.* 2010;**16**(Suppl 3):1–37.
21. Bauer DC, Schwartz A, Palermo L, Cauley J, Hochberg M, Santora A, Cummings SR, Black DM. Fracture prediction after discontinuation of 4 to 5 years of alendronate therapy: the FLEX study. *JAMA Intern Med.* 2014;**174**(7):1126–1134.
22. Hjelle AM, Apalset E, Mielnik P, Bollerslev J, Lundin KE, Tell GS. Celiac disease and risk of fracture in adults—a review. *Osteoporos Int.* 2014;**25**(6):1667–1676.
23. Leffler DA, Green PH, Fasano A. Extraintestinal manifestations of coeliac disease. *Nat Rev Gastroenterol Hepatol.* 2015;**12**(10):561–571.
24. Real A, Gilbert N, Hauser B, Kennedy N, Shand A, Gillett H, Gillett P, Goddard C, Cebolla A, Sousa C, Fraser WD, Satsangi J, Ralston SH, Riches PL. Characterisation of osteoprotegerin autoantibodies in coeliac disease. *Calcif Tissue Int.* 2015;**97**(2):125–133.
25. Phan CM, Guglielmi G. Metabolic bone disease in patients with malabsorption. *Semin Musculoskelet Radiol.* 2016;**20**(4):369–375.

26. Zanchetta MB, Longobardi V, Bai JC. Bone and celiac disease. *Curr Osteoporos Rep.* 2016;**14**(2):43–48.

27. Lindsay R, Nieves J, Formica C, Henneman E, Woelfert L, Shen V, Dempster D, Cosman F. Randomised controlled study of effect of parathyroid hormone on vertebral-bone mass and fracture incidence among postmenopausal women on oestrogen with osteoporosis. *Lancet.* 1997;**350**(9077):550–555.

28. Bone HG, Bolognese MA, Yuen CK, Kendler DL, Miller PD, Yang YC, Grazette L, San Martin J, Gallagher JC. Effects of denosumab treatment and discontinuation on bone mineral density and bone turnover markers in postmenopausal women with low bone mass. *J Clin Endocrinol Metab.* 2011;**96**(4):972–980.

29. Aubry-Rozier B, Gonzalez-Rodriguez E, Stoll D, Lamy O. Severe spontaneous vertebral fractures after denosumab discontinuation: three case reports. *Osteoporos Int.* 2016;**27**(5):1923–1925.

30. Popp AW, Zysset PK, Lippuner K. Rebound-associated vertebral fractures after discontinuation of denosumab-from clinic and biomechanics. *Osteoporos Int.* 2016;**27**(5):1917–1921.

31. Anastasilakis AD, Polyzos SA, Makras P, Aubry-Rozier B, Kaouri S, Lamy O. Clinical features of 24 patients with rebound-associated vertebral fractures after denosumab discontinuation: systematic review and additional cases. *J Bone Miner Res.* 2017;**32**(6):1291–1296.

32. Anastasilakis AD, Yavropoulou MP, Makras P, Sakellariou GT, Papadopoulou F, Gerou S, Papapoulos SE. Increased osteoclastogenesis in patients with vertebral fractures following discontinuation of denosumab treatment. *Eur J Endocrinol.* 2017;**176**(6):677–683.

33. Tsourdi E, Langdahl B, Cohen-Solal M, Aubry-Rozier B, Eriksen EF, Guañabens N, Obermayer-Pietsch B, Ralston SH, Eastell R, Zillikens MC. Discontinuation of denosumab therapy for osteoporosis: a systematic review and position statement by ECTS. *Bone.* 2017;**105**:11–17.

Osteoporosis in Premenopausal Women

M54
Presented, March 23–26, 2019

Carolyn Becker, MD. Division of Endocrinology, Diabetes and Hypertension, Brigham and Women's Hospital, Boston, Massachusetts 02115, E-mail: cbbecker@partners.org

SIGNIFICANCE OF THE CLINICAL PROBLEM

The definition, diagnosis, evaluation, and management of premenopausal osteoporosis are all problematic, and there are no evidence-based guidelines to help the clinician. Given the low incidence of fragility fractures among premenopausal women, ranging from 3/100,000 patient-years in those younger than age 35 years old to 21/100,000 patient-years in those age 35 to 44 years old (1), longitudinal studies linking bone mineral density (BMD) to future fracture risk in the next 5 to 10 years are lacking. In contrast to postmenopausal women, 50% to 90% of premenopausal women with fragility fractures will have a secondary and often reversible cause. For the remaining 10% to 50% of premenopausal women with "idiopathic osteoporosis" (IOP), management issues are very challenging. Importantly, women with a history of premenopausal fracture are 35% more likely to fracture in the postmenopausal years, suggesting that, for some, fracture risk is a lifelong trait (2).

BARRIERS TO OPTIMAL PRACTICE

- There are scant longitudinal data regarding the relationship between low BMD and short-term (5 to 10 years) fracture risk in premenopausal women.
- Low BMD may be due to failure to reach optimal peak bone mass (PBM), ongoing bone loss, or both.
- Clinicians may be unaware of diseases and medications that impact bone health in premenopausal women.
- Clinical trials involving treatment of premenopausal osteoporosis are generally small, short term, and without fracture outcomes.
- Few studies have addressed risks and benefits of antiosteoporosis therapies in premenopausal women.

LEARNING OBJECTIVES

As a result of participating in this session, learners should be able to

- Use the proper terminology to describe premenopausal "osteoporosis"
- Understand the challenges in diagnosing, evaluating, and treating premenopausal osteoporosis
- Carry out an appropriate workup to rule out secondary causes of low BMD or fractures in young women
- Understand the pathophysiology and management of pregnancy-associated osteoporosis
- Understand the pathophysiology and management of IOP

STRATEGIES FOR DIAGNOSIS, THERAPY, AND/OR MANAGEMENT
Definitions and Diagnosis

The International Society for Clinical Densitometry (ISCD) recommends that z scores (comparing a young woman's BMD with the mean of an age-, sex-, and ethnicity-matched reference population) rather than t scores should be used to categorize BMD among premenopausal women (3). In contrast, the International Osteoporosis Foundation (IOF) recommends the use of z scores for women younger than age 30 years old, in whom peak BMD may not have been reached, and t scores for premenopausal women over age 30 years old (4).

In addition, the ISCD recommends that a z score ≤ -2.0 be defined as "low bone density" or BMD "below expected for age" (3). Young women with z scores > -2.0 are defined as having BMD "within the expected range for age." Both the ISCD and the IOF concur on two points: (i) the term "osteoporosis" should not be used to describe premenopausal women with isolated low BMD, and (ii) the term "osteopenia" should be completely avoided in this population.

According to the ISCD, the diagnosis of "osteoporosis" is reserved for two categories of premenopausal women: (i) those with low BMD (z score < -2.0) combined with additional risk factors, such as hypogonadism, chronic glucocorticoids, or hyperparathyroidism, or (ii) those with fragility fractures that occur from a fall from standing height or less, excluding fractures of the digits, face, or skull (3). In contrast, the IOF defines "osteoporosis" in premenopausal women as those with t scores < -2.5 and known secondary causes for bone loss and/or fragility fractures (4).

Concept of PBM

PBM is the major determinant of premenopausal BMD. It is defined as the maximum BMD achieved by age 40 years old as measured by dual energy x-ray absorptiometry (DXA). Low PBM may result from genetic predisposition (accounting for 75% of PBM), illnesses, or medications (5). In healthy girls, 95% to 100% of PBM is achieved by the late teens. Small BMD gains may accrue up until age 30 to 35 years old. Whereas PBM is largely genetically determined, adequate calcium intake and physical activity are key factors in achieving optimal PBM (6).

Low Bone Mass

Low BMD may result from inadequate accrual of PBM or previous or ongoing losses of bone mass. The clinical significance of isolated low bone density (without fracture) in young women is unknown. Some premenopausal women with low BMD, particularly those with known secondary causes of osteoporosis, do indeed have abnormal bone strength and an increased risk of fracture. Other women with IOP (unexplained low BMD and/or low-trauma fracture) seem to have abnormal skeletal microarchitecture when assessed by high-resolution peripheral quantitative computed tomography (HRpQCT) (7) or transiliac bone biopsy (8). In one study, premenopausal women with isolated low BMD had the same abnormal microarchitecture as those with fractures, and both groups differed significantly from normal controls (7). Despite these findings, a longitudinal study of women with IOP showed stable or improved BMD with a very low fracture risk over 3 years of follow-up (9).

Premenopausal Bone Loss
After achieving PBM, healthy premenopausal women experience a gradual loss of BMD ranging from 0.25% to 1% per year, particularly at the femoral neck (10). A number of factors affect the rate and degree of premenopausal bone loss, including hereditary factors, age, weight changes, body mass index (BMI), calcium and vitamin D intake, physical activity, alcohol consumption, family history of osteoporosis, smoking, and number of pregnancies.

Perimenopausal Bone Loss
Bone loss begins before menopause, more often in women with subclinical ovulation disturbances or perimenopausal symptoms (11). In a longitudinal, multiethnic cohort study of 862 women followed for 10 years, the annual rates and cumulative losses of BMD were greater 1 year before through 2 years after the final menstrual period (transmenopause) than those occurring between 2 and 5 years after the final menstrual period (postmenopause) (12). Cumulative 10-year and transmenopause BMD losses were 10.6% and 7.4%, respectively, at the lumbar spine and 9.1% and 5.8%, respectively, at the femoral neck.

Fractures
Premenopausal women have much lower rates of fracture than postmenopausal women, and those who fracture tend to have lower BMD. For example, in premenopausal women with Colles fractures, BMDs at the nonfractured radius (13), lumbar spine, and femoral neck (14) were significantly below age-matched peers. In another study, premenopausal women with distal radius fractures and controls had very similar BMD at the wrist, but trabecular microarchitecture (as measured by HRpQCT) showed deterioration at both the distal radius and distal tibia in the women with fractures (15).

Screening for Low BMD
Routine BMD screening of pre- or perimenopausal women is not recommended unless there is a history of fragility fracture(s) or an ongoing medical disorder or medication exposure

associated with low BMD or bone loss (e.g., estrogen deficiency, glucocorticoid exposure, etc.). Table 1 lists guidelines for BMD testing in premenopausal women.

Secondary Causes of Low BMD and/or Fragility Fractures in Premenopausal Women
When evaluating a young woman presenting with low BMD and/or a fragility fracture, a thorough history, physical examination, and laboratory investigation are needed to rule out secondary causes. The workup should help determine whether the low BMD/fractures are the result of inadequate PBM or ongoing losses of BMD. In 50% to 90% of these young women, a secondary cause will be found that can help direct the therapeutic approach.

Lifestyle choices, including alcohol and tobacco use, dietary habits, calcium and vitamin D intake/exposure, and physical activity, should be discussed. Family history of osteoporosis should be documented. Table 2 lists etiologies of "osteoporosis" in young women, and Table 3 gives an approach to the laboratory evaluation.

Management: General Issues
Because there are no official guidelines regarding management of premenopausal osteoporosis, all recommendations are based on expert opinion (4, 16). Management begins by encouraging healthy lifestyle changes that may help improve PBM and/or slow ongoing bone loss. These recommendations include

- Adequate calcium intake, preferably from dietary sources (1000 to 1200 mg elemental calcium daily)
- Adequate vitamin D intake (400 to 800 IU vitamin D3 daily) to maintain 25-hydroxy-vitamin D levels ~30 ng/mL (75 nmol/L)
- Regular physical activity, particularly weight bearing
- Cessation of smoking
- Avoidance of excess alcohol, caffeine, and phosphorus-containing sodas
- Maintenance of normal body weight and avoidance of extreme thinness or weight cycling

When a secondary etiology for low BMD or fracture is found, therapy should be targeted to that entity. For example, changing to a gluten-free diet in a young woman with celiac disease will lead to increases in BMD. Similarly, parathyroidectomy for primary hyperparathyroidism, reversal of thyrotoxicosis, discontinuation

Table 1. Guidelines for BMD Testing in Premenopausal Women

History of fragility fracture
Diseases/conditions associated with low BMD or bone loss (Table 2)
Medications exposure associated with bone loss (Table 2)
Initiating or monitoring pharmacologic therapy for osteoporosis

Table 2. Secondary Causes of "Osteoporosis" in Premenopausal Women

Diseases or conditions
Anorexia nervosa
Malabsorption (*e.g.*, celiac, postoperative, inflammatory bowel, cystic fibrosis)
Vitamin D and/or calcium deficiency
Thyrotoxicosis
Hyperparathyroidism
Hypercalciuria
Diabetes (types 1 and 2)
Cushing syndrome
Hypogonadism
Rheumatoid arthritis (and other autoimmune/inflammatory conditions)
Alcoholism
Chronic liver disease
Chronic kidney disease
Systemic mastocytosis
Osteogenesis imperfecta and other connective tissue disorders
Marfan syndrome
Homocystinuria
Medications
Glucocorticoids
Depot medroxyprogesterone acetate
Excess thyroid hormone
Immunosuppressants (*e.g.*, cyclosporine)
Anticonvulsants (especially phenobarbital and phenytoin)
Gonadotropin-releasing hormone agonists
Aromatase inhibitors
Cancer cytotoxic chemotherapy
Heparin
Selective serotonin reuptake inhibitors

Table 3. Laboratory Evaluation of Premenopausal Osteoporosis

Highly recommended for all
Complete blood count
Electrolytes, renal function
Calcium, phosphate
Albumin, alkaline phosphatase, liver transaminases
TSH
25-Hydroxy-vitamin D
24-h urine for calcium, creatinine
Optional testing
Estradiol, luteinizing hormone, follicle stimulating hormone, prolactin
PTH
1,25-Dihydroxy-vitamin D
24-h urine for urine free cortisol or 1 mg dexamethasone suppression test (cortisol)
Iron, total iron binding capacity, ferritin
Celiac screen
Serum/urine protein electrophoresis
BTMs (*e.g.*, serum C-telopeptide)
Rheumatoid factor
Erythrocyte sedimentation rate, C-reactive protein
Iliac crest bone biopsy
Genetic testing (*e.g.*, for osteogenesis imperfecta, other rare disorders)
Serial BMD testing (to determine ongoing bone loss)

indicated. If markers of bone turnover are in the lower end of the normal range for premenopausal women, it may be reasonable to treat with calcium, vitamin D, and exercise and repeat a DXA in 1 to 2 years.

Management: Young Women With Fractures or Accelerated Bone Loss

For amenorrheic, hypogonadal women, restoration of menses or treatment with some form of estrogen-progestin therapy may be very beneficial for BMD (17). However, adult women with amenorrhea due to anorexia nervosa do not respond to oral combination estrogen-progestin therapy. In contrast, mature adolescents with anorexia nervosa have substantial BMD improvements with transdermal estrogen (18).

For women who are either unresponsive or unable to take hormonal therapy, other potential therapies that have been studied include bisphosphonates and teriparatide. It should be remembered that long-term efficacy and safety data with pharmaceutical agents as well as fracture data are sparse in premenopausal women. The decision to initiate treatment with a bisphosphonate in any premenopausal woman should be made on a case-by-case basis with consideration of individual fracture risk and potential medication effects. In general, the goal should be to treat with a bisphosphonate for the

of depot medroxyprogesterone acetate, restoration of normal weight in women with anorexia nervosa, or treatment with dopamine agonists or estrogen therapy for hyperprolactinemic women should significantly improve BMD.

In general, pharmacologic therapy for osteoporosis is not recommended, because there are virtually no data on long-term safety or efficacy of these therapies in premenopausal women, particularly in those with IOP. As a result, treatment with medications is reserved for those with fracture(s), accelerated bone loss, and/or known ongoing secondary causes of osteoporosis accompanied by fractures or bone loss.

Management: Young Women Without Fractures or Accelerated Bone Loss

In premenopausal women with low BMD alone (without fractures, known secondary causes for low BMD, or evidence of accelerated bone loss), pharmacotherapy is almost never shortest possible duration, particularly in light of rare potential risks of long-term use, such as osteonecrosis of the jaw or atypical femur fractures. Moreover, bisphosphonates carry a category C rating for safety in pregnancy, because they cross the placenta and have toxic effects in experimental rat models. The long half-life of bisphosphonates in bone is also concerning in reproductive age women.

Teriparatide prevents bone loss in premenopausal women on gonadotropin-releasing hormone agonist therapy for endometriosis (19) or glucocorticoid therapy for any illness (20, 21). It also works well in young women with IOP (22) and anorexia nervosa (23).

Management: Young Women on Glucocorticoids

For premenopausal women with amenorrhea who are initiating or taking glucocorticoids, combination estrogen-progestin contraception (if not contraindicated) is ideal therapy. Glucocorticoids reduce the production of sex steroids, and therefore, it is logical to replace these hormones if the patient has oligo- or amenorrhea.

For women with normal menses, alternatives include bisphosphonates or teriparatide. Both alendronate and risedronate are Food and Drug Administration approved for premenopausal women receiving chronic glucocorticoids. The American College of Rheumatology guidelines suggest oral bisphosphonate treatment of premenopausal women who are taking at least 7.5 mg of prednisone or equivalent per day for ≥6 months and are either high risk (*e.g.*, previous fragility fracture) or moderate risk (*e.g.*, hip or spine BMD z score < −3 and/or bone loss ≥10% over 1 year) as long as there are no near-term plans for pregnancy and effective contraception is used (24).

Teriparatide is an alternative option for such women. Although approved for the treatment of glucocorticoid-induced osteoporosis, no study has been large enough to document fracture risk reduction in premenopausal women. Similar to postmenopausal women, premenopausal women who take teriparatide need antiresorptive treatment after cessation of teriparatide to prevent bone loss (see below).

MAIN CONCLUSIONS

The diagnosis of premenopausal osteoporosis should not be based on BMD alone. Both the ISCD and the IOF emphasize that low BMD must be coupled with ongoing secondary causes of low BMD, accelerated bone loss, and/or presence of fragility fracture(s) to define a young woman as having "osteoporosis." Because a high proportion of these women have secondary causes of low BMD, a thorough history, physical examination, and laboratory evaluation are mandatory. Therapy should be targeted to any secondary causes that can be corrected. In severely affected women with very low BMD, major fractures, or accelerated bone loss with conservative measures, treatment with pharmacologic therapy may be considered.

CASES

Case 1

A 36-year-old white woman is sent to you for evaluation of vertebral fractures. She sustained her first fracture after a motor vehicle accident at age 33 when severe back pain developed. Spinal radiographs revealed a moderate compression fracture at T10. Over time, her symptoms resolved, and she did well. Three years later, she developed back pain after a vigorous yoga class. Repeat radiographs showed new compression fractures at T8, T11, and L1. A DXA revealed z scores of −3.2 at the lumbar spine (L2 to L4), −2.4 at the femoral neck, and −2.0 at the total hip.

You see her 6 weeks after the fractures, do a complete history and detailed physical examination, and find nothing remarkable other than spinal tenderness and mild kyphosis. Her BMI is 23. Family history is positive for osteoporosis in her mother and several maternal aunts. She has normal menses and maintains a very healthy lifestyle. Her only medication is a combination oral contraceptive pill (OCP) containing 35 μg ethinyl estradiol that she started 6 months ago for birth control. Laboratory studies, including complete blood count, renal function, calcium, phosphate, liver enzymes, alkaline phosphatase, 25-hydroxy-vitamin D, PTH, TSH, serum and urine protein electrophoresis, tryptase, and 24-hour urine calcium, are all normal. Genetic testing for osteogenesis imperfecta comes back negative.

What would be your best next step?
A. Obtain fasting serum markers of bone turnover (C-telopeptide and procollagen type 1 N-terminal propeptide)
B. Begin an anabolic agent (teriparatide or abaloparatide)
C. Begin an oral bisphosphonate
D. Refer for tetracycline-labeled iliac crest bone biopsy
E. Switch the OCP to a levonorgestrel-releasing intrauterine device

Case 2

A 31-year-old woman presents with back pain and stiffness 3 months after delivering her first child. She had an uncomplicated pregnancy and delivery and has been breastfeeding ever since. She denies any previous fractures, but her mother has osteoporosis. On examination, she is thin (BMI of 21) with spinal tenderness and paraspinal muscle spasm. Radiographs confirm mild to moderate compression fractures at T11, L1, and L2. On DXA, z scores are −3.5 at the lumbar spine, −2.8 at the femoral neck, and −1.9 at the total hip. An extensive laboratory evaluation is normal except for 25-hydroxy-vitamin D of 21 ng/mL (52.5 nmol/L]).

Which of the following would you advise her about her condition?
A. Cessation of breastfeeding will improve her BMD
B. Over the next 18 months, her BMD will decline further in the absence of pharmacologic intervention
C. Back pain will resolve within the next 2 to 3 months

D. Her risk for fractures in subsequent pregnancies is vanishingly small

E. Treatment with antiresorptive or anabolic therapy now will protect her against future fractures

Case 3

A 40-year-old healthy premenopausal woman undergoes a heel ultrasound at a health fair due to a positive family history of osteoporosis in her mother and an older sister. Results come back abnormal, and therefore, her internist orders a screening DXA. This reveals z scores of -1.8 at the lumbar spine, -2.8 at the left femoral neck, and -1.6 at the left total hip. The patient is referred to you for evaluation and management of osteoporosis.

You do a complete history, physical examination, and laboratory workup, which are unrevealing; 25-hydroxy-vitamin D is 22 ng/mL (55 nmol/L), and a fasting serum C-telopeptide is in the lower one third of the normal premenopausal range. She has never fractured, has regular menses, has a BMI of 24, and has no history of smoking or excess alcohol intake. Her usual diet includes ~750 mg of elemental calcium daily. She does not take any medications, vitamins, or supplements, and she does not exercise. Her same-sex spouse has had two biological children, but the patient herself has no plans for pregnancy.

In addition to optimizing calcium and vitamin D, which of the following would you recommend at this time?

A. Reassurance and repeat DXA in 1 to 2 years
B. Oral bisphosphonate therapy
C. Anabolic therapy (teriparatide or abaloparatide)
D. Regular weight-bearing exercise of moderate intensity
E. A combination OCP containing at least 35 μg of ethinyl estradiol

DISCUSSION
Case 1
The correct answer is B. This case illustrates premenopausal IOP. Women with IOP have fragility fractures in the absence of any identifiable secondary causes, despite an extensive evaluation. IOP primarily affects whites (men and women equally), with mean age in the mid-30s. Multiple fragility fractures, including acute vertebral fractures, may occur over a 5- to 10-year period. Bone biopsy studies have shown microarchitectural disruption, whereas advanced imaging techniques have shown reductions in estimated bone strength and volumetric BMD in women with IOP (7, 8).

Fasting markers of bone turnover (answer A) have not been shown to be particularly useful in IOP, because bone turnover is quite heterogeneous. In some studies, low bone turnover has been associated with the most marked abnormalities in bone density and quality (8). Additionally, all bone turnover markers (BTMs) increase by 50% to 100% within 6 to 12 weeks of a fracture (25). If you want to use BTMs to monitor antiosteoporosis therapy, you have to be aware of this postfracture spike and try to make adjustments. Bone biopsy (answer D) is unlikely to reveal a secondary cause of bone fragility given the

normal findings on history, physical examination, and extensive laboratories. Although combination OCPs have been associated with lower BMD and lower IGF-1 in some studies (26), switching from an OCP to an intrauterine device is unlikely to be useful in the near term given that her exposure to the OCP is only 6 months (answer E).

The real dilemma is whether to treat this young woman with an antiosteoporosis medication. Given the severity of her situation with multiple symptomatic vertebral fractures and very low BMD, pharmacologic intervention seems justified. The choice between anabolic therapy (answer B) or oral bisphosphonate therapy (answer C) is not an easy one. Neither class of drug is approved for use in IOP. However, there are small clinical trials showing improvement in BMD and bone strength in premenopausal women with IOP treated with teriparatide for 18 to 24 months (22, 27). Patient preference is important, and in this case, the patient chose anabolic therapy with teriparatide. However, recent studies have shown that, within 2 years of stopping teriparatide, spinal BMD can decline by a variable amount; therefore, BMD monitoring and possibly, a course of antiresorptive therapy may be needed, even in estrogen-replete women (28).

Case 2
The correct answer is A. This case illustrates "pregnancy-lactation–associated osteoporosis" (PLO), defined as one or more fragility fractures occurring within 6 months of delivery. The majority of cases of PLO occur in primiparous women in their 30s. About two-thirds of patients will have predisposing risk factors for osteoporosis, including positive family history, preexisting illnesses, or pregnancy-related risk factors, such as heparin use or prolonged bedrest. Most fractures occur around the time of delivery or within 2 months postpartum during lactation. The mean number of fractures is 3 to 4, with vertebral fractures being most common (29).

During the first 6 months of lactation, BMD at the spine and hip can decline by 10%; therefore, stopping breastfeeding can have very positive effects on BMD (answer A is correct). Even without pharmacologic treatment, BMD gradually improves within 12 to 18 months after delivery (answer B is wrong). Longitudinal studies have shown that the majority of women with PLO continue to have back pain and disability for 3 or more years after the fractures (answer C is wrong). These studies have also shown an increased risk for fractures both during and independent of subsequent pregnancies, a risk that is not eliminated by treatment with antiosteoporosis agents after the first fracture (answers D and E are wrong). About 25% of women with PLO will sustain subsequent fractures within 6 years of follow-up (29).

In addition to conservative methods, such as cessation of breastfeeding and optimizing calcium plus D, bisphosphonates have been given to women with PLO. In one study, bisphosphonates resulted in a 23% increase in spinal BMD after 2 years compared with an 11% improvement in untreated patients (30). Teriparatide has also been used for PLO. In a group of 27 women from Korea, BMD responses to 12 months of teriparatide ranged greatly from 4.5% to 34%. On average, BMD gains were doubled in the treatment group compared with the control women (15.5% vs 7.5%) (31). Similarly, in a group of 52 women with PLO, treatment with teriparatide increased spinal BMD by ~15% and hip BMD by ~6% in 11 women; untreated women had BMD increases that were about 50% lower over 2.5 years (32).

Case 3

The correct answer is D. This case is an example of a premenopausal healthy woman with isolated low BMD, most likely hereditary. After a complete evaluation comes back negative, it is important to reassure her that she does not have "osteoporosis" but rather, "low bone density, below expected for her age." In the absence of a fragility fracture, accelerated bone loss, or an ongoing secondary cause for low BMD or bone loss, pharmacologic intervention in a patient like this is almost never warranted (therefore, answers B and C are wrong). Because this patient has normal, regular menses, there would be no advantage to starting her on an OCP (answer E is wrong).

Reassurance that she does not have osteoporosis and monitoring her BMD (answer A) are not wrong answers, but they are not adequate. A number of studies suggest that a combination of calcium, vitamin D, and moderate weight-bearing exercise, particularly in sedentary women, can lead to some substantial increases in BMD, particularly at the femoral neck (9, 33, 34). Unfortunately, we do not know if this translates into lower fracture risk, but certainly, exercise has many benefits beyond skeletal health. Thus, the best overall recommendations in this case would be to optimize calcium and vitamin D, prescribe a moderately intense program of weight-bearing exercise, and repeat the BMD in 1 to 2 years.

References

1. Martínez-Morillo M, Grados D, Holgado S. Premenopausal osteoporosis: how to treat? *Reumatol Clin.* 2012;**8**(2):93–97.
2. Hosmer WD, Genant HK, Browner WS. Fractures before menopause: a red flag for physicians. *Osteoporos Int.* 2002;**13**(4):337–341.
3. Schousboe JT, Shepherd JA, Bilezikian JP, Baim S. Executive summary of the 2013 International Society for Clinical Densitometry Position Development Conference on bone densitometry. *J Clin Densitom.* 2013;**16**(4):455–466.
4. Ferrari S, Bianchi ML, Eisman JA, Foldes AJ, Adami S, Wahl DA, Stepan JJ, de Vernejoul MC, Kaufman JM; IOF Committee of Scientific Advisors Working Group on Osteoporosis Pathophysiology. Osteoporosis in young adults: pathophysiology, diagnosis, and management. *Osteoporos Int.* 2012;**23**(12):2735–2748.
5. Chew CK, Clarke BL. Causes of low peak bone mass in women. *Maturitas.* 2018;**111**:61–68.
6. Weaver CM, Gordon CM, Janz KF, Kalkwarf HJ, Lappe JM, Lewis R, O'Karma M, Wallace TC, Zemel BS. The National Osteoporosis Foundation's position statement on peak bone mass development and lifestyle factors: a systematic review and implementation recommendations [published correction appears in Osteoporos Int. 2016; 27(4):1387]. *Osteoporos Int.* 2016;**27**(4):1281–1386.
7. Cohen A, Liu XS, Stein EM, McMahon DJ, Rogers HF, Lemaster J, Recker RR, Lappe JM, Guo XE, Shane E. Bone microarchitecture and stiffness in premenopausal women with idiopathic osteoporosis. *J Clin Endocrinol Metab.* 2009;**94**(11):4351–4360.
8. Cohen A, Dempster DW, Recker RR, Stein EM, Lappe JM, Zhou H, Wirth AJ, van Lenthe GH, Kohler T, Zwahlen A, Müller R, Rosen CJ, Cremers S, Nickolas TL, McMahon DJ, Rogers H, Staron RB, LeMaster J, Shane E. Abnormal bone microarchitecture and evidence of osteoblast dysfunction in premenopausal women with idiopathic osteoporosis. *J Clin Endocrinol Metab.* 2011;**96**(10):3095–3105.
9. Peris P, Monegal A, Martínez MA, Moll C, Pons F, Guañabens N. Bone mineral density evolution in young premenopausal women with idiopathic osteoporosis. *Clin Rheumatol.* 2007;**26**(6):958–961.
10. McLendon AN, Woodis CB. A review of osteoporosis management in younger premenopausal women. *Womens Health (Lond).* 2014; **10**(1):59–77.
11. Seifert-Klauss V, Link T, Heumann C, Luppa P, Haseitl M, Laakmann J, Rattenhuber J, Kiechle M. Influence of pattern of menopausal transition on the amount of trabecular bone loss. Results from a 6-year prospective longitudinal study. *Maturitas.* 2006;**55**(4):317–324.
12. Greendale GA, Sowers M, Han W, Huang MH, Finkelstein JS, Crandall CJ, Lee JS, Karlamangla AS. Bone mineral density loss in relation to the final menstrual period in a multiethnic cohort: results from the Study of Women's Health Across the Nation (SWAN). *J Bone Miner Res.* 2012;**27**(1):111–118.
13. Wigderowitz CA, Cunningham T, Rowley DI, Mole PA, Paterson CR. Peripheral bone mineral density in patients with distal radial fractures. *J Bone Joint Surg Br.* 2003;**85**(3):423–425.
14. Hung LK, Wu HT, Leung PC, Qin L. Low BMD is a risk factor for low-energy Colles' fractures in women before and after menopause. *Clin Orthop Relat Res.* 2005;**&NA;**(435):219–225.
15. Rozental TD, Deschamps LN, Taylor A, Earp B, Zurakowski D, Day CS, Bouxsein ML. Premenopausal women with a distal radial fracture have deteriorated trabecular bone density and morphology compared with controls without a fracture. *J Bone Joint Surg Am.* 2013;**95**(7): 633–642.
16. Cohen A, Shane E. Evaluation and management of the premenopausal woman with low BMD. *Curr Osteoporos Rep.* 2013;**11**(4):276–285.
17. Liu SL, Lebrun CM. Effect of oral contraceptives and hormone replacement therapy on bone mineral density in premenopausal and perimenopausal women: a systematic review. *Br J Sports Med.* 2006;**40**(1):11–24.
18. Robinson L, Aldridge V, Clark EM, Misra M, Micali N. Pharmacological treatment options for low Bone Mineral Density and secondary osteoporosis in Anorexia Nervosa: a systematic review of the literature. *J Psychosom Res.* 2017;**98**:87–97.
19. Finkelstein JS, Klibanski A, Arnold AL, Toth TL, Hornstein MD, Neer RM. Prevention of estrogen deficiency-related bone loss with human parathyroid hormone-(1-34): a randomized controlled trial. *JAMA.* 1998;**280**(12):1067–1073.
20. Saag KG, Shane E, Boonen S, Marín F, Donley DW, Taylor KA, Dalsky GP, Marcus R. Teriparatide or alendronate in glucocorticoid-induced osteoporosis. *N Engl J Med.* 2007;**357**(20):2028–2039.
21. Langdahl BL, Marin F, Shane E, Dobnig H, Zanchetta JR, Maricic M, Krohn K, See K, Warner MR. Teriparatide versus alendronate for treating glucocorticoid-induced osteoporosis: an analysis by gender and menopausal status. *Osteoporos Int.* 2009;**20**(12):2095–2104.
22. Cohen A, Stein EM, Recker RR, Lappe JM, Dempster DW, Zhou H, Cremers S, McMahon DJ, Nickolas TL, Müller R, Zwahlen A, Young P, Stubby J, Shane E. Teriparatide for idiopathic osteoporosis in premenopausal women: a pilot study. *J Clin Endocrinol Metab.* 2013; **98**(5):1971–1981.
23. Fazeli PK, Wang IS, Miller KK, Herzog DB, Misra M, Lee H, Finkelstein JS, Bouxsein ML, Klibanski A. Teriparatide increases bone formation and bone mineral density in adult women with anorexia nervosa. *J Clin Endocrinol Metab.* 2014;**99**(4):1322–1329.
24. Buckley L, Guyatt G, Fink HA, Cannon M, Grossman J, Hansen KE, Humphrey MB, Lane NE, Magrey M, Miller M, Morrison L, Rao M, Robinson AB, Saha S, Wolver S, Bannuru RR, Vaysbrot E, Osani M, Turgunbaev M, Miller AS, McAlindon T. 2017 American College of Rheumatology Guideline for the Prevention and Treatment of

Glucocorticoid-Induced Osteoporosis. *Arthritis Rheumatol.* 2017; **69**(8):1521–1537.

25. Eastell R, Pigott T, Gossiel F, Naylor KE, Walsh JS, Peel NFA. Diagnosis of endocrine disease: bone turnover markers: are they clinically useful? *Eur J Endocrinol.* 2018;**178**(1):R19–R31.

26. Elkazaz AY, Salama K. The effect of oral contraceptive different patterns of use on circulating IGF-1 and bone mineral density in healthy premenopausal women. *Endocrine.* 2015;**48**(1):272–278.

27. Nishiyama KK, Cohen A, Young P, Wang J, Lappe JM, Guo XE, Dempster DW, Recker RR, Shane E. Teriparatide increases strength of the peripheral skeleton in premenopausal women with idiopathic osteoporosis: a pilot HR-pQCT study. *J Clin Endocrinol Metab.* 2014; **99**(7):2418–2425.

28. Cohen A, Kamanda-Kosseh M, Recker RR, Lappe JM, Dempster DW, Zhou H, Cremers S, Bucovsky M, Stubby J, Shane E. Bone density after teriparatide discontinuation in premenopausal idiopathic osteoporosis. *J Clin Endocrinol Metab.* 2015;**100**(11):4208–4214.

29. Kyvernitakis I, Reuter TC, Hellmeyer L, Hars O, Hadji P. Subsequent fracture risk of women with pregnancy and lactation-associated osteoporosis after a median of 6 years of follow-up. *Osteoporos Int.* 2018;**29**(1):135–142.

30. O'Sullivan SM, Grey AB, Singh R, Reid IR. Bisphosphonates in pregnancy and lactation-associated osteoporosis. *Osteoporos Int.* 2006; **17**(7):1008–1012.

31. Hong N, Kim JE, Lee SJ, Kim SH, Rhee Y. Changes in bone mineral density and bone turnover markers during treatment with teriparatide in pregnancy- and lactation-associated osteoporosis. *Clin Endocrinol (Oxf).* 2018;**88**(5):652–658.

32. Laroche M, Talibart M, Cormier C, Roux C, Guggenbuhl P, Degboe Y. Pregnancy-related fractures: a retrospective study of a French cohort of 52 patients and review of the literature. *Osteoporos Int.* 2017; **28**(11):3135–3142.

33. Babatunde O, Forsyth J. Effects of lifestyle exercise on premenopausal bone health: a randomised controlled trial. *J Bone Miner Metab.* 2014; **32**(5):563–572.

34. Zhao R, Zhao M, Zhang L. Efficiency of jumping exercise in improving bone mineral density among premenopausal women: a meta-analysis. *Sports Med.* 2014;**44**(10):1393–1402.

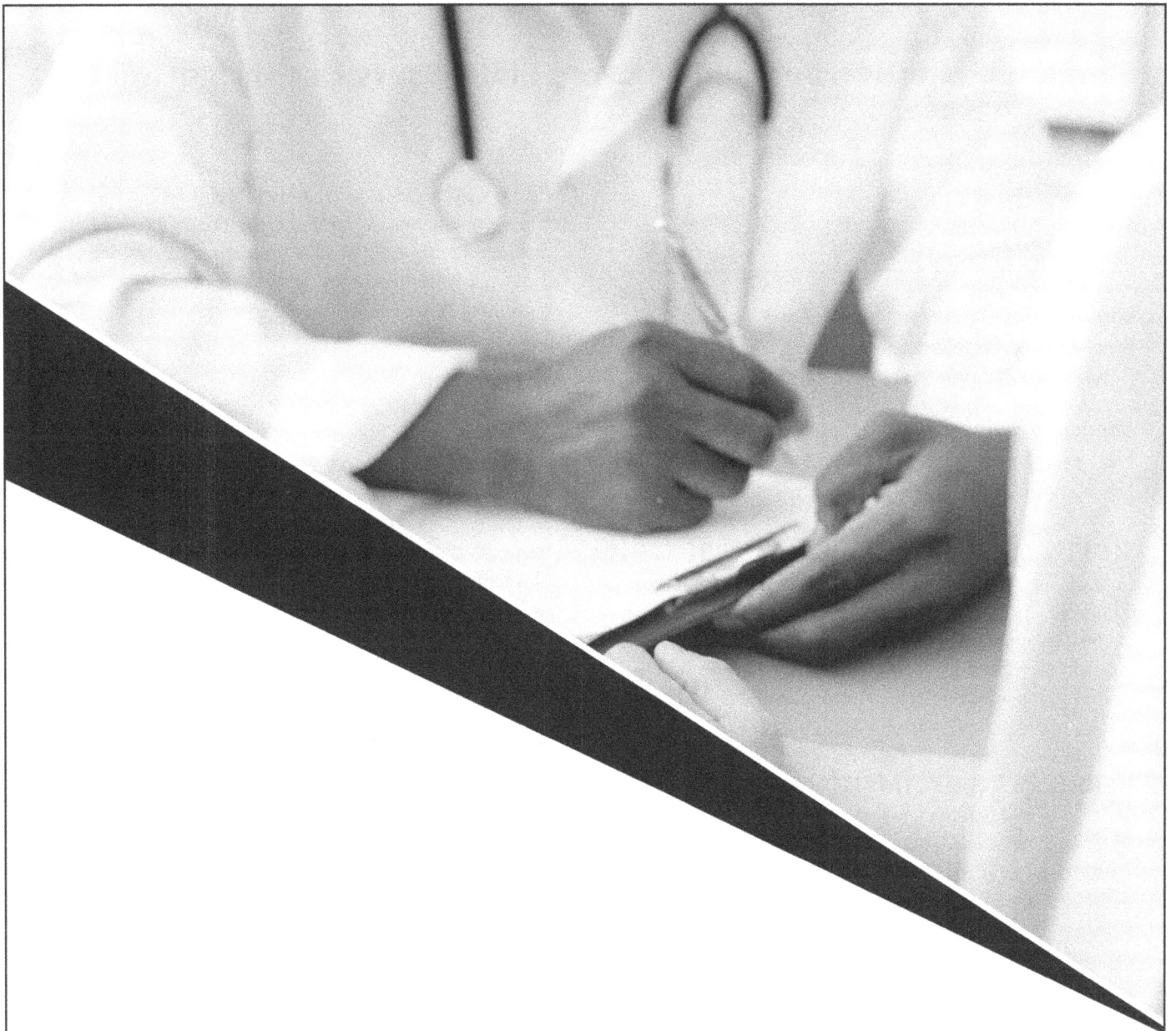

CARDIOVASCULAR ENDOCRINOLOGY

Familial Lipid Disorders: What Every Lipid-Savvy Endocrinologist Needs to Know

M05
Presented, March 23–26, 2019

Sergio Fazio, MD. Center for Preventive Cardiology, Knight Cardiovascular Institute, Oregon Health & Science University, Portland, Oregon, E-mail: fazio@ohsu.edu

Kenneth R. Feingold, MD. University of California, San Francisco, San Francisco, California, E-mail: kenneth.feingold@ucsf.edu

SIGNIFICANCE OF THE CLINICAL PROBLEM

Genetic disorders of lipid metabolism are commonly encountered in clinical practice. For example, familial hypercholesterolemia is estimated to occur in 1 in 200 to 250 individuals. Moreover, it is important to recognize that these disorders cause a great deal of morbidity and mortality, which can be prevented with appropriate diagnosis and treatment.

BARRIERS TO OPTIMAL PRACTICE

Genetic testing is relatively expensive, and the interpretation of genetic tests can often be difficult. Additionally, as discussed below, genetic testing is frequently negative in patients that have familial lipids disorders.

LEARNING OBJECTIVES

As a result of participating in this session, learners should be able to:

- Increase the ability to recognize and diagnose genetic disorders of lipid metabolism
- Develop strategies to reduce the morbidity and mortality associated with genetic disorders of lipid metabolism

STRATEGIES FOR DIAGNOSIS, THERAPY, AND/OR MANAGEMENT

Case 1: Chylomicronemia Syndrome

A 62-year-old male is referred to the clinic after two episodes of acute pancreatitis with admission triglyceride (TG) > 6000 mg/dL (>68 mmol/L). He is concerned as he was never told he had elevated TG levels. He is thin (body mass index, 21.5), exercises regularly, drinks alcohol sporadically, does not take medications that increase TG levels, and does not have conditions that predispose to hypertriglyceridemia, such as prediabetes, diabetes, renal, liver, thyroid, or autoimmune diseases. His TG levels fluctuate from the many thousands to <150 mg/dL (<1.7 mmol/L) without any evident pattern or triggers. He was advised to use a TG meter to monitor TG levels and adjust dietary intake accordingly up to a complete fast for 24 hours if necessary. Treatment regimens have varied from triple combination of fibrate, prescription omega 3 fatty acids, and statin to no drug at all without any obvious differences in TG levels. He has been able to avoid pancreatitis by decreasing food intake when TG levels are high.

Introduction

Chylomicrons are released by enterocytes into the plasma after fat ingestion, but their half-life is short in individuals with reasonably normal lipoprotein lipase activity, which binds to the vascular endothelium and avidly hydrolyzes TG from chylomicrons, which creates chylomicron remnants that are subsequently removed rapidly from the circulation. Thus, fasting plasma concentrations of chylomicrons are low in normal individuals. Chylomicronemia syndrome (CS) is caused by greatly decreased activity of lipoprotein lipase (LPL), which results in greatly delayed TG hydrolysis, leading to the dramatic accumulation of chylomicrons, which raises plasma TG to levels >500 mg/dL (>5.65 mmol/L) even after an overnight fast and often into the several thousands. This, in turn, results in an increased risk for developing acute pancreatitis. Although most TG in plasma is ordinarily carried by liver-derived very-low-density lipoprotein (VLDL) as a result of the much greater flux of TG from dietary fat through the intestine, LPL deficiency results predominantly in a dramatic increase in TG carried by intestinally produced chylomicrons. It is unclear whether the risk of cardiovascular disease is increased by high chylomicron levels as chylomicrons do not easily penetrate the artery wall.

Pathogenesis

The development of CS is secondary to inherited or acquired abnormalities of LPL, which lead to decreased clearance of TG-rich lipoproteins. Several other proteins act on LPL and can affect the activity of LPL. Lipase maturation factor 1 brings LPL from the site of production in parenchymal cells to the endothelial layer, whereas glycosyl-phosphatidyl-inositol high-density lipoprotein (HDL)–binding-protein 1 (GPIHBP1) helps LPL get anchored to the luminal side of the endothelium. Apolipoprotein C2 (apoC2), apoC3, apoA5, and apoE on lipoproteins all modulate the activity of LPL. Thus, severe CS can develop as a consequence of mutations that affect the function of any of these genes. As LPL is an enzyme, inherited disease is a recessive trait and fully manifested only when its function is nearly absent as happens with homozygous LPL mutations. However, as most of the key players in the LPL node are either extracellular or circulating proteins, they are susceptible to the action of autoantibodies, drugs, toxins, and metabolic perturbations. Often a combination of heterozygous genetic variants and acquired conditions (*i.e.*, alcohol abuse, dietary excess, pregnancy, uncontrolled diabetes, estrogen, isotretinoin, or glucocorticoid therapy, *etc.*) determine the escalation from normal or moderately elevated TG levels to frank CS. In addition to clearance abnormalities, the condition is often aggravated by hepatic overproduction of VLDL, a consequence of insulin resistance and dietary indiscretion.

Prevalence
Familial chylomicronemia syndrome as a result of homozygous mutations—or compound heterozygosity—in the genes that control TG metabolism is a rare condition, perhaps affecting fewer than one in 500,000 people. However, acquired issues leading to the development of CS are as frequent as one in 200 people as they represent a complication of common conditions, such as uncontrolled diabetes or dietary excess, in patients with common polymorphisms in genes that affect TG metabolism.

Clinical Manifestations
Lipid Abnormalities. TG levels can vary between 500 (5.68 mmol/L) and >6000 mg/dL (68 mmol/L). Absence or dysfunction of LPL results in elevations primarily in chylomicrons, although VLDL levels are frequently increased as well. HDL cholesterol (HDL-C) levels are generally extremely low, primarily because of the transfer of cholesterol to TG-rich lipoproteins. This is caused by the action of cholesteryl ester transfer protein on a greatly increased substrate of plasma TG. The resulting accelerated exchange of esterified cholesterol from HDL with TG from TG-rich lipoproteins is followed by rapid TG hydrolysis in HDL by normal hepatic lipase activity. This results in a dramatic net loss of core lipid of HDL, along with a loss of surface apolipoproteins and corresponding reductions in the plasma levels of all HDL components. In addition, interference by lipemic plasma with the accuracy of laboratory measurements of HDL-C can occur. Low-density lipoprotein cholesterol (LDL-C) levels are also usually low, in part, because of a similar set of mechanisms that deplete core esterified cholesterol content. In addition, impaired lipolysis of TG causes reduced conversion of VLDL to LDL, which results in decreased LDL production. In contrast, the cholesterol content of chylomicrons and VLDL is greatly increased such that non–HDL-C and total cholesterol levels are elevated. Lipoprotein(a) [Lp(a)] levels are usually low because LDL formation is impaired and apo(a) has little affinity for chylomicrons or VLDL.

Clinical Complications. Patients with severely elevated TG levels can develop eruptive xanthomas, usually as clusters of pimple-like formations on arms, shoulders, buttocks, or legs that develop suddenly and may disappear just as fast, depending on changes in plasma TG levels. Patients often complain of mental fogginess, tingling of hands and feet,

and nonspecific abdominal symptoms, such as bloating and generalized discomfort. With increasing TG levels, patients have a progressively increased risk of developing acute pancreatitis. At admission for TG-induced pancreatitis, TG levels are commonly >3000 mg/dL (34 mmol/L). Whether patients with CS have an increased risk of atherosclerotic cardiovascular disease (ASCVD) depends on the etiology of CS. In addition to the presence of common cardiovascular disease (CVD) comorbidities, such as diabetes, the lipid phenotype of severe hypertriglyceridemia includes both anti- and proatherogenic elements, including large chylomicrons that do not pass through the endothelial barrier, low LDL-C levels, low Lp(a) levels, low HDL-C levels and increased VLDL and chylomicron remnants that are proatherogenic.

Diagnosis
A fasting lipid panel will show elevated TG levels. When TGs are >800 mg/dL (9.04 mmol/L), chylomicrons are present, whereas when TGs are <800 mg/dL, the increase is mostly VLDL. Risk of acute pancreatitis is high for values > 2500 mg/dL (28 mmol/L) and not so high for values hovering around 1000 mg/dL (11.3 mmol/L). Additional lipid testing may include total apoB level (more elevated in cases of overproduction by the liver) or apoB48 level (marker of chylomicrons). A direct LDL-C or β-quantitation is necessary to assess the need for statin treatment. In the presence of even vague abdominal symptoms, it is appropriate to order an amylase/lipase level.

Genetic Testing
Genetic testing for the several genes mentioned above is available but seldom used; there is no insurance coverage for these tests. In addition, the published negative rate (no mutation) is dishearteningly high and there are no clear therapeutic correlates to identifying a specific mutation in any of the genes.

Treatment
Goals of Therapy. The primary goal is to lower fasting TG levels below the range that can trigger pancreatitis (<500 mg/dL; 5.68 mmol/L). Additional goals include the normalization of TG levels (<150 mg/dL; 1.70 mmol/L), treatment of elevated of LDL-C and non–HDL-C if present, and aggressive management of underlying conditions, such as obesity and diabetes.

Lifestyle Recommendations. As most plasma TGs derive from diet, changes in intake are usually the centerpiece of every intervention and range from switching to a low-fat, low-simple sugar diet, to dividing up the daily caloric allowance into several small meals to avoid large postprandial TG peaks, to a full fast for up to 48 hours if prodromic abdominal symptoms develop. Avoidance of alcohol is critical. Regular, prolonged, and strenuous exercise will help, and weight loss in over-weight or obese patients is indicated.

Drug Therapy. If possible, avoid drugs that increase TG levels. Several medications either directly or indirectly decrease TG levels. Antidiabetic agents and weight-loss drugs all have positive effects on TG as long as they are effective on their primary target. Statins lower TG levels and should be used if LDL-C control is needed or CVD risk management mandates it. Niacin is no longer endorsed for treatment of low HDL in patients with high CVD risk on statin, but it is not clear whether it would still help patients with extreme TG elevations. In general, the knowledge that niacin increases the risk of new-onset diabetes and worsens preexisting diabetes is enough to make most providers less enthusiastic to use niacin in these patients. Fibrates and prescription omega 3 fatty acid formulations are the mainstays of therapy, often in combination. Though two generic fibrates are available, preference should be given to fenofibrate over gemfibrozil if statin therapy is likely to be needed. Fenofibrate is usually administered as a nontitrated single dose ranging from 90 to 200 mg/d, depending on formulation. Prescription omega 3 drugs include a generic product that contains both eicosapentaenoic acid (EPA) and docosahexaenoic acid, and one product that contains only EPA. The dose is 4 g/d (2 g twice times per day with food to improve absorption). Omega 3 fatty acid dietary supplements are not recommended for treatment of severe hypertriglyceridemia and plant-source omega-3 fatty acids, which contains α-linolenic acid but not EPA or docosahexaenoic acid, does not lower TG levels.

Back to Our Patient

Though a didactic case is supposed to have a happy ending, with the solution of the diagnostic mystery and resolution of the problem, the main point in this discussion is to make the provider comfortable with the notion that many cases of late-onset, likely acquired CS will not have a cause identified and full metabolic control is only sporadically achieved with the current tools. In the case of our patient, we watched his TG fluctuate from well within normal to nearly 6000 mg/dL (68 mmol/L) with no apparent triggers, despite excellent dietary control, vigorous exercise routine, ideal body weight, and adherence to a regimen that included full-dose fenofibrate, full-dose omega 3 fatty acids, and on/off statin therapy. These unexplained fluctuations suggest the presence of an intermittent endogenous effector. After making sure that the genetic platform was normal—all genes mentioned above showed the absence of functional mutations—the patient's serum was tested for antibodies against LPL and GPIHBP-1, which were undetectable. An additional experimental evaluation showed elevated levels of GPIHBP-1 in serum, perhaps a suggestion that this membrane-anchored protein sheds from its endothelial location under the influence of unknown factors. The patient has been able to avoid markedly elevated TG levels and additional hospital admissions for pancreatitis by carefully monitoring his TG levels at home using a meter (Cardiochek; PTS Diagnostics, Indianapolis, IN) and taking quick action with fasting when TG levels are markedly elevated.

Case 2: Familial Hypercholesterolemia

A 58-year-old female is admitted with an acute myocardial infarction (MI). Three years ago, she experienced an MI followed by coronary bypass surgery. She has a family history of coronary artery disease (CAD), with her mother having died of MI at age 60 years, an uncle and aunt on her mother's side with CAD at a young age, and an older brother with CAD. The patient is currently on atorvastatin 80 mg once per day and ezetimibe 10 mg once per day with an LDL-C of 96 mg/dL (2.48 mmol/L). Before initiating statin/ezetimibe therapy, her LDL-C levels were >250 mg/dL (6.47 mmol/L). HDL-C and TG levels were within normal limits. What disorder does this patient have and what would you do next?

Introduction

Familial hypercholesterolemia (FH), as classically described, is an autosomal-dominant single-gene disorder of lipoprotein metabolism that leads to marked elevations in LDL-C levels that result in premature ASCVD. Classical FH is usually a result of a pathogenetic variant in the LDL receptor, apoB, or PCSK9 gene that leads to a decrease in the clearance of circulating LDL particles and, hence, elevations in LDL-C levels. Heterozygous FH is a result of a single genetic abnormality with a dominant inheritance. Homozygous FH is a result of the presence of two abnormalities and results in extremely high LDL-C levels with the early onset of ASCVD (onset can be as early as age 10 years). Homozygous FH is a rare disorder and given the high LDL-C levels, which are frequently resistant to being lowered with standard cholesterol-lowering drugs, these patients should receive care in specialized lipid clinics; therefore, we will not discuss homozygous FH in this presentation. The information presented below focuses on heterozygous FH. In addition to classical FH, there are other genetic disorders that can lead to an FH phenotype (*e.g.*, polygenic hypercholesterolemia).

Prevalence

FH is a common genetic disorder. Recent studies suggest a prevalence of one in 200 to one in 250 people. Prevalence of FH is even more common in certain ethnic groups and regions, such as Lebanon, South Africa, and Quebec. Of particular note is that most patients with FH have not been diagnosed. In the United States, it has been estimated that <10% of patients with FH carry a diagnosis of FH.

Clinical Manifestations

Lipid Abnormalities. LDL-C levels are frequently >90th percentile for age and gender. The magnitude of LDL-C elevation is affected by the specific mutations that cause FH with mutations in the LDL receptor that lead to greater elevations in LDL-C levels than mutations in apoB or PCSK9. Null mutations in the LDL receptor are more severe than non-null mutations. In addition, other genes that regulate LDL-C levels and environmental factors, such as diet, also influence the magnitude of the elevation in LDL-C levels. It should be recognized that a significant number of patients with genetically diagnosed FH have LDL-C levels < 190 mg/dL (4.92 mmol/L). In some studies, ~50% of patients with genetically diagnosed FH have LDL-C levels < 190 mg/dL (4.92 mmol/L). HDL-C and TG levels are usually normal or only modestly altered. Elevated TG levels and/or low HDL-C levels do not rule out the diagnosis of FH. Lp(a) levels are frequently elevated in patients with FH and may contribute to the increased risk of ASCVD. One should exclude secondary causes of marked elevations in LDL-C, particularly hypothyroidism.

ASCVD. Patients with FH have a 3- to 13-fold higher risk of ASCVD. Untreated males with FH have a 50% risk for a fatal or nonfatal MI by age 50 years, whereas untreated females have a 30% chance by age 60; however, it should be recognized that there is heterogeneity of ASCVD risk. Other cardiovascular risk factors, such as male sex, body mass index, diabetes, hypertension, smoking, low HDL-C levels, and Lp(a) levels modulate the risk of ASCVD. Patients with FH who have corneal arcus or xanthomas are more likely to have ASCVD. Of note, patients with mutations that result in FH have a greater ASCVD risk than do patients with equivalent LDL-C levels. This is likely because of the LDL-C elevations being present from birth—a lifelong exposure to elevated LDL-C.

Other Manifestations. Early-onset corneal arcus (age < 45 years) and tendinous xanthomas, particularly the Achilles tendon and dorsum of hands, are classic abnormalities that occur in patients with FH. Xanthelasma (xanthomas in eyelids) and tuberous xanthoma may also be seen; however, it should be recognized that, in the modern era with increased treatment of elevated LDL-C levels, these abnormalities are no longer frequently observed; only 5% to 20% of patients have xanthoma or corneal arcus currently (Table 1).

Diagnosis

There are three sets of statistically validated criteria that are most commonly used in the diagnosis of FH: the Dutch Lipid Network criteria, Simon Broome Register criteria, and Make Early Diagnosis to Prevent Early Deaths criteria. In the modern era, with widespread statin use, it is often difficult to make a definitive diagnosis of FH using clinical criteria. Lipid-lowering therapy can abort the development of xanthomas and corneal arcus and reduce or delay the occurrence of ASCVD events in

Table 1. When to Suspect FH

1. If LDL-C levels are >190 mg/dL (4.92 mmol/L) or non–HDL-C levels are >220 mg/dL (5.70 mmol/L)
2. Patients with premature ASCVD (age <55 years in males and <65 years in females)
3. Family history of hypercholesterolemia
4. When there is a positive family history of premature ASCVD (age <55 years in males and <65 years in females)
5. When tendon xanthomas or corneal arcus (age < 45 years) are present on physical exam

patients and relatives. Similarly, it is often difficult to know before-treatment LDL-C levels. Thus, without genetic testing, it is often difficult to make a definitive diagnosis of FH in many patients; genetic testing is the gold standard. In patients with genetically diagnosed FH, the ability of the Dutch criteria to indicate a definite or probable diagnosis of FH using clinical criteria is limited (in one study, just 24% of those who were diagnosed genetically met clinical criteria). This indicates that although the specificity of these criteria is good, the sensitivity to diagnose FH is limited and thus the diagnosis of FH will be overlooked in many patients if one just uses clinical criteria.

Genetic Testing

Genetic testing can make a definitive diagnosis of FH. In patients with the clinical diagnosis of FH, detection of mutations ranges from 50% to 80%, depending on the clinical criteria used—the more stringent the criteria, the more likely mutations will be detected—and the genetic testing protocols. When a genetic abnormality is observed, ~90% or more are a result of an LDL receptor variant, 5% to 10% an apoB variant, and < 1% a PCSK9 variant (Table 2).

A negative genetic test result does not exclude the diagnosis of FH. Negative tests could be a result of technical issues, mutations in yet-to-be-identified genes, defects in other genes that are not routinely examined (*e.g.*, apoE, STAP1, LDL receptor adapter protein 1, or cholesterol 7α-hydroxylase), or polygenic variations (Table 3). Patients may have a large number of relatively common LDL-C–raising polymorphisms—high LDL-C level gene score—that can explain the clinical phenotype and hence have polygenic hypercholesterolemia. As discussed above, the presence of a monogenic variant increases the risk of ASCVD even when LDL-C levels are similar and indicates the need for more aggressive lipid

Table 2. Genetic Variants Leading to FH

LDL receptor	Greater than 1000 variants, including nonsense, missense, insertions, deletions, copy number variants, *etc.*
ApoB	Missense variants in the region of apoB that binds to the LDL receptor
PCSK9	Gain-of-function variants leading to increased LDL receptor degradation

Table 3. Rare Genetic Disorders That Can Be Confused With FH

Sitosterolemia	Autosomal-recessive disorder that results from mutations in ABCG5/8. Manifestations include hypercholesterolemia; marked elevations of plasma plant sterols, tendon, and tuberous xanthomas; and premature ASCVD.
Lysosomal acid lipase deficiency	Autosomal-recessive disorder that results from mutations in the LIPA gene, which codes for lysosomal acid lipase. Manifestations include moderate hypercholesterolemia with depressed HDL-C, accelerated atherosclerosis, and progressive liver disease.
Autosomal-recessive hypercholesterolemia	Autosomal-recessive disorder that results from mutations in LDL receptor adapter protein 1. This typically presents with high LDL cholesterol levels.

lowering. Moreover, use of expensive drugs, such as PCSK9 inhibitors, may require a definitive diagnosis of FH, depending on the healthcare system.

Cascade Testing

Classic FH is an autosomal codominant disorder and, therefore, screening close relatives can be an effective approach to identifying additional individuals at risk. Studies have shown that cascade testing using genetic analysis is a cost-effective approach to identify new patients with FH and allows for early treatment to prevent ASCVD. In index patients without a known genetic variant, screening with a lipid panel should be carried out, but the ability to detect affected individuals will be reduced compared with genetic testing.

Treatment

Goals of Therapy. In patients without clinical ASCVD, one should aim for an LDL-C level < 100 mg/dL (2.59 mmol/L). In patients with clinical ASCVD, the goal at a minimum should be an LDL-C level < 70 mg/dL (1.81 mmol/L), with many experts recommending LDL-C levels < 55 mg/dL (1.42 mmol/L), particularly when patients have additional risk factors (acute coronary syndrome, diabetes, polyvascular disease, *etc.*). In patients without ASCVD but who are at high risk because of other risk factors, such as diabetes, Lp(a) > 50 mg/dL, smoking history, a strong family history of premature ASCVD, *etc.*, many experts would recommend an LDL-C goal of <70 mg/dL (1.81 mmol/L).

Lifestyle Recommendations. As with almost all metabolic disorders, we should encourage the patient to follow a lifestyle that will reduce disease manifestations; however, lifestyle changes are rarely sufficient to lower LDL-C levels to the desired range in patients with FH.

Drug Therapy. Intensive statin therapy is the cornerstone of FH treatment. Patients should be treated with atorvastatin 40 to 80 mg once per day or rosuvastatin 20 to 40 mg once per day (*i.e.*, intensive statin therapy). One can anticipate an approximate 50% reduction in LDL-C. Given the high LDL-C levels, this 50% reduction is often not sufficient to lower LDL-C to the desired level. When intensive statin therapy does not result in an LDL-C level in the desired range, additional

therapy should be added. Given that ezetimibe is now generic and relatively inexpensive, this is frequently the next drug used. One can anticipate that ezetimibe 10 mg once per day added to intensive statin therapy will result in an approximate 20% additional reduction in LDL-C level. If this is not sufficient, one can then use a PCSK9 inhibitor to achieve the desired cholesterol goal. Adding a PCSK9 inhibitor will result in an additional 50% to 60% decrease in LDL-C level and in almost all patients will result in LDL-C levels in the desired range. In some instances, if the LDL-C level is far from the goal (>25%) on intensive statin therapy, one can skip treatment with ezetimibe and proceed directly to adding a PCSK9 inhibitor. In certain instances, bile resin binders may be useful in the treatment of FH (*e.g.*, pregnant patients). In our case, addition of a PCSK9 inhibitor to her current therapy of atorvastatin 80 mg once per day and ezetimibe 10 mg once per day is indicated.

Treat Other Risk Factors. One should aggressively control other ASCVD risk factors.

Case 3: Elevated Lp(a)

The patient is a 52-year-old female with coronary heart disease (CHD) and a strong family history of premature CHD—mother, sister, and other relatives had MIs before age 60 years. There are no other CHD risk factors and her initial lipid panel revealed a TG level of 100 mg/dL (1.13 mmol/L), HDL-C 50 mg/dL (1.29 mmol/L), and LDL-C 130 mg/dL (3.37 mmol/L). She was treated with atorvastatin 40 mg, which reduced LDL by only 23%. What disorder might this patient have and what would you do next?

Introduction

Lp(a) is an LDL particle with the addition of the large apo(a) protein linked to apoB on the LDL particle via a disulfide bond. Apo(a) is structurally similar to plasminogen. The molecular weight of apo(a) varies greatly—from 300 to 800 kDa—as a result of a variable number of repeats of one of the kringle domains (kringle IV type 2). Lp(a) is produced by the liver, but the clearance pathways are not well understood. Clearance of Lp(a) is not predominantly regulated by the LDL receptor and, therefore, lowering LDL-C levels with statins or ezetimibe does not lower Lp(a) levels. The kidney seems to play an important role in Lp(a) clearance as renal disease is associated with increased Lp(a) levels. Levels of Lp(a) seem to be regulated primarily by the rate of production of Lp(a).

Epidemiology

Serum levels of Lp(a) are highly skewed, with most individuals having relatively low levels. Concentration of Lp(a) can vary by up to 1000-fold between individuals (<0.1 mg/dL to >200 mg/dL). Approximately 20% of patients have Lp(a) levels > 50 mg/dL and 30% have Lp(a) > 30 mg/dL. Ethnicity greatly affects Lp(a) levels. Levels of Lp(a) in black patients are approximately two- to -threefold higher than in white patients, white and Chinese patients have similar levels, South Asian patients have levels that are between those of black and white patients, and Mexican patients have levels that are less than those of white patients (black > South Asian > white/Chinese > Mexican patients). The serum Lp(a) level is inversely related to the size of the apo(a) protein [*i.e.*, individuals with small apo(a) isoforms have high serum Lp(a) levels, whereas individuals with large apo(a) isoforms have low serum Lp(a) levels]. The size of the apo(a) isoform is inherited, with an individual having two distinct apo(a) isoforms that are derived from apo(a) genes from his or her mother and father. This results in individuals having two different size Lp(a) particles in serum. It is estimated that up to 90% of the variation in Lp(a) levels is determined genetically, with the environment having minimal effect. Lp(a) levels are stable within an individual over his or her lifespan. Inflammation and renal disease increase, whereas severe liver disease decreases Lp(a) levels.

Risk of ASCVD

A large number of studies have shown that elevated serum Lp(a) levels are an independent risk factor for ASCVD in individuals without ASCVD. In patients with preexisting ASCVD, Lp(a) levels predict the risk for new events in most but not all studies. Patients with FH frequently have elevated Lp(a) levels, and the combination of elevated LDL-C levels and high Lp(a) levels markedly exacerbates the risk for ASCVD events. Mendelian randomization studies and genome-wide association studies strongly suggest that an elevated Lp(a) is causal and not just a marker for ASCVD. Additional support for a causal role for Lp(a) is observational studies that show that lipoprotein apheresis in patients with high Lp(a) levels reduces ASCVD events. In addition to ASCVD, elevated Lp(a) levels lead to calcific aortic valve stenosis.

Potential Mechanisms for ASCVD

- Uptake of Lp(a) by macrophages in the arterial wall
- Increased oxidized phospholipids carried on Lp(a), having pro-oxidative and proinflammatory effects

- Lp(a) inhibits the fibrinolytic system

When to Measure LP(a) Levels

- Patients with unexplained premature CHD
- Patients with a strong family history of premature CHD
- Patients with a family history of elevated Lp(a) levels (cascade screening)
- Patients with resistance to LDL-C lowering with statins
- Patients with rapid unexplained progression of atherosclerosis
- Patients with FH
- Patients with aortic valvular stenosis of uncertain cause
- Patients with intermediate risk profiles??

Measuring LP(a) Levels

Standard measurements of LDL-C—either calculated or measured—include Lp(a) cholesterol. When Lp(a) levels are high, they can make a significant contribution to LDL-C levels. Similarly, when LDL-C levels are markedly reduced with treatment, LDL-C measured may include a significant contribution from Lp(a). The contribution of Lp(a) cholesterol to calculated LDL-C is approximately milligrams per deciliter Lp(a) × 0.3 (when both are expressed in milligrams per deciliter). For example, if the Lp(a) level is 100 mg/dL, one can estimate that 30 mg/dL of the calculated LDL level is a result of Lp(a). Accurate measurement of Lp(a) represents a formidable technical challenge, unequalled in the world of biochemical diagnostics. This is because of the extreme length polymorphism of apo(a), whose size can vary more than fivefold. Measuring Lp(a) mass (in milligrams per deciliter) —as it is most often done in commercial clinical laboratories—will not allow for a reliable and consistent way to convert Lp(a) concentration to nmol/L. For example, 50 mg/dL of an Lp(a) with 40 kringle IV type 2 repeats is actually fewer particles than 30 mg/dL of an Lp(a) with 15 kringle IV type repeats. The solution is the adoption of an isoform-independent method that equally identifies each Lp(a) particle. Such a method is currently approximated by the use of a spectrum of isoform-specific calibrators, and providers, if possible, should have Lp(a) measured using this method and reported as concentration in nanomoles per liter.

Lowering LP(a) Levels

Lifestyle changes do not significantly lower Lp(a) levels. Whereas statins and ezetimibe do not lower Lp(a) levels, there are hypolipidemia drugs that do lower Lp(a) (Table 4). Niacin and PCSK9 inhibitors will lower Lp(a) levels by approximately 15% to 30%. In postmenopausal women, estrogens will lower Lp(a) levels (20% to 35%). In development is an antisense oligonucleotide directed at apo(a). Early studies have shown that this antisense can lower Lp(a) by > 75% without affecting other lipoprotein levels. Lipoprotein

Table 4. Effect of Lipid-Lowering Drugs on Lp(a) Levels

Statins	No effect or slight increase
Ezetimibe	No effect or slight increase
Fibrates	No effect
Niacin	Decrease 15%–25%; greatest decrease in patients with highest Lp(a) levels
PCSK9 inhibitors	Decrease 20%–30%
Estrogen	Decrease 20%–35%
Mipomersen[a]	Decrease 25%–30%
Lomitapide[a]	Decrease 15%–20%
Cholesteryl ester transfer protein inhibitors[b]	Decrease ~25%
Apo (a) antisense[b]	Decrease >75%

[a] Only approved for the treatment of homozygous FH.
[b] Not currently available.

apheresis can be used to lower Lp(a) in patients with high Lp(a) levels who continue to have events despite optimal medical management.

Of note, tocilizumab, an antibody against IL-6 used to treat rheumatoid arthritis, has been shown to decrease Lp(a) levels by 30% to 40%. In patients with elevated Lp(a) levels, it is important to aggressively treat other risk factors for ASCVD as we currently do not have treatments that robustly lower Lp(a) levels.

References

1. Chait A, Subramanian S, Brunzell JD. Genetic disorders of triglyceride metabolism. In: De Groot LJ, Chrousos G, Dungan K, Feingold KR, Grossman A, Hershman JM, Koch C, Korbonits M, McLachlan R, New M, Purnell J, Rebar R, Singer F, Vinik A, eds. *Endotext*. South Dartmouth, MA: MDText.com; 2015:26561703.
2. Fong LG, Young SG, Beigneux AP, Bensadoun A, Oberer M, Jiang H, Ploug M. GPIHBP1 and plasma triglyceride metabolism. *Trends Endocrinol Metab*. 2016;**27**(7):455–469.
3. Gryn SE, Hegele RA. Novel therapeutics in hypertriglyceridemia. *Curr Opin Lipidol*. 2015;**26**(6):484–491.
4. Wójcik C, Fazio S, McIntyre AD, Hegele RA. Co-occurrence of heterozygous CREB3L3 and APOA5 nonsense variants and polygenic risk in a patient with severe hypertriglyceridemia exacerbated by estrogen administration. *J Clin Lipidol*. 2018;**12**(5):1146–1150.
5. Lilley JS, Linton MF, Kelley JC, Graham TB, Fazio S, Tavori H. A case of severe acquired hypertriglyceridemia in a 7-year-old girl. *J Clin Lipidol*. 2017;**11**(6):1480–1484.
6. Sturm AC, Knowles JW, Gidding SS, Ahmad ZS, Ahmed CD, Ballantyne CM, Baum SJ, Bourbon M, Carrie A, Cuchel M, de Ferranti SD, Defesche JC, Freiberger T, Hershberger RE, Hovingh GK, Karayan L, Kastelein JJP, Kindt I, Lane SR, Leigh SE, Linton MF, Mata P, Neal WA, Nordestgaard BG, Santos RD, Harada-Shiba M, Sijbrands EJ, Stitziel NO, Yamashita S, Wilemon KA, Ledbetter DH, Rader DJ, for the Familial Hypercholesterolemia Foundation. Clinical genetic testing for familial hypercholesterolemia: JACC Scientific Expert Panel. *J Am Coll Cardiol*. 2018;**72**(6):662–680.
7. Safarova MS, Kullo IJ. My approach to the patient with familial hypercholesterolemia. *Mayo Clin Proc*. 2016;**91**(6):770–786.
8. Berberich AJ, Hegele RA. The complex molecular genetics of familial hypercholesterolaemia [published ahead of print 4 July 2018]. *Nat Rev Cardiol*. doi: 10.1038/s41569-018-0052-6.
9. Levenson AE, de Ferranti SD. Familial hypercholesterolemia (pediatric section). In: De Groot LJ, Chrousos G, Dungan K, Feingold KR, Grossman A, Hershman JM, Koch C, Korbonits M, McLachlan R, New M, Purnell J, Rebar R, Singer F, Vinik A, eds. *Endotext*. South Dartmouth, MA: MDText.com; 2016:27809433.
10. Pendyal A, Fazio S. The severe hypercholesterolemia phenotype: Genes and beyond. In: De Groot LJ, Chrousos G, Dungan K, Feingold KR, Grossman A, Hershman JM, Koch C, Korbonits M, McLachlan R, New M, Purnell J, Rebar R, Singer F, Vinik A, eds. *Endotext*. South Dartmouth, MA: MDText.com; 2015:26844336.
11. McNeal C. Lipoprotein (a). In: De Groot LJ, Chrousos G, Dungan K, Feingold KR, Grossman A, Hershman JM, Koch C, Korbonits M, McLachlan R, New M, Purnell J, Rebar R, Singer F, Vinik A, eds. *Endotext*. South Dartmouth, MA: MDText.com; 2015:27809431.
12. Shapiro MD. Rare genetic disorders altering lipoproteins. In: De Groot LJ, Chrousos G, Dungan K, Feingold KR, Grossman A, Hershman JM, Koch C, Korbonits M, McLachlan R, New M, Purnell J, Rebar R, Singer F, Vinik A, eds. *Endotext*. South Dartmouth, MA: MDText.com; 2015:26561704.
13. Boffa MB, Koschinsky ML. The journey towards understanding lipoprotein(a) and cardiovascular disease risk: Are we there yet? *Curr Opin Lipidol*. 2018;**29**(3):259–267.
14. Enkhmaa B, Anuurad E, Berglund L. Lipoprotein (a): Impact by ethnicity and environmental and medical conditions. *J Lipid Res*. 2016;**57**(7):1111–1125.
15. van Capelleveen JC, van der Valk FM, Stroes ES. Current therapies for lowering lipoprotein (a). *J Lipid Res*. 2016;**57**(9):1612–1618.
16. Tsimikas S, Fazio S, Viney NJ, Xia S, Witztum JL, Marcovina SM. Relationship of lipoprotein(a) molar concentrations and mass according to lipoprotein(a) thresholds and apolipoprotein(a) isoform size. *J Clin Lipidol*. 2018;**12**(5):1313–1323.

Residual Risk: How to Assess Risk Beyond the Atherosclerotic Cardiovascular Disease Risk Calculator

M26
Presented, March 23–26, 2019

Marc-Andre Cornier, MD. Division of Endocrinology, Metabolism and Diabetes, Anschutz Health and Wellness Center, University of Colorado School of Medicine, Aurora, Colorado 80209, E-mail: marc.cornier@ucdenver.edu

SIGNIFICANCE OF THE CLINICAL PROBLEM

Atherosclerotic cardiovascular disease (ASCVD) remains a major cause of death worldwide. Cholesterol is at the core of atherosclerosis development and is one of the major modifiable risk factors. Randomized controlled trials have conclusively shown that cholesterol lowering [specifically low-density lipoprotein cholesterol (LDL-C)] is associated with reductions in ASCVD-related events and mortality. Unfortunately, the reduction in events with LDL-C lowering is often < 50%, which means that some individuals (if not the majority of them) will still have events despite LDL-C lowering. This remaining risk has been coined "residual risk." Residual risk has been attributed to a number of factors, such as LDL-C lowering that is not aggressive enough, starting LDL-C–lowering therapy too late, studies that have not been long enough to see the full effect, and/or other noncholesterol risk factors. Other independent risk factors include age, genetics, sedentary lifestyle, atherogenic diet, obesity, low high-density lipoprotein (HDL)-C, hypertriglyceridemia, metabolic syndrome (MetS), elevated apolipoprotein B (apoB), elevated lipoprotein (a) [Lp(a)], markers of inflammation such as high-sensitivity C-reactive protein (hsCRP), low ankle-brachial index, and evidence of subclinical ASCVD [*e.g.*, coronary artery calcium (CAC)]. When, and in whom, these other markers of risk should be used is not entirely clear, but the new *2018 AHA/ACC/AACVPR/AAPA/ABC/ACPM/ADA/AGS/APhA/ ASPC/NLA/PCNA Guideline on the Management of Blood Cholesterol* offers a reasonable guide, which will be reviewed here (1). Also of controversy is whether treating these other factors results in clinical benefits.

BARRIERS TO OPTIMAL PRACTICE

- The need to better assess a patient's risk for ASCVD to help make decisions on the best treatment goals and options
- Lack of data on the treatment of noncholesterol risk factors

LEARNING OBJECTIVES

As a result of participating in this session, learners should be able to:

- Recognize ASCVD risk factors beyond LDL-C and when to use them appropriately
- Understand recent data regarding treating hypertriglyceridemia as a potential modifiable ASCVD risk factor target
- Be aware of data supporting the use of Lp(a) as an ASCVD risk factor

STRATEGIES FOR DIAGNOSIS, THERAPY, AND/OR MANAGEMENT

Assessment and Goal Setting in Primary Prevention

Before an adequate management plan can be offered to patients for ASCVD risk reduction, a number of steps need to be taken (1).

1. Assessment of risk. Adults 20 years of age or older should undergo assessment of their lipids (preferably in the fasted state) and of other major ASCVD risk factors, including age, sex, family history of premature ASCVD, and personal history of diabetes and hypertension. This should be performed every 4 to 6 years. Individuals with severe hypercholesterolemia (LDL-C $\geq$ 190 mg/dL or $\geq$ 4.9 mmol/L) and those older than 40 years with diabetes should be started on high- or moderate-intensity statin therapy. The 10-year ASCVD risk calculation should be performed in those without severe hypercholesterolemia or diabetes. If the patient is at low risk (< 5%), then lifestyle should be emphasized. If the patient is at high risk ($\geq$ 20%), then high-intensity statin therapy should be initiated. If the risk is $\geq$5% [either borderline (5% to <7.5%) or intermediate ($\geq$7.5% to <20%)], then assessment for ASCVD risk enhancers should be performed.

2. ASCVD risk enhancers. Patients should be assessed for risk enhancers by history, physical examination, and laboratory testing. Historically important factors include family history of premature ASCVD; chronic kidney disease; MetS; inflammatory diseases such as rheumatoid arthritis, psoriasis, and HIV; and ethnicity. Examination findings include blood pressure, waist circumference (assessments for MetS), and ankle-brachial index (<0.9). Laboratory assessments should include looking for elevations in LDL-C (160 to 189 mg/dL or 4.1 to 4.8 mmol/L), triglycerides ($\geq$175 mg/dL or $\geq$2.0 mmol/L), hsCRP ($\geq$2.0 mg/L), and Lp(a) (>50 mg/dL or >125 nmol/L). In patients with hypertriglyceridemia, apoB levels may be helpful as a marker of increased LDL particle number, with apoB levels $\geq$ 130 mg/dL constituting a risk-enhancing factor.

3. CAC. For intermediate-risk individuals ($\geq$ 7.5% to < 20%) in whom the risk decision is uncertain, consideration should be given to obtaining a CAC score. If the score is

elevated (≥100 and/or ≥75th percentile or 1 to 99 in patients older than 55 years), statin therapy should be considered.

4. Goal setting. After a patient's risk has been assessed, goals and treatment options can be discussed. A healthy dietary pattern should be recommended to all individuals. Lifestyle therapy with a goal of maintaining a healthy weight should also be considered, especially in those with MetS. For higher-risk individuals, lipid lowering with statin therapy should be the primary treatment of choice. The goal is to select the appropriate intensity of statin therapy. High-intensity statins typically lower LDL-C by ≥50% and should be used in high-risk individuals. Moderate-intensity statins lower LDL-C by 30% to 49% and should be considered for moderate-risk individuals. Nonstatin therapies such as PCSK9 inhibitors, ezetimibe, and bile acid sequestrants can be considered as add-on treatments to statins in certain circumstances (*e.g.*, patients with severe LDL-C elevations despite statin therapy, as may be seen in cases of familial hypercholesterolemia).

Assessment and Goal Setting in Secondary Prevention

Before an adequate management plan for the prevention of recurrent events can be offered to patients with known ASCVD, a number of steps must be taken (1).

1. Assessment of risk. Individuals with known clinical ASCVD should be assessed for "very high risk." High-risk individuals are those with a history of multiple ASCVD events or those with one major event plus multiple high-risk factors. High-risk factors include age ≥ 65 years, history of coronary artery bypass grafting or percutaneous coronary interventions, diabetes, hypertension, chronic kidney disease, smoking, congestive heart failure, and persistently elevated LDL-C (≥100 mg/dL or ≥2.6 mmol/L).

2. Goal setting. After a patient's risk has been assessed, goals and treatment options can be discussed. Adopting a healthy dietary pattern and lifestyle should be recommended to all individuals. Regardless of risk, it is recommended that all patients with known ASCVD be treated with high-intensity statin therapy unless they are older than 75 years, in which case moderate-intensity statin therapy may be reasonable. For those who are not at very high risk but have persistently elevated LDL-C of ≥ 70 mg/dL, the addition of ezetimibe should be considered. For those who are at very high risk with persistently elevated LDL-C of ≥70 mg/dL, the addition of ezetimibe and/or a PCSK9 inhibitor should be considered.

Residual Risk

The new guidelines support more aggressive LDL-C lowering and potentially starting at a younger age, depending on the risk. More aggressive LDL-C lowering has been shown to reduce the residual risk from 50% to 70% to 40% to 50%. Meta-analyses have shown that more aggressive LDL-C lowering in statin trials is associated with greater reductions in major ASCVD events (2). The JUPITER trial showed that major ASCVD events were further reduced if the LDL-C after reduction was <50 mg/dL (3). Further lowering of LDL-C with nonstatin therapies added to statins has also shown greater ASCVD risk reductions. Specifically, the IMPROVE-IT trial showed that the addition of ezetimibe further lowered risk (4). Both of the recent outcome trials with PCSK9 inhibitors have also shown further reductions in ASCVD events with more aggressive LDL lowering (5, 6). Aggressive LDL-C lowering with PCSK9 inhibitor therapy has also been shown to result in greater regression of atheroma volume (7). Therefore, it is possible that with much more aggressive LDL-C lowering, the residual risk could be reduced to 30% to 40%. Furthermore, longer duration of therapy and initiation at a younger age (before the atherosclerotic process has become severe) may further reduce the residual risk. Long-term follow-up studies suggest that there is continued risk reduction over time (8). But unfortunately, longer-term studies in younger individuals will probably never be performed due to the tremendous cost.

Triglycerides

One potential modifiable risk factor of interest is hypertriglyceridemia. Elevations in triglycerides have been shown to be an independent risk factor for ASCVD (9). That relationship is even stronger in women, and more so in women with diabetes. However, whether triglycerides are causative to the progression of ASCVD and resulting events is not clear. As such, lowering triglycerides as a treatment target is controversial. Early randomized controlled trials have shown that, compared with placebo, fibrate therapy with gemfibrozil results in reduced risk of ASCVD events (10, 11). However, the benefit could not be attributed to triglyceride lowering with the fibrate in either of the studies. Other monotherapy and add-on to statin trials with fenofibrate have not found overall significant benefits in ASCVD events (12, 13). In the ACCORD trial, the subgroup of patients with elevated triglycerides (≥ 204 mg/dL) did experience a 31% reduction in the primary CVD outcomes, but at borderline significance (*P* = 0.057) (13). There has also been mixed results with fish oil therapy. In the JELIS study, 1800 mg of eicosapentaenoic acid (EPA) in addition to statin therapy compared with statin therapy alone resulted in a 19% reduction in major coronary events (14). The recent REDUCE-IT study, with 4000 mg of EPA daily compared with placebo in high-risk individuals receiving statins, showed a 25% reduction in major ASCVD events. Interestingly, the effect was seen regardless of baseline triglyceride levels and degree of triglyceride lowering.

Lp(a)

To further address a patient's risk for ASCVD, the new cholesterol guidelines have adopted Lp(a) as a risk enhancer (1). But, what is Lp(a)? Lp(a) is an LDL particle with an apo(a) protein produced by the liver bound by disulfide linkage to the

LDL-related apoB protein. Soon after its discovery, elevations in Lp(a) were found to be associated with coronary heart disease (15) and atherosclerosis (16). It was then found that apo(a) has 85% homology to plasminogen (17), which may explain the increased risk of thrombosis seen with elevations in Lp(a) (18). More recent reports of the relationship between levels of Lp(a) and ASCVD have been provided from a large number of cohorts (19, 20). A meta-analysis of Lp(a) levels adjusted for age and sex showed a 1.55 relative risk for nonfatal myocardial infarction (MI) and coronary heart disease death (21). Beyond ASCVD, elevated levels of Lp(a) are highly associated with aortic valve disease, including calcification and disease progression including aortic valve replacement (22). Despite the strong evidence of Lp(a) elevations being associated with ASCVD, there is less convincing evidence that lowering Lp(a) reduces ASCVD events. Thus, an important question to address is why should we measure Lp(a)? There are at least three good reasons, which include the following: 1) to better understand familial risk for ASCVD, 2) to be more aggressive in managing other ASCVD risk factors, and 3) to identify individuals who may benefit from new investigational products that target Lp(a). Lifestyle approaches that lower LDL-C have no effect on levels of Lp(a) (23). Historically, niacin at doses up to 3000 mg daily has lowered Lp(a) by up to 30% (24). However, despite the benefit of Lp(a) lowering by nicotinic acid, the AIM-HIGH study showed no benefit on CVD events (25). LDL apheresis performed every 2 weeks not only lowers Lp(a) by approximately 70% but is also associated with reduction in ASCVD event rates. The independent effect of this lowering from that of other apoB-containing lipoproteins, however, remains unclear (26). Nevertheless, patients with recurrent ASCVD events and an Lp(a) > 100 mg/dL should be considered as candidates for apheresis. PCSK9 inhibitors also lower Lp(a) by 25% to 30% (27, 28), but again, the independent benefit on ASCVD events has not been demonstrated. An investigational antisense oligonucleotide targeting apo(a) has been shown to reduce Lp(a) by up to 70% in early-phase trials (29). Inclisiran, an investigational PCSK9 RNA interference agent, also reduces Lp(a) in a dose-dependent manner, with reductions of up to 40% (30).

CONCLUSIONS

LDL-C lowering is associated with substantial reductions in ASCVD outcomes and remains a mainstay in the treatment and prevention of ASCVD. However, despite LDL-C lowering, some individuals are still at risk for ASCVD events. This residual risk may be caused by a number of factors. One factor that can be addressed and is supported by data is to be more aggressive with LDL-C lowering than in the past. Residual risk can be further minimized by starting treatment earlier and treating patients longer. The benefits are not as clear for other targets, such as lowering triglyceride or Lp(a) levels. New data suggest that high-dose EPA-based fish oil may further lower residual risk, although the mechanisms are not clear.

CASES WITH ANSWERS AND DISCUSSIONS
Case 1

A 56-year-old man is seeking ongoing care for hypertension. Besides being overweight and fairly sedentary, he considers himself to be healthy. He does not take any medications. His father had an MI at the age of 54 years. He does not exercise but tries to eat healthily. He was a smoker but quit a number of years ago. He feels well overall. His physical examination is notable for central adiposity. His blood pressure is 132/80 mm Hg, his body mass index is 28 mg/kg^2, and he has a waist circumference of 44 inches. Fasting laboratory results reveal total cholesterol 209 mg/dL, triglycerides 220 mg/dL, LDL-C 128 mg/dL, HDL-C 37 mg/dL, glucose 108 mg/dL, and HbA$_{1c}$ 5.9%.

Questions

1. What is this patient's risk for ASCVD—should there be concern?

Because the patient does not have known clinical ASCVD, severe hypercholesterolemia, or diabetes, his 10-year risk of ASCVD should be calculated using the "Pooled Cohort Equations" (1). Based on his history, physical examination, and untreated lipid levels, he has a 10-year ASCVD risk of 8.7%, which puts him in the intermediate-risk category.

2. How can his risk be further assessed?

An assessment of risk enhancers should be performed. In addition to his known risk factors (a family history of premature ASCVD, MetS, and hypertriglyceridemia), other markers could be measured to assist in the decision making. An elevated hsCRP, Lp(a), and/or apoB would be associated with increased risk. If the decision is still unclear, then further assessment could be made by measuring his CAC.

3. How should this patient be treated to prevent ASCVD?

In light of his intermediate risk and the presence of other risk enhancers (especially the family history of premature ASCVD), strong consideration should be given to initiating at least moderate-intensity statin therapy in addition to making healthy lifestyle recommendations. Other markers of risk [e.g., hsCRP, Lp(a), apoB (because he has hypertriglyceridemia), and/or CAC] could be considered to guide the intensity of statin therapy, i.e., high-intensity therapy would be considered if any of these factors are elevated.

Case 2

A 66-year-old woman comes in for follow up of her hyperlipidemia. She had a non–ST-elevation MI with coronary stent placement a few years ago. She is doing well, without any evidence of recent symptoms of ischemia or heart failure. She takes atorvastatin 80 mg (since her MI), metoprolol, aspirin, levothyroxine, and omeprazole. She follows a heart-healthy dietary pattern, walks 45 minutes every day, and does not smoke. Her physical examination is unremarkable. Her blood pressure is 134/82 mm Hg, and her body mass index is 26 mg/kg^2. Results of a fasting lipid panel reveal total cholesterol 189 mg/dL, triglycerides 155 mg/dL, LDL-C 121 mg/dL, and HDL-C 37 mg/dL.

Questions

1. What is this patient's risk for ASCVD?

The new cholesterol guideline recommends determining if secondary prevention patients are at very high risk (1). Because she is older than 65 years, had a percutaneous coronary intervention, and has an LDL-C level that is persistently ≥100 mg/dL, this patient should be considered very high risk. Although not necessarily endorsed by the new guideline, if she did not have any high-risk conditions, it might be reasonable to measure other markers of risk [e.g., hsCRP and Lp(a)] and treat as very high risk if these markers are elevated.

2. What should our goals be to prevent recurrent ASCVD events in this high-risk patient?

Initial treatment goals should include a healthy lifestyle and high-intensity statin therapy. This patient is following a heathy lifestyle and is taking atorvastatin 80 mg daily (high-intensity statin). Although the new guideline does not recommend setting LDL-C goals *per se*, they do recommend the addition of nonstatin therapies in patients who have an LDL-C level that is still ≥70 mg/dL despite maximal statin therapy.

3. How should we treat this patient to prevent ASCVD?

Because this patient's LDL-C level is 121 mg/dL and thus significantly >70 mg/dL, it would be reasonable to be more aggressive with her LDL-C lowering. The atorvastatin 80 mg could be switched to rosuvastatin 40 mg daily, but this would probably reduce her LDL-C level by only a few percentage points. The addition of ezetimibe is recommended by the new guideline and is often required by insurers before moving on to a PCSK9 inhibitor. However, ezetimibe would probably reduce her LDL-C level by only 18% on average, thus unlikely to get her LDL-C level to ≤ 70 mg/dL. A PCSK9 inhibitor would probably be necessary to achieve such a reduction goal. Another intriguing option would be to consider pure EPA-based high-dose fish oil. With known clinical ASCVD and a triglycerides level > 150 mg/dL, she meets criteria set by the REDUCE-IT trial.

References

1. Grundy SM, Stone NJ, Bailey AL, Beam C, Birtcher KK, Blumenthal RS, Braun LT, de Ferranti S, Faiella-Tommasino J, Forman DE, Goldberg R, Heidenreich PA, Hlatky MA, Jones DW, Lloyd-Jones D, Lopez-Pajares N, Ndumele CE, Orringer CE, Peralta CA, Saseen JJ, Smith SC aJr, Sperling L, Virani SS, Yeboah J. 2018 AHA/ACC/AACVPR/AAPA/ABC/ACPM/ADA/AGS/APhA/ASPC/NLA/PCNA guideline on the management of blood cholesterol: executive summary: a report of the American College of Cardiology/American Heart Association Task Force on Clinical Practice Guidelines [published online ahead of print 3 November 2018]. *J Am Coll Cardiol.* doi:10.1016/j.jacc.2018.11.002.
2. Boekholdt SM, Hovingh GK, Mora S, Arsenault BJ, Amarenco P, Pedersen TR, LaRosa JC, Waters DD, DeMicco DA, Simes RJ, Keech AC, Colquhoun D, Hitman GA, Betteridge DJ, Clearfield MB, Downs JR, Colhoun HM, Gotto AM Jr, Ridker PM, Grundy SM, Kastelein JJ. Very low levels of atherogenic lipoproteins and the risk for cardiovascular events: a meta-analysis of statin trials. *J Am Coll Cardiol.* 2014;**64**(5): 485–494.
3. Hsia J, MacFadyen JG, Monyak J, Ridker PM. Cardiovascular event reduction and adverse events among subjects attaining low-density lipoprotein cholesterol <50 mg/dl with rosuvastatin. The JUPITER trial (Justification for the Use of Statins in Prevention: an Intervention Trial Evaluating Rosuvastatin). *J Am Coll Cardiol.* 2011;**57**(16): 1666–1675.
4. Cannon CP, Blazing MA, Giugliano RP, McCagg A, White JA, Theroux P, Darius H, Lewis BS, Ophuis TO, Jukema JW, De Ferrari GM, Ruzyllo W, De Lucca P, Im K, Bohula EA, Reist C, Wiviott SD, Tershakovec AM, Musliner TA, Braunwald E, Califf RM; IMPROVE-IT Investigators. Ezetimibe added to statin therapy after acute coronary syndromes. *N Engl J Med.* 2015;**372**(25):2387–2397.
5. Sabatine MS, Giugliano RP, Keech AC, Honarpour N, Wiviott SD, Murphy SA, Kuder JF, Wang H, Liu T, Wasserman SM, Sever PS, Pedersen TR; FOURIER Steering Committee and Investigators. Evolocumab and clinical outcomes in patients with cardiovascular disease. *N Engl J Med.* 2017;**376**(18):1713–1722.
6. Schwartz GG, Steg PG, Szarek M, Bhatt DL, Bittner VA, Diaz R, Edelberg JM, Goodman SG, Hanotin C, Harrington RA, Jukema JW, Lecorps G, Mahaffey KW, Moryusef A, Pordy R, Quintero K, Roe MT, Sasiela WJ, Tamby JF, Tricoci P, White HD, Zeiher AM; ODYSSEY OUTCOMES Committees and Investigators. Alirocumab and cardiovascular outcomes after acute coronary syndrome. *N Engl J Med.* 2018;**379**(22): 2097–2107.
7. Nicholls SJ, Puri R, Anderson T, Ballantyne CM, Cho L, Kastelein JJ, Koenig W, Somaratne R, Kassahun H, Yang J, Wasserman SM, Scott R, Ungi I, Podolec J, Ophuis AO, Cornel JH, Borgman M, Brennan DM, Nissen SE. Effect of evolocumab on progression of coronary disease in statin-treated patients: the GLAGOV Randomized Clinical Trial. *JAMA.* 2016;**316**(22):2373–2384.
8. Zhao XQ, Phan BA, Davis J, Isquith D, Dowdy AA, Boltz S, Neradilek M, Monick EA, Brockenbrough A, Hus-Frechette EE, Albers JJ, Brown BG. Mortality reduction in patients treated with long-term intensive lipid therapy: 25-year follow-up of the Familial Atherosclerosis Treatment Study-Observational Study. *J Clin Lipidol.* 2016;**10**(5):1091–1097.
9. Miller M, Stone NJ, Ballantyne C, Bittner V, Criqui MH, Ginsberg HN, Goldberg AC, Howard WJ, Jacobson MS, Kris-Etherton PM, Lennie TA, Levi M, Mazzone T, Pennathur S; American Heart Association Clinical Lipidology, Thrombosis, and Prevention Committee of the Council on Nutrition, Physical Activity, and Metabolism Council on Arteriosclerosis, Thrombosis and Vascular Biology Council on Cardiovascular Nursing Council on the Kidney in Cardiovascular Disease. Triglycerides and cardiovascular disease: a scientific statement from the American Heart Association. *Circulation.* 2011;**123**(20):2292–2333.
10. Rubins HB, Robins SJ, Collins D, Fye CL, Anderson JW, Elam MB, Faas FH, Linares E, Schaefer EJ, Schectman G, Wilt TJ, Wittes J; Veterans Affairs High-Density Lipoprotein Cholesterol Intervention Trial Study Group. Gemfibrozil for the secondary prevention of coronary heart disease in men with low levels of high-density lipoprotein cholesterol. *N Engl J Med.* 1999;**341**(6):410–418.
11. Frick MH, Elo O, Haapa K, Heinonen OP, Heinsalmi P, Helo P, Huttunen JK, Kaitaniemi P, Koskinen P, Manninen V, Mäenpää H, Mälkönen M, Mänttäri M, Norola S, Pasternack A, Pikkarainen J, Romo M, Sjöblom T, Nikkilä EA. Helsinki Heart Study: primary-prevention trial with gemfibrozil in middle-aged men with dyslipidemia. Safety of treatment, changes in risk factors, and incidence of coronary heart disease. *N Engl J Med.* 1987;**317**(20):1237–1245.
12. Keech A, Simes RJ, Barter P, Best J, Scott R, Taskinen MR, Forder P, Pillai A, Davis T, Glasziou P, Drury P, Kesäniemi YA, Sullivan D, Hunt D, Colman P, d'Emden M, Whiting M, Ehnholm C, Laakso M; FIELD study investigators. Effects of long-term fenofibrate therapy on cardiovascular events in 9795 people with type 2 diabetes mellitus (the FIELD study): randomised controlled trial. *Lancet.* 2005;**366**(9500): 1849–1861.
13. ACCORD Study Group, Ginsberg HN, Elam MB, Lovato LC, Crouse JR 3rd, Leiter LA, Linz P, Friedewald WT, Buse JB, Gerstein HC, Probstfield J, Grimm RH, Ismail-Beigi F, Bigger JT, Goff DC Jr, Cushman WC, Simons-Morton DG,

Byington RP. Effects of combination lipid therapy in type 2 diabetes mellitus. *N Engl J Med.* 2010;**362**(17):1563–1574.

14. Yokoyama M, Origasa H, Matsuzaki M, Matsuzawa Y, Saito Y, Ishikawa Y, Oikawa S, Sasaki J, Hishida H, Itakura H, Kita T, Kitabatake A, Nakaya N, Sakata T, Shimada K, Shirato K; Japan EPA Lipid Intervention Study (JELIS) Investigators. Effects of eicosapentaenoic acid on major coronary events in hypercholesterolaemic patients (JELIS): a randomised open-label, blinded endpoint analysis. *Lancet.* 2007;**369**(9567):1090–1098.

15. Berg K, Dahlén G, Frick MH. Lp(a) lipoprotein and pre-beta1-lipoprotein in patients with coronary heart disease. *Clin Genet.* 1974;**6**(3):230–235.

16. Walton KW, Hitchens J, Magnani HN, Khan M. A study of methods of identification and estimation of Lp(a) lipoprotein and of its significance in health, hyperlipidaemia and atherosclerosis. *Atherosclerosis.* 1974;**20**(2):323–346.

17. McLean JW, Tomlinson JE, Kuang WJ, Eaton DL, Chen EY, Fless GM, Scanu AM, Lawn RM. cDNA sequence of human apolipoprotein(a) is homologous to plasminogen. *Nature.* 1987;**330**(6144):132–137.

18. Hancock MA, Boffa MB, Marcovina SM, Nesheim ME, Koschinsky ML. Inhibition of plasminogen activation by lipoprotein(a): critical domains in apolipoprotein(a) and mechanism of inhibition on fibrin and degraded fibrin surfaces. *J Biol Chem.* 2003;**278**(26):23260–23269.

19. Suk Danik J, Rifai N, Buring JE, Ridker PM. Lipoprotein(a), measured with an assay independent of apolipoprotein(a) isoform size, and risk of future cardiovascular events among initially healthy women. *JAMA.* 2006;**296**(11):1363–1370.

20. Bennet A, Di Angelantonio E, Erqou S, Eiriksdottir G, Sigurdsson G, Woodward M, Rumley A, Lowe GD, Danesh J, Gudnason V. Lipoprotein(a) levels and risk of future coronary heart disease: large-scale prospective data. *Arch Intern Med.* 2008;**168**(6):598–608.

21. Lee SR, Prasad A, Choi YS, Xing C, Clopton P, Witztum JL, Tsimikas S. LPA gene, ethnicity, and cardiovascular events. *Circulation.* 2017;**135**(3):251–263.

22. Capoulade R, Chan KL, Yeang C, Mathieu P, Bossé Y, Dumesnil JG, Tam JW, Teo KK, Mahmut A, Yang X, Witztum JL, Arsenault BJ, Després JP, Pibarot P, Tsimikas S. Oxidized phospholipids, lipoprotein(a), and progression of calcific aortic valve stenosis. *J Am Coll Cardiol.* 2015;**66**(11):1236–1246.

23. Kelly E, Hemphill L. Lipoprotein(a): a lipoprotein whose time has come. *Curr Treat Options Cardiovasc Med.* 2017;**19**(7):48.

24. Guyton JR. Extended-release niacin for modifying the lipoprotein profile. *Expert Opin Pharmacother.* 2004;**5**(6):1385–1398.

25. Albers JJ, Slee A, O'Brien KD, Robinson JG, Kashyap ML, Kwiterovich PO Jr, Xu P, Marcovina SM. Relationship of apolipoproteins A-1 and B, and lipoprotein(a) to cardiovascular outcomes: the AIM-HIGH trial (Atherothrombosis Intervention in Metabolic Syndrome with Low HDL/High Triglyceride and Impact on Global Health Outcomes). *J Am Coll Cardiol.* 2013;**62**(17):1575–1579.

26. Pokrovsky SN, Afanasieva OI, Ezhov MV. Lipoprotein(a) apheresis. *Curr Opin Lipidol.* 2016;**27**(4):351–358.

27. Raal FJ, Giugliano RP, Sabatine MS, Koren MJ, Langslet G, Bays H, Blom D, Eriksson M, Dent R, Wasserman SM, Huang F, Xue A, Albizem M, Scott R, Stein EA. Reduction in lipoprotein(a) with PCSK9 monoclonal antibody evolocumab (AMG 145): a pooled analysis of more than 1,300 patients in 4 phase II trials. *J Am Coll Cardiol.* 2014;**63**(13):1278–1288.

28. Gaudet D, Kereiakes DJ, McKenney JM, Roth EM, Hanotin C, Gipe D, Du Y, Ferrand AC, Ginsberg HN, Stein EA. Effect of alirocumab, a monoclonal proprotein convertase subtilisin/kexin 9 antibody, on lipoprotein(a) concentrations (a pooled analysis of 150 mg every two weeks dosing from phase 2 trials). *Am J Cardiol.* 2014;**114**(5):711–715.

29. Viney NJ, van Capelleveen JC, Geary RS, Xia S, Tami JA, Yu RZ, Marcovina SM, Hughes SG, Graham MJ, Crooke RM, Crooke ST, Witztum JL, Stroes ES, Tsimikas S. Antisense oligonucleotides targeting apolipoprotein(a) in people with raised lipoprotein(a): two randomised, double-blind, placebo-controlled, dose-ranging trials. *Lancet.* 2016;**388**(10057):2239–2253.

30. Fitzgerald K, White S, Borodovsky A, Bettencourt BR, Strahs A, Clausen V, Wijngaard P, Horton JD, Taubel J, Brooks A, Fernando C, Kauffman RS, Kallend D, Vaishnaw A, Simon A. A highly durable RNAi therapeutic inhibitor of PCSK9. *N Engl J Med.* 2017;**376**(1):41–51.

Pharmacotherapy for Lipid Disorders: Which Drugs for Which Disease

M46
Presented, March 23–26, 2019

Robert H. Eckel, MD. Division of Endocrinology, Metabolism, and Diabetes and Division of Cardiology, University of Colorado Anschutz Medical Campus, Aurora, Colorado 80045, E-mail: robert.eckel@ucdenver.edu

SIGNIFICANCE OF THE CLINICAL PROBLEM

Managing disorders of lipid and lipoprotein metabolism includes but extends far beyond lifestyle. Historic, more recent, and ongoing cardiovascular disease (CVD) outcome trials (CVOTs) provide increasing evidence for what drugs should be considered for which disorders.

BARRIERS TO OPTIMAL PRACTICE

Barriers to the optimal treatment of disorders related to lipid and lipoprotein include multiple guidelines, adverse effects, and cost.

LEARNING OBJECTIVES

As a result of participating in this session, learners should be able to

- Simplify guideline recommendations into evidence-based pharmacological therapy of lipid and lipoprotein disorders
- More effectively treat patients with statin intolerance
- Know when to implement PCSK9 therapy
- Consider when and how to treat patients with moderate and severe hypertriglyceridemia

STRATEGIES FOR PHARMACOLOGICAL THERAPY

To be discussed in the following three cases.

CASE 1: HYPERCHOLESTEROLEMIA

V.K. is a 69-year-old woman S/P acute myocardial infarction with "combined hyperlipidemia," hypertension, prediabetes, and a well-documented intolerance to four statins, including high intensity and low intensity at infrequent intervals. She is now taking ezetimibe 10 mg daily and omega-3 fatty acids 930 mg twice a day (BID). The physical exam revealed blood pressure (BP) 140/70 mm Hg, heart rate 78 beats/min, and body mass index (BMI) 28.5 kg/m^2. Her laboratories on presentation are as follows: cholesterol 254 mg/dL, triglycerides (TG) 192 mg/dL, high-density lipoprotein cholesterol (HDL-C) 58 mg/dL, low-density lipoprotein cholesterol (LDL-C) 158 mg/dL, lipoprotein (a) 14 mg/dL, hs-CRP 1.8 mg/L, and HbA$_{1c}$ 5.8%.

What is the best next step in the management of V.K.'s lipid profile?
- A. Colesevelam, 1875 mg BID
- B. Evolocumab 140 mg every 2 weeks
- C. Alirocumab 75 mg every 2 weeks
- D. Reevaluate her response to a statin

Statins

Current and most recently updated statin guidelines recommend a high-intensity statin, 20 or 40 mg rosuvastatin or 40 or 80 mg atorvastatin, to reduce LDL-C by ≥50% (1–3). Although some controversy persists regarding the use of LDL-C goals, clearly on-treatment LDL-C levels are very important and I personally feel that the American Association of Clinical Endocrinologists (AACE) guidelines, with an LDL-C goal of <55 mg/dL for extreme-risk patients such as this one, are most applicable (2) (Table 1). In addition, data from FOURIER (and meta-analyses of statin trials) suggest that an on-treatment LDL-C <40 mg/dL is likely to be of further benefit. CVOTs of LDL-lowering therapy clinical trials show that atherosclerotic CVD (ASCVD) risk reduction is greatest in the highest-risk patients (secondary prevention and primary prevention when LDL-C ≥190 mg/dL or diabetes is present). In addition to aggressive LDL-lowering treatment, a heart-healthy lifestyle including diet and physical activity is always warranted (4). Overall, statins are well tolerated, and major serious adverse effects are rare, including hepatic transaminase elevation greater than three times the normal level in <0.3% of patients and rhabdomyolysis in 0.01% of patients. Although memory loss is listed in the package insert, this is extremely rare in clinical trials, and some studies demonstrate a lower risk of cognitive impairment in patients treated with statins. In primary care clinics, myopathy defined as myalgias and/or elevations in creatine phosphate kinase occurs in ~10% of statin-treated patients. There is a higher risk of these complications when a statin is combined with other lipid-lowering medications, such as fibrates or niacin, or when combined with drugs that inhibit their metabolism, e.g., CYP3A4 inhibitors such as ketoconazole or protease inhibitors. Finally, statins are also associated with an ~10% risk of new-onset type 2 diabetes mellitus (T2DM), especially in patients with prediabetes, such as this one. Preexisting glucose intolerance and/or a positive family history of T2DM predispose to this outcome. Despite new-onset diabetes, these patients benefit greatly from ASCVD risk reduction and so the net risk-benefit ratio in a patient at high risk for future ASCVD events, such as this one, is virtually always strongly favorable. Many patients with statin-induced adverse effects can be reinitiated on statin therapy with a low and/or infrequent dose increased as tolerated slowly (5). Figure 1 provides an algorithm of approach (5).

Table 1. The AACE LDL-C Guideline

Risk Category	Risk Factors/10-Year Risk	LDL-C Goal
Extreme	ASCVD, multiple risk factors	<55 mg/dL <40 mg/dL (FOURIER)[RHE]
Very high	ASCVD, ≥1 risk factor, 10-year risk >20%	<70 mg/dL
High	≥2 risk factors, diabetes, chronic kidney disease	<100 mg/dL
Moderate	≤2 risk factors, 10-year risk <10%	<100 mg/dL
Low	No risk factors	<130 mg/dL

Adapted with permission from the American Association of Clinical Endocrinologists: Garber AJ, Abrahamson MJ, Barzilay JI, et al. Concensus statement by the American Association of Clinical Endocrinologists and American College of Endocrinology on the comprehensive type 2 diabetes management algorithm—2017 executive summary. *Endocr Prac.* 2017;23(2):207–238. ©2017 AACE.

Ezetimibe

Ezetimibe lowers cholesterol by selectively inhibiting intestinal cholesterol absorption by inhibiting the cholesterol transport protein NPC1L1. Because less cholesterol reaches the liver, intrahepatic cholesterol is reduced, LDL receptors are increased, and LDL-C levels are decreased. Like bile acid sequestrants (BAS), ezetimibe is not typically used as monotherapy, but it is additive in combination with a statin to further reduce LDL-C levels and ASCVD risk in high-risk patients (6), and particularly in patients with T2DM (7). Ezetimibe has virtually no side effects and does not increase the risk of new-onset T2DM.

BAS

BAS were the first class of cholesterol-lowering medications shown to decrease ASCVD events in a CVOT (8). Beyond this very early trial, however, BAS have fallen on "tough times" in that statins and PCSK9 inhibitors lower LDL-C much more and are associated with far fewer adverse effects. BAS reduce the enterohepatic circulation of bile acids. Because bile acids are synthesized in the liver from cholesterol, BAS result in reduction in the intrahepatic pool of cholesterol and reduce circulating LDL-C (by 10% to 30%) by increasing hepatic LDL receptors. BAS side effects are primarily gastrointestinal (bloating, abdominal pain, and constipation) and reduced drug absorption (*e.g.*, estrogen, warfarin, β-blockers, digoxin, and thyroid hormone).

PCSK9 Inhibitors

This class of drugs binds circulating PCSK9 and blocks the adverse effect of PCSK9 on LDL receptor recycling. PCSK9 inhibitors, alirocumab and evolocumab, are injected every 2 to

4 weeks and lower LDL-C by up to 60%. Two recent CVOTs (FOURIER and ODYSSEY Outcomes) (9, 10) have shown an added benefit of evolocumab (140 mg every 2 weeks or 420 mg monthly) and alirocumab (75 or 150 mg every 2 weeks) to reduce ASCVD events in high-risk patients already on statins. This drug class is Food and Drug Administration (FDA) approved as adjuncts to diet and maximally tolerated statin therapy for the treatment of adults with heterozygous familial hypercholesterolemia or clinical ASCVD who require additional lowering of LDL-C, and evolocumab for ASCVD event reduction. The only adverse effect is injection site reactions.

CASE 2: HYPERTRIGLYCERIDEMIA

A 49-year-old woman is referred for hypertriglyceridemia. She is a nonsmoker, and her family history includes a mother with T2DM and myocardial infarction at age 55 years. She is on no medications. Her physical exam reveals the following: BMI 32 kg/m^2 and BP 135/80 mm Hg. Her laboratories are as follows: cholesterol 240 mg/dL, TG 511 mg/dL, HDL-C 39 mg/dL, direct LDL-C 101 mg/dL, non–HDL-C 201 mg/dL, fasting glucose 104 mg/dL, HbA$_{1c}$ 6.7%, estimated glomerular filtration rate 86 mL/min, trace urine protein, thyrotropin (TSH) 2.1 mIU/L, aspartate aminotransferase (10-40) 32 units/L, alanine aminotransferase (7-56) 58 U/L, lipoprotein (a) 12 mg/dL, and Apo B 115 mg/dL.

What is the most reasonable and evidence-based goal for this patient?
A. TG <200 mg/dL, LDL-C <130 mg/dL
B. TG <150 mg/dL, LDL-C <130 mg/dL
C. TG <200 mg/dL, LDL-C <100 mg/dL, Apo B <90 mg/dL
D. TG <150 mg/dL, LDL-C <100 mg/dL, Apo B <80 mg/dL
E. TG <200 mg/dL, LDL-C <70 mg/dL, Apo B <80 mg/dL

The best choice of pharmacological management would be:
A. High-intensity statin alone
B. Moderate intensity statin + fibrate
C. Moderate intensity statin + omega-3 fatty acids
D. Moderate intensity statin + ezetimibe + fibrate
E. High-intensity statin + fibrate and/or omega-3 fatty acids

Current guidelines for treatment of hypertriglyceridemia are tentative due to the lack of evidence for ASCVD efficacy based on CVOTs published as of October 2018 (1–3). Table 2 is from the 2018 American College of Cardiology/American Heart Association/National Lipid Association Cholesterol Guidelines (1), which, unfortunately, covered hypertriglyceridemia only briefly and made no mention of prescription omega-3 fatty acids. Further, it was published simultaneously with the REDUCE-IT CVOT (11); therefore, it did not take those results into account.

Fibrates

Fibrates work by inducing PPARα-related gene expression, which leads to increases in intrahepatic fatty acid oxidation

Step #1:
Patient
Assessment

Symptomatic patient[a]

Perform history and physical exam to determine potential causes[b]. Check CK level and review prior labs[c].

| Normal CK (myalgia) | CK <10x ULN | CK >10x ULN (rule out rhabdomyolysis[d]) |

Step #2:
Modification
of Statin
Therapy
and Statin
Rechallenge

Lower statin dose or discontinue statin depending on symptom severity

Discontinue statin, consider intensive treatment (fluids), and monitor patient closely

In patients with moderate to severe symptoms weekly reports back to the prescribing physician or her/his staff should follow.

If symptoms resolve: rechallenge with statin if initial muscle injury was not severe

If symptoms persist: consider expert consultation with lipid specialist, neurology, rheumatology, or endocrinology.

Symptoms resolved but initial muscle injury was severe therefore statin rechallenge is not appropriate in most cases

If statin rechallenge is appropriate and acceptable to the patient:
Switch to different statin at guideline recommended dose or use alternative statin dose strategy; examples of starting doses:
- Rosuvastatin 5 mg QWK
- Fluva- or pravastatin 10mg QOD or QD
- Atorvastatin 10 mg QWK
- Red yeast rice, 600 mg BID

Step #3:
Reassess
Patient

Reassess patient within 6 weeks of restarting or changing statin[e]. Clarify patient's lipid-lowering goal based on their individualized ASCVD risk.

Not tolerating low-dose statin

Tolerating statin, but not reaching individualized lipid-lowering goal

Tolerating statin and goals met --> continue current therapy and evaluate patient at appropriate intervals for adherence and tolerability

Step #4:
Alternative
Therapies

Consider non-statin LDL-C lowering agents:
1) Ezetimibe
2) Bile acid sequestrants
3) PCSK9 inhibitors[f]

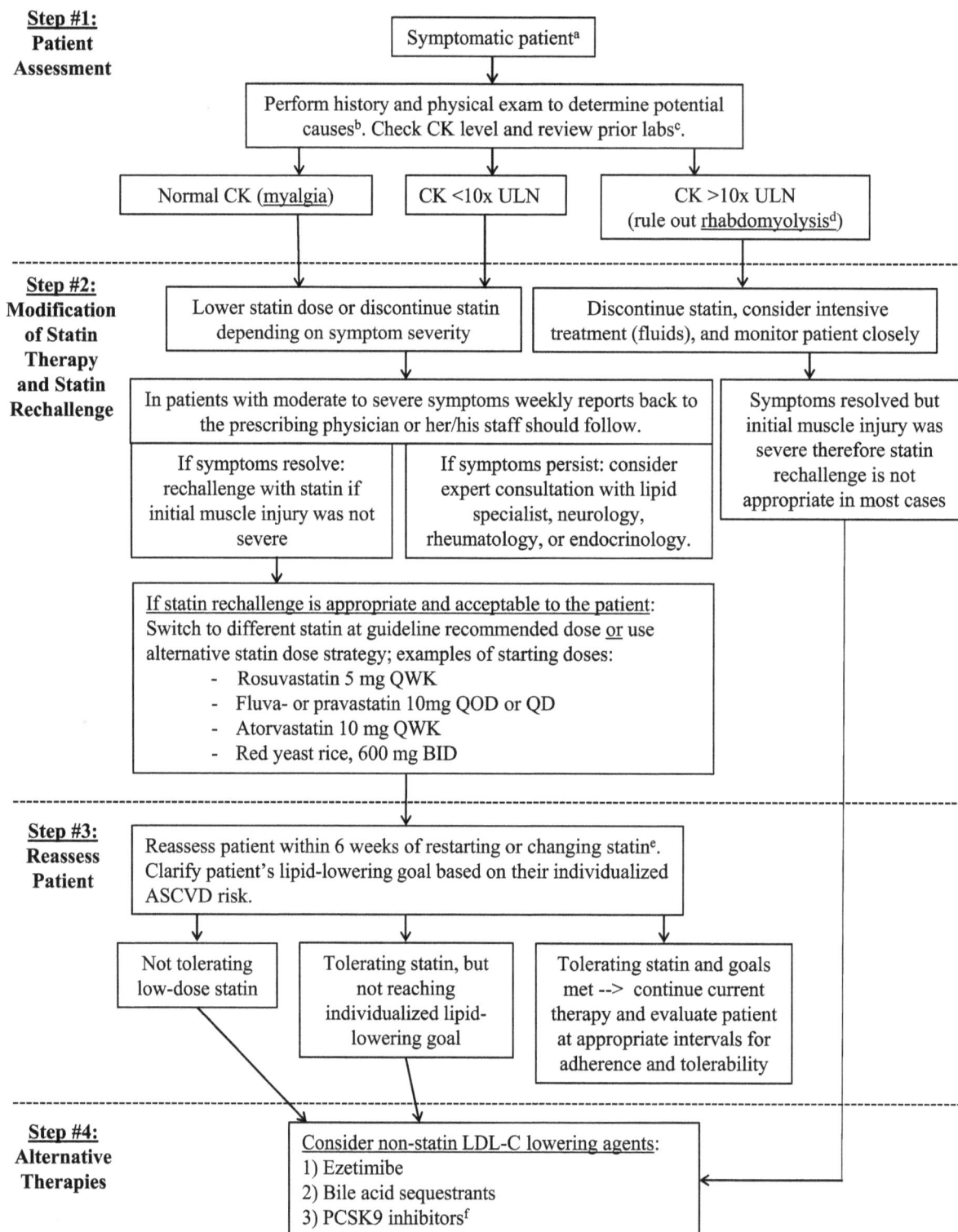

Figure 1. Summary of management approach to statin-related muscle problems. [a]Per 2013 ACC/AHA Cholesterol Guidelines, CK should only be checked in asymptomatic patients at high risk of developing myopathy. Statin should be continued if asymptomatic and CK <10× the upper limit of normal. [b]To help determine whether symptoms are related to statin therapy, consider using statin myalgia clinical index score. [c]If recent labs are not available, consider checking creatinine, TSH, 25-vitamin D, and inflammatory markers depending on the clinical scenario. [d]Check creatinine and check urine for myoglobin. [e]Close follow-up is critical to improving long-term adherence to statin therapy. [f]If a PCSK9 inhibitor is not approved or patient is not appropriate for this therapy, then niacin and fibrates should be considered. Reproduced with permission from Saxon DR, Rasouli N, Eckel RH. Pharmacological prevention of cardiovascular outcomes in diabetes mellitus: established and emerging agents. *Drugs.* 2018;78(2):203–214.

Table 2. Recommendations for Hypertriglyceridemia

COR	LOE	Recommendations
I	B-NR	1. In adults 20 years of age or older with moderate hypertriglyceridemia [fasting or nonfasting TG 175–499 mg/dL (1.9–5.6 mmol/L)], clinicians should address and treat lifestyle factors (obesity and metabolic syndrome), secondary factors (diabetes mellitus, chronic liver or kidney disease and/or nephrotic syndrome, hypothyroidism), and medications that increase TG.
IIa	B-R	2. In adults 40–75 years of age with moderate or severe hypertriglyceridemia and ASCVD risk of 7.5% or higher, it is reasonable to reevaluate ASCVD risk after lifestyle and secondary factors are addressed and to consider a persistently elevated TG level as a factor favoring initiation or intensification of statin therapy.
IIa	B-R	3. In adults 40–75 years of age with severe hypertriglyceridemia [fasting TG ≥500 mg/dL (≥5.6 mmol/L)] and ASCVD risk of 7.5% or higher, it is reasonable to address reversible causes of high TG and to initiate statin therapy.
IIa	B-NR	4. In adults with severe hypertriglyceridemia [fasting TG ≥500 mg/dL (≥5.7 mmol/L), and especially fasting TG ≥1000 mg/dL (11.3 mmol/L)], it is reasonable to identify and address other causes of hypertriglyceridemia, and if TG are persistently elevated or increasing, to further reduce TG by implementation of a very-low-fat diet, avoidance of refined carbohydrates and alcohol, consumption of omega-3 fatty acids, and, if necessary to prevent acute pancreatitis, fibrate therapy.

Reproduced with permission from the American Association of Clinical Endocrinologists: Jellinger PS, Handelsman Y, Rosenblit PD, et al. American Association of Clinical Endocrinologists and American College of Endocrinology Guidelines for Management of Dyslipidemia and Prevention of Cardiovascular Disease. *Endocr Pract.* 2017;23(Suppl 2):1–87. ©2017 AACE.
Abbreviations: COR, class of recommendation; LOE, level of evidence; NR, not randomized; R, randomized.

and reductions in TG synthesis and very-low-density lipoprotein (VLDL) secretion as well as increases in lipoprotein lipase (LPL) activity. Fibrates lower TG by 20% to 50% (strongly proportional to baseline TG) and raise HDL-C by 5% to 15%. Because fenofibrate is renally cleared and usually also modestly raises serum creatinine, caution is needed in patients with chronic kidney disease; however, this increase is most often reversible once the drug is stopped. Gemfibrozil should be avoided when statins are coadministered, related to a higher risk of myopathy (with all statins except fluvastatin). Before statins were available, fibrates were shown to be beneficial in primary prevention of ASCVD (10). More recent CVOT evidence has failed to show ASCVD benefit with fenofibrate added to a statin in a general dyslipidemic population, although subgroup analysis suggests that fenofibrate may be beneficial as a statin adjunct in secondary prevention in patients with diabetes or with existing ASCVD who are hypertriglyceridemic (>200 mg/dL) and have lower levels of HDL-C (<40 mg/dL) (12).

Omega-3 Fatty Acids

High-dose omega-3 fatty acids (purified from fish oil) lower TG by 15% to 50% (generally comparable to fibrates and also proportional to baseline TG). Dietary supplement fish oil varies widely in stated purity and content of the major active ingredients, eicosapentaenoic acid (EPA) ± docosahexaenoic acid (DHA), and frequently contains large amounts of saturated and/or oxidized fatty acids. Dietary supplements are neither regulated by the FDA nor approved for treatment of disease, and there are no over-the-counter (nonprescription but FDA regulated) omega-3 products, at present. The approved dose of prescription omega-3 for TG lowering is 4 g/d,

and the two currently available products are omega-3-acid-ethyl-esters (465 mg EPA and 375 mg DHA per 1-g capsule) and icosapent ethyl (pure EPA, ≥960 mg per 1-g capsule). Both are recommended to be taken 2 g twice daily with food (to increase absorption). Similar to the fibrates, the major pharmacological effect is to reduce TG synthesis and VLDL secretion as well as to increase LPL activity. Presently, prescription omega-3 fatty acids are only approved for patients with fasting TG >500 mg/dL; however, there are two large CVOTs, REDUCE-IT and STRENGTH, assessing the ASCVD effects of prescription icosapent ethyl and prescription omega-3 carboxylic acid (with 550 mg EPA and 200 mg DHA per 1-g capsule, Epanova®, not yet available clinically), respectively. Of importance, baseline TG had to be 135 to 500 mg/dL for REDUCE-IT and 180 to 500 mg/dL for STRENGTH; thus, these are the first CVOTs ever to recruit subjects for elevated TG levels. REDUCE-IT demonstrated that icosapent ethyl reduced major ASCVD events by a surprising 25% in addition to a statin (11), and of interest, the degree of benefit did not appear to relate to on-treatment TG above or below 150 mg/dL.

Summary

So how should patients with TG between 150 and 500 mg/dL be assessed and treated? Let's begin by modifying the many acquired causes of hypertriglyceridemia, *e.g.*, poorly controlled diabetes and TG-altering medications (13). Next, most of these patients should be statin treated, and high-intensity statins produce the most TG reduction. Subgroup analyses of fenofibrate CVOTs suggest a possible decrease in ASCVD risk with the addition of fenofibrate to patients with TG 200 to 500 mg/dL with CVD or at high risk on maximally treated statin.

The REDUCE-IT trial, however, proves the ASCVD benefit in similar patients (although, paradoxically, the degree of TG-lowering effect did not appear to predict the benefit), and a prior CVOT of a lower dose of icosapent ethyl also showed ASCVD benefit, although with much lower background statin therapy and in subjects selected for high baseline cholesterol. Let's await STRENGTH to determine whether a full dose of a DHA-containing prescription omega-3 treatment can also reduce ASCVD. Also, does measuring Apo B in these patients help direct decisions to follow?

CASE 3: SEVERE HYPERTRIGLYCERIDEMIA

The patient is a 45-year-old man with known coronary heart disease, S/P multiple percutaneous coronary interventions and stents, and recently found to be severely hyper-triglyceridemic. The patient has had T2DM for 20 years and hypertension for >20 years. He was hospitalized 5 months previously for chest pain, but an acute myocardial infarction was ruled out. During his admission, the TG level was 2509 mg/dL and the HbA$_{1c}$ 10.2%. His prescriptions on that admission are as follows: gemfibrozil 600 mg BID, dietary supplement DHA + EPA 2.5 g/d, atorvastatin 20 mg, glipizide 10 mg, and metformin 850 mg BID. The patient was discharged on medications, a low-fat diet, and an escalating dose of insulin glargine beginning at 10 units daily. Blood glucose recordings at home have been 100 to 150 mg/dL. At the time of his clinic visit, medications included glargine 70 units daily, metformin 1 g BID, glipizide 10 mg BID, rosuvastatin 20 mg daily, gemfibrozil 600 mg BID, omega-3 fatty acids 1.6 g BID, clopidogrel 75 mg, and aspirin 81 mg daily. The physical exam reveals a BMI 30.8 kg/m^2 and BP 138/76 mm Hg. His laboratories are as follows: cholesterol 259 mg/dL, TG 1965 mg/dL, HDL-C 35 mg/dL, HbA$_{1c}$ 7.8%, normal aspartate aminotransferase/alanine aminotransferase, creatinine 1.0 mg/dL, TSH 1.6 mIU/L, and urine microalbumin 789 mg/g creatinine.

After changing gemfibrozil to fenofibrate 150 mg/d (to reduce myopathy risk), what is your best recommendation?

A. Increase insulin dose and measure TG in 1 month
B. Increase atorvastatin dose to 80 mg daily and measure TG in 1 month
C. Continue all existing medications/doses, reduce dietary fat to <20%, and measure TG in 1 week
D. Continue all existing medications/doses, reduce dietary fat to <5%, and measure TG in 1 week
E. Stop all lipid-lowering medications, reduce dietary fat to <5%, and measure TG in 3 days

The chylomicronemia syndrome occurs when TG levels are severely elevated (by definition, starting with a TG >880 mg/dL, usually >1500 mg/dL) and is characterized by clinical features such as abdominal pain, acute pancreatitis, eruptive xanthomas, and lipemia retinalis (13). It can result from (i) deficiency in the enzyme LPL and some associated proteins,

termed the familial chylomicronemia syndrome (FCS), or (ii) the presence of secondary forms of hypertriglyceridemia concurrently with genetic etiologies of hypertriglyceridemia, termed the multifactorial chylomicronemia syndrome (MFCS). FCS is very rare, the diagnosis frequently is missed, and most cases of the chylomicronemia syndrome are due to MFCS. In all conditions with fasting chylomicronemia, TG-rich lipoproteins (chylomicrons and VLDL) accumulate due to their greatly impaired clearance from plasma and can lead to acute pancreatitis, the most dangerous consequence of severe hypertriglyceridemia. Increased ASCVD risk is also present in MFCS but does not directly relate to chylomicron accumulation. In these cases, a diet consisting of <5% of calories from fat is critical and needed until fasting TG is <1000 mg/dL (14), at which point the risk of acute pancreatitis is dramatically reduced. Subsequently, a fibrate, high-intensity statin, and/or prescription omega-3 fatty acids will lower TG to <500 mg/dL. The best therapeutic approach to TG lowering beyond strict limitation of dietary fat varies with the cause of the chylomicronemia, with exciting new therapeutic approaches on the horizon. Treatment of ASCVD prevention should be undertaken independently after lowering plasma TG below about 500 mg/dL to prevent pancreatitis.

CORRECT ANSWERS FOR CASES

Case 1

An LDL-C goal of <55 mg/dL is reasonable. Although a statin rechallenge is an option, the most efficacious next step would be a PCSK9 inhibitor, either alirocumab 150 mg or evolocumab 140 mg every 2 weeks. Alirocumab 75 mg every 2 weeks (~45% LDL-C reduction) would not likely achieve this level of LDL-C.

Case 2

The best answer to the first question is debatable, but I would choose TG <200 mg/dL, LDL-C <100 mg/dL, and Apo B <80 mg/dL. Presently no data exist to target TG to <150 versus <200 mg/dL, and in this patient with T2DM and moderate CVD risk, an LDL-C goal of at least <70 mg/dL is reasonable and Apo B <80 rather than <90 mg/dL is a reduction in proatherogenic particle number. Regarding the second question, a high-intensity statin should accomplish the LDL-C goal; however, the addition of a fibrate and/or high-dose omega-3 fatty acid will likely be needed to reduce TG to <200 mg/dL. (REDUCE-IT results strongly favor the latter to reduce ASCVD risk.)

Case 3

Patients with severe hypertriglyceridemia need major reductions in dietary fat to remove saturation kinetics of TG-rich lipoprotein removal, a process dependent on LPL. I typically stop TG-lowering drugs for two reasons: (i) drugs do not work on chylomicron production, and (ii) once TG are approximately <1000 mg/dL, TG-lowering drugs now reduce VLDL and total TG. Because fasting TG falls by ~25% daily on <5%

dietary fat, the best answer is E. Stop existing lipid-lowering medications, reduce dietary fat to <5%, and measure TG in 3 days. This assures dietary compliance and the best time for reinitiating TG-lowering drugs.

References

1. Grundy SM, Stone NJ, Bailey AL, Beam C, Birtcher KK, Blumenthal RS, Braun LT, de Ferranti S, Faiella-Tommasino J, Forman DE, Goldberg R, Heidenreich PA, Hlatky MA, Jones DW, Lloyd-Jones D, Lopez-Pajares N, Ndumele CE, Orringer CE, Peralta CA, Saseen JJ, SmithSC Jr, Sperling L, Virani SS, Yeboah J. 2018 AHA/ACC/AACVPR/AAPA/ABC/ACPM/ADA/AGS/APhA/ASPC/NLA/PCNA guideline on the management of blood cholesterol: a report of the American College of Cardiology/American Heart Association Task Force on Clinical Practice Guidelines [published online ahead of print 8 November 2018]. *J Am Coll Cardiol*. doi:10.1016/j.jacc.2018.11.003.

2. Jellinger PS, Handelsman Y, Rosenblit PD, Bloomgarden ZT, Fonseca VA, Garber AJ, Grunberger G, Guerin CK, Bell DSH, Mechanick JI, Pessah-Pollack R, Wyne K, Smith D, Brinton EA, Fazio S, Davidson M. American Association of Clinical Endocrinologists and American College of Endocrinology guidelines for management of dyslipidemia and prevention of cardiovascular disease. *Endocr Pract*. 2017; **23**(Suppl 2):1–87.

3. Soran H, Adam S, Durrington PN. Optimising treatment of hyperlipidaemia: quantitative evaluation of UK, USA and European guidelines taking account of both LDL cholesterol levels and cardiovascular disease risk. *Atherosclerosis*. 2018;**278**:135–142.

4. Eckel RH, Jakicic JM, Ard JD, de Jesus JM, Houston Miller N, Hubbard VS, Lee IM, Lichtenstein AH, Loria CM, Millen BE, Nonas CA, Sacks FM, Smith SC, Jr, Svetkey LP, Wadden TA, Yanovski SZ, Kendall KA, Morgan LC, Trisolini MG, Velasco G, Wnek J, Anderson JL, Halperin JL, Albert NM, Bozkurt B, Brindis RG, Curtis LH, DeMets D, Hochman JS, Kovacs RJ, Ohman EM, Pressler SJ, Sellke FW, Shen WK, Smith SC, Jr, Tomaselli GF; American College of Cardiology/American Heart Association Task Force on Practice Guidelines. 2013 AHA/ACC guideline on lifestyle management to reduce cardiovascular risk: a report of the American College of Cardiology/American Heart Association Task Force on Practice Guidelines. *Circulation*. 2014 **129**(25, Suppl 2):S76–S99.

5. Saxon DR, Rasouli N, Eckel RH. Pharmacological prevention of cardiovascular outcomes in diabetes mellitus: established and emerging agents. *Drugs*. 2018;**78**(2):203–214.

6. Cannon CP, Blazing MA, Giugliano RP, McCagg A, White JA, Theroux P, Darius H, Lewis BS, Ophuis TO, Jukema JW, De Ferrari GM, Ruzyllo W, De Lucca P, Im K, Bohula EA, Reist C, Wiviott SD, Tershakovec AM, Musliner TA, Braunwald E, Califf RM; IMPROVE-IT Investigators. Ezetimibe added to statin therapy after acute coronary syndromes. *N Engl J Med*. 2015;**372**(25):2387–2397.

7. Bonaca MP, Gutierrez JA, Cannon C, Giugliano R, Blazing M, Park JG, White J, Tershakovec A, Braunwald E. Polyvascular disease, type 2 diabetes, and long-term vascular risk: a secondary analysis of the IMPROVE-IT trial. *Lancet Diabetes Endocrinol*. 2018;**6**(12):934–943.

8. LRC-CPPT Trialists. The Lipid Research Clinics Coronary Primary Prevention Trial results. II. The relationship of reduction in incidence of coronary heart disease to cholesterol lowering. *JAMA*. 1984; **251**(3):365–374.

9. Sabatine MS, Giugliano RP, Keech AC, Honarpour N, Wiviott SD, Murphy SA, Kuder JF, Wang H, Liu T, Wasserman SM, Sever PS, Pedersen TR; FOURIER Steering Committee and Investigators. Evolocumab and clinical outcomes in patients with cardiovascular disease. *N Engl J Med*. 2017;**376**(18):1713–1722.

10. Schwartz GG, Steg PG, Szarek M, Bhatt DL, Bittner VA, Diaz R, Edelberg JM, Goodman SG, Hanotin C, Harrington RA, Jukema JW, Lecorps G, Mahaffey KW, Moryusef A, Pordy R, Quintero K, Roe MT, Sasiela WJ, Tamby JF, Tricoci P, White HD, Zeiher AM; ODYSSEY OUTCOMES Committees and Investigators. Alirocumab and cardiovascular outcomes after acute coronary syndrome. *N Engl J Med*. 2018;**379**(22): 2097–2107.

11. Bhatt DL, Steg PG, Miller M, Brinton EA, Jacobson TA, Ketchum SB, Doyle RT, Jr, Juliano RA, Jiao L, Granowitz C, Tardif JC, Ballantyne CM; REDUCE-IT Investigators. Cardiovascular risk reduction with icosapent ethyl for hypertriglyceridemia. *N Engl J Med*. 2019;**380**(1):11–22.

12. Wang D, Liu B, Tao W, Hao Z, Liu M. Fibrates for secondary prevention of cardiovascular disease and stroke. *Cochrane Database Syst Rev*. 2015;**10**:CD009580.

13. Donahoo WT, Kosmiski LA, Eckel RH. Drugs causing dyslipoproteinemia. *Endocrinol Metab Clin North Am*. 1998;**27**(3):677–697.

14. Brown WV, Brunzell JD, Eckel RH, Stone NJ. Severe hypertriglyceridemia. *J Clin Lipidol*. 2012;**6**(5):397–408.

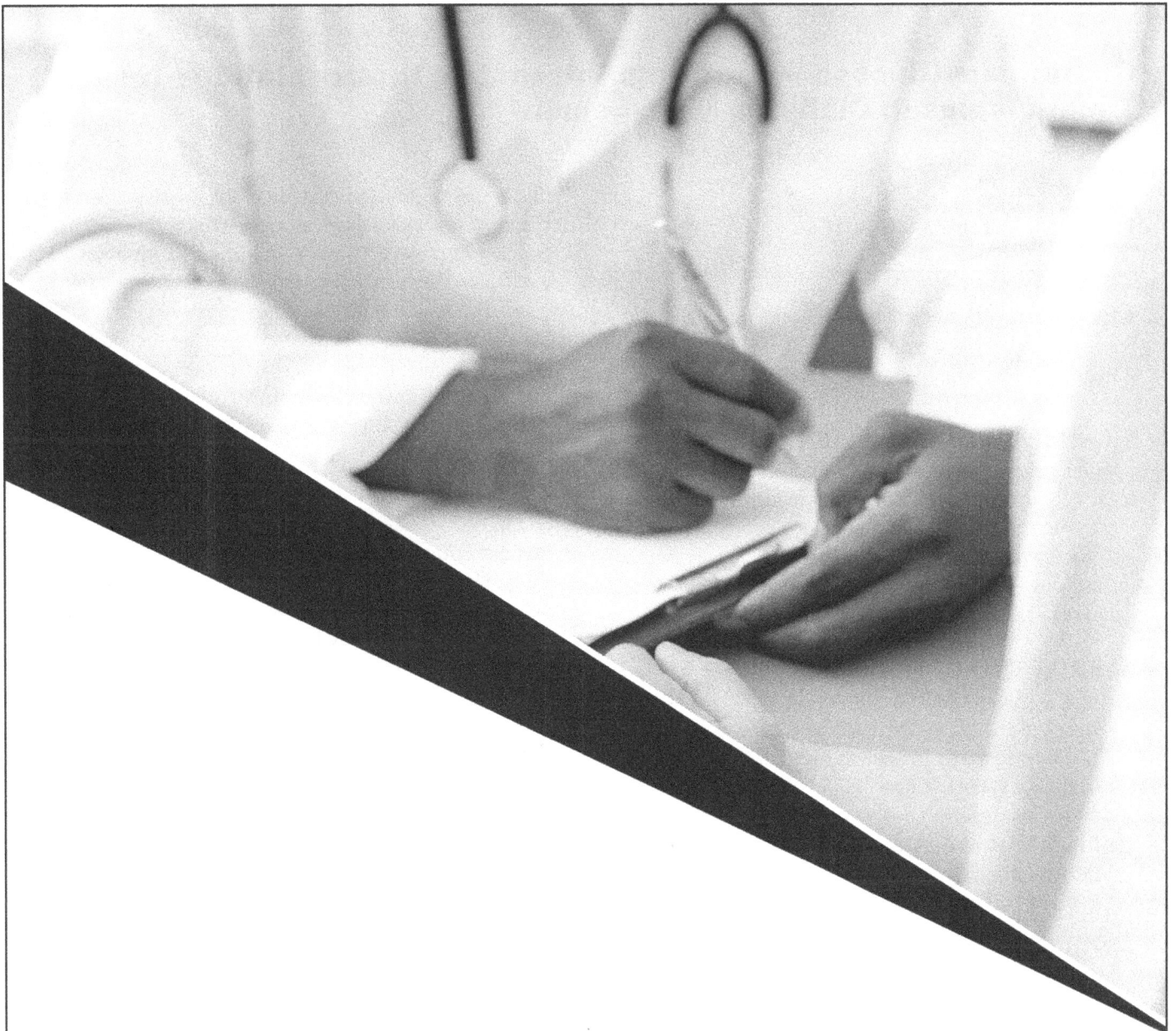

DIABETES MELLITUS AND GLUCOSE METABOLISM

Continuous Glucose Monitoring: Interactive Interpretation—New Technologies in Diabetes Management

M06
Presented, March 23–26, 2019

Anne Peters, MD. Keck School of Medicine, University of Southern California, Los Angeles, California 90033, E-mail: annepete@med.usc.edu

SIGNIFICANCE OF THE CLINICAL PROBLEM

Continuous glucose monitoring (CGM) is a tool that has increasingly become part of diabetes management. However, there is much to learn about how to interpret the data and integrate them into clinical care. This session will discuss the retrospective evaluation of CGM data as well as how to teach patients to react to their own data in real time.

BARRIERS TO OPTIMAL PRACTICE

Barriers to using CGM in practice include the following:
- A lack of the ability to download the devices
- The time required to analyze the data, which often translates to not having a method for interpreting data in a systematic fashion
- Insufficient knowledge on how to train patients to use the devices/troubleshoot, which leads to frustration in both patients and providers

LEARNING OBJECTIVES

As a result of participating in this session, learners should be able to:
- Develop an approach for using the average glucose profile (AGP) in their practice
- Create a stepwise plan for training patients on how to maximize use of CGM
- Teach troubleshooting techniques to enhance patient adherence to CGM use

STRATEGIES FOR MANAGEMENT

The main strategies for using CGM effectively come from understanding the data downloaded from the devices. Ideally, all data would be provided in the same format. The AGP is a helpful tool (1). It provides such information as time in range, glucose variability, and percentage of time in high and low ranges. These parameters have been associated increasingly with the risk of complications and may be more important than the HbA_{1c} (2–6). A new concept—glucose management indicator—has been developed for summarizing CGM data (7).

The AGP heading provides the immediate data, which often are most quickly interpreted by looking at time in range (ideally ≥75%), coefficient of variation (ideally ≤33%), and

time spent <54 mg/dL. This assessment, plus a glance at the graph, can provide a quick ascertainment of how well a patient is doing. If patients are largely in range with a low level of variability, they generally are doing well. When more detail is needed for adjusting insulin doses, the day-by-day graphs can be analyzed. Usually, the past 2 weeks are the most useful in terms of adjusting/assessing the patient's status, but date ranges can be expanded or contracted as needed (8). Although displaying the AGP is not standardized across all devices, a general sense of the patient's data can be obtained from that provided in the device printouts (Figs. 1 and 2).

Patient Education Regarding CGM

When starting a patient on CGM, it is important to set appropriate expectations and provide education in a way that the patient prefers. Knowing how to set the alarms and alerts so that patients (and their spouses) do not develop alarm fatigue also is important. An example of all possible alarms (9) is provided in Figure 3. Initially, patients may need only low alarms to get them used to CGM and then advance to high alarms. The predicted low alerts tend to be helpful, simply falling or rising blood glucose alerts potentially less so. The alert profile can be set by time of day on some devices.

Steps for Starting and Following Patients on CGM

I generally follow these steps. To begin, discuss CGM with the patient and set appropriate expectations, and if the patient is a prior user, explore reasons for stopping. To prepare the patient for using the CGM, note that some will start on their own, but others may prefer meeting with a trainer. In all cases, advise the patient on initial alarm settings:
- Consider very high or no high alarm
- Set low alarm based on patient preference
- Set falling glucose alert

Counsel on the need to avoid stacking, and set the initial goal to reduce hypoglycemia.

Review data with patient within 2 to 4 weeks of initial use. At follow-up, discuss any issues with device wear and troubleshoot as indicated. Adjust insulin doses by first looking for patterns of lows, especially at night. Next, assess periods of hyperglycemia. Finally, teach the patient trend arrow adjustments (10, 11) and how to use reports for self-analysis of data and how to transmit data to the clinic.

Be sure to download and analyze CGM data at every clinic visit and to check skin sites and help patients to deal with sensor wear issues/allergic reactions to the adhesive (12–14). Often, these issues can be overcome, although it may take trial and error.

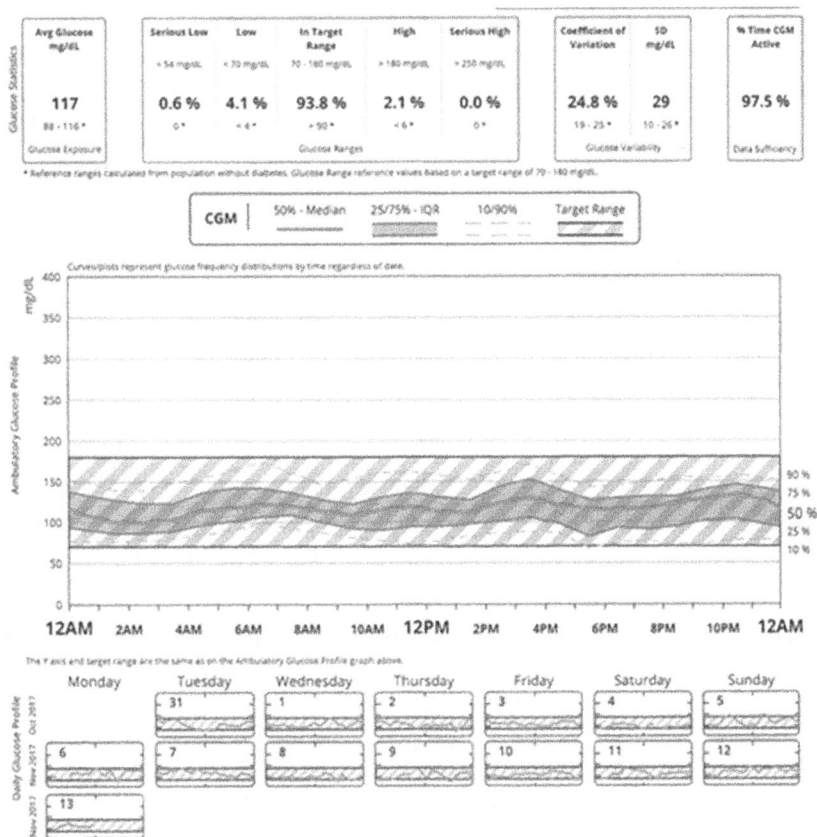

Figure 1. Example AGP display. Reading from Dexcom glucose monitor. Avg, average; IQR, interquartile range.

MAIN CONCLUSIONS

The use of the AGP can help in the management of patients with diabetes; however, the data must be interpreted and feedback provided to patients. Key features for analysis include evaluation of time in range, coefficient of variation, and interpretation of patterns of highs and lows. These data may be as important (or more important) than following HbA$_{1c}$s.

Barriers to successful use of CGM must be discussed with patients. Initial settings should be managed to avoid over-alarming and then advanced based on individual patient needs. Skin reactions and difficulty keeping the sensor in place

should be addressed and solutions provided to enhance long-term adherence.

DISCUSSION OF CASES AND ANSWERS
Case 1

Angie is a 32-year-old female with type 1 diabetes. She recently has been trying hard to manage her diabetes, including more-detailed carbohydrate counting and correcting. Her point-of-care HbA$_{1c}$ in your office is 8.1%, and she is discouraged. Her AGP over the past 2 weeks shows a time in range of 65%, a coefficient of variation of 30%, mean glucose

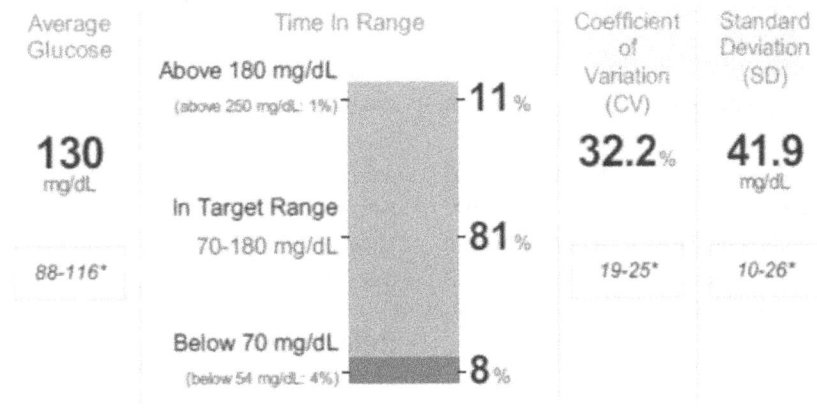

Figure 2. Printout from flash glucose monitoring system. Reading from an Abbott FreeStyle Libre glucose monitor.

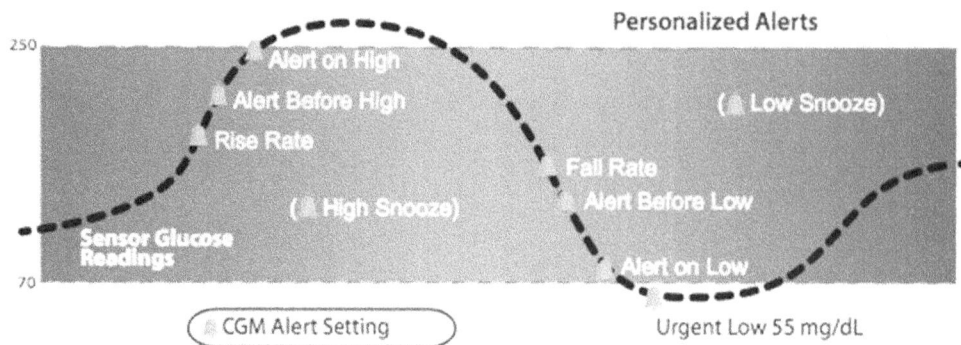

The **glucose alerts** in the Guardian Connect system are listed below:

Alert type	Description
High Sensor Glucose	Your sensor glucose level has gone above the high limit you set.
High Predicted	Your sensor glucose is predicted to go above the high limit you set, within a period of time that you set (up to 60 minutes ahead).
Rise Alert	Your sensor glucose is rising faster than a rate you set (corresponding to the rising arrows displayed next to your sensor glucose level).
Low Sensor Glucose	Your sensor glucose level has gone below the low limit you set.
Low Predicted	Your sensor glucose is predicted to go below the low limit you set, within a period of time that you set (up to 60 minutes ahead).
Fall Alert	Your sensor glucose is falling faster than a rate you set (corresponding to the falling arrows displayed next to your sensor glucose level).
Urgent Low Sensor Glucose	Your sensor glucose level has gone below 55 mg/dL.

Figure 3. Example of possible alerts on a CGM system. Reproduced from https://www.medtronicdiabetes.com/sites/default/files/library/download-library/user-guides/GuardianT%20Connect%20CGM%20System%20User%20Guide.PDF.

of 150 mg/dL, SD of 46 mg/dL, time <54 mg/dL at 0.8%, and time >180 mg/dL of 7%.

Which value do you use to discuss most effectively Angie's improved carbohydrate counting/insulin dosing efforts?

A. Mean glucose levels

B. Time in range

C. SD

D. HbA$_{1c}$

The correct answer is B, time in range. The average mean glucose level is not the most helpful in terms of her glucose control because a good average glucose level can consist of many highs and lows that balance out to a reasonable number. Time in range will provide a good sense of whether she is routinely swinging too high or too low and will best reflect her recent improvement in her control. The SD depends on the mean; coefficient of variation is more useful to look at variability in her blood glucose values. HbA$_{1c}$ is a 3-month average and will not reflect her recent improvements.

Case 2

Joe is an active 46-year-old male who works out daily. He has type 1 diabetes and was started on CGM. He stopped wearing it

after a few weeks because he said it kept falling off when he exercises.

What would you tell Joe to do next?

A. Stop using CGM

B. Apply deodorant on the insertion site

C. Use an adherent flexible over-bandage

D. Apply fluticasone nasal spray on the insertion site

The correct answer is C, use an adherent flexible over-bandage. Stopping use of the CGM is not an option, although it often happens if patients cannot keep the device attached. Applying deodorant on the insertion site would not help, although sometimes application of an antiperspirant can help in cases of excessive sweating. Use of an adherent flexible over-bandage is a good first step because it can help to prevent the sensor from falling off during exercise. Application of fluticasone nasal spray on the insertion site is helpful if there is an allergic reaction to the adhesive.

References

1. Bergenstal RM, Ahmann AJ, Bailey T, Beck RW, Bissen J, Buckingham B, Deeb L, Dolin RH, Garg SK, Goland R, Hirsch IB, Klonoff DC, Kruger DF, Matfin G, Mazze RS, Olson BA, Parkin C, Peters A, Powers MA, Rodriguez H, Southerland P, Strock ES, Tamborlane W, Wesley DM. Recommendations for standardizing glucose reporting and analysis to

optimize clinical decision making in diabetes: the ambulatory glucose profile. *J Diabetes Sci Technol.* 2013;**7**(2):562–578.

2. Beck RW, Connor CG, Mullen DM, Wesley DM, Bergenstal RM. The fallacy of average: how using HbA$_{1c}$ alone to assess glycemic control can be misleading. *Diabetes Care.* 2017;**40**(8):994–999.

3. Agiostratidou G, Anhalt H, Ball D, Blonde L, Gourgari E, Harriman KN, Kowalski A, Madden P, McAufliffe-Fogarty AH, McElwee-Malloy M, Peters A, Raman S, Reifschneider K, Rubin K, Weinzimer SA. Standardizing clinically meaningful outcomes measures beyond HbA$_{1c}$ for type 1 diabetes: a consensus statement of the American Association of Clinical Endocrinologists, the American Association of Diabetes Educators, the American Diabetes Association, the Endocrine Society, JDRF International, the Leona M. and Harry B. Helmsley Charitable Trust, the Pediatric Endocrine Society and the T1D Exchange. *Diabetes Care.* 2017;**40**:1622–1630.

4. Beck RW, Bergenstal RM, Riddlesworth TD, Kollman C, Li Z, Brown AS, Close KL. Validation of time in range as an outcome measure for diabetes clinical trials [published ahead of print on 23 October 2018]. *Diabetes Care.* doi:10.1002/dc18-144.

5. Chiang JI, Jani BD, Mair FS, Nicholl BI, Furler J, O'Neal D, Jenkins A, Condron P, Manski-Nankervis JA. Associations between multimorbidity, all-cause mortality and glycaemia in people with type 2 diabetes: a systematic review. *PLoS One.* 2018;**13**(12): e0209585.

6. Lachin JM, Bebu I, Bergenstal RM, Pop-Busui R, Service FJ, Zinman B, Nathan DM for the DCCT/EDIC Research Group. Association of glycemic variability in type 1 diabetes with progression of microvascular outcomes in the Diabetes Control and Complications Trial. *Diabetes Care.* 2017;**40**(6):777–783.

7. Bergenstal RM, Beck RW, Close KL, Grunberger G, Sacks DB, Kowalski A, Brown AS, Heinemann L, Aleppo G, Ryan DB, Riddlesworth TD, Cefalu WT. Glucose management indicator (GMI): a new term for estimating A1C from continuous glucose monitoring. *Diabetes Care.* 2018;**41**(11):2275–2280.

8. Riddlesworth TD, Beck RW, Gal RL, Connor CG, Bergenstal RM, Lee S, Willi SM. Optimal sampling duration for continuous glucose monitoring to determine long-term glycemic control. *Diabetes Technol Ther.* 2018;**20**(4):314–316.

9. Medtronic. Guardian Connect System User Guide, page 32. Available at: www.medtronicdiabetes.com/sites/default/files/library/download-library/user-guides/GuardianT%20Connect%20CGM%20System%20User%20Guide.PDF. Accessed 27 December 2018.

10. Aleppo G, Laffel LM, Ahmann AJ, Hirsch IB, Kruger DF, Peters A, Weinstock RS, Harris DR. A practical approach to using trend arrows on the Dexcom G5 CGM system for the management of adults with diabetes. *J Endocr Soc.* 2017;**1**(12):1445–1460.

11. Kudva YC, Ahmann AJ, Bergenstal RM, Gavin JR III, Kruger DF, Midyett LK, Miller E, Harris DR. Approach to using trend arrows in the FreeStyle Libre flash glucose monitoring systems in adults. *J Endocr Soc.* 2018;**2**(12): 1320–1337.

12. Englert K, Ruedy K, Coffey J, Caswell K, Steffen A, Levandoski L for the Diabetes Research in Children (DirecNet) Study Group. Skin and adhesive issues with continuous glucose monitors: a sticky situation. *J Diabetes Sci Technol.* 2014;**8**(4):745–751.

13. Messer LH, Berget C, Beatson C, Polsky S, Forlenza GP. Preserving skin integrity with chronic device use in diabetes. *Diabetes Technol Ther.* 2018;**20**(S2):S254–S264.

14. Berg AK, Nørgaard K, Thyssen JP, Zachariae C, Hommel E, Rytter K, Svensson J. Skin problems associated with insulin pumps and sensors in adults with type 1 diabetes: a cross-sectional study. *Diabetes Technol Ther.* 2018;**20**(7):475–482.

Metformin or Glyburide for Treatment of Gestational Diabetes: Time to Hit the Pause Button?

M17
Presented, March 23–26, 2019

Linda A. Barbour, MD, MSPH, FACP. Department of Medicine and Obstetrics and Gynecology, Divisions of Endocrinology, Metabolism, and Diabetes and Maternal-Fetal Medicine, University of Colorado School of Medicine and Anschutz Medical Campus, Aurora, Colorado 80045, E-mail: lynn.barbour@ucdenver.edu

SIGNIFICANCE OF THE PROBLEM

In parallel with the increase in obesity in women of child-bearing age, gestational diabetes (GDM) affected ~14% of women globally in 2017 (1) or approximately one in seven women. The prevalence is even higher in high-risk ethnicities in which the International Association of the Diabetes and Pregnancy Study Groups (adopted by the World Health Organization) diagnostic criteria are used rather than that of Coustan and Carpenter [American College of Obstetrics and Gynecology (ACOG)] (2). In addition to increasing the risk of large-for-gestational age (LGA) infants (≥90th percentile for gestational age), birth injury, cesarean delivery, preeclampsia, neonatal hypoglycemia, and pulmonary distress, excess maternal nutrients and the resulting fetal hyperinsulinemia in GDM can cause enlargement of the fetal pancreas, heart, liver, and fat stores (3). Additional alterations in appetite regulation and mitochondrial function may place offspring at risk for future metabolic disease (4, 5). A significant number of women with GDM experience failure with diet therapy alone (20% to 40%), and alternatives for medical treatment include insulin, glibenclamide (glyburide), and metformin. Although insulin negligibly crosses the placenta, and many consider it the safest and most effective choice (6), it is often expensive, poorly received by the patient, and associated with hypoglycemia. Guidelines from the Society of Maternal-Fetal Medicine (SMFM) published in 2018 support the conclusion that metformin is an equal alternative to insulin (7). In 2018, ACOG supported insulin as a first-line therapy when diet fails, with metformin as a second alternative (8). The 2018 American Diabetes Association (ADA) literature supports insulin as a first-line drug and either metformin or glyburide as a second-line drug, recognizing that metformin has a higher rate of failure (9). Although a future update is planned, 2013 guidelines from the Endocrine Society (ES) state that metformin could be considered for women who decline or who cannot use insulin or glyburide (10).

With up to one in five women diagnosed with GDM, a significant number who experience failure with diet therapy, rising costs of insulins, and more intensive efforts required from both providers and patients to determine effective and safe insulin doses, oral agents have increased in popularity as easier and less costly options to treat this rapidly growing population of pregnant women (11). There is intense debate and a lack of consensus as to whether metformin and glyburide produce similar pregnancy outcomes, with a preference by some toward metformin, especially given its neutral weight gain effect and absence of hypoglycemia. Although both glyburide and metformin seem both to be safe with regard to the risk of teratogenicity and not to cause unexpected adverse short-term outcomes (12–14), both drugs cross the placenta, with metformin crossing to a greater degree than glyburide. Given the growing recognition that intrauterine exposures can increase the risk for future metabolic, cardiovascular, and neurodevelopmental disorders in offspring, there are concerns about safety and adverse long-term intrauterine programming effects (6, 15).

BARRIERS TO OPTIMAL PRACTICE

- There is no consensus from experts, meta-analyses, or guidelines from SMFM, ACOG, ADA, or ES about the risks and benefits of oral agents in pregnancy with regard to pregnancy outcomes and potential long-term effects on offspring.
- GDM, like type 2 diabetes (T2DM), is a heterogeneous disorder with variability in hepatic, adipose tissue, and skeletal muscle insulin resistance, as well as β-cell dysfunction, that results in a wide distribution of glycemic patterns that are not all effectively targeted by the same agent (16).
- The rapidly growing number of women with GDM, rising costs of insulins, difficulties and time intensiveness in effectively titrating insulin throughout pregnancy, and patient preference for oral therapies are promoting widespread use of oral agents.
- Use patterns of oral agents tend to be governed by local provider practices and personal experience rather than on the basis of differences in patients' metabolic profiles and attention to their pharmacokinetic properties.

LEARNING OBJECTIVES

As a result of participating in this session, learners should be able to:
- Appreciate differences in 2018 guidelines on the pharmacologic treatment of GDM from major medical organizations as well as the data on which these guidelines are based
- Compare the relative efficacy and safety of insulin, metformin, and glyburide for the treatment of GDM and recognize the potential for long-term programming effects on offspring

- Discuss the pharmacology and optimal dosing of metformin and/or glyburide in GDM, including placental transfer
- Describe a personalized approach to the discussion of the use of oral glucose-lowering medications with pregnant patients

STRATEGIES FOR THERAPY AND MANAGEMENT: METFORMIN RISKS AND BENEFITS

Metformin is relatively simple to use, does not cause maternal hypoglycemia, causes less maternal weight gain than insulin, and is usually well tolerated in most women. In addition, ample data support its short-term safety and the fact that it is not a major teratogen (11–14). Metformin may also have some beneficial effects, specifically by promoting angiogenesis and possibly preventing preeclampsia, at least in some studies (17). Although metformin would be expected to improve maternal insulin sensitivity and prevent GDM, there were no differences in the rate of LGA, prevention of GDM, or a decrease in miscarriage in obese women in the Metformin in Obese Pregnancy randomized controlled trial (RCT) (18) and EMPOWaR RCT (19) or in women with polycystic ovarian syndrome (PCOS) (20); therefore, it should not be administered for the prevention of these outcomes. In a 2018 Cochrane review (21) of three RCTs that randomly assigned ~1100 obese women to metformin or placebo, there was no statistical difference in LGA, gestational hypertension, pre-eclampsia, GDM, cesarean delivery, or preterm birth, but a slightly lower weight gain (mean, ~2.6 kg). Metformin has a high rate of failure and in the Metformin in Pregnancy (MiG) RCT, 46% of women experienced failure with metformin, which resulted in the need to add insulin therapy (22). As a result, pregnancy outcome effects reported with metformin are often in women who received both insulin and metformin and not necessarily with metformin alone. The MiG RCT demonstrated that mothers who were randomly assigned to metformin—often supplemented with insulin—vs. insulin alone had less weight gain and gestational hypertension, but there was no difference in LGA and the number of preterm births were increased. Metformin alone was associated with increased maternal triglycerides (TGs) compared with insulin. TGs and free fatty acids, which result from their hydrolysis, are increasingly recognized as a substrate for fetal fat accretion, and maternal TGs correlate with infant adiposity, especially in pregnancies with obesity (23). Maternal TGs in the MiG study (24) were correlated with LGA and infant adiposity despite lower maternal gestational weight gain. Metformin is transported across the placenta so that fetal levels are at least as high as maternal levels. There are also concerns about the use of metformin if the fetus is at risk for an ischemic environment—placental insufficiency, maternal hypertension, pre-eclampsia, or growth restriction. Metformin was not used in these conditions in the MiG trial. The utility of metformin in women with T2DM to reduce insulin requirements and weight gain is limited but is the focus of two ongoing RCTs—the

Metformin in Women with Type 2 Diabetes in Pregnancy trial (25) and the Medical Optimization of Management of Type 2 Diabetes Complicating Pregnancy trial, the results of which should be available soon.

As a result of metformin's transport by organic cation transporters into mitochondrial membranes, which are present abundantly in both the fetus and placenta, metformin has the potential to act on placental and fetal tissues. Metformin has multiple effects and is currently the focus of investigation in nonpregnant individuals as a result of its anticancer effects, growth inhibitory properties, ability to suppress mitochondrial respiration, and effects on gluconeogenic responses, which have the potential to affect both fetal and childhood development. During early gestation, the embryo has few—and relatively immature—mitochondria because of the low rates of aerobic vs. anaerobic metabolism and express low levels of organic cation transporters (15); therefore, metformin exposure is likely safe in the first trimester. In contrast, the placenta and fetus express metformin transporters, exhibit high rates of aerobic metabolism, and depend on mature mitochondrial activity in the second and third trimesters, which are critical for fetal growth, nutrient and oxygen transport, and placental hormone production. Metformin inhibits mitochondrial respiratory complex I of the electron transport chain, which leads to decreased ATP production and increased AMP:ATP ratios. Metformin activates AMP kinase and inhibits the mammalian target of the rapamycin (mTOR) pathway (6, 13, 15), which results in a decrease in proliferation and an increase in apoptosis and cell-cycle arrest. mTOR is the primary nutrient sensor in the placenta and its inhibition may directly attenuate nutrient flux and fetal growth (26). Metformin has an abundance of effects that could affect fetal metabolic health, including impairment of glycolysis and the tricarboxylic acid cycle, impairment of one-carbon metabolism and antifolate properties, inhibition of thiamine uptake and B_{12} deficiency, inhibition of mTOR with suppression of protein synthesis, and impairment of histone acetylation and epigenetic modifications (13, 15). It is unclear whether pregnant women who take metformin should be screened for B_{12} deficiency or may need supplementation. There is no evidence that metformin causes small-for-gestational age infants and it is unknown if it causes these fetal effects in humans; however, metformin has the potential to inhibit mitochondrial activity and adversely affect function, growth, or differentiation of fetal or placental tissues. Although inadequately studied in pregnancy, metformin also has microbiome effects that could alter gut serotonin levels, increase lactate delivery to the liver, increase glucagon-like polypeptide-1, and increase the use of gut glucose, decreasing serum glucose levels even when not absorbed.

Exposure of prenatal mice to metformin at doses that achieved concentrations that were similar to those used in humans resulted in lower birth weights compared with non-exposed mice; however, metformin-exposed offspring that were fed a Western-style diet postweaning have demonstrated conflicting findings for adipose tissue development and glucose intolerance (13). In a number of animal models and human epidemiologic studies, relative nutrient restriction *in utero* followed by an environment of nutrient excess post-natally in infancy and childhood predisposed offspring to later obesity and metabolic disease (6, 13, 15). Offspring in the MiG trial at age 2 years demonstrated evidence of higher sub-cutaneous fat mass without evidence of a decrease in visceral fat (27), but there were no differences in neurodevelopmental outcomes. Of high clinical relevance, two long-term follow-up analyses from earlier RCTs were published after the SMFM, ACOG, and ADA statements were released. MiG investigators reported longer-term outcomes from a subset of offspring at age 7 years (60% of the Adelaide subgroup) and age 9 years (25% of the Auckland subgroup), which were analyzed sep-arately (28). Although the total cohort in the MiG index trial showed no differences in rates of LGA, when stratified into Adelaide and Auckland subgroups the metformin-exposed offspring from Adelaide demonstrated a higher rate of LGA compared with insulin alone (20.7 *vs.* 5.9%) and maternal fasting glucoses were higher compared with those exposed to insulin alone. However, at age 7 years, there were no differ-ences in offspring weight or body composition among the Adelaide subgroup. In contrast, patients in the Auckland subgroup demonstrated no differences in LGA rates compared with insulin, but at age 9 years the metformin-exposed group was heavier, had greater arm and waist circumference and waist:height ratio (<0.05), and trended toward a higher body mass index (BMI), triceps skinfold, and abdominal fat volume by MRI (all $P = 0.05$). There was no difference in glucose, lipids, insulin resistance, or liver function test measures in the metformin-exposed offspring compared with insulin from either subgroup. Interpretation of these results is complicated, especially by the fact that only 25% of the offspring in the Auckland group received long-term follow-up and postnatal influences on the risk of childhood obesity are unclear. In RCT studies that examined offspring of women with PCOS who were treated with metformin *vs.* placebo, there were no differ-ences in rates of LGA or GDM in the metformin-treated group (20); however, offspring weighed more at age 1 year. In a limited study of 25 offspring who were observed at age 8 years, researchers found higher fasting glucoses and systolic blood pressures in the metformin-exposed group, despite insignificant differences in growth or body composition. At age 4 years, 182 offspring were analyzed (55% of the total cohort) from the two RCTs in which women with PCOS were randomly assigned to metformin. Off-spring exposed to metformin *in utero* had higher weight and BMI z-scores and were at twice the risk of being overweight and obese compared with those who received placebo (29).

Although not definitive, data from these follow-up trials from the 9-year MiG offspring follow-up of women who were treated with metformin for GDM and the 4-year offspring follow-up of women who were treated with metformin for PCOS raise concerns that the use of metformin during pregnancy could increase the risk of later childhood obesity. The increased risk for childhood obesity among the offspring of some mothers with PCOS and GDM is consistent with fetal developmental programming by metformin, which may place the exposed offspring at later risk for metabolic disease, especially when exposed to an obesogenic postnatal environment (6).

STRATEGIES FOR THERAPY AND MANAGEMENT: GLYBURIDE RISKS AND BENEFITS

Glyburide is metabolized by the liver and effluxed from the fetal to the maternal compartment against a concentration gradient by protein binding so that glyburide levels are less than those achieved by metformin but still as high as 50% to 70% of maternal levels (6, 12, 30). If levels are high enough to stimulate fetal β-cells, this could directly contribute to fetal hyperinsulinemia in addition to the fetal hyperinsulinemia that occurs as a result of inadequate maternal glucose control. Recent data suggest that glyburide may increase placental GLUT1 expression, potentially increasing glucose delivery (31). In a 2015 meta-analysis, Balsells *et al.* (32) concluded that metformin—often used with insulin—was associated with less maternal weight gain, lower birth weight, less macro-somia, and less LGA, but the number of preterm births was increased compared with glyburide. Another meta-analysis that used a network approach suggested that metformin has the highest probability of being the most effective treatment compared with insulin or glyburide (33); however, two Cochrane meta-analyses concluded that the evidence comparing insulin with oral agents was of low to moderate quality and there were no clear differences among the agents (34, 35).

Although the SMFM and ACOG statements endorsed the superior safety and efficacy of metformin over glyburide, differences in pregnancy outcomes and failures among oral agents are likely influenced by physician or maternal pref-erence, the availability of agents, the severity of GDM, and the fact that glyburide dosing is often not administered according to its pharmacokinetic properties. The overall failure rate of glyburide (~25%) is less than that of metformin, but often unrecognized is that glyburide's peak is at 2 to 3 hours and the peak of insulin stimulated by glyburide is 3 to 4 hours after administration. Although glyburide may have active metab-olites, the effect of glyburide is greater if administered 1 hour before meals (36). Given that the peak of glyburide is similar to that of regular insulin, the pharmacokinetic properties of glyburide do not support the practice of administering it before bedtime to treat fasting hyperglycemia. Taking gly-buride immediately before a meal or at bedtime, which is a common clinical practice, is likely to result in significant maternal hypoglycemia 3 to 4 hours later and an inability to effectively up-titrate the dose. This can result in inadequately treated 1-hour postprandial (PP) hyperglycemia, fetal hyperinsulinemia, excess fetal growth, and neonatal hypo-glycemia. It has also been shown that lower glyburide levels are achieved in pregnancy compared with nonpregnant individuals, which raises questions about insufficient dosing, but there are no data on doses >20 mg in pregnancy (6, 12, 36). Glyburide failures were examined in a retrospective trial (37) and the higher rates of failure were observed with a diagnosis at <25 weeks, multiparity, older maternal age, and fasting hyperglycemia >10 mg/dL (6.1 mmol/L). A recent multi-institutional RCT that included 809 women (38) that was designed to investigate whether treatment with glyburide was noninferior to insulin for preventing a composite outcome of macrosomia (>4000 g) or LGA, neonatal hypoglycemia, and/or hyperbilirubinemia reported the composite outcome in 23.4% of infants in the insulin group compared with 27.6% of infants in the glyburide group using a per-protocol analysis. Although the difference between groups in adverse outcomes was only 4.2% (one-sided 97.5% CI, 0% to 10.5%), the upper confidence limit of 10.5% exceeded the prespecified 7% upper limit of the difference; therefore, the authors concluded that their study did not demonstrate that glyburide was non-inferior to insulin for the prevention of perinatal complications. However, glyburide was started at 2.5 mg once per day irrespective of fasting or PP hyperglycemia and could only be increased every 4 days. The mean dose received was only 5.4 mg. No information was provided on the timing of glyburide administration or titration regimen, and 18% of patients were switched to insulin. Conversely, insulin could be initiated using multiple injections per day that target both fasting and PP hyperglycemia and self-titrated every 2 days. Despite the greater flexibility of the insulin regimen, there was actually a tendency for the patients receiving glyburide to be in better control in the per-protocol analysis, although it caused more hypoglycemia (39). At this time, there are no RCTs reporting any long-term offspring outcomes in fetuses exposed to glyburide.

There are limited RCTs that directly compare glyburide with metformin, and although most observed a lower birthweight with metformin, the studies were limited by small sample sizes (12, 35). Nachum *et al.* (40) randomized metformin *vs.* glyburide first (in which glyburide was taken before bedtime for fasting hyperglycemia) and added the other agent if glycemia was not controlled. The authors concluded that using both drugs reduced the need for insulin from 32% to 11%. Neither drug clearly performed better than the other, and although the authors advocated for their combined efficacy, prescribing two drugs that cross the placenta to avoid insulin raises significant concerns.

MAIN CONCLUSIONS

Although the ACOG and SMFM statements take the position of metformin being superior to glyburide as an oral agent for short-term perinatal outcomes, common misuse of glyburide according to its pharmacokinetic properties deserves consideration. Angiogenic properties of metformin may be found to prevent preeclampsia. Although metformin does have beneficial antiproliferative, mitochondrial, and hepatocellular effects in nonpregnant adults with prediabetes, T2DM, and

cancer, these same effects cannot be presumed to be beneficial to a fetus. Recent follow-up data suggest that metformin may create an intrauterine environment that places the fetus at risk for developmental programming that could promote an obesogenic phenotype, especially when exposed to a postnatal environment of nutritional excess. No long-term data are available for glyburide and follow-up studies are needed given the possibility of β-cell stimulation and potential promotion of β-cell fatigue over the long-term.

This speaker concurs with both the ADA and ACOG recommendations that insulin is the preferred treatment for GDM; however, individualizing therapy is suggested rather than recommending one agent over another in all patients. For patients who are unwilling or unable to administer multiple insulin injections appropriately and safely, who are unable to afford insulin, or who are at high risk of hypoglycemia, choosing an oral agent should be based on his or her individual glucose profile, carefully considering benefits and risks. Failure rates for oral hypoglycemic agents are highest when a patient receives a diagnosis of GDM at an earlier gestation, has higher fasting glucose >110 mg/dL (6.1 mmol/L), higher maternal BMI, older age, and a history of GDM. Patients with primarily fasting hyperglycemia—frequent in Hispanic Americans—are not good candidates for glyburide and may benefit from a single dose of neutral protamine Hagedorn (NPH) insulin immediately before bedtime. If PP hyperglycemia warrants treatment and there are barriers to using multiple insulin injections, glyburide administered 30 minutes to 1 hour before breakfast and dinner may successfully lower 2-hour PP glucose (6). Combination NPH at night and glyburide preprandially deserves additional study for these candidates. Metformin might be particularly useful in women who are unwilling to use insulin and who are extremely fearful of hypoglycemia, especially in those with mild hyperglycemia and predominantly fasting hyperglycemia. Both agents may be used in mothers who wish to breast feed as a result of extremely low concentrations in breast milk.

Carefully controlled studies that appropriately target the use of oral agents according to individual patterns of hyperglycemia and optimize drug administration according to pharmacodynamic and pharmacokinetic properties are essential. A personalized approach should be used to better meet the biologic, psychosocial, and socioeconomic needs of individual patients. If oral therapy is used in patients with mild GDM, patients should be counseled on the limited long-term safety data and potential for adverse childhood metabolic effects with both oral agents; however, inadequately controlled hyperglycemia poses even greater risks.

Case 1

A 30-year-old gravida 1, para 1 (G1P0) woman with a BMI of 32 and history of PCOS and prediabetes who takes 1000 mg metformin two times per day discovers she is 6 weeks pregnant. Her HbA_{1c} is 5.9, fasting blood glucose (FBG) is <95 mg/dL (5.3 mmol/L), and 1-hour PP glucose is <135 mg/dL (7.5 mmol/L).

You recommend the following:

A. Continue metformin through the first trimester because of reassuring data in early pregnancy

B. Continue metformin because it will decrease her risk of GDM

C. Continue metformin because it will decrease her chance of having an LGA infant

D. Stop metformin for 2 weeks, then perform appropriate screening and/or diagnosis to asses for GDM and, if so, switch her to insulin

Case 2

A 27-year-old G3P2 woman at 26 weeks had newly diagnosed GDM on a 3-hour oral glucose tolerance test with an FBG of 115 mg/dL (6.4 mmol/L) and 1-hour PP glucose of 206 mg/dL (11.4 mmol/L). After diet, her glucometer shows consistent fasting hyperglycemia up to 112 mg/dL (6.2 mmol/L) and elevated 1-hourr PP glucose up to 155 mg/dL (8.6 mmol/L) at breakfast, lunch, and dinner. The patient's FBG goal is ≤95 mg/dL (5.3 mmol/dL), 1-hour PP glucose goal is ≤140 mg/dL (7.8 mmol/L), and 2-hour PP glucose goal is ≤120 mg/dL (6.7 mmol/L). She is reticent to use insulin.

You advise:

A. Metformin for her FBG and glyburide two times per day for her PP hyperglycemia

B. Glyburide in the morning before breakfast and every night at bedtime for her fasting hyperglycemia

C. Start multiple-dose insulin because she already meets the criteria for T2DM

D. Start NPH every night at bedtime and glyburide before breakfast and dinner

DISCUSSION OF CASES AND ANSWERS

Case 1

The answer is A. Case 1 illustrates the importance of pre-conception counseling for women on oral agents. Abundant data indicate that metformin is not a major teratogen, but that hyperglycemia is. Therefore, stopping metformin during the time of organogenesis when fetal organs are forming (~5 to 8 weeks after last menstrual period) could result in high maternal glucose levels during this critical window and may actually increase the risk of malformations. Thus, answer D is not a good strategy. Furthermore, mitochondrial activity and cation transporters in the embryo are low and there are no data to suggest that metformin poses any risk in the first trimester. Answer A is the best option as it would be safe to continue metformin until after organogenesis is complete and then evaluate the patient for GDM using either International Association of the Diabetes and Pregnancy Study Groups (preferred by the World Health Organization and ES) or ACOG criteria (preferred by the National Institutes of Health consensus panel; either is recommended by the ADA). Women who are found to have GDM and who experience failure with diet or those women who have preexisting diabetes could then switch to insulin and be tapered off metformin after the first trimester. Metformin has not been shown to decrease LGA, GDM, or miscarriage in RCTs where it has been administered to women with obesity or PCOS; therefore, answers B and C are incorrect.

Case 2

The answer is D. Case 2 underscores how preexisting diabetes is diagnosed for the first time during pregnancy and the importance of individualizing therapy according to an agent's pharmacokinetic properties and the patient's glycemic patterns. Diagnosis of preexisting diabetes during pregnancy is identical to that made outside of pregnancy, especially given that both fasting glucose and HbA$_{1c}$ normally fall in pregnancy. An FBG of >125 mg/dL (7.0 mmol/L), a random glucose level ≥200 mg/dL (11.1 mmol/L), or an HbA$_{1c}$ ≥6.5 is required to diagnose preexisting (overt) diabetes in pregnancy, so answer C is incorrect. Administering glyburide before bedtime to treat fasting hyperglycemia places the patient at risk for nocturnal hypoglycemia given that the insulin from glyburide, in a manner similar to regular insulin, peaks at ~3 to 4 hours after the dose and should be administered at least 30 minutes to 1 hour before meals. Therefore, answer B is likely to be less efficacious and to result in maternal hypoglycemia. Administering two oral agents that both cross the placenta is a strategy that should be reserved for patients who are unwilling or unable to take insulin and who are not controlled on a single agent, given the potential long-term programming risks of both agents. This makes answer A a less attractive choice. Many women may be unwilling, financially limited, or unable to safely take multiple doses of insulin but are receptive to taking one dose of NPH immediately before bedtime, which typically peaks at ~7 to 8 hours and usually effectively controls fasting hyperglycemia. Therefore, answer D is the best option; combination NPH immediately before bedtime controls FBG and glyburide 30 minutes to 1 hour before breakfast and dinner may target both fasting and PP hyperglycemia in women unwilling to take multiple doses of insulin. NPH every night at bedtime can also be used to treat women with primarily fasting hyperglycemia—common in Hispanic women who primarily experience failure with their oral glucose tolerance test by their fasting glucose. It is uncommon for patients with insulin-resistant GDM to develop nocturnal hypoglycemia if NPH is titrated carefully and it is much less expensive than many other insulins.

References

1. International Diabetes Federation. *IDF Diabetes Atlas.* 8th ed. Brussels, Belgium: International Diabetes Federation; 2017.

2. Vandorsten JP, Dodson WC, Espeland MA, Grobman WA, Guise JM, Mercer BM, Minkoff HL, Poindexter B, Prosser LA, Sawaya GF, Scott JR, Silver RM, Smith L, Thomas A, Tita AT. NIH consensus development conference: diagnosing gestational diabetes mellitus. *NIH Consens State Sci Statements.* 2013;**29**(1):1–31.

3. Barbour LA. Unresolved controversies in gestational diabetes: implications on maternal and infant health. *Curr Opin Endocrinol Diabetes Obes.* 2014;**21**(4):264–270.

4. Catalano PM, Shankar K. Obesity and pregnancy: mechanisms of short term and long term adverse consequences for mother and child. *BMJ.* 2017;**356**:j1.

5. Barbour LA. Changing perspectives in pre-existing diabetes and obesity in pregnancy: maternal and infant short- and long-term outcomes. *Curr Opin Endocrinol Diabetes Obes.* 2014;**21**(4): 257–263.

6. Barbour LA, Scifres C, Valent AM, Friedman JE, Buchanan TA, Coustan D, Aagaard K, Thornburg KL, Catalano PM, Galan HL, Hay WW, Jr., Frias AE, Shankar K, Simmons RA, Moses RG, Sacks DA, Loeken MR. A cautionary response to SMFM statement: pharmacological treatment of gestational diabetes. *Am J Obstet Gynecol.* 2018;**219**(4): 367.e1–367.e7.

7. Society of Maternal-Fetal Medicine (SMFM) Publications Committee. SMFM statement: pharmacological treatment of gestational diabetes. *Am J Obstet Gynecol.* 2018;**218**(5):B2–B4.

8. Committee on Practice Bulletins—Obstetrics. ACOG practice bulletin No. 190: gestational diabetes mellitus. *Obstet Gynecol.* 2018;**131**(2): e49–e64.

9. American Diabetes Association. Management of Diabetes in pregnancy: *Standards of Medical Care in Diabetes—2018. Diabetes Care.* 2018;**41**(Suppl 1):S137–S143.

10. Blumer I, Hadar E, Hadden DR, Jovanovič L, Mestman JH, Murad MH, Yogev Y. Diabetes and pregnancy: an endocrine society clinical practice guideline. *J Clin Endocrinol Metab.* 2013;**98**(11): 4227–4249.

11. Johns EC, Denison FC, Norman JE, Reynolds RM. Gestational diabetes mellitus: mechanisms, treatment, and complications. *Trends Endocrinol Metab.* 2018;**29**(11):743–754.

12. Feghali MN, Scifres CM. Novel therapies for diabetes mellitus in pregnancy. *BMJ.* 2018;**362**:k2034.

13. Priya G, Kalra S. Metformin in the management of diabetes during pregnancy and lactation. *Drugs Context.* 2018;**7**:212523.

14. Hyer S, Balani J, Shehata H. Metformin in pregnancy: mechanisms and clinical applications. *Int J Mol Sci.* 2018;**19**(7):1954.

15. Lindsay RS, Loeken MR. Metformin use in pregnancy: promises and uncertainties. *Diabetologia.* 2017;**60**(9):1612–1619.

16. Powe CE, Allard C, Battista M-C, Doyon M, Bouchard L, Ecker JL, Perron P, Florez JC, Thadhani R, Hivert MF. Heterogeneous contribution of insulin sensitivity and secretion defects to gestational diabetes mellitus. *Diabetes Care.* 2016;**39**(6):1052–1055.

17. Romero R, Erez O, Hüttemann M, Maymon E, Panaitescu B, Conde-Agudelo A, Pacora P, Yoon BH, Grossman LI. Metformin, the aspirin of the 21st century: its role in gestational diabetes mellitus, prevention of preeclampsia and cancer, and the promotion of longevity. *Am J Obstet Gynecol.* 2017;**217**(3):282–302.

18. Syngelaki A, Nicolaides KH, Balani J, Hyer S, Akolekar R, Kotecha R, Pastides A, Shehata H. Metformin versus placebo in obese pregnant women without diabetes mellitus. *N Engl J Med.* 2016;**374**(5): 434–443.

19. Chiswick C, Reynolds RM, Denison F, Drake AJ, Forbes S, Newby DE, Walker BR, Quenby S, Wray S, Weeks A, Lashen H, Rodriguez A, Murray G, Whyte S, Norman JE. Effect of metformin on maternal and fetal outcomes in obese pregnant women (EMPOWaR): a randomised, double-blind, placebo-controlled trial. *Lancet Diabetes Endocrinol.* 2015;**3**(10):778–786.

20. Vanky E, Stridsklev S, Heimstad R, Romundstad P, Skogøy K, Kleggetveit O, Hjelle S, von Brandis P, Eikeland T, Flo K, Berg KF, Bunford G, Lund A, Bjerke C, Almås I, Berg AH, Danielson A, Lahmami G, Carlsen SM. Metformin versus placebo from first trimester to delivery in polycystic ovary syndrome: a randomized, controlled multicenter study. *J Clin Endocrinol Metab.* 2010;**95**(12):E448–E455.

21. Dodd JM, Grivell RM, Deussen AR, Hague WM. Metformin for women who are overweight of obese during pregnancy for improving maternal and infant outcomes. *Cochrane Database Syst Rev.* 2018;**7**: CD010564.

22. Rowan JA, Hague WM, Gao W, Battin MR, Moore MP, for the MiG Trial Investigators. Metformin versus insulin for the treatment of gestational diabetes. *N Engl J Med.* 2008;**358**(19):2003–2015.

23. Barbour LA, Farabi SS, Friedman JE, Hirsch NM, Reece MS, Van Pelt RE, Hernandez TL. Postprandial triglycerides predict newborn fat more strongly than glucose in women with obesity in early pregnancy. *Obesity (Silver Spring).* 2018;**26**(8):1347–1356.

24. Barrett HL, Dekker Nitert M, Jones L, O'Rourke P, Lust K, Gatford KL, De Blasio MJ, Coat S, Owens JA, Hague WM, McIntyre HD, Callaway L, Rowan J. Determinants of maternal triglycerides in women with gestational diabetes mellitus in the Metformin in Gestational Diabetes (MiG) study. *Diabetes Care.* 2013;**36**(7):1941–1946.

25. Feig DS, Murphy K, Asztalos E, Tomlinson G, Sanchez J, Zinman B, Ohlsson A, Ryan EA, Fantus IG, Armson AB, Lipscombe LL, Barrett JF, for the MiTy Collaborative Group. Metformin in women with type 2 diabetes in pregnancy (MiTy): a multi-center randomized controlled trial. *BMC Pregnancy Childbirth.* 2016;**16**(1):173.

26. Jansson N, Rosario FJ, Gaccioli F, Lager S, Jones HN, Roos S, Jansson T, Powell TL. Activation of placental mTOR signaling and amino acid transporters in obese women giving birth to large babies. *J Clin Endocrinol Metab.* 2013;**98**(1):105–113.

27. Lau SM. Comment on: Rowan et al. Metformin in Gestational Diabetes: The Offspring Follow-Up (MiG TOFU): body composition at 2 years of age. Diabetes Care 2011;34:2279-2284. *Diabetes Care.* 2012;**35**(3): e29.

28. Rowan JA, Rush EC, Plank LD, Lu J, Obolonkin V, Coat S, Hague WM. Metformin in Gestational Diabetes: The Offspring Follow-Up (MiG TOFU): body composition and metabolic outcomes at 7-9 years of age. *BMJ Open Diabetes Res Care.* 2018;**6**(1):e000456.

29. Hanem LGE, Stridsklev S, Juliusson PB, Salvesen Ø, Roelants M, Carlsen SM, Ødegård R, Vanky E. Metformin use in PCOS pregnancies increases the risk of offspring overweight at 4 years of age: follow-up of two RCTs. *J Clin Endocrinol Metab.* 2018;**103**(4):1612–1621.

30. Schwartz RA, Rosenn B, Aleksa K, Koren G. Glyburide transport across the human placenta. *Obstet Gynecol.* 2015;**125**(3):583–588.

31. Díaz P, Dimasuay KG, Koele-Schmidt L, Jang B, Barbour LA, Jansson T, Powell TL. Glyburide treatment in gestational diabetes is associated with increased placental glucose transporter 1 expression and higher birth weight. *Placenta.* 2017;**57**:52–59.

32. Balsells M, García-Patterson A, Solà I, Roqué M, Gich I, Corcoy R. Glibenclamide, metformin, and insulin for the treatment of gestational diabetes: a systematic review and meta-analysis. *BMJ.* 2015;**350**(14): h102.

33. Farrar D, Simmonds M, Bryant M, Sheldon TA, Tuffnell D, Golder S, Lawlor DA. Treatments for gestational diabetes: a systematic review and meta-analysis. *BMJ Open.* 2017;**7**(6):e015557.

34. Brown J, Grzeskowiak L, Williamson K, Downie MR, Crowther CA. Insulin for the treatment of women with gestational diabetes. *Cochrane Database Syst Rev.* 2017;**11**:CD012037.

35. Brown J, Martis R, Hughes B, Rowan J, Crowther CA. Oral anti-diabetic pharmacological therapies for the treatment of women with gestational diabetes. *Cochrane Database Syst Rev.* 2017;**1**:CD011967.

36. Caritis SN, Hebert MF. A pharmacologic approach to the use of glyburide in pregnancy. *Obstet Gynecol.* 2013;**121**(6):1309–1312.

37. Kahn BF, Davies JK, Lynch AM, Reynolds RM, Barbour LA. Predictors of glyburide failure in the treatment of gestational diabetes. *Obstet Gynecol.* 2006;**107**(6):1303–1309.

38. Sénat MV, Affres H, Letourneau A, Coustols-Valat M, Cazaubiel M, Legardeur H, Jacquier JF, Bourcigaux N, Simon E, Rod A, Héron I, Castera V, Sentilhes L, Bretelle F, Rolland C, Morin M, Deruelle P, De Carne C, Maillot F, Beucher G, Verspyck E, Desbriere R, Laboureau S, Mitanchez D, Bouyer J, for the Groupe de Recherche en Obstétrique et Gynécologie (GROG). Effect of glyburide vs subcutaneous insulin on perinatal complications for women with gestational diabetes: a randomized clinical trial. *JAMA.* 2018;**319**(17):1773–1780.

39. Coustan DR, Barbour L. Insulin vs glyburide for gestational diabetes. *JAMA.* 2018;**319**(17):1769–1770.

40. Barbour LA, Davies JK. Comment on Nachum et al. Glyburide versus metformin and their combination for the treatment of gestational diabetes mellitus: a randomized controlled study. Diabetes Care 2017; 40:332–337. *Diabetes Care.* 2017;**40**(8):e115.

Diabetic Nephropathy

M42
Presented, March 23–26, 2019

Robert C. Stanton, MD. Kidney and Hypertension Section, Joslin Diabetes Center, Boston, Massachusetts 02215, E-mail: robert.stanton@joslin.harvard.edu

SIGNIFICANCE OF THE CLINICAL PROBLEM

Diabetic kidney disease (DKD) has become the leading cause of kidney disease in the United States, Canada, Europe, and Australia and is becoming the most common cause of kidney disease and end-stage renal disease (ESRD) throughout the world. China and India will have the most people with DKD and eventually ESRD because the number of people with diabetes mellitus (DM) in these countries continues to rise. Other areas of the world, such as the Middle East, also are affected greatly due to the high number of people with DM. Thus, DKD is a major worldwide public health issue primarily because of the dramatic rise in the number of people with DM (especially type 2 DM). One of the best ways to illustrate how this epidemic of kidney disease has affected global health is to look at the number of people with ESRD over time (Fig. 1). It is most valuable to look at ESRD data because there is no debate over the accuracy of ESRD numbers, yet one could argue over the accuracy of the definition of chronic kidney disease (CKD), which usually is described as a glomerular filtration rate (GFR) of <60 mL/min per 1.73 m^2 and/or an increase in the urine albumin/creatinine ratio (ACR) >30 mg/g. This definition likely overestimates CKD numbers because, for example, normal aging will lead to a GFR of <60 mL/min per 1.73 m^2 as a result of the normal rate of decline being 0.5 to 1 mL/min per year (GFR at birth varies from 100 to 140 mL/min per 1.73 m^2). However, the number of people with CKD must be very high for the following reasons: First, most patients with CKD will not make it to ESRD because they will die as a result of a cardiac event, and second, the US death rates of patients on dialysis are 15% to 20% per year. In the United States, the prevalent number of people with ESRD in 1980 (people either on dialysis or who have received a kidney transplant) was 56,435; by 2016, the number was 726,331, showing a 13-fold increase (2). Most of this epidemic increase is due to DM, and the rest primarily is due to hypertension. As of 2015, there were about 700,000 people in the United States with ESRD (about 0.2% of the population). About half of these people had kidney failure due to DM. The federal government spent 7.3% of the Medicare budget on this population (about $38 billion) in 2015. When taking into account all CKD and associated comorbidities (especially cardiovascular disease, which increases dramatically as kidney function declines), it is estimated that an additional $50 billion was spent on CKD and ESRD for a total of about $90 billion. The biggest impact on the health of people with DM and on controlling health care costs that can be made at this time is to prevent development of DKD or to slow progression of CKD.

Furthermore, it is important to know that certain groups have substantially higher rates of CKD and DKD than others and to keep this in mind when considering the risk of development and progression of CKD in specific individuals. From US Renal Data System data, the highest risk groups on the basis of rates are the Pacific Islander/Hawaiian population followed by African American, Native American Indian, Hispanic, and Asian compared with the white population, which has the lowest risk (2) (Figs. 2 and 3). Worldwide, the South Asian community has a high rate of DKD as well.

Current interventions do not cure the disease, but if implemented properly and early, they can either dramatically slow the rate of decline or, in some people, stop progression of the disease. Early recognition and early intervention are critical. Goals are suggestions, and the individualization of goals must be done for each patient. The groups of health care providers that can have the biggest impact on this epidemic are endocrinologists and primary care physicians (PCPs) because they see people with DM early in the disease process. Therefore, endocrinologists and PCPs have the unique opportunity to diagnose and treat at an early stage of the disease process and make a major change in public health.

BARRIERS TO OPTIMAL PRACTICE

Barriers to the diagnosis and management of DKD are lack of awareness in the PCP and endocrinology community to check routinely for declining GFR and increasing urine ACR. Most clinicians have many other medical problems and diagnoses to consider in their patients, and it is common for these tests to not be checked routinely. Moreover, GFR decline or ACR increase in DKD can be gradual. The physician may not even realize that there has been a continual decline in GFR or rise in ACR because it has been occurring slowly over years. I strongly urge all practices to look routinely at graphs showing the changes in GFR and urine ACR over time. This will greatly enhance the likelihood of recognizing declining kidney function so that proper interventions can be done.

LEARNING OBJECTIVES

As a result of participating in this session, learners should be able to:
- Know when to look for diseases other than DKD in a person with DM
- Know optimal strategies aimed at preventing the development of DKD
- Know current optimal strategies for the treatment of DKD

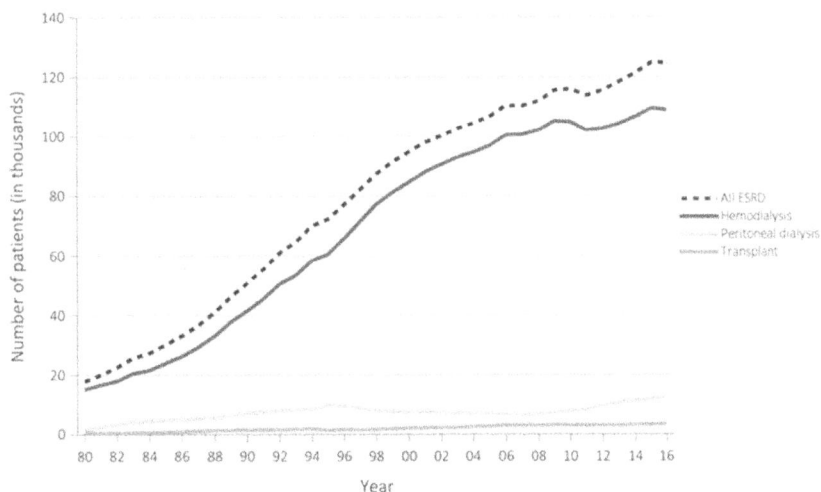

Figure 1. Trends in the annual number of ESRD incident cases, by modality, in the US population, 1980 to 2016. Data source: Reference Table D1 and special analysis of US Renal Data System ESRD database. Persons with uncertain dialysis were included in the All ESRD total but are not represented separately (1). Reproduced from United States Renal Data System. 2018 USRDS annual data report: epidemiology of kidney disease in the United States. National Institutes of Health, National Institute of Diabetes and Digestive and Kidney Diseases, Bethesda, MD, 2018.

STRATEGIES FOR DIAGNOSIS, THERAPY, AND/OR MANAGEMENT

In management of patients with DM and kidney disease, it is very important to remember that just because someone has DM and kidney disease does not always mean that they have DKD. Indeed, any cause of kidney disease may occur (3). Most

of the time, people with DM and kidney disease will have DKD, but being aware that any kidney disease may present in someone with DM is important to recognize when considering kidney diseases other than DKD. Kidney disease usually is diagnosed by a decrease in GFR and/or an increase in urine albumin level. The first and most important initial test in a patient with

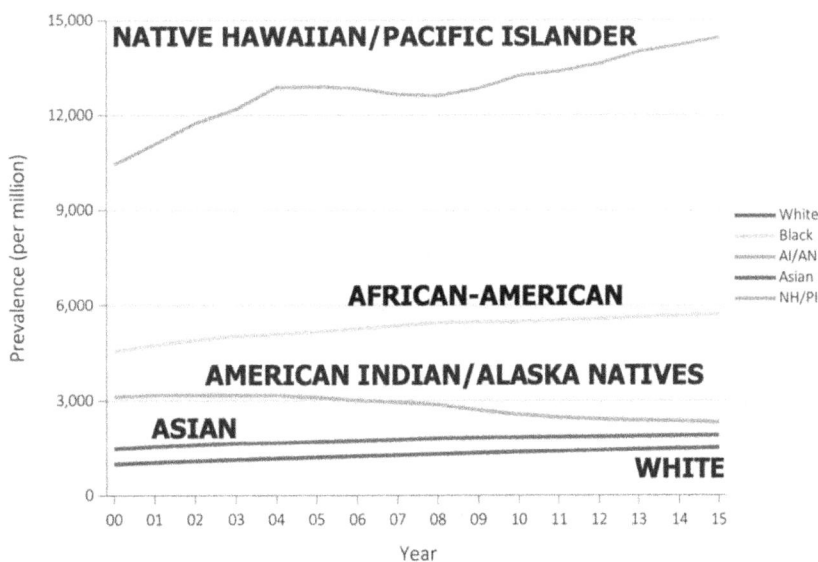

Figure 2. Trends in adjusted prevalence of ESRD, by race, in the US population, 2000 to 2015. Data source: Reference Table B.2(2) and special analyses, US Renal Data System ESRD database. Point prevalence on December 31 of each year. Standardized for age and sex. The standard population was the US population in 2011. AI/AN, American Indian/Alaska Native; NH/PI, Native Hawaiian/Pacific Islander (2). Reproduced from United States Renal Data System. 2017 USRDS annual data report: Epidemiology of kidney disease in the United States. National Institutes of Health, National Institute of Diabetes and Digestive and Kidney Diseases, Bethesda, MD, 2017.

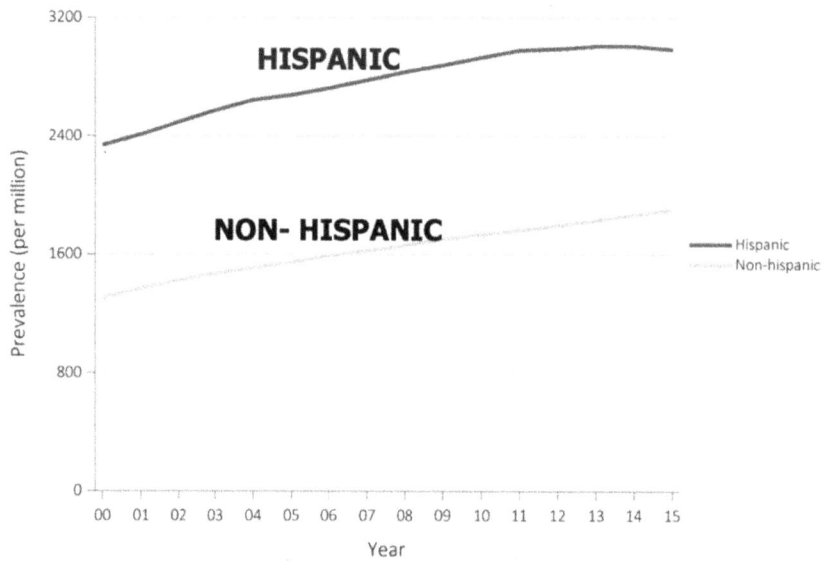

Figure 3. Trends in the adjusted prevalence of ESRD, by Hispanic ethnicity, in the US population, 2000 to 2015. Data source: Reference Tables B.1 and B.2(2). Point prevalence on December 31 of each year. Standardized for age, sex, and race. The standard population was the US population in 2011 (2). Reproduced from United States Renal Data System. 2017 USRDS annual data report: Epidemiology of kidney disease in the United States. National Institutes of Health, National Institute of Diabetes and Digestive and Kidney Diseases, Bethesda, MD, 2017.

suspected DKD is urinalysis with urine microscopic sediment analysis (not just a dipstick urinalysis). In general, patients with DKD have relatively bland microscopic urinalyses. That is, the urinalysis either has no cells or casts or has relatively few red blood cells, white blood cells, or casts. A large number of any of these might reflect an acute or chronic process that suggests a disease other than DKD. In that situation, further testing (*e.g.,* serologies, kidney ultrasound, possibly a kidney biopsy) might be indicated to determine whether there is another kidney disease. Of note, other kidney diseases also have relatively bland microscopic sediments (*e.g.,* the diseases that may be associated

with nephrotic syndrome, such as minimal change disease, membranous glomerulonephritis, focal and segmental glomeruloclerosis). If any question exists, then referral to a nephrologist would be indicated. It is also important to be aware that a new kidney disease may develop in a person with established DKD. An unexpected decrease in GFR or increase in ACR may reflect another kidney disease, which should stimulate a search for another cause of kidney disease.

An estimated 10% to 40% of people with DM will develop DKD, which also means that 60% to 90% of people with DM will not develop kidney disease. It is relatively easy to miss the

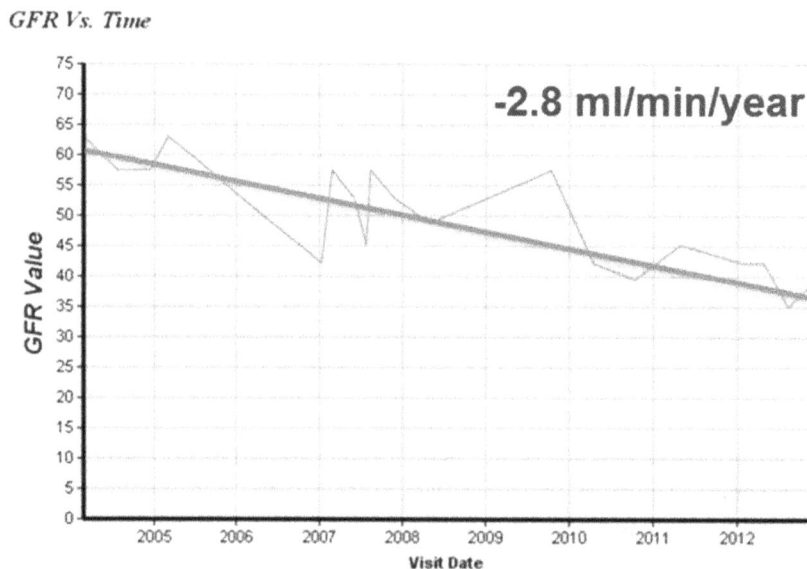

Figure 4. Example of graph showing change in eGFR over time.

onset of DKD when most patients will not develop DKD. Thus, GFR and ACR need to be used routinely to assure that the diagnosis is made early. To that end, routine uses of graphs of estimated GFR (eGFR) and urine ACR over time are invaluable. An example of a graph is shown in Figure 4. At many time periods, it appears as if this patient's GFR is stable, but there has been a relatively steady decline of about 3 mL/min per year. The recognition of the steady decline in eGFR was not noticed until the eGFR was <40 mL/min per 1.73 m^2, even though it had been steadily declining for almost 7 years. At this time, more aggressive blood pressure and blood sugar control was done. eGFR should be calculated using the CKD-Epidemiology Collaboration equation, which has been shown to be the most accurate at all levels of GFR (4). ACRs also should be measured by nephelometry and not by dipstick. The dipstick is qualitative and not sensitive to low-level increases in ACR. If the ACR is elevated, it should be rechecked about 1 month later. Transient elevations in ACR can occur due to such factors as exercise, pregnancy, urinary tract infections, and other reasons.

To prevent DKD, it is necessary to treat all patients as if they are going to develop DKD. This should not be a problem because the main goals for prevention of DKD are the same as for the prevention of other DM complications. One active area of research is determining markers to indicate who will likely develop DKD and who will have progressive DKD. Such markers as TNF-α and KIM-1 have shown promise. Many possible new markers exist, although their clinical utility remains to be determined (5). The main goals for prevention of DKD are blood pressure control and blood sugar control. Studies in type 1 and type 2 DM have shown the utility of achieving blood pressure and blood sugar control (6). In particular, in type 1 DM, the Diabetes Control and Complications Trial/Epidemiology of Diabetes Interventions and Complications has firmly established that controlling blood sugar (goal of 7%) as early as possible has both primary prevention and secondary treatment benefits for as long as 25 years later (7). There are similar results for people with type 2 DM, although there has not been as long a follow-up. Blood pressure goals have fluctuated in recent years and will be discussed in more detail in the cases. In addition, smoking cessation is indicated. There have never been and never will be randomized control trials with smoking, but epidemiologic analyses have indicated a reasonably strong association between smoking and DKD (8).

Treatment goals for established DKD are blood pressure control, blood sugar control, smoking cessation, and lowering of the urine albumin level. The goals of blood pressure and blood sugar control are similar to the prevention goals. A separate goal is the lowering of the urine ACR level. Urine ACR levels fluctuate normally, so it is important to routinely follow the levels over time. A one-time unexpected elevation may be transient, so a repeat test is indicated before making any changes. Blood pressure control and blood sugar control will lower urine ACR levels effectively. But in addition to blood pressure and blood sugar control, many studies have shown

that blockers of the renin-angiotensin-aldosterone system (RAAS) are effective in lowering urine ACR (6). Most physicians are well aware of the utility of angiotensin-converting enzyme inhibitors (ACE-Is) and angiotensin receptor blockers (ARBs), but recent studies have shown that aldosterone antagonists (*e.g.*, spironolactone, eplerenone) are also effective in lowering urine ACR levels (9). A number of companies are producing new nonsteroidal mineralocorticoid inhibitors to address this therapeutic need (*e.g.*, finerenone, which is in phase 3 trials). In addition to RAAS blockade, small studies have suggested that the nondihydropyridine calcium channel blockers (CCBs) diltiazem and verapamil have a modest effect on lowering urine ACR (10). Thus, one can use any of these to lower urine ACR. The goal of lowering urine ACR is to achieve as-low-as-possible levels, even back to normal (<30 mg/g), or if this is not achievable, then to <300 mg/g. A question that often arises is when to stop RAAS inhibition. There is no clear answer. In my practice, I tend to continue RAAS inhibition for as long as the rate of decline in GFR is steady (even at low levels of GFR). An ongoing study is addressing this issue wherein participants will either continue or stop their ACE-I or ARB when their eGFR is <30 mL/min per 1.73 m^2 (11). Perhaps this study will answer the question about whether to continue or stop RAAS inhibitors. Finally, new drugs are on the market that can be taken daily to lower serum potassium (patiromer and sodium zirconium cyclosilicate) (12). These drugs have been studied for up to 1 year and offer the possibility of maintaining patients who become considerably hyperkalemic on RAAS inhibitors longer.

MAIN CONCLUSIONS

Recognition of DKD at as early a stage as possible by routinely evaluating eGFR (using the CKD-Epidemiology Collaboration equation) and by routinely checking urine ACR is essential to slow the development and progression of DKD. Patients with DKD usually have a relatively bland urine microscopic sediment analysis. Hence, if the urinalysis is not relatively bland, a nondiabetic cause for kidney disease should be considered. In addition, if a patient with established DKD has an unexpected decrease in eGFR or increase in urine ACR, then one should consider that another kidney disease may have developed. Prevention of DKD is achieved by blood sugar control [goal glycohemoglobin A_{1c} (HbA$_{1c}$) of 7%], blood pressure control (<130/80 mm Hg), and smoking cessation. Treatment of DKD is achieved by the same method as prevention and the use of RAAS inhibitors to lower urine albumin level.

DISCUSSIONS OF CASES AND ANSWERS
Case 1

J.H. is a 22-year-old man with type 1 DM diagnosed at age 17 years. In October 2003, he had a urine ACR of 1380 mg/g (previous value in June 2003 was 528 mg/g). His eGFR was 120 mL/min per 1.73 m^2 [serum creatinine, 0.9 mg/dL (79.56 μmol/L)]. The patient did not report any other symptoms. He had no other diabetic complications. Blood pressure was 120/70 mm Hg. HbA_{1c} was 7.8%. Urinalysis showed no red blood cells/high power field, no white blood cells, and no casts. His medications included lisinopril 20 mg/d, atorvastatin 40 mg/d, insulin glargine 40 units at bedtime, and insulin lispro as needed. Physical examination was unremarkable. He felt well and reported that he lifted weights at the gym routinely.

Question 1

What is the next best therapeutic intervention?

A. Increase lisinopril
B. Lower HbA_{1c}
C. Do nothing at this time
D. Evaluate dietary protein intake

At this point, the most likely intervention to make a difference is A, increase lisinopril. Even if the blood pressure is normal, it is valuable to lower urine ACR to both reduce the risk of progression of kidney disease (this has been shown for both DKD and non-DKD) and reduce cardiovascular risk. In the situation where the blood pressure is excellent (as in this patient), the blood pressure–lowering effect is now the side effect. I would add 5 mg (or 10 mg at most) and monitor blood pressure; serum potassium; serum creatinine; and of course, change in urine ACR. You can gradually increase the lisinopril up to its maximal dose to achieve the maximal benefits of the ACE-I. Dose changes are likely best made every 4 to 6 weeks. It is important to check the serum creatinine and potassium levels about 1 week later to be sure that there is not too big a change in these parameters. Of note, ACE-Is and ARBs will lower eGFR (raise serum creatinine) by inhibiting the actions of angiotensin II. Indeed, an analysis of the Reduction of Endpoints in Non-Insulin-Dependent Diabetes Mellitus With the Angiotensin II Antagonist Losartan study, which explored the effects of losartan on the progression of DKD in people with type 2 DM (13), revealed that participants with the largest initial decrease in GFR had the slowest long-term decline in GFR. Therefore, a decline in eGFR is expected when using ACE-Is and ARBs. (Up to 25% is likely acceptable; it should be stable after the initial lowering of eGFR.) Lowering J.H.'s HbA_{1c} may have a modest effect on lowering his urine albumin level because he is already at a good level for slowing progression of DKD. As for protein intake, studies in animals with diabetes in the 1980s showed that low-protein diets were protective of kidney function. The low-protein diets had similar actions to RAAS blockade: lowering of intraglomerular pressures. Many human studies since have not been similarly positive. Although some studies have shown benefits of low-protein diets, most have not. In general, the recommended dietary intake of protein is 0.8 to 1.0 g/kg per day. On the other hand, high-protein intake may not be a good idea for people with CKD (>1.5 g/kg per day). High-protein intake in animals with DKD greatly enhances kidney function decline. Only suggestive studies have been done on the deleterious effects of high-protein intake, but in considering the animal data, I would discourage my patients

with kidney disease from being on a high-protein diet. This is especially relevant in J.H.'s case because he is an avid weightlifter and may well be ingesting a lot of protein to build muscle.

Question 2

All of the following are reasons to suspect a non-DKD in J.H. except:

A. Lack of diabetic retinopathy
B. HbA_{1c} of 7.8%
C. Increasing levels of urine ACR
D. Normal urine sediment analysis

The answer is D, normal urine sediment analysis. Most patients with DKD are expected to have a normal urinalysis and bland urine sediment. Patients with DKD can have a few red blood cells or a few white blood cells or some casts but not a large number of these. Other reasons to consider non-DKD are relatively well-controlled blood sugar, rapid unexpected increase in urine ACR and/or decrease in eGFR, and development of kidney disease signs in a person with <5 years of type 1 DM. In general, it takes 5 to 10 years to see either an increase in urine ACR or a decrease in eGFR due to diabetes. Because the length of time one has type 1 DM is well known, the development of kidney disease early in the course of type 1 DM should lead to a search for other causes of kidney disease. This is not true for people with type 2 DM because they may have had DM for ≥10 years before the diagnosis and may present with DKD. The final reason is lack of diabetic retinopathy, especially in people with type 1 DM. The reasons for this association are not clear. It is a relative issue but should be taken into account when considering whether a particular patient may have a nondiabetic cause of kidney disease (Table 1).

In J.H., further analysis led to a kidney biopsy because his urine ACR rose to 6000 mg/g. The biopsy revealed that he had Alport syndrome. Genetic analysis confirmed the diagnosis. When asked about hearing problems, he told me that he had been reading lips for a few years but was too embarrassed to tell anyone. Over the next 11 years J.H. gradually lost kidney function. He received a kidney transplant in 2014 and has done very well since. J.H. is still lifting weights at the gym.

Table 1.   Reasons to Consider Non-DKD in a Person With DM and Kidney Disease

Type 1 DM duration <5 years
Active urine sediment
Many red blood cells/high power field
Many casts
Many white blood cells/high power field
Rapidly declining eGFR
Rapidly increasing or very high urine ACR or urine protein/ creatinine level
No retinopathy in a person with type 1 DM

Case 2

L.K. is a 30-year-old woman with type 1 DM for 8 years, HbA_{1c} of 8.2%, blood pressure of 130/70 mm Hg, urine ACR of 25 mg/g, and eGFR of 87 mL/min per 1.73 m^2. Her current medications are amlodipine 5 mg/d and hydrochlorothiazide 12.5 mg/d. She uses a continuous glucose monitor and an insulin pump.

Question

L.K. should be started on an ACE-I or ARB to prevent the development of DKD.

    A. True
    B. False

The answer is B, false. Many people believe that RAAS inhibitors prevent the development of DKD. Although there have been studies showing beneficial effects of RAAS inhibition on the prevention of DKD, in my view, the evidence against using RAAS inhibitors routinely to prevent DKD is stronger. First, in 2009, a study by Mauer *et al.* (14) evaluated the effect of losartan, enalapril, or placebo on the development of albuminuria in a cohort of 285 people with type 1 DM over 5 years. There was no statistical difference among the three groups. In addition, all patients had a kidney biopsy at the start of the study and 5 years later. As assessed by an early sign of DKD (mesangial fractional volume), there were no differences among the three groups, suggesting no prevention benefit from ACE-I or ARB. For people with type 2 DM, no biopsy studies have been done, but an analysis of the studies that appear to show a benefit in reducing urine ACR compared with those with no benefit of ACE-I or ARB showed that the starting blood pressures in the positive studies were much higher than in the negative studies (15). Hence, it appears that blood pressure control is a good intervention for the development of albuminuria but that there likely is no unique role for ACE-I or ARB in primary prevention.

Case 3

A 48-year-old man with type 2 DM has an eGFR of 34 mL/min per 1.73 m^2 and a serum creatinine of 2.5 mg/dL (221 μmol/L). His ACR was 1020 mg/g, HbA_{1c} 8.4%, and blood pressure 140/85 mm Hg. He takes a maximal dose of olmesartan as well as 20 mg of furosemide and 1000 mg metformin twice a day. The patient has no history of cardiovascular disease. He does have occasional numbness in his toes and nonproliferative diabetic retinopathy.

Question 1

What should the blood pressure goal be?

    A. <140/90 mm Hg
    B. <120/80 mm Hg
    C. <150/90 mm Hg
    D. <130/80 mm Hg

The correct answer is D, <130/80 mm Hg. Blood pressure goals have been in flux in recent years. The Action to Control

Cardiovascular Risk in Diabetes (ACCORD) study (16) and similar studies from about 10 years ago reported that there is no cardiovascular benefit from lowering the blood pressure from a systolic of 135 to 120 mm Hg. This led many guidelines committees to change recommendations to <140/80 or <140/90 mm Hg as the goal for blood pressure. ACCORD evaluated people with type 2 DM who were at high risk for cardiovascular disease. It did not address risk for kidney disease. Studies over many years, including recently, have suggested that lower blood pressure is better for slowing progression of kidney disease. A few years ago, the Systolic Blood Pressure Intervention Trial (17) showed that cardiovascular risk was substantially decreased by lowering systolic blood pressure to 120 mm Hg, even in people >75 years old; however, the study did not include people with DM. A reanalysis of ACCORD using the Systolic Blood Pressure Intervention Trial criteria showed a similar benefit (18). The American Heart Association has changed its guidelines back to <130/80 mm Hg as the goal blood pressure. At this time, the best goal blood pressure (with the safest risk because blood pressure can be too low for certain patients) for the prevention and treatment of diabetic complications is <130/80 mm Hg.

Question 2

To lower urine ACR, which of the following would be the most appropriate intervention to start next?

    A. Lisinopril
    B. Spironolactone
    C. Low-protein diet
    D. Diltiazem

The correct answer is B, spironolactone. Blockade of aldosterone has been shown to have substantial effects on lowering urine ACR (11). The combination of an ACE-I or ARB with an aldosterone blocker appears to be safe. It is important to check potassium (and serum creatinine) levels about 1 week after using a combination of an ACE-I or ARB with aldosterone blockade. There only have been short-term studies with the combination of ACE-I or ARB with aldosterone blockade. Long-term studies on this combination for both efficacy and safety remain to be done. On the other hand, there have been two major studies on the combination of ACE-I and ARB: Ongoing Telmisartan Alone and in Combination with Ramipril Global Endpoint Trial and Veterans Affairs Nephropathy in Diabetes Trial. These trials did not report a benefit of the combination and even reported an increased incidence of acute kidney injury (AKI) and hyperkalemia. This led to a consensus view that ACE-Is and ARBs should not be used in combination. Similar poor outcomes were reported with the renin inhibitor aliskiren in combination with ACE-I and ARB in the Aliskiren Trial in Type 2 Diabetes Using Cardiovascular and Renal Disease Endpoints (Core and Extension Phases). Since the publication of these studies, however, further analyses have suggested that the combination may be beneficial in certain patients (*e.g.*, those with high levels of proteinuria and with congestive heart failure). But for now, the recommendation is to not use the ACE-I/ARB combination or only in specific circumstances. Of course, if one does use this combination to lower urine ACR, close monitoring of serum creatinine and serum potassium are necessary. The low-protein diet (which is considered to have a similar effect as the ACE-Is or ARBs), as discussed in an earlier case, appears to have either no effect or a modest effect on urine ACR. This intervention certainly can be considered but is likely to have only a modest therapeutic impact. Finally, diltiazem and verapamil (non-dihydropyridine CCBs) have a modest effect on lowering urine ACR. This effect of the nondihydropyridine CCBs has been seen only in small, short-term studies. It is reasonable to add these medications for blood pressure control and for their modest effects on urine ACR, but I believe that the better alternative at this time is aldosterone blockade for the following reasons: i) Inhibition of RAAS has been shown in many studies to have clear benefits for patients with DKD and elevated urine ACR; ii) there have been a number of studies in animals and humans with the addition of aldosterone blockade (albeit with relatively few patients and of short duration) that have shown likely beneficial effects of aldosterone blockade, whereas very few studies have shown the beneficial effects of the nondihydropyridine CCBs; and iii) there is a concern that the addition of aldosterone antagonists might increase potassium too much, and this has to be monitored. But in consideration of the likelihood that aldosterone antagonists are more directly targeted to a known pathophysiological mechanism underlying DKD, I believe that the benefits outweigh the risks. Nondihydropyridine CCBs certainly have few side effects but are not clearly directed toward a known pathophysiological mechanism. Indeed, it is unclear how renoprotective nondihydropyridine CCBs are.

Question 3

The patient is on metformin with a serum creatinine of 2.5 mg/dL (eGFR of 34 mL/min per 1.73 m^2). What should be done with the metformin?

A. Do nothing
B. Stop the metformin
C. Decrease the dose to 500 mg twice a day
D. Decrease the dose to 500 mg once a day

The answer is C, decrease the dose to 500 mg twice a day. Answer D, decrease the dose to 500 mg once a day, also is a reasonable answer. Metformin dosing has undergone major changes in the past 5 years. The main risk of metformin in the patient with CKD is the development of lactic acidosis. A number of studies have suggested that the risk of metformin-associated lactic acidosis is very low (19), even at lower levels of eGFR. This led to a change in the guideline recommendation

in 2016 by the Food and Drug Administration to suggest that metformin 1000 mg twice a day is reasonable in CKD for eGFR >45 mL/min per 1.73 m^2. When the eGFR is between 45 and 60 mL/min per 1.73 m^2, then more frequent checking of eGFR should be done (every 3 to 6 months). Between eGFR of 30 and 45 mL/min per 1.73 m^2, a dose reduction to 500 mg twice a day should be considered. The Food and Drug Administration recommends not initiating metformin in someone with an eGFR of <45 mL/min per 1.73 m^2, and metformin is contraindicated in people with an eGFR of <30 mL/min per 1.73 m^2. Close monitoring of serum creatinine should be done about every 3 months. The main risk for metformin-associated lactic acidosis is a sudden decline in eGFR. Thus, metformin should be held in any situation that may lead to a decrease in eGFR, such as contrast dye studies where AKI is a risk and other conditions that lead to AKI (*e.g.*, surgery, dehydration). Reasonable alternatives to metformin in patients with CKD are dipeptidyl peptidase 4 inhibitors, glucagon-like peptide 1 agonists (*e.g.*, the Liraglutide Effect and Action in Diabetes: Evaluation of Cardiovascular Outcome Results—A Long Term Evaluation trial showed that liraglutide reduced urine ACR), sulfonylureas [although hypoglycemic risk increases significantly as eGFR declines, sulfonylureas are likely best to avoid (*e.g.*, glyburide is very likely to cause hypoglycemia) in patients with CKD with an eGFR <30 mL/min per 1.73 m^2], and possibly sodium–glucose cotransporter 2 (SGLT2) inhibitors. SGLT2 inhibitors have been shown to have an important cardiovascular benefit. Analyses of these cardiovascular trials suggest renoprotection. But as of this writing, the only kidney trial CREDENCE (Effects of Canagliflozin on Renal and Cardiovascular Outcomes in Participants With Diabetic Nephropathy), was stopped early, but no detailed report about why it was stopped has been released. SGLT2 inhibitors appear to be excellent medications in that they have been shown to lower blood pressure, lower HbA$_{1c}$, cause weight loss, reduce cardiovascular events, and appear to stop or dramatically reduce the decline in eGFR. My personal concern, though, is that allowing high levels of glucose to pass through the nephrons for many years may well lead to kidney damage years later. Therefore, I am personally cautious about using these drugs. I am awaiting the detailed report from CREDENCE about efficacy and for future DKD clinical trials before routinely using SGLT2 inhibitors in patients with DKD.

References

1. United States Renal Data System. *Annual Data Report 2018: Epidemiology of Kidney Disease in the United States.* Bethesda, MD: National Institutes of Health, National Institute of Diabetes and Digestive and Kidney Diseases; 2018.
2. United States Renal Data System. *2017 USRDS Annual Data Report: Epidemiology of Kidney Disease in the United States.* Bethesda, MD: National Institutes of Health, National Institute of Diabetes and Digestive and Kidney Diseases; 2017.
3. Jin Kim Y, Hyung Kim Y, Dae Kim K, Ryun Moon K, Ho Park J, Mi Park B, Ryu H, Eun Choi D, Ryang Na K, Sun Suh K, Wook Lee K, Tai Shin Y.

Nondiabetic kidney diseases in type 2 diabetic patients. *Kidney Res Clin Pract.* 2013;**32**(3):115–120.

4. Matsushita K, Mahmoodi BK, Woodward M, Emberson JR, Jafar TH, Jee SH, Polkinghorne KR, Shankar A, Smith DH, Tonelli M, Warnock DG, Wen CP, Coresh J, Gansevoort RT, Hemmelgarn BR, Levey AS for the Chronic Kidney Disease Prognosis Consortium. Comparison of risk prediction using the CKD-EPI equation and the MDRD study equation for estimated glomerular filtration rate. *JAMA.* 2012; **307**(18):1941–1951.

5. Looker HC, Colombo M, Hess S, Brosnan MJ, Farran B, Dalton RN, Wong MC, Turner C, Palmer CN, Nogoceke E, Groop L, Salomaa V, Dunger DB, Agakov F, McKeigue PM, Colhoun HM for the SUMMIT Investigators. Biomarkers of rapid chronic kidney disease progression in type 2 diabetes. *Kidney Int.* 2015;**88**(4):888–896.

6. Stanton RC. Clinical challenges in diagnosis and management of diabetic kidney disease. *Am J Kidney Dis.* 2014; **63**(2, Suppl 2)S3–S21.

7. de Boer IH, DCCT/EDIC Research Group. Kidney disease and related findings in the diabetes control and complications trial/epidemiology of diabetes interventions and complications study. *Diabetes Care.* 2014;**37**(1):24–30.

8. Go AS, Yang J, Tan TC, Cabrera CS, Stefansson BV, Greasley PJ, Ordonez JD for the Kaiser Permanente Northern California CKD Outcomes Study. Contemporary rates and predictors of fast progression of chronic kidney disease in adults with and without diabetes mellitus. *BMC Nephrol.* 2018;**19**(1):146.

9. Sun LJ, Sun YN, Shan JP, Jiang GR. Effects of mineralocorticoid receptor antagonists on the progression of diabetic nephropathy. *J Diabetes Investig.* 2017;**8**(4):609–618.

10. Bakris GL, Weir MR, Secic M, Campbell B, Weis-McNulty A. Differential effects of calcium antagonist subclasses on markers of nephropathy progression. *Kidney Int.* 2004;**65**(6):1991–2002.

11. Bhandari S, Ives N, Brettell EA, Valente M, Cockwell P, Topham PS, Cleland JG, Khwaja A, El Nahas M. Multicentre randomized controlled trial of angiotensin-converting enzyme inhibitor/angiotensin receptor blocker withdrawal in advanced renal disease: the STOP-ACEi trial. *Nephrol Dial Transplant.* 2016;**31**(2):255–261.

12. Bakris GL, Pitt B, Weir MR, Freeman MW, Mayo MR, Garza D, Stasiv Y, Zawadzki R, Berman L, Bushinsky DA for the AMETHYST-DN Investigators. Effect of patiromer on serum potassium level in patients with hyperkalemia and diabetic kidney disease: the AMETHYST-DN randomized clinical trial [published correction appears in *JAMA.* 2015;314(7):731]. *JAMA.* 2015;**314**(2):151–161.

13. Holtkamp FA, de Zeeuw D, Thomas MC, Cooper ME, de Graeff PA, Hillege HJ, Parving HH, Brenner BM, Shahinfar S, Lambers Heerspink HJ. An acute fall in estimated glomerular filtration rate during treatment with losartan predicts a slower decrease in long-term renal function. *Kidney Int.* 2011;**80**(3):282–287.

14. Mauer M, Zinman B, Gardiner R, Suissa S, Sinaiko A, Strand T, Drummond K, Donnelly S, Goodyer P, Gubler MC, Klein R. Renal and retinal effects of enalapril and losartan in type 1 diabetes. *N Engl J Med.* 2009;**361**(1):40–51.

15. Bilous R, Chaturvedi N, Sjølie AK, Fuller J, Kein R, Orchard T, Porta M, Parving HH. Effect of candesartan on microalbuminuria and albumin excretion rate in diabetes: three randomized trials. *Ann Intern Med.* 2009;**151**(1):11–20, W3–W4.

16. Cushman WC, Evans GW, Byington RP, Goff DC Jr, Grimm RH Jr, Cutler JA, Simons-Morton DG, Basile JN, Corson MA, Probstfield JL, Katz L, Peterson KA, Friedewald WT, Buse JB, Bigger JT, Gerstein HC, Ismail-Beigi F for the ACCORD Study Group. Effects of intensive blood-pressure control in type 2 diabetes mellitus. *N Engl J Med.* 2010; **362**(17):1575–1585.

17. Cheung AK, Rahman M, Reboussin DM, Craven TE, Greene T, Kimmel PL, Cushman WC, Hawfield AT, Johnson KC, Lewis CE, Oparil S, Rocco MV, Sink KM, Whelton PK, Wright JT Jr, Basile J, Beddhu S, Bhatt U, Chang TI, Chertow GM, Chonchol M, Freedman BI, Haley W, Ix JH, Katz LA, Killeen AA, Papademetriou V, Ricardo AC, Servilla K, Wall B, Wolfgram D, Yee J for the SPRINT Research Group. Effects of intensive BP control in CKD. *J Am Soc Nephrol.* 2017;**28**(9): 2812–2823.

18. Buckley LF, Dixon DL, Wohlford GF IV, Wijesinghe DS, Baker WL, Van Tassell BW. Intensive versus standard blood pressure control in SPRINT-eligible participants of ACCORD-BP [published correction appears in *Diabetes Care.* 2018;41(9):2048]. *Diabetes Care.* 2017; **40**(12):1733–1738.

19. Stanton RC. Metformin use in type 2 diabetes mellitus with CKD: Is it time to liberalize dosing recommendations? *Am J Kidney Dis.* 2015; **66**(2):193–195.

Prevention of T1D: Where Are We in 2019?

M59
Presented, March 23–26, 2019

Desmond Schatz, MD. Department of Pediatrics, University of Florida, Gainesville, Florida 32605, E-mail: schatda@peds.ufl.edu

SIGNIFICANCE OF THE CLINICAL PROBLEM

The incidence of type 1 diabetes (T1D) continues to rise by 3% each year, affecting between 1 and 2 million Americans. Yet the ability to prevent this disease remains elusive. Hybrid closed loop devices, artificial pancreas systems, and continuous glucose monitoring technology have helped to ease the daily burden for many with T1D. However, the artificial pancreas is not a cure; more research is needed to achieve our ultimate goal of preventing T1D. The preceding decades have generated a wealth of information regarding the natural history of pre-T1D. Islet autoimmunity in the form of multiple autoantibodies is highly predictive of progression to disease (1, 2). Staging systems have been devised to better characterize pre-T1D, the mechanistic understanding of disease, and to guide the design of prevention studies. However, there are no evidence-based recommendations for practitioners caring for patients with positive autoantibodies other than to encourage enrollment in research studies. Close monitoring of high-risk patients markedly reduces diabetic ketoacidosis rates at diagnosis, and research participation is critical to finding a means of preventing T1D. The discovery of an effective preventative strategy for T1D will justify universal risk screening for all children.

BARRIERS TO OPTIMAL PRACTICE

There is no proven therapy to successfully cure or prevent T1D.

LEARNING OBJECTIVES

As a result of participating in this session, learners should be able to:

- Enhance their understanding of the natural history of pre-T1D
- Be aware of worldwide efforts, past and present, to prevent T1D
- Screen at-risk individuals and enroll them in prevention trials

BACKGROUND

Identification of At-Risk Individuals

To prevent T1D, our understanding of the natural history of pre-T1D and the mechanisms culminating in the autoimmune destruction of β cells is critical. Large international cohorts have been studied from birth in both relatives of patients with T1D and members of the general population who are at high genetic risk. These studies have selected infants based on high-risk HLA alleles, most commonly HLA-DR3/4, DQB1*0201/DQB1*0302. Monozygotic twins have a lifetime 50% to 70% risk of developing T1D. In the United States, the risk of developing T1D is 1 in 20 in first-degree relatives and 1 in 300 in the general population. Islet autoantibodies develop in 90% to 95% of those destined to develop T1D. These include islet cell autoantibodies, insulin autoantibodies, glutamic acid decarboxylase (GAD) autoantibodies, insulinoma associated-2 autoantibodies, and zinc transporter 8 autoantibodies.

The risk of progression to T1D varies based on the age of appearance of autoimmunity and number of autoantibodies. Young cohorts of genetically high-risk children with one autoantibody have a 10-year risk of progression to diabetes of ~15%. Children with two or more autoantibodies have a markedly increased risk of progression to T1D at 5 years (~45%), 10 years (70%), and 15 years (85%). Overall, the rate of progression is ~11%/y (3, 4).

Staging of Pre-T1D

The American Diabetes Association (ADA), JDRF, and Endocrine Society released a joint position statement for the staging of pre-T1D (5). Stage 1 is defined by the presence of two or more islet autoantibodies with normoglycemia (normal glucose tolerance on 2-hour oral glucose tolerance test). Stage 2 shows progression to dysglycemia (impaired glucose tolerance) in the setting of two or more islet autoantibodies, and stage 3 occurs when a patient meets ADA criteria for the diagnosis of diabetes.

Why is this distinction important? The overall goal of all those who care for children and adults with T1D is to cure the disease (obviously preventing its recurrence) as well as prevention of the disease in those at risk and destined to subsequently develop clinical onset. Those found to be genetically at risk for developing islet autoimmunity are targeted with primary prevention strategies that are typically of low risk. Secondary prevention studies aim to slow down or halt the destruction of β cells in those who have islet autoantibodies.

PREVENTION STRATEGIES

1. Past Strategies of Limited Success

Multiple approaches have been used with limited success to date. These include dietary changes, antigen-based therapy, and immunomodulatory and immunosuppression therapies. Primary dietary prevention strategies beginning in the mid-1990s included the Trial to Reduce IDDM in the Genetically at Risk (TRIGR), which evaluated the role of a hydrolyzed casein-based formula (free of intact bovine insulin) compared with cow's milk–based formula; BABYDIET, which looked at a gluten-free diet in the first year of life; the Finnish Dietary

Intervention Trial for the Prevention of Type 1 Diabetes (FINDIA) with insulin-free bovine formula; and the TrialNet Nutritional Intervention to Prevent (NIP) Type 1 Diabetes study with docosahexaenoid acid. All studies failed to show efficacy.

Antigen therapy was established with the hope of inducing peripheral tolerance by exposure of the naive immune system to an antigen found in the target organ (β cell) or through induction of anergy of already present autoreactive T cells. The Type 1 Diabetes Prediction and Prevention (DIPP) study in Finland screened cord blood samples for high-risk HLA genotypes and followed children for the subsequent development of autoantibodies. Children were treated with intranasal insulin or placebo, and the outcome was no different between groups. In Germany, the Primary Oral/Intranasal Insulin Trial (Pre-POINT) administered different doses of oral insulin (and intranasal insulin) to high-risk HLA individuals prior to the development of autoantibodies. This small study demonstrated potential mechanistic/immunological effects. In the early 1990s, two insulin-based therapies were conducted in the Diabetes Prevention Trial–Type 1 network. In separate studies, oral insulin and intravenous/subcutaneous insulin were administered to those with intermediate and high risk, respectively. No difference was seen except in an ad hoc analysis of a subgroup (those with positive islet cell autoantibodies, elevated insulin autoantibody titers, and normal glucose tolerance); a projected delay of 4.8 years in onset was observed. The large TrialNet Oral Insulin Study (2007 to 2016), however, showed no overall benefit; although a delay was noted in a stratum of high-risk subjects (with loss of first-phase insulin response). GAD, another islet autoantigen, used as a vaccine both in new onset and as a potential prevention has failed to provide preservation of β-cell function or effective delay in T1D onset, respectively. The use of GAD together with an aluminum adjuvant (Diamyd®) in the Diabetes Prevention–Immune Tolerance (DIAPREV-IT) study showed increases in GAD autoantibody titers but no delayed onset of disease. The addition of high-dose vitamin D to Diamyd® for the DIAPREV-IT2 study is ongoing. A non–antigen-based therapy, the European Nicotinamide Diabetes Intervention Trial (ENDIT), in which relatives who had developed islet cell antibodies were randomized to 5 years of nicotinamide, showed no difference in the rate of diabetes development.

2. Current Studies

In addition to oral insulin and GAD-alum studies, there are other ongoing antigen-based prevention (and intervention) trials, including those using multiple peptide mixtures from known islet autoantigens, with the aim of inducing immunological tolerance to β cells. Recently, there has been a focus on immunologic modulation in prevention studies after promising efficacy results in new-onset studies. Attempts to restore self-tolerance, promote regulatory T cells, and reduce effector

T cells have been evaluated with several different classes of drugs. Based on data from well-designed new-onset studies using anti-CD3 T-cell antibodies [Protégé and AbATE (Autoimmunity-Blocking Antibody for Tolerance in Recently Diagnosed Type 1 Diabetes)], TrialNet just completed enrollment in a high-risk population of relatives with two or more autoantibodies and dysglycemia (stage 2 disease) using anti-CD3 (tepiluzimab). Abatacept (CTLA-4, costimulation blockade) was chosen for transition from intervention to prevention trials after it demonstrated a slowed rate of β-cell decline that was maintained 1 year after therapy cessation. The TrialNet Abatacept prevention study is underway and close to completion.

A cellular therapy approach seeking the promotion of tolerizing regulatory T cells using autologous cord blood is underway in Australia (The CoRD Study). This open-label pilot study is recruiting multiple islet autoantibody-positive first-degree relatives.

3. Future Studies

Once efficacy, safety, and feasibility (and hopefully mechanism) are demonstrated in patients with new-onset T1D receiving immune and other therapies, they should be moved into the prevention arena. The successful (preservation of c-peptide) low-dose anti-thymocyte globulin study in patients with new-onset T1D as well as patients with established T1D opens the path or its use in prevention trials. Due to the number of potential therapeutic targets (both immune and nonimmune), multiagent (cocktail) therapy targeting multiple aspects of this disease is likely to be needed.

Type 1 Diabetes TrialNet has recently expanded to other therapeutics that have been approved and tested safe in other conditions and populations. One is the use of methyldopa to inhibit the communication between antigen-presenting cells through MHC class II signaling in susceptible HLA-DQ8 haplotypes. This focused, small mechanistic study will enroll participants with HLA-DQ8, one or more autoantibodies, and stage 1 or stage 2 disease. Hydroxychloroquine, after its success in rheumatoid arthritis, will be tested in stage 1 individuals. The rationale for this therapeutic, historically used to treat malaria, includes modulation of T cells and interleukins, specifically reductions in Th17 cells in the non-obese diabetic mouse model of T1D. Hydroxychloroquine also has been shown to improve glucose metabolism and insulin sensitivity in type 2 diabetes.

In Germany, the Fr1da study, performing general population screening for islet autoantibodies, will also be conducting the Fr1da Insulin Intervention looking at oral insulin in multiple autoantibody–positive subjects enrolled in the natural history study and progression to dysglycemia. This study serves many important purposes, mainly the feasibility of population screening and seamless enrollment into a prevention study.

Many exciting trials will finish enrollment and follow-up in the next couple of years. As is the challenge with prevention trials, waiting for a clinical end point is costly and time-consuming. Large numbers of patients need to be screened, and well-powered studies require large numbers of participants, which limit the number of studies able to be performed. Other clinically relevant end points are being explored, and small, brief studies are being designed to test mechanistic outcomes.

MAIN CONCLUSIONS

Be it through targeted screening of relatives for autoanti-bodies or population-based screening for high-risk HLA genes, we must continue to study the natural history of T1D and identify patients with β-cell autoimmunity. These patients should be identified and encouraged to participate in research so as to ultimately prevent and reverse T1D.

References

1. Jacobsen, LJ, Haller MJ, Schatz DA. Understanding pre-type 1 diabetes: the key to prevention. *Front Endocrinol (Lausanne).* 2018;**9**:70.
2. Simmons KM, Michels AW. Type 1 diabetes: a predictable disease. *World J Diabetes.* 2015;**6**(3):380–390.
3. Krischer JP, Lynch KF, Schatz DA, Ilonen J, Lernmark Å, Hagopian WA, Rewers MJ, She JX, Simell OG, Toppari J, Ziegler AG, Akolkar B, Bonifacio E; TEDDY Study Group. The 6 year incidence of diabetes-associated autoantibodies in genetically at-risk children: the TEDDY study. *Diabetologia.* 2015;**58**(5):980–987.
4. Ziegler AG, Rewers M, Simell O, Simell T, Lempainen J, Steck A, Winkler C, Ilonen J, Veijola R, Knip M, Bonifacio E, Eisenbarth GS. Seroconversion to multiple islet autoantibodies and risk of progression to diabetes in children. *JAMA.* 2013;**309**(23):2473–2479.
5. Insel RA, Dunne JL, Atkinson MA, Chiang JL, Dabelea D, Gottlieb PA, Greenbaum CJ, Herold KC, Krischer JP, Lernmark Å, Ratner RE, Rewers MJ, Schatz DA, Skyler JS, Sosenko JM, Ziegler AG. Staging pre-symptomatic type 1 diabetes: a scientific statement of JDRF, the Endocrine Society, and the American Diabetes Association. *Diabetes Care.* 2015;**38**(10):1964–1974.

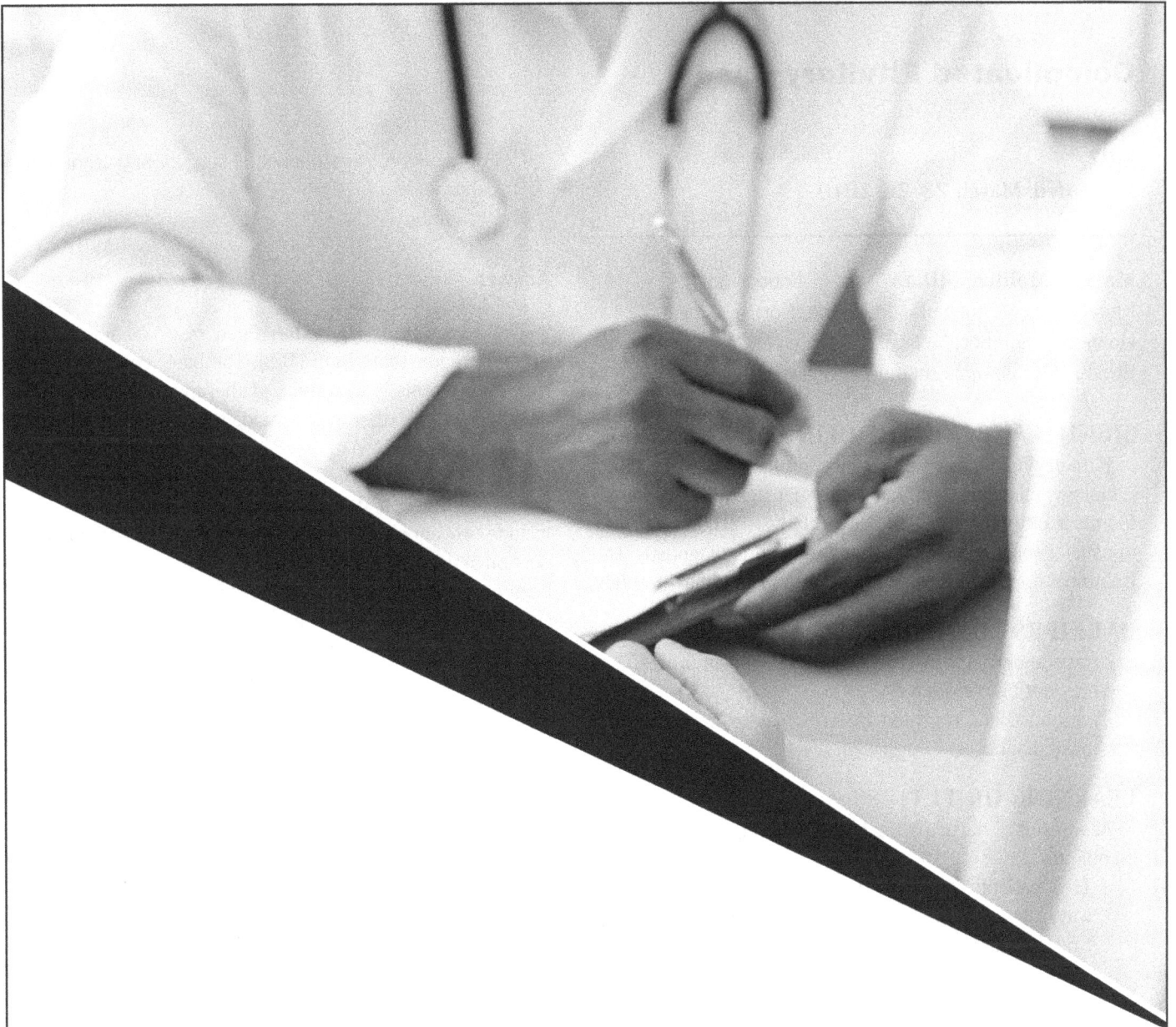

NEUROENDOCRINOLOGY AND PITUITARY

Complicated Pituitary Cases

M07
Presented, March 23–26, 2019

Mark E. Molitch, MD. Division of Endocrinology, Metabolism & Molecular Medicine, Northwestern University Feinberg School of Medicine, Chicago, Illinois 60611, E-mail: molitch@northwestern.edu

SIGNIFICANCE OF THE CLINICAL PROBLEM

Pituitary adenomas are common problems seen by endocrinology clinicians. Although the management strategies for most pituitary adenomas are relatively straightforward, unusual clinical presentations may require diagnostic and treatment approaches that differ from conventional methods.

BARRIERS TO OPTIMAL PRACTICE

- Nonstandard approaches to unusual clinical problems may not be considered.
- Continued and repeated analyses may be necessary to make diagnoses.

LEARNING OBJECTIVES

As a result of participating in this session, learners should be able to:
- Treat patients with prolactinomas who present in unusual ways
- Understand the importance of critical review of MRI scans

STRATEGIES FOR DIAGNOSIS, THERAPY, AND/OR MANAGEMENT AND CONCLUSIONS
Case 1

A 17-year-old woman was evaluated by her pediatrician for primary amenorrhea. She had no headaches, visual complaints, galactorrhea, or other symptoms. Her examination was normal, including Tanner Stage IV breast and pubic hair development. Laboratory testing showed levels of prolactin (PRL) 35.1 μg/L, free thyroxine (FT$_4$) 1.08 ng/dL (0.8 to 2.3) (13.9 pmol/L), LH 0.25 IU/L, FSH 1.5 IU/L, IGF-1 164 ng/mL (176 to 452) (21.5 nmol/L), and cortisol 16.3 μg/dL (450 nmol/L). An MRI showed a very large, irregular tumor encasing (but not compressing) both internal carotid arteries and extending almost to the surface of the right temporal lobe. The optic chiasm could not be visualized, but formal visual field testing was normal. Upon dilution, her PRL level was 48,600 μg/L.

Question

What is the best choice of initial therapy for a patient with a giant prolactinoma?
- A. Transsphenoidal surgery
- B. Craniotomy
- C. Combination transsphenoidal surgery and craniotomy
- D. Cabergoline
- E. Irradiation

Answer

D. Cabergoline

The appellation "giant" has been reserved for pituitary tumors greater than 4 cm (1–3). The basic controversy in a case such as this is what type of therapy to try first. Before deciding upon the therapeutic modality, the goals of treatment need to be specified. With respect to PRL levels, these must be reduced to near normal in order to restore normal reproductive function. With respect to tumor size, however, goals include prevention of further tumor growth in addition to reduction of tumor size. For a tumor this size, which has probably been growing for many years, substantial reduction of tumor size may not reverse visual field defects or hypopituitarism. A reasonable goal may be to prevent further growth. The benefits of therapy designed to achieve these goals must be balanced against the risks of such therapy.

The primary consideration in this patient is whether to use surgery or a dopamine agonist as initial treatment. In this patient, given the size of the tumor and its wrapping around the internal carotid arteries, surgery certainly could not be curative. Furthermore, surgery for such giant tumors has a high complication rate. In a series of 77 patients with giant tumors reported by Pia *et al.*, complications included eight deaths, four patients with visual loss, eight with oculomotor palsies, 15 with diabetes insipidus (DI), 14 with mental deterioration, and five with cerebrospinal fluid (CSF) fistulas (1). In a similar series of 21 cases reported by Guidetti *et al.*, there were two deaths, four patients with DI, one with hemiparesis, and one with hypothalamic failure (2). In contrast, cabergoline has been successful in normalizing PRL levels and causing marked tumor size reduction in many patients with giant prolactinomas (3). In some cases of prolactinomas that continue to grow and are refractory to high doses of cabergoline and even subsequent surgery and irradiation, the alkylating agent temozolomide can be beneficial (4). Rarely, prolactinomas can be malignant, but to diagnose malignancy, intra- or extracranial metastases must be demonstrated (5). Temozolomide has also been found to be beneficial in some patients with malignant prolactinomas (6). This patient responded extremely well to cabergoline.

Case 2

A 35-year-old man presented with erectile dysfunction and decreased libido. His examination was normal, and he was well virilized. Testing revealed a testosterone level of 153 ng/dL (280 to 1000) (5.31 nmol/L) and a PRL level of 58.2 μg/L. An MRI showed a large macroadenoma wrapped around the left internal carotid artery. The PRL test was rerun at a 1:100 dilution and was still only minimally abnormal. Transsphenoidal surgery was performed but left a considerable amount of residual tumor extending superiorly and wrapped around the internal carotid artery. The tumor stained positive for PRL.

Question

What should be the next step in management of this patient with considerable residual tumor after surgery?

- A. Repeat surgery
- B. Conventional irradiation
- C. Stereotactic irradiation (stereotactic radiosurgery, linear accelerator, proton beam)
- D. Cabergoline

Answer

D. Cabergoline

Approximately two-thirds of clinically nonfunctioning pituitary adenomas actually do produce pituitary hormones, and most of those are gonadotroph adenomas. Only 1% to 2% are lactotroph adenomas (7). By definition, they are clinically silent (*i.e.*, cause no clinical syndrome). Although blood hormone levels are usually normal in such patients, that is not always the case. In this patient, his PRL levels were modestly elevated—certainly not commensurate with the size of his tumor—and perhaps were due to stalk effect rather than having been directly secreted by the tumor.

The risk of regrowth of a large tumor remnant is close to 50% (8, 9). Treatment of this patient's residual tumor could have been by a second surgery, irradiation, or medical therapy. Given the location of the residual tumor, surgery was not an option. Irradiation can reduce this risk to 11% (8). Another approach is to use a dopamine agonist, such as cabergoline, which has been shown to reduce the regrowth of nonfunctioning tumors in most patients (10). Because this patient had a silent lactotroph adenoma, we decided to try this. It has been very successful in preventing regrowth of his tumor remnant. Had there been evidence of continued growth, irradiation would have been performed.

Case 3

A 31-year-old woman initially presented with 4 to 5 weeks of intractable headaches. CT scans of her sinuses and brain were normal. She was known to have a family history positive for thyroiditis, rheumatoid arthritis, and vitiligo. On July 1, 2018, she presented to the emergency department with a very severe headache, fever, and neck stiffness. Her vital signs were temperature of 101.6° F, blood pressure 125/82 mm Hg, pulse rate 142 beats/min, respiratory rate 24 breaths/min, and weight 126.6 kg. Her examination was normal except for mild distress and delirium. Routine laboratory tests were normal. A lumbar puncture showed aseptic meningitis with a glucose level of 70 mg/dL, protein 118 mg/dL, white blood count 1239 (78% polymorphonuclear leukocytes), red blood count 0, clear fluid,

and bacteria culture negative. PCR was negative for West Nile virus, herpes simplex virus, respiratory syncytial virus, *Cryptococcus*, human parechovirus, cytomegalovirus, and enterovirus. CSF angiotensin-converting enzyme was negative, and serum antineutrophil cytoplasmic antibodies were negative. An MRI showed an enlarged sella with a cystic component and a thickened stalk. No bone lesions were found on imaging. A QuantiFERON-TB Gold test for tuberculosis was negative. Results of endocrine testing included the following: thyrotropin 0.09 mU/L (0.4 to 4.0), FT_4 0.52 ng/dL (0.7 to 1.5) (6.69 pmol/L), ACTH 2.9 ng/L (5 to 50), cortisol 3 µg/L (82.8 nmol/L) (time of day, 2:20 PM), PRL 22.1 µg/L, FSH 1.81 IU/L, LH 0.3 IU/L, IGF-1 101 ng/dL (53 to 331) (13.2 nmol/L), GH < 0.1 µg/L, serum osmolality 301 mOsm/kg, and urine osmolality 75 mOsm/kg.

Question

What is the probable cause of this patient's severe headache, stiff neck, and fever?

- A. Meningitis
- B. West Nile encephalitis
- C. Lymphocytic hypophysitis
- D. Pituitary apoplexy

Answer

D. Pituitary apoplexy

Pituitary apoplexy is a clinical syndrome consisting of severe headache, stiff neck, nausea, vomiting, and often neurologic symptoms such as ophthalmoplegia, cranial nerve palsies, visual field defects, ptosis, or altered mental status (11, 12). These symptoms are related to rapid expansion of the contents of the sella into the parasellar and suprasellar spaces due to hemorrhage into or hemorrhagic infarction of an adenoma (11, 12). Clinically, apoplexy may resemble meningitis and subarachnoid hemorrhage; the CSF may be abnormal, showing increased protein and pleocytosis in all three conditions (11, 12). Varying degrees of hypopituitarism are found in up to three-quarters of such patients (11, 12). It is thought that apoplexy essentially only occurs in tumors and not in normal pituitary tissue. The enlarged sella in this patient would be consistent with this.

The other unusual feature in this patient was the marked stalk thickening on MRI. Inflammatory causes of stalk thickening include lymphocytic hypophysitis, Langerhans cell histiocytosis (although this could also be classified as a neoplastic lesion), sarcoidosis, tuberculosis, Whipple's disease, and neoplastic lesions such as infundibuloma, dysgerminoma, metastasis, and lymphoma (13, 14). This patient was treated with hormone replacement including thyroxine, desmopressin, an oral contraceptive (continued from pre-event), and high-dose prednisone. Her symptoms, signs, and stalk thickening resolved over the next 3 months, but her hypopituitarism and DI remained. She did not have a tissue biopsy. However, based on her family history of autoimmune disorders and her stalk thickening and response to high-dose steroids, a presumptive diagnosis of infundibulo- and anterior pituitary hypophysitis was made. On the other hand, this does not explain her apoplexy. It is possible that the stalk thickening may have been some sort of reactive inflammation that subsequently resolved.

Case 4

A 31-year-old woman presented to her gynecologist with secondary amenorrhea and infertility. She denied any vision problems, headaches, or galactorrhea. There was no history suggestive of either acromegaly or Cushing's disease. However, she did state that her shoe size had increased from 8 to 9, more because of a need for increased width rather than length. She denied any changes in ring or glove size. She had slowly gained approximately 10 pounds over the past 8 years, but she was not overweight. She did not think that she had any changes in her facial appearance. Her physical examination was completely normal. Laboratory results obtained by the gynecologist showed PRL 8.4 μg/L, AM (morning) cortisol 8.4 ng/dL (231.8 nmol/L), FSH 2.1 IU/L, LH 0.9 IU/L, and estradiol < 15 pg/mL (< 55.1 pmol/L). An MRI showed a 1.9-cm pituitary adenoma compressing the optic chiasm. She was referred to Endocrinology and did not have any evidence of acromegaly or Cushing's disease on examination. Visual fields were normal. Further testing for hypopituitarism because of the macroadenoma showed PRL' 10.5 μg/L, AM (morning) cortisol 9.9 ng/dL (273 nmol/L), FT_4 0.9 ng/dL (0.7 to 1.5) (11.6 pmol/L), and IGF-1 569 ng/mL (53 to 331) (74.5 nmol/L).

Question

What should be the next step in this patient's management?
  A. Refer for transsphenoidal surgery
  B. Refer for stereotactic radiotherapy
  C. Perform an oral glucose tolerance test measuring glucose and growth hormone
  D. Start cabergoline 0.5 mg twice weekly

Answer

  C. Perform an oral glucose tolerance test measuring glucose and growth hormone

This patient had no clinical evidence of acromegaly. However, she had an elevated IGF-1 during the evaluation for hypopituitarism, which was performed because of this large tumor. Because the presence of a GH-producing tumor might alter subsequent treatment (*i.e.*, the possibility of using a somatostatin analog rather than performing surgery), it would be important to know if she had nonsuppressible GH levels during an oral glucose tolerance test (15). In fact, this did turn out to be the case. As noted in Case 1, two-thirds of clinically nonfunctioning adenomas actually produce hormones without any clinical syndrome (7). In most such cases, a full hormonal evaluation for hypersecretion had not been done because of the lack of clinical symptoms and signs. Measurement of GH/IGF-1 preoperatively in this setting is not clinically necessary, because no treatment would be instituted

preoperatively if a deficiency was found. Such testing was done in this case more for the sake of completeness than for any clinical indication. To our surprise, after surgery, she noted clinical improvement in ring size, facial appearance, and skin oiliness. Thus, she had symptoms and signs of acromegaly that she had not been aware of and were not appreciated by an experienced pituitary endocrinologist.

Case 5

A 58-year-old woman presented with increasing headaches over 6 to 8 weeks. She also had felt fatigued and had noticed polyuria and polydipsia. An MRI showed a 1.7-cm sellar mass with suprasellar extension and a thickened stalk. Visual fields were normal. Her examination was unremarkable. Laboratory testing revealed an LH level of 5 IU/L, FSH 3 IU/L, PRL 28.7 μg/L, and AM (morning) cortisol 18 ng/dL (497 nmol/L). Serum osmolality was 293 mOsm/kg, and urine osmolality was 154 mOsm/kg. Surgery was advised, but the patient declined. She preferred to drink when thirsty rather than take medications for what seemed to be DI. A repeat MRI 3 months later showed that the mass had increased to 2.1 cm, and there was bitemporal hemianopsia.

Question

What is the most probable diagnosis in this patient?
  A. Prolactinoma
  B. Clinically nonfunctioning adenoma
  C. Metastasis
  D. Meningioma
  E. Craniopharyngioma

Answer

  C. Metastasis

The key here is rapid growth of the tumor over 3 months. None of the other lesions would have grown that quickly. DI is common in this setting, occurring in more than 50% of cases, with varying degrees of hypopituitarism in close to 50% of cases (16, 17). Other signs and symptoms include headache, visual field deficits, and cranial nerve palsies (16, 17). DI is thought to occur due to hematogenous spread through the inferior hypophyseal artery, which directly supplies the posterior lobe. Anterior pituitary involvement is probably due to direct contiguous spread from the posterior pituitary, because the anterior pituitary has no direct arterial supply. Anterior pituitary involvement could also be due to spread from the hypothalamus, which is supplied by the superior hypophyseal artery (17).

Case 6

A 56-year-old woman presented to her physician with progressive fatigue over the last 2 years and amenorrhea of 3-year duration. Her physical examination was unremarkable. Laboratory testing showed normal chemistries and complete blood count. Because her physician suspected that her symptoms might be due to menopause, he obtained an FSH test, the result of which was 2.1 IU/L. This prompted a test for her PRL level, which was 91.7 µg/L (84.5 µg/L upon a 1:100 dilution). An MRI showed a sellar mass extending into the left cavernous sinus, with encasement and compression of the left internal carotid artery.

Question

How should this patient be treated?

A. Start cabergoline 0.5 mg twice weekly
B. Refer for transsphenoidal surgery
C. Repeat scan in 6 months
D. Refer for stereotactic radiotherapy

Answer

B. Refer for transsphenoidal surgery

This patient had a low FSH level and a mildly elevated PRL level, essentially compatible with any large mass in the sella, especially one with suprasellar extension. The key finding in this case is compression of the internal carotid artery by the mass. In an analysis of 85 cases with tumors extending into the cavernous sinus and encasing the internal carotid arteries, only one of 58 (1.7%) pituitary adenomas caused such compression, whereas seven of 25 (28%) nonpituitary adenomas (two meningiomas, one paraganglioma, one Wegener's granuloma, and three metastatic cancers of other primary sites) did so ($P < 0.0007$) (18). Thus, when carotid compression is seen on MRI, lesions other than pituitary adenomas are probably the cause, albeit this is not the case 100% of the time. In this particular case, it proved to be a meningioma. Meningiomas are the most common benign tumors that invade the cavernous sinus and commonly cause stenosis of the internal carotid artery (19).

References

1. Pia HW, Grote E, Hildebrandt G. Giant pituitary adenomas. *Neurosurg Rev.* 1985;**8**(3-4):207–220.
2. Guidetti B, Fraioli B, Cantore GP. Results of surgical management of 319 pituitary adenomas. *Acta Neurochir (Wien).* 1987;**85**(3-4): 117–124.
3. Corsello SM, Ubertini G, Altomare M, Lovicu RM, Migneco MG, Rota CA, Colosimo C. Giant prolactinomas in men: efficacy of cabergoline treatment. *Clin Endocrinol (Oxf).* 2003;**58**(5):662–670.
4. Neff LM, Weil M, Cole A, Hedges TR, Shucart W, Lawrence D, Zhu JJ, Tischler AS, Lechan RM. Temozolomide in the treatment of an invasive prolactinoma resistant to dopamine agonists. *Pituitary.* 2007;**10**(1): 81–86.
5. Kars M, Roelfsema F, Romijn JA, Pereira AM. Malignant prolactinoma: case report and review of the literature. *Eur J Endocrinol.* 2006; **155**(4):523–534.
6. Halevy C, Whitelaw BC. How effective is temozolomide for treating pituitary tumours and when should it be used? *Pituitary.* 2017;**20**(2): 261–266.
7. Saeger W, Lüdecke DK, Buchfelder M, Fahlbusch R, Quabbe HJ, Petersenn S. Pathohistological classification of pituitary tumors: 10 years of experience with the German Pituitary Tumor Registry. *Eur J Endocrinol.* 2007;**156**(2):203–216.
8. Molitch ME. Nonfunctioning pituitary tumors. *Handb Clin Neurol.* 2014;**124**:167–184.
9. Lelotte J, Mourin A, Fomekong E, Michotte A, Raftopoulos C, Maiter D. Both invasiveness and proliferation criteria predict recurrence of nonfunctioning pituitary macroadenomas after surgery: a retrospective analysis of a monocentric cohort of 120 patients. *Eur J Endocrinol.* 2018;**178**(3):237–246.
10. Greenman Y, Cooper O, Yaish I, Robenshtok E, Sagiv N, Jonas-Kimchi T, Yuan X, Gertych A, Shimon I, Ram Z, Melmed S, Stern N. Treatment of clinically nonfunctioning pituitary adenomas with dopamine agonists. *Eur J Endocrinol.* 2016;**175**(1):63–72.
11. Capatina C, Inder W, Karavitaki N, Wass JA. Article I. Management of endocrine disease: pituitary tumour apoplexy. *Eur J Endocrinol.* 2015; **172**(5):R179–R190.
12. Briet C, Salenave S, Bonneville JF, Laws ER, Chanson P. Pituitary apoplexy. *Endocr Rev.* 2015;**36**(6):622–645.
13. Rupp D, Molitch M. Pituitary stalk lesions. *Curr Opin Endocrinol Diabetes Obes.* 2008;**15**(4):339–345.
14. Sbardella E, Joseph RN, Jafar-Mohammadi B, Isidori AM, Cudlip S, Grossman AB. Pituitary stalk thickening: the role of an innovative MRI imaging analysis which may assist in determining clinical management. *Eur J Endocrinol.* 2016;**175**(4):255–263.
15. Katznelson L, Laws ER Jr, Melmed S, Molitch ME, Murad MH, Utz A, Wass JAH; Endocrine Society. Acromegaly: an Endocrine Society clinical practice guideline. *J Clin Endocrinol Metab.* 2014;**99**(11): 3933–3951.
16. Morita A, Meyer FB, Laws ER Jr. Symptomatic pituitary metastases. *J Neurosurg.* 1998;**89**(1):69–73.
17. Castle-Kirszbaum M, Goldschlager T, Ho B, Wang YY, King J. Twelve cases of pituitary metastasis: a case series and review of the literature. *Pituitary.* 2018;**21**(5):463–473.
18. Molitch ME, Cowen L, Stadiem R, Uihlein A, Naidich M, Russell E. Tumors invading the cavernous sinus that cause internal carotid artery compression are rarely pituitary adenomas. *Pituitary.* 2012; **15**(4):598–600.
19. Shaffrey ME, Dolenc VV, Lanzino G, Wolcott WP, Shaffrey CI. Invasion of the internal carotid artery by cavernous sinus meningiomas. *Surg Neurol.* 1999;**52**(2):167–171.

Diagnosis and Management Strategies for Two Unusual Pituitary/Parasellar Lesions: Rathke's Cleft Cyst and Craniopharyngioma

M11
Presented, March 23–26, 2019

Kevin O. Lillehei, MD. Department of Neurosurgery, University of Colorado Anschutz Medical Center, Aurora, Colorado 80045, E-mail: kevin.lillehei@ucdenver.edu

SIGNIFICANCE OF THE PROBLEM

Differentiation of lesions of the sellar nd parasellar region often poses a diagnostic dilemma to neurosurgeons, endocrinologists, radiologists, and pathologists involved in treating patients with these entities. As a result of the pattern of embryological development of the adenohypophysis, as well as subsequent inflammatory, metaplastic, and neoplastic processes that can occur, the potential exists for the formation of a variety of cystic and solid lesions in the sellar and parasellar region. The spectrum of pathology occurring in the sellar region includes benign solid or cystic adenomas, craniopharyngiomas (CPs), Rathke's cleft cysts (RCCs), arachnoid cysts, xanthogranulomas, epidermoid cysts, dermoid cysts, and rarely, metastatic tumors. CPs and RCCs represent two relatively uncommon lesions in this area that often present with both neurologic and endocrinologic dysfunction. Diagnosis is often not straightforward, creating a dilemma in management. Establishing an accurate working diagnosis for sellar region pathology is critical in formulating appropriate treatment goals (*i.e.*, surgery vs medical management vs radiation therapy), predicting the likelihood of lesion recurrence, and guiding postoperative adjunctive management. In this presentation, we will discuss the clinical presentation, diagnosis, pathophysiology, and management of these two discrete entities.

BARRIERS TO OPTIMAL PRACTICE

- Difficulty in making initial diagnosis, often based on the experience and familiarity with the disease entity of the interpreting radiologist
- Understanding the natural history of the disease entity
- Knowledge of the short- and long-term sequelae of treatment

LEARNING OBJECTIVES

As a result of participating in this session, learners should be able to:
- Have familiarity with the radiologic presentation of each disease entity
- Understand the underlying etiology and natural history of each disease entity
- Be familiar with the endocrine abnormalities associated with each disease entity
- Identify a treatment strategy appropriate to each disease entity

STRATEGIES FOR DIAGNOSIS, THERAPY, AND MANAGEMENT
RCC
Diagnosis

Symptomatic RCCs account for approximately 6% to 10% of patients who present with sellar and suprasellar lesions in neurosurgical series (1, 2). Most studies show a mean age of onset in the 30s and an associated female predominance. Occasionally, RCCs become sufficiently large to cause mass effects on the pituitary gland and its surrounding structures. These lesions typically arise in the area between the anterior and posterior pituitary gland and histologically are composed of either a single or pseudostratified layer of cuboidal or columnar epithelium with an underlying layer of connective tissue (3–6). They range in size from a few millimeters to as large as 50 mm (7). They are often discovered incidentally and have been identified in up to 22% of the population, according to routine autopsy studies. Indications for treatment generally include headaches, visual disturbances, and/or pituitary hormonal deficiencies.

Endocrine dysfunction has been described in approximately 30% to 60% of patients with RCC, with hyperprolactinemia being the most common abnormality. Panhypopituitarism and diabetes insipidus (DI) also occur in an estimated 5% to 15% of patients. In the author's experience, 56% of patients had a pituitary hormone abnormality, with hypogonadism and hyperprolactinemia being the most common (in 31% and 20% of patients, respectively). Further analysis revealed preoperative hypogonadism in 26% of premenopausal women tested and in 38% of males tested. These hormone abnormalities were followed, in relative frequency, by hypothyroidism (12%), panhypopituitarism (10%), DI (9%), and isolated adrenal insufficiency (3%) (8). Following surgery, as reported in most series, hyperprolactinemia improved in most patients (77% to 100%), but the recovery of other hormones varied as a function of the extent of surgical resection and the degree of preoperative panhypopituitarism. In the author's experience, 64% of patients had an overall improvement in pituitary hormone dysfunction, with resolution or improvement in hyperprolactinemia, hypothyroidism, hypopituitarism, DI, and adrenal insufficiency observed in 93.8%, 90.0%, 50.0%, 33.3%, and 67.0% of patients, respectively (8).

Radiologic Appearance

Radiographically, these lesions arise most commonly within the sella and extend into the suprasellar region, with lesions occasionally occurring along the pituitary stalk, above the diaphragma. Magnetic resonance imaging (MRI) is the radiologic study of choice; the sagittal view shows the lesion occupying the region of the pars intermedia, displacing the anterior lobe forward, often in a wedge-shaped fashion (Fig. 1a). Patients often have an unusual ledge posteriorly, overlying the posterior lobe of the pituitary gland (shelf sign), which is not typically seen in pituitary adenomas. There is no associated contrast enhancement seen within the lesion. A pathognomonic radiology finding, observed on sagittal imaging, is reversal of the imaging intensity of the lesion, from hyperintense to hypointense, seen with contrast administration (Fig. 1b and 1c).

Treatment

Transnasal transsphenoidal surgery remains the treatment of choice for symptomatic RCCs. At the present time, cyst drainage without an attempt to aggressively strip the cyst wall is recommended. Aggressive cyst wall resection has been associated with a decreased recurrence rate but is associated with increased postoperative endocrine dysfunction, including a high rate of postoperative diabetes insipidus. With surgery, postsurgical improvement in headache is observed in most patients (>80%). Vision problems, including disturbances of acuity and perimetry (which occur in an estimated 20% to 49% of patients), improve in a reported 64% to 100% of cases.

In the literature, RCC recurrence rates of between 2.3% and 33% are reported. The variance in published recurrence rates may be attributable to numerous factors, including study design, period of follow up, patient cohort number, surgical approach, as well as the definition of recurrent RCC (radiologic vs symptomatic). Although risk factors associated with RCC recurrence are relatively unknown, proposed factors include the presence of squamous metaplasia and/or inflammation seen on histologic evaluation when evaluating primary vs recurrent RCC. The presence of squamous metaplasia has been related to chronic inflammation, possibly secondary to cyst contents such as mucin. Additional risk factors described include cyst size, enhancement on MRI, the use of a fat graft at the time of surgery, presence of a solid lesion within the cyst, and extent of surgical

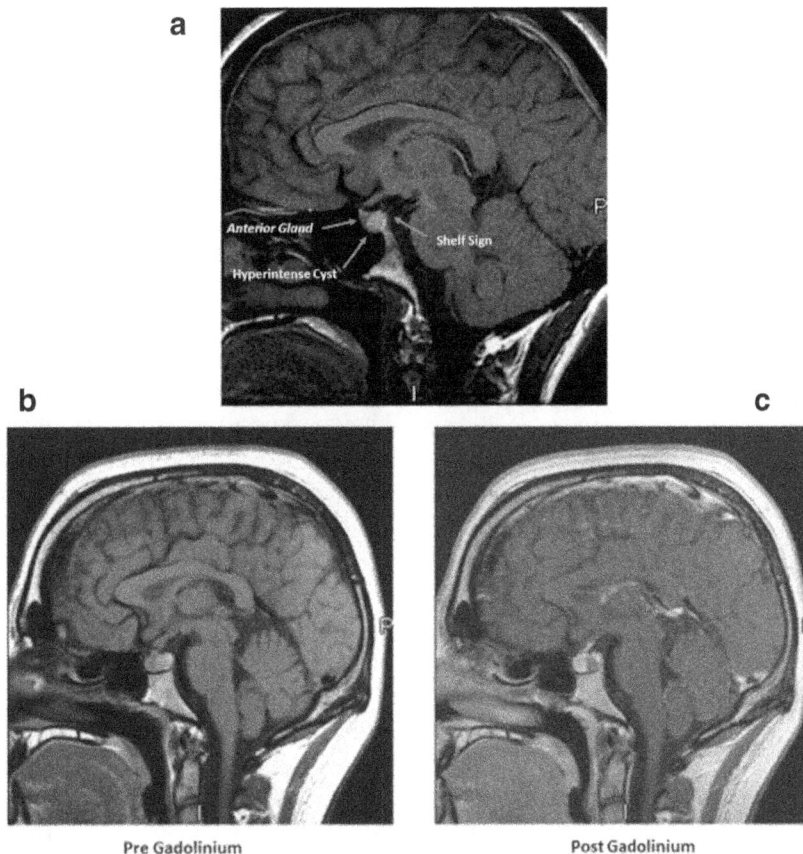

Figure 1. (a) Sagittal MRI scan of Rathke's Cleft cyst. Lesion is most commonly hyperintense on T1-weighted imaging (prior to gadolinium administration), occurring in the pars intermedia, with the normal anterior pituitary gland displaced forward. Often seen is a "shelf sign" over the top edge of the posterior pituitary gland. (b and c) Pathognomonic reversal of cyst intensity seen on sagittal MRI before and after gadolinium administration.

resection of the cyst wall. Unfortunately, few treatment options exist for the treatment of recurrent RCC other than surgery. Although radiation therapy is often used as a last resort, there are limited data delineating the long-term efficacy of this approach. Furthermore, the use of intra-cystic alcohol as a method of chemical epithelial cauter-ization has been previously described by our group and has demonstrated limited efficacy in minimizing cyst re-currence (8). The recent use of intracystic bleomycin, ad-ministered at the time of surgical re-exploration, seems to offer an effective and safe adjuvant treatment strategy aimed at preventing radiographic and symptomatic RCC recurrence (9, 10). Further studies are needed to assess the overall therapeutic potential of this promising therapy.

CP
Diagnosis

CPs are benign World Health Organization grade 1 tumors, comprising approximately 3% of all intracranial tumors. This proportion is notably higher in the pediatric pop-ulation (10% of all pediatric brain tumors). The estimated incidence of CPs is 0.13 per 100,000 cases per year (12). Historically, CPs present in a bimodal age distribution, with peak ages at the time of presentation of 5 to 14 years and then at 50 to 74 years. However, these lesions may present in patients of all ages. CPs can arise anywhere along the vestiges of the stomodeal diverticulum, but they most frequently originate in the region of the infundibulum, where squamous epithelial rests are known to occur. In rare cases, CPs arise in less typical locations along the remnants of the primitive craniopharyngeal duct (including the naso-pharynx and sphenoid bone) or as primary intraventricular lesions.

The clinical presentation of CPs at any age frequently includes headache, vision loss, and hypopituitarism. In children, growth and sexual retardation, obesity, and hydrocephalus are frequently observed as well. Many patients with CPs suffer from chronic obesity, more com-monly in children, which is thought to develop secondary to hypothalamic dysfunction (11, 12). Memory loss and cognitive deficits are more common findings in older pa-tients (13). Diabetes insipidus is seen on presentation in 6% to 38% of new cases. The two major pathological subtypes of CP are the adamantinomatous (ACP) and squamous-papillary (PCP) varieties. ACPs, but not PCPs, are seen in children, whereas both ACPs and PCPs are seen in adults.

Typical Imaging Features of CPs

From an imaging standpoint, CPs are typically described as calcified, solid, and/or cystic lesions, typically with a lob-ular shape and a diameter of 20 to 40 mm (Fig. 1). The majority of CPs involve the suprasellar space, with 40% to

53% of cases exhibiting some intrasellar involvement. CPs occasionally extend into the anterior, middle, or posterior fossa and may invade the floor or walls of the third ven-tricle. Hydrocephalus is observed in up to 38% of cases and is a more common finding in children. On standard CT scanning, calcification is evident in 60% of tumors and is more common in pediatric cases and the ACP subtype. The majority of ACPs are mixed solid–cystic or predominantly cystic tumors with a lobulated appearance (Fig. 1). On MRI, the solid elements are usually isointense or hypointense on T1-weighted images, exhibit inhomogeneous high in-tensity on T2-weighted images, and heterogeneously en-hance following gadolinium administration. The cystic elements of ACPs typically display a high intensity on T1-weighted images, high or mixed intensity on T2-weighted images, and contrast enhancement of the cyst wall. The PCP subtype is found in approximately one-third of adult CP cases and rarely shows calcification. The majority of PCPs are predominantly solid or mixed solid-cystic tumors with a spherical shape, and usually exhibit low intensity on T1-weighted images, high intensity on T2-weighted images, and enhancement of the cyst wall after addition of gadolinium. The MRI appearance of the solid regions is frequently similar to those of the ACP variety.

Typical Histopathological Features of CPs

Histologically, ACPs are thought to arise from squamous embryonic rests and bear similarity to adamantinomas or ameloblastomas of the jaw with the potential for enamel production. The epithelium is often stratified squamous or adamantinoid type, frequently with evidence of wet keratin nodules. The cystic components are often described as having a characteristic "machine oil" interior, containing desquamated squamous epithelium and comprised mainly of keratin and cholesterol. The papillary subtype of CP is known to occur more commonly in adults than in children (14% to 50% of CPs in adults compared with only 2% of CPs in children). PCPs usually bear similarity to oropharyngeal mucosa and rarely exhibit calcification. The cyst contents are typically yellow and viscous. Histopathological analysis frequently demonstrates squamous epithelium forming pseudopapillae, without discrete nodules of wet keratin or calcium.

Exome sequencing of CPs has revealed that >90% of PCPs have *BRAF* V600E mutations and that >90% of ACPs have *CTNNB1* mutations (14, 15). Of note, these mutations were found to be clonal, with no other recurrent mutations or genomic aberrations noted in either subtype. In addi-tion, these mutations were noted to be mutually exclusive. These findings have important implications for the di-agnosis and treatment of these neoplasms and have opened the door for potential medical therapy with BRAF and MEK inhibitors.

Treatment

Historically, the treatment of CP has ranged from aggressive surgical resection to biopsy alone, followed by radiation therapy. Due to the location of the tumor and its proximity to vital structures (*i.e.*, optic nerves and chiasm, pituitary stalk, and hypothalamus), substantial surgical morbidity had been noted. Major advances in neurosurgical techniques, however, have significantly decreased the morbidity and mortality associated with resection, making aggressive resection feasible in more cases. At the same time, improvements in radiation therapy techniques have permitted more accurate delivery of radiation to the tumor target, while minimizing radiation damage to normal structures. *Surgery.* At present, surgery is recommended for favorably located CPs (*i.e.*, without hypothalamic involvement), with an attempt at radical surgical resection with preservation of visual, pituitary, and hypothalamic functionality. For unfavorably located tumors (*i.e.*, with contact or infiltration of the hypothalamus and optic structures), a radical surgical approach is not recommended. Cyst and/or tumor decompression followed by radiation therapy is the treatment of choice. In children, hypothalamic obesity occurs in 40% to 66% of patients, often as a result of surgery. This is a significant and debilitating complication and a major factor in a patient's long-term quality of life.

Irradiation. Standard fractionated photon beam radiotherapy is the current gold standard for treatment of CPs. This modality has been shown to be effective in prevention and treatment of progression and recurrence. The current use of proton beam therapy in patients with CPs is promising, especially for CPs located in proximity to optic structures, pituitary gland, or hypothalamus. Proton beam therapy offers a more protective radio-oncological treatment modality compared with conventional external photon radiation. Stereotactic radiosurgery is also a potential treatment option, preferably in low-volume CPs.

PRESENTATION OF CASES

Case 1

An 81-year-old woman has a 6-year history of adrenal insufficiency and hypothyroidism and is on replacement therapy. She presents with a 6-month history of visual deterioration (> in the left eye than the right). Visual field examination reveals evidence of a bitemporal hemianopsia. Endocrine work-up reveals prolactin (PRL) 14 ng/mL (normal range, 3 to 20 ng/mL), luteinizing hormone (LH) <0.2 mIU/mL (normal range, 15.9 to 54.0 mIU/mL), follicle-stimulating hormone (FSH) 1 mIU/mL (normal range, 23 to 116 mIU/mL), estradiol 25 pg/mL (normal range, <20 to 32 pg/mL), insulin-like growth factor (IGF)-1 30 ng/mL (normal range, 17 to 167 ng/mL), thyrotropin (TSH) 1.51 mIU/L (normal range, 0.34 to 5.60 mIU/L), free T$_4$ 0.54 ng/dL (normal range, 0.89 to 1.76 ng/dL), and adrenocorticotrophic hormone (ACTH) <5 pg/mL (normal range, 6 to 58 pg/mL). An MRI scan, before and after gadolinium administration, is shown in Figure 2.

An MRI Scan Suggests Which of the Following Diagnoses?

    A. CP
    B. RCC
    C. Cystic prolactinoma
    D. Pituitary arachnoid cyst

Discussion

This patient presents with adrenal insufficiency and hypothyroidism. A review of the MR image (Fig. 2) shows that the cyst contents are slightly hyperintense precontrast and lower intensity postcontrast, favoring an RCC vs an arachnoid cyst. A normal prolactin level argues against a cystic prolactinoma. A purely cystic CP cannot be ruled out, but is less likely with no clear involvement of the stalk or hypothalamus. The presence of a shelf sign makes a diagnosis of RCC highly likely.

The patient underwent an uneventful transsphenoidal surgery with the finding of clear mucoid liquid filling the cyst cavity. There was no communication with cerebrospinal fluid. The cyst wall was biopsied. Pathology revealed flattened cuboidal epithelium, which is consistent with an RCC.

Case 2

A 40-year-old woman presents with a 1-year history of progressive headaches (HAs) (now occurring five times per week),

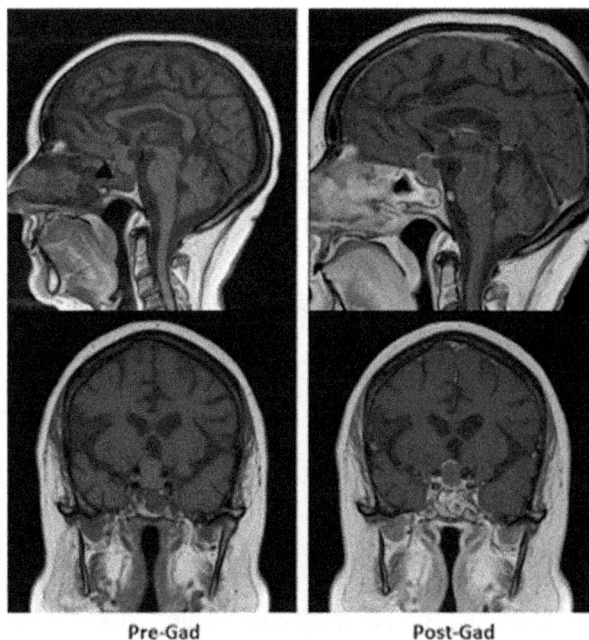

Pre-Gad   Post-Gad

Figure 2. Case 1. Preoperative MRI scan before and after gadolinium administration.

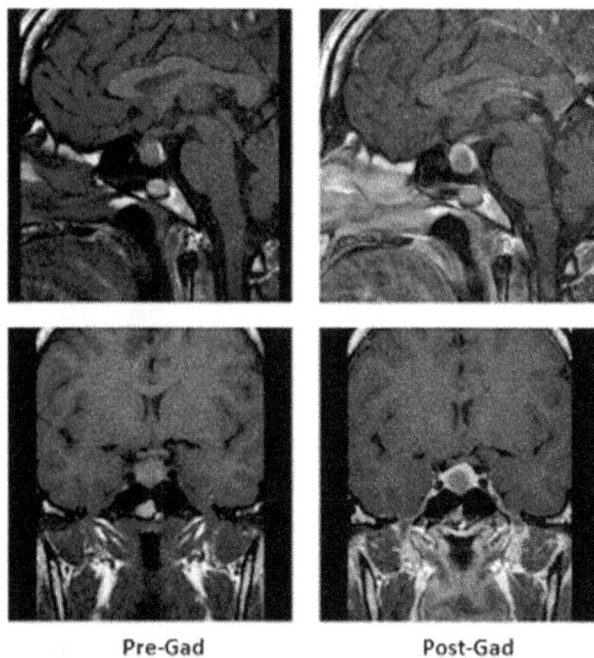

Pre-Gad   Post-Gad

Figure 3. Case 2. Preoperative MRI scan before and after gadolinium administration.

increasing visual blurring, and polyuria/polydipsia. She is noted to have normal menses, with no galactorrhea.

Endocrine work-up revealed cortisol 6 μg/dL (normal range, 3.0 to 22.4 μg/dL), ACTH 52 pg/mL (normal range, 6 to 50 pg/mL), dihydroepiandrosterone 124 μg/dL (normal range, 32 to 240 μg/dL), estradiol 23 pg/mL (normal range, 20 to 214 pg/mL), IGF-1 122 ng/mL (normal range, 76 to 271 ng/mL), PRL 45 ng/mL (normal range, 3 to 27 ng/mL), LH 3.1 mIU/mL (normal range, 0.7 to 5.6 mIU/mL), FSH 6 mIU/mL (normal range, 2 to 10 mIU/mL), TSH 1.15 mIU/L (normal range, 0.34 to 5.60 mIU/L), and free T_4 1.15 ng/dL (normal range, 0.89 to 1.76 ng/dL). An MRI scan, before and after gadolinium administration, is shown in Figure 3.

An MRI Scan Suggests Which of the Following Diagnoses?

A. CP
B. RCC
C. Cystic prolactinoma
D. Pituitary arachnoid cyst

Discussion

The patient presents with HAs, visual blurring, and symptoms of DI. MRI (Fig. 3) shows a cystic pituitary lesion that is somewhat off center to the right, with the pituitary stalk displaced to the left. The cyst contents are slightly hyperintense precontrast, suggesting a possible RCC. There is no shelf sign. The

cyst appears noncomplex, without septations or secondary cysts, arguing against a CP. The prolactin level is slightly elevated, consistent with either stalk effect or a poorly secreting prolactinoma. There is a suggestion of enhancing tissue within the sella, more so than would be expected from a displaced normal gland.

The patient underwent transsphenoidal surgery and upon opening the cyst, dark "motor oil"–like fluid was encountered, consistent with liquefied hematoma. Curetting within the cyst cavity revealed soft abnormal tissue lining the cyst walls, consistent with adenoma. Pathology was consistent with a benign adenoma, positive on immunohistochemical staining for prolactin only. Postoperatively, the patient's HAs, visual blurring, and symptoms of DI resolved, and her prolactin level was normal 2 years after surgery.

Case 3

A 22-year-old female, with a history of normal growth and pubertal development, presents with a 12-month history of headaches, vision changes, amenorrhea, and progressive weight gain (60 pounds).

Endocrine work-up revealed ACTH 40 pg/mL (normal range, 6 to 50 pg/mL), random cortisol 12.4 μg/dL (normal range, 3.0 to 22.4 μg/dL), 8:00 AM cortisol following 1 mg dexamethasone 0.9 μg/dL, 17-hydroxyprogesterone 14 ng/dL (normal < 207 ng/dL), PRL 17.9 ng/mL (normal range, 3 to 27 ng/mL), IGF-1 159 ng/mL (normal range, 105 to 337 ng/mL), FSH 3.1 mIU/mL (normal range, 1.5 to 33.4 mIU/mL), LH 0.6 mIU/mL (normal range, 0.5 to 76 mIU/mL), total testosterone 14 ng/dL (normal range, 2 to 45 ng/dL), free testosterone 1.7 ng/dL (normal range, 0.1 to 6.4 ng/dL), estradiol 14.5 pg/mL (normal range, 20 to 214 pg/mL), TSH 2.43 mIU/L (normal range, 0.35 to 5.5 mIU/L), free T_4 1.2 ng/dL (normal range, 0.8 to 1.8 ng/dL, serum sodium 143 mmol/L (normal range, 133 to 145 mmol/L), serum osmolality 291 mOs/kg (normal range, 275 to 303 mOs/kg), and urine osmolality 727 mOs/kg (normal range, 50 to 800 mOs/kg).

MRI (Fig. 4) of the brain demonstrated a 2.6- × 1.7- × 1.8-cm suprasellar, predominantly cystic mass with distortion of the third ventricle.

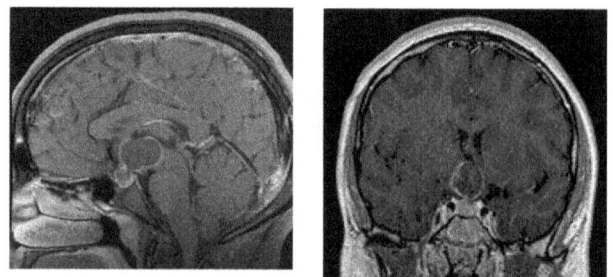

Figure 4. Case 3. Preoperative MRI scan; sagittal and coronal images after gadolinium administration.

BMI Change and Weight Loss Efforts

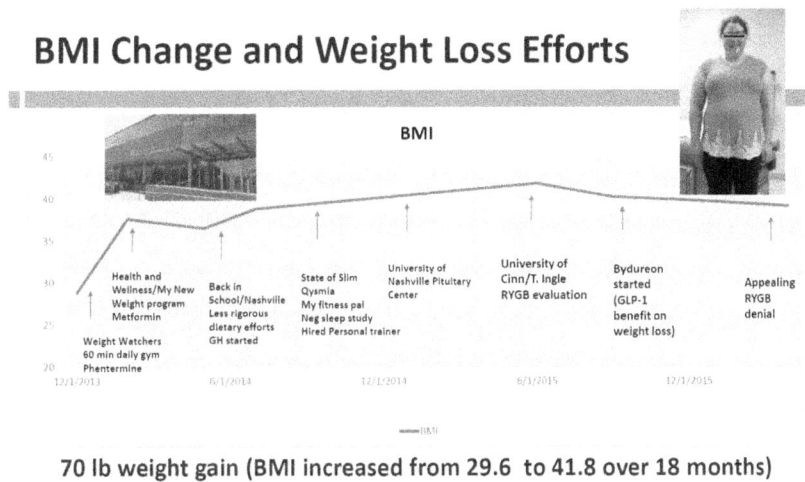

70 lb weight gain (BMI increased from 29.6 to 41.8 over 18 months)

Figure 5. Case 3. Treatment timeline with tracking of postoperative body mass index (BMI).

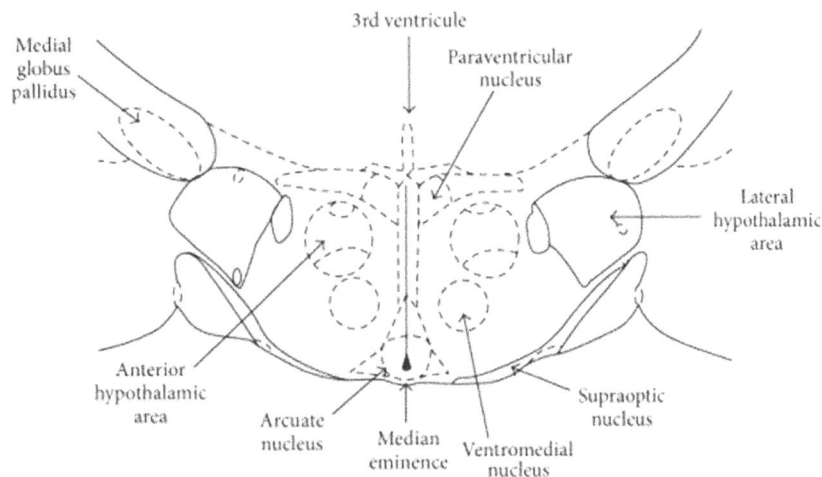

Figure 6. Coronal view of hypothalamic nuclei. Note proximity of ventromedial nucleus to the wall of the third ventricle. Reproduced from the National Library of Medicine Open-i archive. https://openi.nlm.nih.gov/ detailedresult.php?img=PMC4737468_NP2016-3276383.001&req=4.

Which Should Be the Treatment of Choice?

A. Observation
B. Surgery with limited resection and irradiation
C. Surgery with attempt at gross total resection
D. Treatment with a BRAF inhibitor (vemurafenib)

Discussion

The patient underwent an endoscopic transnasal tumor resection. The pathology was consistent with an adamantinomatous CP, with a gross total resection obtained. This required, however, sacrifice of the pituitary stalk and removal of tumor from within the third ventricle. Postoperatively, the patient suffered the expected panhypopituitarism and DI, which was managed appropriately without difficulty. The major postoperative morbidity was weight gain, with an increase in the patient's body mass index from 29.6 to 41.8 kg/m^2 (Fig. 5).

Using the lesion grading system (0 to 2) from the KRANIOPHARYNGEOM 2000 European study (15), the lesion extended posterior to the mammillary bodies, well into the posterior hypothalamus adjacent to the ventromedial nucleus (Fig. 6), giving her a +2.7 body mass index standard deviation score at 36 months. She is without recurrence 5 years after surgery. The factors predicting long-term morbidity, including injury to the ventromedial nucleus of the hypothalamus, balanced against tumor recurrence, will be discussed.

References

1. Benveniste RJ, King WA, Walsh J, Lee JS, Naidich TP, Post KD. Surgery for Rathke cleft cysts: technical considerations and outcomes. *J Neurosurg.* 2004;**101**(4):577–584.
2. Ross DA, Norman D, Wilson CB. Radiologic characteristics and results of surgical management of Rathke's cysts in 43 patients. *Neurosurgery.* 1992;**30**(2):173–178, discussion 178–179.
3. Kleinschmidt-DeMasters BK, Lillehei KO, Stears JC. The pathologic, surgical, and MR spectrum of Rathke cleft cysts. *Surg Neurol.* 1995; **44**(1):19–26, discussion 26–27.

4. Mukherjee JJ, Islam N, Kaltsas G, Lowe DG, Charlesworth M, Afshar F, Trainer PJ, Monson JP, Besser GM, Grossman AB. Clinical, radiological and pathological features of patients with Rathke's cleft cysts: tumors that may recur. *J Clin Endocrinol Metab.* 1997;**82**(7):2357–2362.

5. Shin JL, Asa SL, Woodhouse LJ, Smyth HS, Ezzat S. Cystic lesions of the pituitary: clinicopathological features distinguishing craniopharyngioma, Rathke's cleft cyst, and arachnoid cyst. *J Clin Endocrinol Metab.* 1999;**84**(11):3972–3982.

6. Voelker JL, Campbell RL, Muller J. Clinical, radiographic, and pathological features of symptomatic Rathke's cleft cysts. *J Neurosurg.* 1991;**74**(4):535–544.

7. Roux FX, Constans JP, Monsaingeon V, Meder JF. Symptomatic Rathke's cleft cysts; clinical and therapeutic data. *Neurochirurgia (Stuttg).* 1988;**31**(1):18–20.

8. Lillehei KO, Widdel L, Astete CA, Wierman ME, Kleinschmidt-DeMasters BK, Kerr JM. Transsphenoidal resection of 82 Rathke cleft cysts: limited value of alcohol cauterization in reducing recurrence rates. *J Neurosurg.* 2011;**114**(2):310–317.

9. Landolt A. Commentary on (Demasters et al. "The pathologic, surgical, and MR spectrum of Rathke cleft cysts"). *Surg Neurol.* 1995;**44**(1): 26–27.

10. Ung TH, Yang M, Wang M, Harland T, Lillehei KO. Benefit of intracystic bleomycin for symptomatic recurrent Rathke cleft cyst [published online ahead of print 16 November 2018]. *Oper Neurosurg (Hagerstown).* doi:10.1093/ons/opy361.

11. Elowe-Gruau E, Beltrand J, Brauner R, Pinto G, Samara-Boustani D, Thalassinos C, Busiah K, Laborde K, Boddaert N, Zerah M, Alapetite C, Grill J, Touraine P, Sainte-Rose C, Polak M, Puget S. Childhood craniopharyngioma: hypothalamus-sparing surgery decreases the risk of obesity. *J Clin Endocrinol Metab.* 2013;**98**(6): 2376–2382.

12. Müller HL, Gebhardt U, Teske C, Faldum A, Zwiener I, Warmuth-Metz M, Pietsch T, Pohl F, Sörensen N, Calaminus G; Study Committee of KRANIOPHARYNGEOM 2000. Post-operative hypothalamic lesions and obesity in childhood craniopharyngioma: results of the multi-national prospective trial KRANIOPHARYNGEOM 2000 after 3-year follow-up. *Eur J Endocrinol.* 2011;**165**(1):17–24.

13. Karavitaki N, Brufani C, Warner JT, Adams CB, Richards P, Ansorge O, Shine B, Turner HE, Wass JA. Craniopharyngiomas in children and adults: systematic analysis of 121 cases with long-term follow-up. *Clin Endocrinol (Oxf).* 2005;**62**(4):397–409.

14. Brastianos PK, Taylor-Weiner A, Manley PE, Jones RT, Dias-Santagata D, Thorner AR, Lawrence MS, Rodriguez FJ, Bernardo LA, Schubert L, Sunkavalli A, Shillingford N, Calicchio ML, Lidov HG, Taha H, Martinez-Lage M, Santi M, Storm PB, Lee JY, Palmer JN, Adappa ND, Scott RM, Dunn IF, Laws ER Jr, Stewart C, Ligon KL, Hoang MP, Van Hummelen P, Hahn WC, Louis DN, Resnick AC, Kieran MW, Getz G, Santagata S. Exome sequencing identifies BRAF mutations in papillary craniopharyngiomas. *Nat Genet.* 2014;**46**(2):161–165.

15. Hussain I, Eloy JA, Carmel PW, Liu JK. Molecular oncogenesis of craniopharyngioma: current and future strategies for the development of targeted therapies. *J Neurosurg.* 2013;**119**(1):106–112.

Health Outcomes in Acromegaly: Comorbidity and Cancer Surveillance Beyond IGF-1

M18
Presented, March 23–26, 2019

Asha Pathak, MD. Cedars Sinai Medical Center, Los Angeles, California 90048, E-mail: asha.pathak@cshs.org

Shlomo Melmed, MB, ChB. Cedars-Sinai Pituitary Center, Los Angeles, California 90048, E-mail: melmed@csmc.edu

SIGNIFICANCE OF THE CLINICAL PROBLEM

Acromegaly results from excessive pituitary adenoma secretion of GH and, consequently, IGF-1. Disease progression is usually slow and insidious, with an average interval from symptom onset to diagnosis of ~5 to 10 years. Acromegaly is associated with increased morbidity and decreased life expectancy. Systemic complications include musculoskeletal, endocrine, and metabolic disorders; cardiovascular disease; respiratory compromise; and soft tissue neoplasms.

BARRIERS TO OPTIMAL PRACTICE

Features of acromegaly are commonly encountered in clinical practice (*e.g.*, headaches, joint pains, diabetes), yet the disorder is rare. Hence, practitioners may miss the diagnosis. Furthermore, symptoms may take many years to manifest, and the slow onset may mask patient and/or family awareness.

LEARNING OBJECTIVES

As a result of participating in this session, learners should be able to:

- Understand the comorbidities associated with acromegaly outcomes
- Identify appropriate screening, management, and surveillance measures

STRATEGIES FOR DIAGNOSIS, THERAPY, AND/OR MANAGEMENT

Musculoskeletal and Soft Tissue

Excess GH and IGF-1 stimulate growth of connective tissue, cartilage, and bone. Synovial tissue and cartilage enlarge, causing macrognathia, frontal bossing, enlarged and swollen hands and feet, and hypertrophic arthropathy. Increased edema of the median nerve may lead to paresthesias and carpal tunnel syndrome. Macroglossia, craniofacial deformities, and swelling of pharyngeal and laryngeal soft tissues are associated with development of sleep apnea.

Anabolic effects of excess GH and IGF-1 on bone and increased bone turnover lead to osteopathy. Vertebral fracture risk is increased and positively correlated with duration of active disease. Interpretation of dual-energy x-ray absorptiometry results may be challenging due to the presence of osteophytes and facet joint hypertrophy. Screening x-rays or vertebral fracture assessment should be obtained in patients with newly diagnosed acromegaly and during follow-up. Bone density may improve within 6 to 12 months of biochemical control, but an increased risk of vertebral fracture risk can persist. Treatment with antiresorptives may be indicated in addition to addressing GH levels, hypogonadism, and other risk factors.

Endocrine

Patients with acromegaly may present with hypopituitarism as a result of compression of normal pituitary tissue by tumor. The gonadal axis is most commonly affected, and hypogonadism may be exacerbated by increased prolactin levels, from stalk effect (serum prolactin level usually <200 ng/mL), or from a cosecreting somatomammotroph adenoma (serum prolactin level usually >200 ng/mL). Thyroid function is usually normal, although patients may demonstrate subclinical hyperthyroidism or central hypothyroidism. GH deficiency may develop after surgical resection of the adenoma or, more commonly, after radiation treatment, although reported prevalence and time to development are variable. Signs and symptoms of GH deficiency include decreased exercise tolerance and endurance, reduced quality of life, and development of central obesity and dyslipidemia. Diagnosis of GH deficiency is supported by an IGF-1 level <2 standard deviations below the age-adjusted mean or by results of an insulin tolerance test, which is considered the gold standard. Consideration may be given to GH replacement, and a low-dose approach and cautious titration should be undertaken. Before initiating GH replacement therapy, patients should be up to date on cancer screening and evaluated for cardiovascular disease risk, including a lipid profile.

Glucose and Lipid Homeostasis

Patients with acromegaly may demonstrate insulin resistance and hyperglycemia, and the prevalence of diabetes mellitus may be 50% or higher. However, the net effect of elevated GH and IGF-1 levels on glucose homeostasis differs between patients and may be influenced by age, BMI, and family history of diabetes. Elevated GH levels cause insulin resistance, associated with increased lipolysis, lipid oxidation, elevated free fatty acid levels. Lipoprotein lipase may be suppressed, but insulin secretion may be increased. Elevated IGF-1 levels promote lipogenesis, fatty acid uptake, glucose uptake, and insulin sensitivity.

Treatment with somatostatin receptor ligands or GH receptor antagonists can also affect glucose homeostasis. In particular, pasireotide, with its higher affinity for SST5 (which is most highly expressed in β-cells), has been associated with elevated glucose levels and reduced insulin, incretin, and gastric inhibitory polypeptide secretion. Pasireotide-associated hyperglycemia occurs in approximately one half of patients but can be reversed with drug discontinuation. Pegvisomant, a GH receptor antagonist, may confer reduced free fatty acid concentration and increased insulin sensitivity and is an alternative option for patients with pasireotide-associated hyperglycemia. Combined treatment with pasireotide and pegvisomant may allow for a decrease in pasireotide dose but may not resolve impaired glucose metabolism.

Elevated GH levels may result in hypertriglyceridemia and lower high-density lipoprotein levels. Although low-density lipoprotein may be normal or only slightly elevated, lipoprotein (a) and oxidized low-density lipoprotein levels may be increased, contributing to cardiovascular disease risk. Lipid profiles may improve with biochemical control, although many patients require treatment with lipid-lowering medications.

At time of presentation with acromegaly, practitioners should assess fasting glucose, HbA_{1c}, and lipid profile. These parameters should be monitored at least annually in patients with active disease. Patients receiving pasireotide should be followed closely for development of hyperglycemia or worsening from baseline. Suggested medications for glucose control include metformin, incretin agents, or insulin. Sodium-glucose cotransporter-2 (SGLT-2) inhibitors should be avoided in the setting of uncontrolled GH levels, as free fatty acid levels may be elevated and risk of ketoacidosis increased.

Cardiovascular

Cardiovascular disease is the leading cause of premature mortality in acromegaly. Elevated GH levels are associated with many cardiovascular sequelae, including sodium retention, hypervolemia, cardiomyocyte growth, increased valve root diameter and valvular regurgitation, and collagen and mucopolysaccharide deposition on cardiac structures. Hypertension is present in 30% to 60% of patients with acromegaly. Valvulopathy may be identified in up to 75% of patients on presentation, with aortic and mitral valves most commonly affected. Left ventricular hypertrophy and reduced ejection fraction also can be present, with diastolic dysfunction more common than systolic dysfunction. Patients may experience arrhythmias related to structural cardiac abnormalities. There may be an increased risk of ischemic heart disease in the setting of elevated GH/IGF-1 levels, although this has not been definitively established.

Early recognition and treatment of acromegaly may interrupt progression of cardiovascular disease and potentially reverse abnormalities. On initial evaluation, ambulatory blood pressure, electrocardiogram, and echocardiogram are recommended, as well as evaluation for other cardiac risk factors such as signs or symptoms of ischemic heart disease, diabetes, hyperlipidemia, lifestyle habits, and family history. In the setting of uncontrolled acromegaly, surveillance echocardiogram is indicated.

Prior to initiation of pharmacologic therapy for acromegaly, an EKG should be obtained, followed by periodic monitoring during treatment. Somatostatin receptor ligands may cause bradycardia or AV node dysfunction. QT prolongation has been observed with pasireotide use, which may be compounded by underlying electrolyte abnormalities or concurrent use of other medications with QT-prolonging effects.

Respiratory

Elevated GH levels are associated with soft tissue changes of the upper airway and hypertrophy of pulmonary tissues and may lead to sleep apnea syndrome or generalized respiratory insufficiency. Sleep apnea syndrome is diagnosed in ~50% to 70% of patients, and a component of central sleep apnea also may be present. Predictive factors include severity and duration of GH excess, obesity, older age, smoking, and male sex. A sleep study is recommended in all patients at diagnosis as well as continued monitoring for signs or symptoms of sleep apnea or respiratory complications during follow-up. There is variable improvement with normalization of GH levels, and sleep apnea is an additional risk factor for cardiovascular complications.

Oncologic

Patients with acromegaly may have an increased risk of developing cancer compared with the general population. Proposed mechanisms include trophic effects of IGF-1, increased cellular proliferation and differentiation, angiogenesis, and inhibition of apoptosis and tumor suppressor mechanisms. In one study, standardized cancer incidence ratios were slightly elevated across all cancer types compared with the general population (1.41; 95% CI, 1.18 to 1.68) as well as individually for colorectal cancer (1.67; 95% CI, 1.07 to 2.58), thyroid cancer (3.99; 95% CI, 2.32 to 6.87), and kidney cancer (2.87; 95% CI, 1.55 to 5.34). A recent meta-analysis again identified an increased cancer risk (standardized incidence ratio, 1.5; 95% CI, 1.2 to 1.8) compared with the general population, especially for colorectal, thyroid, urinary tract, gastric, and breast cancers. However, in interpreting these findings, the effects of selection and surveillance bias should be considered. Colorectal and thyroid cancers are the most commonly diagnosed subtypes among patients with acromegaly.

Increased incidence of adenomatous and hyperplastic colon polyps occurs particularly in patients age >50 years, men, those with three or more skin tags, or those with a family history of colon cancer. Up to 20% of patients age <40 years have colon polyps at the time of diagnosis. Increased mortality from colon cancer has not been firmly established, but colonoscopy should be performed at diagnosis in patients age >40 years. If colonoscopy is normal, and acromegaly is biochemically controlled, patients can be screened every 10 years per guidelines. Among patients with polyps or uncontrolled disease, screening every 3 to 5 years is indicated.

Thyroid cancer in acromegaly is usually of the differentiated subtypes, with a natural history similar to that in the general population. Clinical thyroid exam is recommended at time of presentation and annually thereafter. Nodular goiter occurs in ~60% of patients and equally in men and women. Thyroid ultrasound should be obtained if there are palpable nodules.

Quality of Life

Patients require careful follow-up and care for quality-of-life challenges, including fertility counseling; appropriate need for cosmetic surgery for self-awareness and sensitivity; discussion of informed risks and benefits of available treatment options, including potential side effects and cost challenges; support in interpreting laboratory results; and reduction of potential economic burden of chronic illness.

MAIN CONCLUSIONS

Emphasis is placed on early diagnosis and treatment of acromegaly to minimize long-term effects of associated comorbidities, especially those that may be reversible. With achievement of biochemical control, mortality rate can be returned to that of the general population. Comorbidities associated with acromegaly may improve with treatment but could persist, especially skeletal and arthritic changes and hypertension, requiring continued monitoring and follow-up.

Long-term outcomes may be predetermined by functional classification of the disorder. Patients with type 3 acromegaly (*i.e.*, those with sparsely granulated macroadenomas, younger age, poor responsiveness to somatostatin receptor ligands, and higher IGF-1 levels at diagnosis) are more likely to exhibit long-term comorbidities and more adverse outcomes. These patients require more-rigorous long-term surveillance and often repeat surgery and/or radiation in addition to combination medical therapy.

DISCUSSION OF CASES AND ANSWERS

Case 1

A 63-year-old woman returns for follow-up after incomplete resection of an invasive GH-secreting pituitary macroadenoma 1 year ago. Pasireotide was initiated postoperatively for persistently elevated IGF-1 levels. She subsequently demonstrated hyperglycemia and began taking metformin for glucose control. Metformin dose has been increased to 1500 mg daily, but glucose levels are not controlled. IGF-1 level is improved but remains elevated, and you plan to increase pasireotide dose. Renal function is normal. You discuss adjustment of antidiabetic medication regimen. Which of the following should be avoided?
- A. Increasing metformin dose
- B. Glucagon-like peptide-1 agonist
- C. Dipeptidyl peptidase-4 inhibitor
- D. Insulin
- E. SGLT-2 inhibitor

Answer

E, SGLT-2 inhibitor. Treatment with pasireotide, a somatostatin receptor ligand with higher affinity for SST5, may be contributing to poorly controlled glucose in this patient. Antihyperglycemic medications should be managed carefully in patients with acromegaly. Elevated GH levels are associated with increased lipolysis, lipid oxidation, and elevated free fatty acid levels. SGLT-2 inhibitors can promote fat oxidation, glucosuria, and decreased glucose uptake by α-cells, leading to an increased glucagon-to-insulin ratio and reduced renal clearance of ketone bodies. The combined effects of elevated circulating GH levels and SGLT-2 inhibition increase the risk of ketoacidosis.

Case 2

A 57-year-old male with a history of a 1.7-cm GH-secreting pituitary macroadenoma was treated with surgical resection followed by radiation 5 years ago. He presents to the clinic to discuss bothersome symptoms. For the past few months, he has noticed increased difficulty with keeping up with his peers at their rather competitive weekly baseball games. Despite dietary changes and exercising more, he has noted a continued decline in energy level, inability to maintain his previous physique, and an increase in his waist size. An IGF-1 level 2 weeks ago at an outside laboratory was 55 ng/mL (range, 51 to 194 ng/mL). A concurrent chemistry panel was within normal limits. He does not have a history of hypertension, dyslipidemia, or hyperglycemia. On physical exam, weight is 6 kg higher than at last visit, BMI is 32 kg/m^2, and heart rate and blood pressure are normal. He does not have a goiter or abnormal skin findings. Cardiopulmonary and abdominal examinations are unremarkable. Which of the following would you recommend?
- A. Reassurance
- B. Repeat IGF-1 level in 3 months
- C. GH stimulation test
- D. Initiation of GH replacement
- E. Evaluation of pituitary axes, including GH stimulation test

Answer

E, evaluation of pituitary axes, including GH stimulation test. Patients treated with sellar radiation are at an increased risk of developing hypopituitarism, which may take years to manifest. This patient has nonspecific symptoms that could be related to various pituitary deficiencies. Although his IGF-1 level is just above the lower limit of normal for his age group, GH deficiency cannot be ruled out by a single IGF-1 level in the setting of concerning symptoms. A GH stimulation test should be performed for additional evaluation. If GH deficiency is confirmed, a trial of GH replacement may be considered. Prior to initiating GH replacement, a baseline lipid panel should be obtained along with reassessment of cardiovascular disease risk factors, and colon cancer screening should be up to date.

Case 3

A 50-year-old male with newly diagnosed acromegaly presents for evaluation. You appreciate large hands with fleshy palms on greeting handshake. The patient complains of diffuse joint pains, sweating, shoes fitting more tightly, and not feeling rested in the morning. He admits to diminished libido. He reports a recent diagnosis of prediabetes and hypertension. On physical examination his blood pressure is 150/92 mm Hg, and he has frontal bossing, macroglossia, and jaw malocclusion. Heart rate is regular, but he has a murmur over the aortic valve. GH and IGF-1 levels are unequivocally elevated. On MRI, a 1.6-cm pituitary adenoma is observed. What additional laboratory testing is indicated?

A. Pituitary axis evaluation with prolactin, fasting chemistry panel, and lipid panel
B. ECG, echocardiogram, and sleep study
C. Vertebral fracture assessment and 25-hydroxy vitamin D level
D. Colonoscopy
E. All of the above

Answer

E, all of the above. This patient demonstrates many classic findings associated with acromegaly. Pituitary axes should be evaluated, with attention to gonadal axis and prolactin level. Cardiovascular evaluation should entail an ECG in the clinic and echocardiogram for concern for valvulopathy and left ventricular hypertrophy given hypertension and murmur. Lipid profile and family history should be obtained to account for other risk factors for cardiovascular disease. Obtaining a vertebral fracture assessment is appropriate given increased risk of fractures, and vitamin D should be replete. Polysomnography is recommended due to concern for sleep apnea. Colonoscopy is indicated given his age and increased risk of polyps and colorectal cancer.

Recommended Reading

Ben-Shlomo A, Sheppard MC, Stephens JM, Pulgar S, Melmed S. Clinical, quality of life, and economic value of acromegaly disease control. *Pituitary.* 2011;**14**(3):284–294.

Cuevas-Ramos D, Carmichael JD, Cooper O, Bonert VS, Gertych A, Mamelak AN, Melmed S. A structural and functional acromegaly classification. *J Clin Endocrinol Metab.* 2015;**100**(1):122–131.

Dal J, Leisner MZ, Hermansen K, Farkas DK, Bengtsen M, Kistorp C, Nielsen EH, Andersen M, Feldt-Rasmussen U, Dekkers OM, Sørensen HT, Jørgensen JOL. Cancer incidence in patients with acromegaly: a cohort study and meta-analysis of the literature. *J Clin Endocrinol Metab.* 2018;**103**(6):2182–2188.

Davi' MV, Dalle Carbonare L, Giustina A, Ferrari M, Frigo A, Lo Cascio V, Francia G. Sleep apnoea syndrome is highly prevalent in acromegaly and only partially reversible after biochemical control of the disease. *Eur J Endocrinol.* 2008;**159**(5):533–540.

Gadelha MR, Bronstein MD, Brue T, Coculescu M, Fleseriu M, Guitelman M, Pronin V, Raverot G, Shimon I, Lievre KK, Fleck J, Aout M, Pedroncelli AM, Colao A for the Pasireotide C2402 Study Group. Pasireotide versus continued treatment with octreotide or lanreotide in patients with inadequately controlled acromegaly (PAOLA): a randomised, phase 3 trial. *Lancet Diabetes Endocrinol.* 2014;**2**(11):875–884.

Gadelha MR, Kasuki L, Lim DS, Fleseriu M. Systemic complications of acromegaly and the impact of the current treatment landscape: an update [published online ahead of print 31 August 2018]. *Endocr Rev.* doi:10.1210/er.2018-00115.

Katznelson L, Laws ER Jr, Melmed S, Molitch ME, Murad MH, Utz A, Wass JA for the Endocrine Society. Acromegaly: an Endocrine Society clinical practice guideline. *J Clin Endocrinol Metab.* 2014;**99**(11):3933–3951.

Mazziotti G, Marzullo P, Doga M, Aimaretti G, Giustina A. Growth hormone deficiency in treated acromegaly. *Trends Endocrinol Metab.* 2015;**26**(1):11–21.

Melmed S. Medical progress: acromegaly. *N Engl J Med.* 2006;**355**(24):2558–2573.

Melmed S, Bronstein MD, Chanson P, Klibanski A, Casanueva FF, Wass JAH, Strasburger CJ, Luger A, Clemmons DR, Giustina A. A consensus statement on acromegaly therapeutic outcomes. *Nat Rev Endocrinol.* 2018;**14**(9):552–561.

Pivonello R, Auriemma RS, Grasso LF, Pivonello C, Simeoli C, Patalano R, Galdiero M, Colao A. Complications of acromegaly: cardiovascular, respiratory and metabolic comorbidities. *Pituitary.* 2017;**20**(1):46–62.

Quarella M, Walser D, Brändle M, Fournier JY, Bilz S. Rapid onset of diabetic ketoacidosis after SGLT2 inhibition in a patient with unrecognized acromegaly. *J Clin Endocrinol Metab.* 2017;**102**(5):1451–1453.

Terzolo M, Reimondo G, Berchialla P, Ferrante E, Malchiodi E, De Marinis L, Pivonello R, Grottoli S, Losa M, Cannavo S, Ferone D, Montini M, Bondanelli M, De Menis E, Martini C, Puxeddu E, Velardo A, Peri A, Faustini-Fustini M, Tita P, Pigliaru F, Peraga G, Borretta G, Scaroni C, Bazzoni N, Bianchi A, Berton A, Serban AL, Baldelli R, Fatti LM, Colao A, Arosio M for the Italian Study Group of Acromegaly. Acromegaly is associated with increased cancer risk: a survey in Italy. *Endocr Relat Cancer.* 2017;**24**(9):495–504.

van Bunderen CC, van Varsseveld NC, Heymans MW, Franken AA, Koppeschaar HP, van der Lely AJ, Drent ML. Effect of long-term GH replacement therapy on cardiovascular outcomes in GH-deficient patients previously treated for acromegaly: a sub-analysis from the Dutch National Registry of Growth Hormone Treatment in Adults. *Eur J Endocrinol.* 2014;**171**(6):717–726.

Approach to the Diagnosis of Pituitary and Ectopic ACTH-Secreting Tumors

M23
Presented, March 23–26, 2019

Lynnette K. Nieman, MD. Diabetes, Endocrinology and Obesity Branch, National Institute of Diabetes and Digestive and Kidney Diseases, National Institutes of Health, Bethesda, Maryland 20892, E-mail: lynnette. nieman@gmail.com

Katherine Araque Triana, MD. Diabetes, Endocrinology and Obesity Branch, National Institute of Diabetes and Digestive and Kidney Diseases, National Institutes of Health, Bethesda, Maryland 20892, E-mail: katherine. araque@nih.gov

SIGNIFICANCE OF THE CLINICAL PROBLEM

Endogenous Cushing's syndrome (CS) is caused by chronic hypercortisolism that results from either excessive ACTH production or primary adrenal disorders. If untreated, it can lead to fatal complications, including pulmonary embolism, cardiovascular disease, and opportunistic infections. The rarity of this disease [0.7 to 2.4 cases per 10,000,000 individuals per year (1)] complicates its recognition and management.

BARRIERS TO OPTIMAL PRACTICE

Optimal care for patients with ACTH-dependent CS requires an experienced multidisciplinary team of endocrinologists, radiologists, and surgeons who work together to establish the diagnosis, manage multiple comorbidities, and normalize cortisol levels. Many patients do not have access to a center with such expertise, leading to missed diagnoses, reduced access to screening tests, and inappropriate interpretation of test results. Physicians need more familiarity with the nuances of CS.

LEARNING OBJECTIVES
- Understand the basic approach to interpretation of tests to establish ACTH-dependent CS and its causes, including inferior petrosal vein sampling (IPSS) and pituitary MRI
- Know how to best identify an ectopic ACTH-secreting (EAS) tumor

STRATEGIES FOR DIAGNOSIS OF ACTH-DEPENDENT CS

Diagnosis of CS

The clinical presentation of CS, regardless of its cause, is variable, and there is a lack of pathognomonic clinical symptoms or signs (2–4). Features that occur at an unusual age or accumulate over time are more likely to reflect underlying hypercortisolism.

Biochemical screening is indicated when features consistent with CS are not explained by other comorbidities, exogenous glucocorticoid exposure, or physiologic hypercortisolism [e.g., severe obesity, alcoholism, depression, anorexia nervosa or bulimia, pregnancy, or glucocorticoid resistance (5)]. The Endocrine Society recommends the use of two of three different screening tests, considering the assay limitations and caveats regarding test interpretation (4).

Diagnosis of ACTH-Dependent CS

Once CS is established, tests for the differential diagnosis are initiated, beginning with ACTH measurement. Chronic hypercortisolism suppresses normal corticotrope ACTH production. In ACTH-independent CS, ACTH is usually subnormal (undetectable or <10 pg/mL, 2.2 pmol/L). Conversely, values within the reference range (>20 pg/mL, 4.4 pmol/L) or frankly elevated are seen in ACTH-dependent CS. Intermediate values (10 to 20 pg/mL) can be seen with both causes.

Caveat

In cyclic CS (*i.e.*, intermittent hypercortisolism followed by normal values), the exposure to cortisol may not be sufficient to suppress the normal corticotropes. The danger here is that a patient with a non–ACTH-dependent cause will be misdiagnosed as ACTH dependent.

Differential Diagnosis of ACTH-Dependent CS

Biochemical and radiologic localization studies to identify the source of the ACTH production [pituitary, Cushing's disease (CD) vs ectopic, ectopic ACTH syndrome, EAS] should be performed only after confirmation of ACTH-dependent CS.

Noninvasive Tests

Depending on the criteria used for interpretation, ~90% of CD and 10% of EAS patients increase ACTH and/or cortisol after administration of ovine CRH (oCRH; 1 μg/kg; maximum, 100-μg dose). National Institutes of Health criteria for response are: a cortisol increase ≥20% (from mean −5- and 0-minute values to mean 30- and 45-minute values) and/or an increase in ACTH ≥35% (from mean baseline to mean 15- and 30-minute values) (6). The 8-mg overnight dexamethasone suppression test (DST) is less helpful. When measured at 0830 hours before and 0900 hours after administration of dexamethasone at midnight, serum cortisol will suppress >69% in 77% of CD patients and ~18% of EAS patients (7, 8).

A mass ≥6 mm on T1-weighted spin echo pituitary MRI has a high predictive value for CD. This cutoff point considers that an incidental mass <6 mm is present in 10% of healthy individuals (9). When patients fulfill criteria for CRH, DST, and

MRI, CD is 100% confirmed, in our experience; however, when results are conflicting, IPSS should be performed.

IPSS

IPSS is the gold-standard test (10). When performed in experienced centers (*e.g.*, at National Institutes of Health, >1000 procedures), the sensitivity and specificity are as high as 98% and 97%, respectively. False-negative IPSS results in CD are associated with abnormal venous anatomy, anomalous venous drainage, and technical problems in achieving catheter placement. False-positive results in EAS occur with cyclic CS and insufficient corticotrope suppression or when a noncorticotrope tumor drains into the petrosal sinuses. When performing IPSS, consider this stepwise approach:

- Perform the test after confirmed hypercortisolemia Normalization of cortisol as a result of medical therapy or cyclic CS can give a false-positive result for CD
- Evaluate venogram to confirm accurate catheterization and normal venous drainage
- Measure prolactin (PRL) in all samples to confirm adequate catheterization; a baseline PRL inferior petrosal sinus/peripheral (IPS/P) ratio (ipsilateral to the highest post-CRH ACTH IPS/P ratio) ≥1.8 suggests successful catheterization during IPSS (11)
- Review ACTH IPS/P ratios; if basal ACTH IPS/P ≥2 or post-CRH ACTH IPS/P ≥3, CD diagnosis is likely, regardless of venography or PRL (assuming that point 1 above is followed)
- If ACTH IPS/P ratios do not meet criteria for CD, PRL-normalized ACTH IPS/P ratios can be used to differentiate between a pituitary and ectopic source of ACTH; values ≤0.7 suggest EAS, and those ≥1.3 suggest CD. Indeterminate values (0.7 to 1.3) need further study (11)

Identification of Ectopic ACTH-Secreting Tumors

In 80% of cases, the tumor is located in the chest, including pulmonary carcinoids or tumorlets, mediastinal or thymic neuroendocrine tumors, or small-cell lung cancers. Other possibilities are pheochromocytomas, paragangliomas, rare NETs (appendix, prostate), ovarian teratomas, or medullary thyroid cancers. A cost-effective approach is first to obtain anatomic (CT and/or MRI) and functional (F-DOPA, 68-Ga-DOTATATE) imaging of the thorax. Results should be correlated to eliminate false-positive targets.

Overview of Treatment Modalities

Surgery is the first-line therapeutic option after IPSS suggests CD or IPSS/imaging identifies a probable EAS target (12). If surgery is precluded by comorbidities or unresectable or metastatic disease, medical therapy or bilateral adrenalectomy is an alternative treatment choice .

CASES

Case 1

A 22-year-old white man presented with 3 months of lower back pain not relieved by over the counter painkillers. On evaluation, vertebral fractures were identified between L1 and L4. He was admitted for pain management. He also reported 6 months of multiple symptoms, including facial fullness, increased dorsocervical fat, central obesity, easy bruising, violaceous striae on the abdomen, acne, temporal balding, proximal muscle weakness, and fatigue.

Physical examination: afebrile; blood pressure, 142/80; RR, 18; and oxygen saturation, 99% as well as facial plethora, dorsocervical fat pad, acne, temporal balding, central adiposity, 2-cm violaceous striae on the back, and 1+ pedal edema. He was unable to stand up from a chair without using his arms.

Biochemical and endocrine evaluation: K+, 2.8 mEq/L (normal range, 3 to 5) with metabolic alkalosis; hemoglobin A_{1c} (HbA$_{1c}$), 4.9%; urine free cortisol (UFC), 1800 to 2219 μg/24 h (normal range, 3.5 to 45); 1-mg DST cortisol, 16.3 μg/dL; basal ACTH, 360 to 439 pg/mL (normal range, 3.5 to 45); oCRH test, increased cortisol by 10% and ACTH by 20%; pituitary MRI was unremarkable; IPSS venogram, unremarkable (Table 1).

What is the next best step in this patient's management?

A. Perform imaging to identify an ectopic ACTH-secreting tumor
B. Refer for transsphenoidal surgery (TSS)
C. Treat with octreotide
D. Treat with bisphosphonates, potassium, ketoconazole, and metyrapone

Table 1. IPSS Results: Case 1

Time (min)	Hormone Concentrations and Sampling Sites									
	ACTH Concentration (pg/mL)					PRL Concentration (ng/dL)				
	RP	LP	P	RP/P	LP/P	RP	LP	P	RP/P	LP/P
−5	156	161	152	1.02	1.05	34.5	52.6	18.6	1.85	2.8
0	161	162	160	1.00	1.01	38.3	48.6	18.7	2.04	2.59
3	146	154	139	1.05	1.10	41.7	52.2	16.5	2.52	3.16
5	142	144	145	0.97	0.99	36.9	55.7	16.5	2.23	3.37
10	155	162	143	1.08	1.13	36.9	55.7	16.9	2.18	3.29

Abbreviations: LP, left petrosal sinus; RP, right petrosal sinus; P, peripheral vein.

The best answer is A. The biochemical testing is consistent with EAS. The next step is to identify the source. TSS is not correct, because this patient does not have CD. Treatment of EAS/CS is an off-label use for octreotide, ketoconazole, and metyrapone. These are not correct, because imaging to find the ACTH-secreting tumor should be done first. Medications also are costly, cause adverse reactions, and may not normalize cortisol. However, if imaging fails to identify a potential tumor or if a patient is too ill to undergo surgery immediately or surgery is delayed, it is important to initiate medical therapy promptly.

Case 2

A 54-year-old white woman presents with a 50-lb weight gain (to 200 lbs; body mass index, 30 kg/m^2) in 5 weeks, lower extremity edema, weakness with difficulty climbing stairs, facial acne, and temporal balding. Physical examination: skin atrophy, purplish striae on the breast, chest, and abdomen, and hirsutism on the chin and sideburns. Laboratory evaluation: HbA$_{1c}$, 7.1%; UFC, 7000 to 7800 μg/24 h (normal range, 3.5 to 45); AM serum cortisol, 56 to 97 μg/dL (normal, <25); AM ACTH, 114 to 400 pg/mL (normal range, 5 to 46). Imaging did not reveal an ACTH-secreting tumor. She received 600 mg mifepristone per day for 7.5 months.

Three weeks after discontinuation of mifepristone, she was admitted to a specialized CS referral center for evaluation. She reported weight loss and significant improvement in her symptoms. Diagnostic testing: mean 2330- and 0000-hour serum cortisol, 3.9 μg/dL (normal, <7.5); AM serum cortisol, 24 to 29 μg/dL; AM ACTH, 90 to 156 pg/mL (normal range, 5 to 46); PM ACTH, 15 pg/mL; oCRH stimulation test, 5% increase in cortisol and 141% increase in ACTH; cortisol pre- and post-8-mg DST, 24.3 to 1 μg/dL (95%); pituitary MRI unremarkable.

What is the best next step in management?
A. Perform IPSS
B. Start treatment with metyrapone
C. Discharge the patient and measure UFC and bedtime salivary cortisol
D. Discharge the patient and refer her to a weight-management clinic

The best answer is C. This patient has evidence of cyclic CS (13). Initial evaluation found clinical and biochemical hypercortisolemia with elevated ACTH levels, confirming

ACTH-dependent CS. Upon referral to a specialized center after 7.5 months of mifepristone and a 3-week washout, her symptoms had improved, and late-night cortisol and ACTH were normal. Biochemical testing during eucortisolemia can result in an erroneous diagnosis of CD, if the corticotropes cells have been disinhibited. Therefore, the best option is to discharge her, repeat UFC and bedtime salivary cortisol measurements, and readmit her when hypercortisolism recurs. Performing IPSS (answer A) will result in a false-positive diagnosis of CD and potentially lead to unnecessary treatment. Starting treatment with metyrapone (answer B) during eucortisolism can lead to adrenal insufficiency. Answer D is incorrect because it does not address the question of CS.

This patient had recurrent hypercortisolism. Biochemical evaluation was consistent with EAS, and she underwent successful resection of a left bronchial carcinoid followed by remission (14).

Case 3

A 47-year-old black man had a 6-year history of type 2 diabetes and hypertension, central weight gain, irritability, abnormal fat distribution, facial flushing, facial swelling, hair thinning, fatigue, abdominal distension, proximal muscle weakness, abdominal striae, and central hypogonadism. Biochemical evaluation: UFC, 180 to 1223.2 μg/24 h (normal range, 3.5 to 45); bedtime salivary cortisol, 3.21 to 4.34 μg/dL (normal, <0.228); ACTH, 71 to 158 pg/mL (normal range, 5 to 46); CRH stimulation test consistent with CD; 8-mg DST consistent with EAS; pituitary MRI, 8 × 6 mm lesion without mass effect on adjacent structures; IPSS venogram unremarkable (Table 2).

What is the best management?
A. Perform TSS
B. Complete torso CT and 68-Ga-DOTATATE to identify the source of EAS
C. Perform bilateral adrenalectomy
D. Start ketoconazole and metyrapone and check AM serum cortisol and UFC in 8 to 10 weeks

The best answer is B. This patient has evidence of EAS by the DST and IPSS, but evidence for CD based on MRI and CRH test. In cases of conflicting biochemical testing results during an episode of hypercortisolemia, IPSS is the gold-standard test to discriminate between CD and EAS. In this case, a 1-cm

Table 2. IPSS Results: Case 3

	Hormone Concentrations and Sampling Sites									
	ACTH Concentration (pg/mL)					PRL Concentration (ng/dL)				
Time (min)	RP	LP	P	RP/P	LP/P	RP	LP	P	RP/P	LP/P
−5	72.5	70.6	73.4	0.98	0.96	136	113	32	4.25	3.53
0	65.5	68.9	65.7	0.99	1.04	135	110	31.5	4.28	3.49
3	69.7	71.6	64.2	1.08	1.11	130	98.1	30.5	4.26	3.21
5	72.9	74.6	69.2	1.05	1.07	155	148	32.7	4.74	4.52
10	65.5	63.1	59.4	1.10	1.06	115	126	28.8	3.99	4.37

pulmonary carcinoid was identified on imaging and resected, with subsequent remission. Because structural imaging may reveal false-positive lesions, functional imaging with F-DOPA or a somatostatin analog (octreotide or DOTATATE) is extremely useful to confirm a lesion on CT/MRI or to point to an area for additional scrutiny on structural imaging.

Because this patient has EAS, he will not benefit from TSS (answer A). A bilateral adrenalectomy (answer C) is reserved for cases of occult CS, cases where surgery is not curative or is precluded by comorbidities or tumor location, cases of metastatic disease, or cases of intolerance to medical therapy. Starting medical therapy and following up in several weeks (answer D) exposes the patient unnecessarily to the effects of hypercortisolemia and adverse reactions to medical therapy.

Case 4

A 54-year-old woman presents with weight gain, proximal muscle weakness, violaceous striae, easy bruising, decreased memory, and dorsocervical and supraclavicular fat pads. Biochemical workup: 3 weeks before IPSS, 24-hour UFC was 8116 μg/24 h. No additional tests were done until admission, when the following results were seen: 0000-hour serum cortisol, <7.5 μg/dL; AM ACTH, 34.5 pg/mL; UFC, 27 μg/24 h. Prescheduled IPSS: peak ACTH IPS/P ratio, 9.5 (normal ratio, 212:22.4); baseline PRL IPS/P, 1.7 (normal ratio, 4.2:2.5); ACTH/PRL IPS/P, 5.6. Within 1 week, UFC was 755 μg/24 h (normal range, 3.5 to 45), CRH stimulation test and 8-mg DST results were consistent with EAS, and pituitary MRI was unremarkable.

What is the best management option for this patient?
A. Perform TSS
B. Perform chest CT and 68-Ga-DOTATATE positron emission tomography/CT to locate the ectopic EAS tumor
C. Repeat IPSS the next day
D. Repeat CRH stimulation test and HD DST

The best answer is B. The peak ACTH IPS/P ratio of 9.5 during IPSS cannot be trusted, because it was done during eucortisolism. Because this is potentially a false-positive result for CD, TSS (answer A) should not be done immediately. Baseline ipsilateral PRL IPS/P ratio was 1.7, suggesting unsuccessful catheterization, and normalized ACTH/PRL IPS/P ratio was 5.6, indicative of a pituitary source. Laboratory results subsequently confirmed cyclic CS.

Within a week, UFC = 755 μg/24 hr (n = 3.5 to 45), and the CRH stimulation test and 8-mg DST results were consistent with EAS. Pituitary MRI was unremarkable. Imaging revealed a 1.4-cm retrocardiac lesion that was an ACTH-positive pulmonary

carcinoid. Postoperatively, ACTH levels were undetectable, and hypercortisolemia resolved. Repeating IPSS during eucortisolemia will lead to a false-positive diagnosis of CD (answer C is incorrect). There is no indication to repeat the biochemical testing at this time; the current data are sufficient to establish a final diagnosis (answer D is incorrect).

References

1. Lindholm J, Juul S, Jørgensen JO, Astrup J, Bjerre P, Feldt-Rasmussen U, Hagen C, Jørgensen J, Kosteljanetz M, Kristensen L, Laurberg P, Schmidt K, Weeke J. Incidence and late prognosis of cushing's syndrome: a population-based study. *J Clin Endocrinol Metab*. 2001; **86**(1):117–123.
2. Wagner-Bartak NA, Baiomy A, Habra MA, Mukhi SV, Morani AC, Korivi BR, Waguespack SG, Elsayes KM. Cushing syndrome: diagnostic workup and imaging features, with clinical and pathologic correlation. *AJR Am J Roentgenol*. 2017;**209**(1):19–32.
3. Nieman LK. Recent updates on the diagnosis and management of Cushing's syndrome. *Endocrinol Metab (Seoul)*. 2018;**33**(2): 139–146.
4. Nieman LK, Biller BM, Findling JW, Newell-Price J, Savage MO, Stewart PM, Montori VM. The diagnosis of Cushing's syndrome: an Endocrine Society clinical practice guideline. *J Clin Endocrinol Metab*. 2008;**93**(5):1526–1540.
5. Sharma ST, Nieman LK, Feelders RA. Cushing's syndrome: epidemiology and developments in disease management. *Clin Epidemiol*. 2015;**7**:281–293.
6. Nieman LK, Oldfield EH, Wesley R, Chrousos GP, Loriaux DL, Cutler GB Jr. A simplified morning ovine corticotropin-releasing hormone stimulation test for the differential diagnosis of adrenocorticotropin-dependent Cushing's syndrome. *J Clin Endocrinol Metab*. 1993;**77**(5): 1308–1312.
7. Dichek HL, Nieman LK, Oldfield EH, Pass HI, Malley JD, Cutler GB Jr. A comparison of the standard high dose dexamethasone suppression test and the overnight 8-mg dexamethasone suppression test for the differential diagnosis of adrenocorticotropin-dependent Cushing's syndrome. *J Clin Endocrinol Metab*. 1994;**78**(2):418–422.
8. Findling JW, Nieman L, Tabarin A. Diagnosis and differential diagnosis of Cushing's syndrome. *N Engl J Med*. 2017;**377**(2):e3.
9. Hall WA, Luciano MG, Doppman JL, Patronas NJ, Oldfield EH. Pituitary magnetic resonance imaging in normal human volunteers: occult adenomas in the general population. *Ann Intern Med*. 1994;**120**(10): 817–820.
10. Oldfield EH, Doppman JL, Nieman LK, Chrousos GP, Miller DL, Katz DA, Cutler GB, Jr, Loriaux DL. Petrosal sinus sampling with and without corticotropin-releasing hormone for the differential diagnosis of Cushing's syndrome. *N Engl J Med*. 1991;**325**(13):897–905.
11. Sharma ST, Raff H, Nieman LK. Prolactin as a marker of successful catheterization during IPSS in patients with ACTH-dependent Cushing's syndrome. *J Clin Endocrinol Metab*. 2011;**96**(12):3687–3694.
12. Nieman LK, Biller BM, Findling JW, Murad MH, Newell-Price J, Savage MO, Tabarin A; Endocrine Society. Treatment of Cushing's syndrome: an Endocrine Society clinical practice guideline. *J Clin Endocrinol Metab*. 2015;**100**(8):2807–2831.
13. Meinardi JR, Wolffenbuttel BH, Dullaart RP. Cyclic Cushing's syndrome: a clinical challenge. *Eur J Endocrinol*. 2007;**157**(3):245–254.
14. Carmichael JD, Zada G, Selman WR. Making the diagnosis of cyclic Cushing's syndrome: a position statement from the topic editors. *Neurosurg Focus*. 2015;**38**(2):E8.

Optimizing Hormone Treatment in the Patient With Hypopituitarism

M32
Presented, March 23–26, 2019

Laurence Katznelson, MD. Division of Endocrinology, Gerontology and Metabolism, Stanford University School of Medicine, Stanford, California 94304, E-mail: katznels@stanford.edu

Laura Dichtel, MD, MHS. Neuroendocrine Unit, Massachusetts General Hospital, Boston, Massachusetts 02114, E-mail: ldichtel@mgh.harvard.edu

SIGNIFICANCE OF THE CLINICAL PROBLEM

Hypopituitarism refers to complete or partial deficiency in pituitary hormones. Anterior pituitary hormone deficiency includes adrenal insufficiency (AI; due to adrenocorticotropic hormone deficiency), hypogonadism [due to luteinizing hormone (LH)/follicle-stimulating hormone (FSH) deficiency or hyperprolactinemia], hypothyroidism [due to thyrotropin (TSH) deficiency], and growth hormone deficiency (GHD; due to hypothalamic GHRH or pituitary gland GHD). Posterior gland deficiency primarily involves diabetes insipidus [DI; due to antidiuretic hormone (ADH) deficiency]. Appropriate awareness of pituitary function testing as well as therapeutic strategies is critical for accurate management of hypopituitarism. In this review, we focus on several clinical scenarios that offer impactful lessons on management of hypopituitarism, including perioperative management following pituitary surgery and traumatic brain injury (TBI). Although not extensively covered in this session, patients treated with cranial radiotherapy for both pituitary and nonpituitary tumors must be monitored and treated for hypopituitarism. Finally, opiate use or abuse is an often-unrecognized cause of central AI and hypogonadism. In these settings, there is a range of approaches and, in the case of TBI and opiate use, limited awareness of the impact on pituitary function. This Meet-the-Professor session will focus on the issues involved to help facilitate a more focused approach to the treatment of the patient with hypopituitarism.

BARRIERS TO OPTIMAL PRACTICE

- Effective management of a patient who undergoes pituitary surgery; identifying appropriate perioperative, postoperative, and chronic treatment strategies
- Awareness of hypopituitarism following TBI and understanding an appropriate strategy for diagnosis and management of such patients

LEARNING OBJECTIVES

As a result of participating in this session, learners should be able to:

- Perform the appropriate pituitary function tests and endocrine management for a patient undergoing pituitary surgery
- Demonstrate the correct clinical approach to diagnosis and treatment of hypopituitarism in a patient with a history of TBI

STRATEGIES FOR DIAGNOSIS, THERAPY, AND/OR MANAGEMENT

I. Basic Pituitary Function Testing (1)

1. Hypothyroidism

Caused by insufficient TSH stimulation of thyroid gland function due to inadequate production of either TSH and/or TRH.

Diagnosis

Low free T_4 level in the setting of a low, normal, or mildly elevated TSH level in the setting of pituitary disease.

2. AI

Inadequate cortisol secretion due to inadequate adrenocorticotropic hormone and/or CRH production.

Diagnosis

i. Low morning serum cortisol (<3 μg/dL).
ii. Inadequate serum cortisol response (<18 μg/dL) following 250-μg cosyntropin injection IV/IM at 30 or 60 minutes. The cosyntropin stimulation test assesses the adrenal gland response (but not the hypothalamus or pituitary gland response) to exogenous cosyntropin. A normal response assumes integrity of the entire axis, but this supposition may be incorrect, especially with acute trauma (<6 weeks) to the pituitary gland.
iii. Test should be performed at least 18 to 24 hours after the last hydrocortisone dose.
iv. Total cortisol levels should be interpreted with caution in women who are taking oral contraceptive pills (OCPs), because oral estrogen leads to a variable and at times robust increase in cortisol-binding globulin and an overestimation of adrenal function.

3. Central Hypogonadism

Caused by inadequate secretion of LH and FSH.

Diagnosis

i. In men, low morning serum testosterone should be demonstrated on at least two occasions (2).
ii. In women, the presence of amenorrhea or oligomenorrhea, with low estradiol in a premenopausal woman. In a postmenopausal woman, the absence of high FSH and LH levels.

iii. A normal prolactin level should be documented to exonerate hyperprolactinemia as a potentially treatable cause of central hypogonadism.

4. GHD
Caused by inadequate GH secretion by the pituitary or GHRH production by the hypothalamus.

Diagnosis
i. Low IGF-1 level in the setting of three other anterior pituitary hormone axis deficiencies is diagnostic of GHD.
ii. It is important to note that a normal IGF-1 level does not rule out GHD. In addition, due to the pulsatile nature of GH secretion, single, unstimulated GH levels are not useful.
iii. Provocative GH stimulation testing is often required, with appropriate selection of stimulation testing based on patient comorbidities. Food and Drug Administration–approved testing options that are available in the United States include glucagon, insulin, and macimorelin. GHRH, which is not available in the United States but is still available elsewhere, can be used as a combined GHRH–arginine test.
iv. Multiple studies have demonstrated that obesity leads to a reduction in peak-stimulated GH levels, and body mass index–stratified GH cutoffs should be used whenever possible for any given test (3–5).
v. Interactions: GH administration may result in a reduction in both free T_4 and cortisol values; therefore, adjustment of levothyroxine and glucocorticoids may be necessary.
vi. Oral estrogens in women may lead to a state of relative GH resistance, and the GH dose may need to be increased if oral estrogens are initiated, and likewise reduced if oral estrogens are removed.

5. Central DI
Caused by inadequate secretion of ADH.

Diagnosis
i. Determination of polyuria: >3.5 L/d in a person weighing 70 kg.
ii. Simultaneous measurement of serum and urine osmolarity, with finding of relatively dilute urine compared with serum osmolality, especially in the setting of dehydration.
iii. Of note, DI can be unmasked by initiation of steroids in patients with AI.

II. Approach to a Patient Undergoing Pituitary Surgery
Hypopituitarism may occur in the setting of a pituitary adenoma or result from the associated surgical and radiation treatments. Surgery may lead to pituitary axis recovery or dysfunction. Surgery for any form of sellar mass may lead to pituitary

dysfunction. Transsphenoidal surgery has traditionally been performed using the microscopic method, but has been increasingly performed using an endonasal endoscopic technique, often with both a neurosurgeon and an otolaryngologist present. There are insufficient data on whether the different techniques have different impacts on pituitary function. Either way, it is imperative that pituitary function is monitored and that deficiency is replaced appropriately, both during and after pituitary surgery. The hormones monitored mostly closely during and immediately after surgery are cortisol and ADH, because AI and sodium derangements must be closely assessed peri- and postoperatively (6, 7). In general, thyroid, GH, and gonadal axes may be measured 6 weeks or longer after surgery.

a. Preoperative Evaluation
A thorough evaluation is necessary to determine whether hormone replacement should be administered before and during surgery.

i. Baseline Endocrine Testing
1. Assessment of hypercortisolism and acromegaly.
2. Prolactin level to rule out prolactinoma. Prolactin in serial dilution can rule out interference by the hook effect in the setting of a macroadenoma.
3. Hypofunction
   a. If AI, then glucocorticoids should be administered preoperatively and stress-dose steroids given during surgery.
   b. DI is usually not caused by pituitary adenomas, but may be present with cystic sellar masses, neoplastic diseases, or infiltrative diseases. If DI is present, DDAVP may be started preoperatively with judicious use of isotonic intraoperative fluids and close monitoring of urine output.
   c. Hypothyroidism: If mild, replacement is not necessary and surgery does not need to be postponed, because there is no clear evidence for major associated adverse outcomes. For moderate hypothyroidism, surgery should be performed if there is urgency, such as in the setting of local mass effects. If elective, then thyroid hormone replacement should be initiated first and appropriate free T_4 levels achieved. For severe hypothyroidism, levothyroxine therapy should be initiated before surgery, although this decision will be dictated by urgency for neurosurgical intervention. Assessment of the adrenal axis and treatment of coexisting AI should always precede thyroid hormone replacement to avoid precipitation of adrenal crisis.
   d. Gonadal insufficiency and GHD do not need replacement before surgery and should not be assessed in the acute setting.

b. Peri- and Postoperative Management

    i. If the patient has AI preoperatively, then appropriate stress doses of steroids should be administered during surgery, with postoperative taper and reassessment of adrenal function.

    ii. If the patient has normal adrenal function preoperatively, an individualized approach can be taken. In some centers, steroids are administered to all subjects to cover for possible AI, with subsequent assessment of adrenal reserve following taper. In other centers, steroids are withheld during surgery and postoperatively, and morning cortisol levels are measured and postoperative steroids instituted if the serum cortisol is <5 μg/dL, or if it is between 5 and 10 μg/dL and there are symptoms of AI. This method has been shown to be safe and can reduce unnecessary steroid management in approximately half of subjects (6).

    iii. Some centers perform routine outpatient sodium monitoring in the first 2 postoperative weeks to monitor for the development of hyponatremia with syndrome of inappropriate antidiuretic hormone secretion (SIADH). The onset of DI is generally clinically apparent, because patients report substantial polyuria, polydipsia, and thirst.

    iv. DDAVP is administered using either subcutaneous aqueous or oral dosing as needed for DI, without prescheduled dosing given the risk of potentiation of hyponatremia with SIADH several days later (part of the triphasic response).

    v. Pituitary axes should be retested starting at 6 weeks postoperative.

c. Management of Chronic Hypopituitarism

    i. Patients with AI should be counseled on use of a medical alert bracelet and stress-dose steroid instructions for illness and procedures.

    ii. Patients with central hypothyroidism should be instructed that levothyroxine may be erroneously down titrated based on a low TSH level. Because levothyroxine should be titrated to maintain a normal free T_4 value, we recommend that patients contact their endocrinologists for input regarding any proposed change to thyroid hormone replacement dosing.

    iii. Patients with central hypogonadism should be started on gonadal replacement unless contraindicated.

        1. In men with hypogonadism, testosterone can be replaced using injections, gels, patches, and longer-term implantable pellets. Safety monitoring includes routine prostate-specific antigen and hematocrit measurements per Endocrine Society Guidelines (2).

        2. Premenopausal women with an intact uterus require combined hormone replacement with both estrogen and progesterone. Of note, oral estrogen will falsely elevate total cortisol levels and affect any ongoing reassessment of the adrenal axis.

    iv. Adult GHD should be treated in the absence of contraindications, such as history of malignancy or considerable glucose intolerance. IGF-1 levels should be titrated to the age-appropriate normal range, per Endocrine Society Guidelines (5).

III. Management of Patients With TBI

Hypopituitarism occurs following both penetrating and blunt head trauma in approximately 25% of subjects, with a range from 15% to 68% of subjects. The pathophysiology of hypopituitarism in patients with TBI includes direct injury to the gland, vasospasm of the hypothalamo-hypophyseal blood supply, and compression of the hypothalamus and pituitary gland by edema, hemorrhage, or elevated intracranial pressure (8). Genetic factors, including certain apolipoprotein E haplotypes, may affect this risk. Also, there are studies showing that antipituitary and antihypothalamic antibodies are found in patients with TBI, although the pathogenic role is unclear. Autopsy series have shown necrotic glands in up to 80% of fatal cases. GHD is the most common deficiency found, and this has critical implications because GHD may have an impact on full convalescence.

All patients with moderate to severe TBI should be evaluated for hypopituitarism during the acute and chronic course of their recovery (9). Immediately following the TBI, emphasis on care during the first 2 weeks post-TBI should be on the adrenal axis and posterior pituitary function. The adrenal axis must be assessed by random cortisol levels in the setting of recent TBI, because cosyntropin stimulation testing will be falsely reassuring in the setting of acute central AI. In the months after injury, the entire anterior and posterior pituitary hormonal axes should be assessed. In addition, symptomatic patients with mild TBI (including those with repetitive mild TBI) and impaired quality of life are also at risk for hypopituitarism and should be considered for neuroendocrine testing.

Testing for chronic hypopituitarism following TBI is usually performed at least 6 to 12 months after the event. Hormone replacement should be administered accordingly (10).

MAIN CONCLUSIONS

    1. Evaluation of pituitary function following pituitary surgery should be performed using a step-wise approach that incorporates preoperative function data with postoperative management. This approach involves assessment of individual pituitary hormones in a temporal fashion following surgery. GHD and central hypogonadism can be treated after 6-week postoperative hormone reassessment.

    2. TBI is associated with hypopituitarism, and assessment and treatment should be performed both immediately and at least 6 months after the event.

Case 1

A 28-year-old man with hypopituitarism has been doing well following surgery for craniopharyngioma 5 years earlier. However, at the current visit, he describes having experienced 2 months of progressive fatigue. He admits cold intolerance and constipation. His internist had recently noted a low TSH level and reduced the levothyroxine dose. Current medications include oral levothyroxine 50 μg daily, oral hydrocortisone 15 mg daily, depot testosterone 200 mg IM every 2 weeks, and oral DDAVP 0.3 mg three times per day.

His laboratory results were as follows: TSH 0.09 uIU/mL (normal, 0.45 to 4.5 uIU/mL), free T_4 0.7 ng/dL (normal, 0.9 to 1.8 ng/dL), serum testosterone 295 ng/dL (normal, 250 to 840 ng/dL), and IGF-1 87 ng/mL (age-appropriate normal, 63 to 373 ng/mL).

Question 1

What should be the first step to improve his energy?
- A. Perform glucagon stimulation test to determine if he has GHD
- B. Increase levothyroxine to target a normal free T_4 level
- C. Raise the glucocorticoid dose
- D. Increase the testosterone IM dose

Answer: B

Case 2

A 33-year-old woman has hypopituitarism following surgery and received radiation therapy for a nonfunctioning pituitary macroadenoma 8 years earlier. She has been taking GH replacement therapy at a dose of 1.2 mg subcutaneous injection daily and has been tolerating it well. She has noted improvements in energy, memory capacity, and exercise tolerance with the GH replacement. She also takes levothyroxine 125 μg and hydrocortisone 15 mg daily. She has amenorrhea, and upon the recommendation of her gynecologist, she started taking an OCP for estrogen replacement approximately 8 weeks ago. Over the past month, she notes progressive fatigue and weight gain.

Question 2

What is the likely cause of her fatigue?
- A. Excessive hydrocortisone dosing
- B. Inadequate estradiol dosage in the OCP
- C. Relative GH resistance due to oral estrogen
- D. Progressive hypothyroidism

Answer: C

Case 3

A 34-year-old woman has been diagnosed with a 2.5-cm clinically nonfunctioning pituitary macroadenoma that has caused chiasmal compression. She is being scheduled for surgery. Her history is notable for oligomenorrhea and bilateral galactorrhea, but is otherwise adequate. She underwent testing, with the following results: prolactin 43 ng/mL (normal, <25 ng/mL), TSH 2.1 uIU/mL (normal, 0.45 to 4.5 uIU/mL), free T_4 1.2 ng/dL (normal, 0.9 to 1.8 ng/dL), LH 6 IU/L, FSH 30 IU/L, IGF-1 87 ng/mL (age-appropriate normal, 53 to 331 ng/mL), cosyntropin stimulation test (250 μg), and peak cortisol 25 μg/dL (normal, >18 μg/dL). The patient underwent surgery. On postoperative day 1, she had polyuria and polydipsia, nocturia (five times), and a sodium level of 154 mEq/L.

Question 3

Which of the following management options should be used for treating the DI?
- A. DDAVP scheduled dosing, one spray intranasally twice daily
- B. Dehydration test
- C. 1 L fluid restriction
- D. DDAVP 0.1 to 0.2 mg orally, as needed

Answer: D

Case 4

A 28-year-old man initially presented to the intensive care unit (ICU) after suffering severe head trauma during a motor vehicle accident. He was in a coma for 10 days with cerebral edema and a small cerebral hemorrhage on imaging. He had DI that was managed with intermittent subcutaneous DDAVP doses as needed for breakthrough polyuria and sodium elevations. Random cortisol of 24 μg/dL (normal, >18 μg/dL) proved adrenal sufficiency while he was in the ICU. The DI was transient, and no DDAVP was required by the end of the patient's ICU stay. He did well and was transferred to a rehabilitation facility. He has since undergone inpatient and outpatient physical rehabilitation. He returned to see the physician approximately 6 months after the initial accident. He denied having polyuria and polydipsia. Because of fatigue, he had been placed on Provigil. He was referred to an endocrinologist, and the following laboratory results were noted: TSH 1.4 uIU/mL (normal, 0.45 to 4.5 uIU/mL), free T_4 1.0 ng/dL (normal, 0.9 to 1.8 ng/dL), serum testosterone 130 ng/dL (normal, 250 to 840 ng/dL), IGF-1 65 ng/mL (age-appropriate normal, 63 to 373 ng/mL), cosyntropin stimulation test (250 μg), and peak cortisol 25 μg/dL (normal, >18 μg/dL).

Question 4

Which of the following tests should be performed next?
- A. Morning plasma cortisol
- B. Glucagon stimulation test
- C. Reverse T_3
- D. Plasma ADH

Answer: B

Case 4 (Continued)

Following a glucagon stimulation test with a peak GH level of 0.5 ng/mL (goal, >3 ng/mL), GHD was diagnosed and GH replacement was initiated. The patient's testosterone level was confirmed to be low on a second morning sample, and a transdermal testosterone gel was initiated at two pumps daily. There was an overall improvement in energy and vitality. However, he continued to have chronic pain. He returned to see his physician 1 year after the TBI. He had been taking escalating doses of short- and long-acting opiates for his accident-related pain and reported substantial fatigue, arthralgias, and occasional dizziness on standing. His testosterone and GH levels on replacement were checked. Results were as follows: serum testosterone 300 ng/dL (normal, 250 to 840 ng/dL) and IGF-1 275 ng/mL (age-appropriate normal, 53 to 331 ng/mL).

Question 5

What is the next step in this patient's plan of care?

    A. Increase testosterone replacement

    B. Increase GH replacement

    C. Retest thyroid axis

    D. Perform a cosyntropin stimulation test

Answer: D

A cosyntropin stimulation test (250 μg) was performed, and the peak cortisol level was 8 μg/dL (normal, >18 μg/dL). Prednisone 4 mg was initiated, and the patient was instructed to obtain a medical alert bracelet. He was provided with printed stress-dose steroid instructions. The patient called his doctor 1 week later, and although he was feeling significantly better, he noted that he had developed polyuria and polydipsia that was affecting his ability to sleep. A morning sodium level was 146 mEq/L (normal, 135 to 145 mEq/L) with urine osmolarity of 250 mOsm/kg (expected, >600 mOsm/kg).

Question 6

What is the cause of the patient's new-onset polyuria and polydipsia?

    A. Initiation of levothyroxine

    B. Initiation of prednisone

    C. Initiation of testosterone

    D. New-onset DI from motor vehicle accident 12 months earlier

Answer: B

DISCUSSION OF CASES AND ANSWERS

Question 1

In patients with central hypothyroidism, the replacement dose of levothyroxine should target a normal free T_4 level. The TSH value is not useful in determining adequacy of the replacement dose, because TSH levels are usually suppressed in the setting of pituitary insufficiency. Therefore, the appropriate first step would be to increase the levothyroxine dose with the goal of targeting a mid-normal free T_4 value. The patient probably had GHD, and it would be appropriate to evaluate this as a next step. The glucocorticoid dose was

adequate and was not the problem in this case. His testosterone dose was likewise adequate and did not need to be addressed.

Question 2

This patient had been feeling well, and then developed more fatigue following initiation of an oral contraceptive agent. Oral estrogen treatment causes a relative resistance to GH effect, resulting in a reduction in serum IGF-1. In women with GHD, oral estrogens may lead to the need for a GH replacement dose up to 50% higher compared with women or men who are not receiving estrogen. Of note, this effect does not occur with transdermally administered estrogen.

Question 3

If a patient has early postoperative central DI, then DDAVP should be administered (either by subcutaneous injection or oral tablets) on an as needed basis. The concern is that overdosing of DDAVP may exaggerate hyponatremia, particularly if SIADH kicks in a few days later as part of the triphasic response. Therefore, scheduled DDAVP dosing should not be administered at this time. A dehydration test is important for evaluating DI in a patient with polyuria but is not useful for a patient in this clinical setting, where the risk of DI is relatively high. Fluid restriction is part of the management of SIADH, not DI.

Question 4

This patient had history of a TBI and was at risk for hypopituitarism. He had evidence of a low serum testosterone level, as well as a very low IGF-1 level. GHD is the most common deficient pituitary axis, and the low IGF-1 level is suggestive of this diagnosis. A provocative test, such as a glucagon stimulation test, should be performed as the next step to confirm this diagnosis. The cosyntropin stimulation test was normal, so there was no need to obtain an additional cortisol level. The thyroid tests were sufficient, and there was no benefit to obtaining a reverse T_3 value in this case. Plasma ADH was not useful. In this case, there was no clinical evidence to support DI, so that did not add to the diagnosis.

Question 5

Per question 4, in the case of this patient with a TBI, there was evidence of hypogonadism and GHD due to the TBI. Although he initially felt better upon receiving testosterone and GH replacement, he reported having continued fatigue, arthralgias, and orthostasis, suggesting AI. He had been receiving increasing doses of opiates for chronic pain, which can lead to central AI. In addition, because GH suppresses the conversion of cortisone to cortisol, patients may become relatively hypoadrenal while taking GH. Thus, assessment should be performed for new-onset AI. Therefore, a cosyntropin stimulation test should be performed. The testosterone replacement could be increased concurrently in this patient, although this was not the cause of his current symptoms. Likewise, increasing the GH dose would not address these symptoms.

Question 6

This patient had extensive polyuria and hypernatremia requiring treatment with DDAVP while unconscious in the ICU immediately after his acute TBI. However, his DI seemed transient and resolved before discharge from the ICU. He did not report notable polyuria and polydipsia before hormone replacement for his panhypopituitarism. However, AI impairs excretion of free water; thus the initiation of glucocorticoids for AI can unmask DI. The other hormone replacements are not expected to affect free water excretion. DI is most severe immediately after the TBI and is not expected to worsen 12 months after the acute event.

References

1. Fleseriu M, Hashim IA, Karavitaki N, Melmed S, Murad MH, Salvatori R, Samuels MH. Hormonal replacement in hypopituitarism in adults: an Endocrine Society clinical practice guideline. *J Clin Endocrinol Metab.* 2016;**101**(11):3888–3921.
2. Bhasin S, Brito JP, Cunningham GR, Hayes FJ, Hodis HN, Matsumoto AM, Snyder PJ, Swerdloff RS, Wu FC, Yialamas MA. Testosterone therapy in men with hypogonadism: an Endocrine Society clinical practice guideline. *J Clin Endocrinol Metab.* 2018;**103**(5): 1715–1744.
3. Dichtel LE, Yuen KC, Bredella MA, Gerweck AV, Russell BM, Riccio AD, Gurel MH, Sluss PM, Biller BM, Miller KK. Overweight/obese adults with pituitary disorders require lower peak growth hormone cutoff values on glucagon stimulation testing to avoid overdiagnosis of growth hormone deficiency. *J Clin Endocrinol Metab.* 2014;**99**(12): 4712–4719.
4. Hamrahian AH, Yuen KC, Gordon MB, Pulaski-Liebert KJ, Bena J, Biller BM. Revised GH and cortisol cut-points for the glucagon stimulation test in the evaluation of GH and hypothalamic-pituitary-adrenal axes in adults: results from a prospective randomized multicenter study. *Pituitary.* 2016;**19**(3):332–341.
5. Molitch ME, Clemmons DR, Malozowski S, Merriam GR, Vance ML; Endocrine Society. Evaluation and treatment of adult growth hormone deficiency: an Endocrine Society clinical practice guideline. *J Clin Endocrinol Metab.* 2011;**96**(6):1587–1609.
6. Jia X, Pendharkar AV, Loftus P, Dodd RL, Chu O, Fraenkel M, Katznelson L. Utility of a glucocorticoid sparing strategy in the management of patients following transsphenoidal surgery. *Endocr Pract.* 2016;**22**(9):1033–1039.
7. Woodmansee WW, Carmichael J, Kelly D, Katznelson L; AACE Neuroendocrine and Pituitary Scientific Committee. Article I. American Association of Clinical Endocrinologists and American College of Endocrinology disease state clinical review: postoperative management following pituitary surgery. *Endocr Pract.* 2015;**21**(7):832–838.
8. Tritos NA, Yuen KC, Kelly DF; AACE Neuroendocrine and Pituitary Scientific Committee. Article I. American Association of Clinical Endocrinologists and American College of Endocrinology disease state clinical review: a neuroendocrine approach to patients with traumatic brain injury. *Endocr Pract.* 2015;**21**(7):823–831.
9. Klose M, Feldt-Rasmussen U. Chronic endocrine consequences of traumatic brain injury—what is the evidence? *Nat Rev Endocrinol.* 2018;**14**(1):57–62.
10. Giuliano S, Talarico S, Bruno L, Nicoletti FB, Ceccotti C, Belfiore A. Growth hormone deficiency and hypopituitarism in adults after complicated mild traumatic brain injury. *Endocrine.* 2017;**58**(1): 115–123.

Optimizing Clinical Management of Patients With Acromegaly

M44
Presented, March 23–26, 2019

Andrea Giustina, MD. Endocrinology, Università Vita-Salute San Raffaele, 20132 Milan, Italy; and Division of Endocrinology, IRCCS San Raffaele Hospital, 20132 Milan, Italy, E-mail: giustina.andrea@hsr.it

SIGNIFICANCE OF THE PROBLEM

Acromegaly is a chronic disorder characterized by growth hormone (GH) hypersecretion and consequently high levels of insulin-like growth factor-I (IGF-I), caused by a pituitary adenoma in a majority of the cases (>98%) (1). GH-secreting pituitary adenoma is still considered a rare disease, even if recent findings suggested an increasing prevalence and incidence, reported to be between 2.8 and 13.7 cases per 100,000 people and between 0.2 and 1.1 cases per 100,000 people per year, respectively (2).

Acral and soft tissue overgrowth, particularly of hands, feet, and face, is a pathognomonic feature of acromegaly. However, the quality of life as well as survival of affected patients is conditioned by the systemic complications of the disease, because GH excess may negatively affect many organs and tissues (3). In fact, as a result of the persistently delayed diagnosis of acromegaly (2), patients may already present with vertebral fractures at diagnosis because of a specific osteopathy (4), ventricular hypertrophy and hypertension (3), sleep apnea (5), or obstructive and restrictive lung diseases and several metabolic dysfunctions, such as dyslipidemia, insulin resistance, and diabetes mellitus, which are related to an increased risk of cardiovascular events (6). Acromegaly patients have also been reported to be at increased risk of cancer (7). Moreover, taking into account the frequent diagnostic delay, acromegaly patients in a large majority of cases present at diagnosis with a pituitary macroadenoma. Therefore, they may also experience tumor mass effects, such as headache, visual disturbance from optic chiasm compression, and cranial nerve palsy (8). In addition, they may present with early signs and symptoms of hypopituitarism, particularly hypogonadism (3).

Therefore, effective treatment of the disease is crucial to improve quality of life (9) and increase survival (10) of the patients. However, management of acromegaly and the comorbidities of the disorder is complex and requires a comprehensive and coordinated approach by a multidisciplinary team (MDT) of physician experts in the treatment of pituitary adenomas, aimed mainly but not only at normalizing GH and IGF-I levels (3).

BARRIERS TO OPTIMAL PRACTICE

- The need to integrate new treatment options into the therapeutic algorithm of acromegaly
- The need to implement treatment guidelines into clinical practice
- The need to consider the whole clinical picture (not only biochemical parameters) in the therapeutic decision making process

LEARNING OBJECIVES

As a result of participating in this session, learners should be able to:

- Summarize the available medical treatments for patients with acromegaly
- Identify clinical features that may guide treatment choices in patients with acromegaly
- Identify how new treatment guidelines of acromegaly may help clinicians in optimizing management of their patients

THERAPEUTIC APPROACH TO ACROMEGALY

In a majority of patients with acromegaly, the first therapeutic choice is transsphenoidal surgery (11), which is the only therapeutic option potentially leading, in the hands of an experienced neurosurgeon, to a rapid cure of acromegaly by removing a GH-secreting adenoma (12). However, persistent GH hypersecretion after neurosurgery may be observed in >15% and 50% of patients harboring micro- and macro-adenomas, respectively (13, 14).

In these latter patients, medical therapy, particularly first-generation somatostatin receptor ligands (SRLs; *i.e.*, octreotide and lanreotide, which mainly interact with subtype 2 of the somatostatin receptor), plays a key role in the management of acromegaly. In fact, besides the effects on GH hypersecretion, octreotide LAR and lanreotide ATG were shown to be effective in determining the shrinkage of a pituitary adenoma (15). It is noteworthy that clinical pivotal trials provided discrepant data, as compared with observational studies in nonselected cohorts of patients, on efficacy of SRLs; 25% to 60% of patients treated with first-generation SRLs achieved safe levels of GH and age- and sex-normalized IGF-I levels (16).

Defining and adequately treating patients resistant to conventional SRLs are major challenges in the management of patients with acromegaly. Interestingly, there are emerging data concerning the safety and efficacy of the GH antagonist pegvisomant from large real-life observational studies, reporting biochemical control of acromegaly in approximately two thirds of patients (17). Moreover, pasireotide, a novel SRL with a broader spectrum of affinity for the somatostatin receptor (mainly subtypes 2 and 5), has recently become available on the market (18). These recent developments are great advancements, because they offer more options to better personalize the clinical approach; however, they may paradoxically complicate management, because criteria for prioritizing this therapeutic choice are still not universally accepted. In August 2018, an updated consensus statement was published (19) to tackle the emerging challenges in the medical treatment of acromegaly and optimize and harmonize clinical management of the disease. The following case-based discussion will focus on optimization of the clinical management of acromegaly patients, whose disease is not adequately controlled by conventional SRLs based on the conclusions of this consensus statement (19).

CASES WITH QUESTIONS AND ANSWERS
Case 1
S.F. was a 22-year-old woman who was referred to a local general hospital by a private practice gynecologist because of oligomenorrhea (menses every 80 to 90 days), obesity, and headache nonresponsive to common analgesics. At presentation, she also reported increased perspiration, and she had typical signs of acromegaly (acral growth, acromegaloid facie, and macroglossia).

Table 1 lists the baseline biochemical data of the patient. The pituitary MRI reported an invasive giant pituitary adenoma (maximal diameter, 4.2 cm) infiltrating the temporal lobe and encasing the whole cavernous sinus and its structures. The patient was referred to a specialized regional hospital in which a Pituitary Tumor Center of Excellence (PTCOE) was operating (20). The case was discussed at the joint endocrine-neurosurgical meeting.

Question 1
What was decided as the next step?
   A. Surgery
   B. Medical treatment with conventional SRLs

Table 1. Baseline Biochemical Data in Case 1

Characteristic	No.
Random GH, ng/mL	18.7
GH nadir during OGTT, ng/mL	12.3
IGF-I, ng/mL	956
Normal range	80–230
LH, UI/L	<0.4
FSH, UI/L	<0.4
E2, pg/mL	<5
TSH, mUI/L	0.35
Free T_4, pg/mL	8.9
Normal range	8–17
Free T_3, pg/mL	2.1
Normal range	2–4.35
ACTH, pg/mL	9
Morning serum cortisol, mg/dL	10.9
Fasting blood glucose, mg/dL	102
Serum insulin, mUI/L	12.3

Abbreviation: OGTT, oral glucose tolerance test.

   C. Medical treatment with pegvisomant
   D. Radiosurgery

Answer A
Preoperative medical treatment with octreotide at 30 mg monthly was considered in this case because of the low probability of cure through a surgical approach, as suggested by international guidelines and clinical trials (16, 21, 22).

After 6 months, there was a mild reduction of biochemical parameters of somatotropic axis activity (random GH, 14.1 ng/mL; IGF-I, 764 ng/mL), and a 10% shrinkage was reported on MRI (maximal diameter, 3.8 cm); improvements in headache and persistent amenorrhea were also noted. Therefore, the decision of the MDT was to send the patient to the neurosurgeon for a debulking procedure, which may also improve subsequent response to SRLs (23). S.F. underwent pituitary surgery that was not able to resolve GH hypersecretion, as expected. Considering the young age and symptoms of the patient, she continued octreotide at incremental doses (40 mg monthly) and estrogens (24).

Six months later, the patient still presented with active disease but with a better biochemical profile as compared with presurgical treatment [GH, 4.5 ng/mL; IGF-I, 431 ng/mL; normal glycemic control (fasting blood glucose, 96 mg/dL)]. Neither the adenoma nor the surgical procedure negatively influenced other pituitary axes, except for gonadal function. The residual pituitary adenoma was stable on successive MRI controls (maximal diameter, 2 cm), confirming the encasement of the carotid artery.

Question 2
What was the decision of the MDT?
   A. No change in treatment
   B. Reoperation
   C. Switch to pasireotide
   D. Switch to pegvisomant

Answer C
A recently published consensus paper (19) recommended that patients not controlled by high-dose SRLs and with clinically relevant residual tumor mass should be switched to pasireotide LAR. Pasireotide targets four of five somatostatin receptor subtypes, with higher affinity for somatostatin receptor subtypes 2 and 5, which are widely expressed by pituitary adenoma cells (25). In a phase 3 study, a significantly greater number of patients experienced biochemical control when treated with pasireotide LAR vs octreotide LAR (26). Recent findings also suggest that pasireotide LAR may have a similar or even greater shrinkage effect on the GH-secreting adenoma as compared with conventional SRLs (27).

As suggested by a study enrolling healthy volunteers, pasireotide may cause hyperglycemia through a significant reduction in insulin and incretin secretion, with no effect on insulin resistance (28). In fact, the most serious and peculiar adverse effect of pasireotide is hyperglycemia, and all patients receiving this treatment should be closely monitored for possible blood glucose derangement. However, as reported by Schmid *et al.* in a posthoc analysis of the PAOLA trial (29), patients at high risk of developing relevant worsening of blood glucose metabolism are those (~30% of acromegaly patients at diagnosis) with preexisting diabetes mellitus.

We switched our patient to pasireotide at 40 mg monthly via IM injection.

Question 3

Which safety biochemical parameters should be more carefully monitored during pasireotide vs conventional SRL treatment?

A. Glucose metabolism
B. Liver enzyme
C. Bilirubin
D. Creatine kinase

Answer A

Fasting blood glucose initially slightly increased (7 days, 104 mg/dL; 14 days, 107 mg/dL) but remained stable thereafter (28 days, 105 mg/dL); GH and IGF-I had already decreased at the 3-month follow-up visit (2.8 and 325 ng/mL, respectively) and then normalized at the 6-month visit (0.9 and 238 ng/mL, respectively). Pituitary MRI showed a decrease by 30% in maximal diameter to 1.4 cm, without additional changes in fasting blood glucose. Therefore, as shown in previous studies, pasireotide may control acromegaly in ~20% of patients resistant to octreotide or lanreotide as reported by Gadehla *et al.* (27). In the same report, a further shrinkage effect of pasireotide as compared with conventional SRLs was reported.

Case 2

L.A. was a 54-year-old man who was referred to the endocrine unit of a general hospital by the hospital pneumologist because of persistent sleep apnea and feet and hand enlargement. The patient was obese [body mass index (BMI), 31 kg/m^2] and had diabetes mellitus, for which he was receiving metformin plus repaglinide treatment, and arterial hypertension. Oral glucose tolerance test was not performed because of the baseline diabetic status (30).

Table 2 lists the baseline biochemical data of the patient. Pituitary MRI showed a pituitary macroadenoma (maximal diameter, 1.5 cm) with minimal extrasellar extension and without optic chiasm compression as shown by absence of alterations at campimetric evaluations.

L.A. was referred to the regional PTCOE for the therapeutic decision.

Question 1

What was decided as the next step?

A. Surgery

Table 2. Baseline Biochemical Data in Case 2

Characteristic	No.
Random GH, ng/mL	24.7
IGF-I, ng/mL	778
Normal range	150–320
LH, UI/L	<0.4
FSH, UI/L	<0.4
Total testosterone, ng/dL	2.8
TSH, mUI/L	1.35
Free T$_4$, pg/mL	9.9
Normal range	8-17
Free T$_3$, pg/mL	2.7
Normal range	2–4.35
ACTH, pg/mL	29
Morning serum cortisol, μg/dL	12
Fasting blood glucose, mg/dL	202
Serum HbA$_{1c}$, %	7.8

Abbreviation: HbA$_{1c}$, hemoglobin A$_{1c}$.

B. Medical treatment with conventional SRLs
C. Medical treatment with pegvisomant
D. Radiosurgery

Answer A

The MDT decided on pituitary surgery, which according to published results (13) may offer a relevant chance to definitively cure the disease at this stage. The patient underwent pituitary surgery that seemed successful in entirely removing the adenoma. However, GH and IGF-I levels at discharge were 8.7 and 688 ng/mL, respectively. Three months after surgery, biochemical data were stable, and MRI was negative for residual tumor. The patient was started on lanreotide ATG at 120 mg every 28 days. After 6 months, GH was 8.3 ng/mL and

Table 3. Baseline Biochemical Data in Case 3

Characteristic	No.
Random GH, ng/mL	14.7
IGF-I, ng/mL	1078
Normal range	54–185
LH, UI/L	14
FSH, UI/L	24
TSH, mUI/L	0.95
Free T$_4$, pg/mL	7.9
Normal range	8-17
Free T$_3$, pg/mL	2.0
Normal range	2–4.35
ACTH, pg/mL	12
Morning serum cortisol, μg/dL	10
24-hour urinary cortisol, μg/dL	20
Fasting blood glucose, mg/dL	222
HbA$_{1c}$, %	8.1

IGF-I was 660 ng/mL. The patient had a slight improvement in sleep apnea but not remission, as expected based on literature findings (5). Serum hemoglobin A$_{1c}$ (HbA$_{1c}$) was slightly worse (8.2%). Lanreotide ATG dose was increased to 180 mg/d (31). Six months later, GH was 7.3 ng/mL and IGF-I was 580 ng/ml. Blood glucose and sleep apnea were stable. The patient was reevaluated at the weekly meeting of the MDT.

Question 2
What did the MDT decide as the next step?
   A. No change in treatment
   B. Reoperation
   C. Switch to pasireotide
   D. Switch to pegvisomant

Answer D
A recently published consensus article (19) advised for a switch to pegvisomant in acromegaly patients with diabetes mellitus whose disease is not controlled by SRLs. In fact, as shown in clinical trials, pegvisomant can control acromegaly in most patients (32, 33). Moreover, improvement in blood glucose control during pegvisomant treatment is often observed (34). This likely happens because of an improvement in IGF-I levels (35), whereas with pasireotide, a worsening of glucose metabolism may occur, particularly in those patients with pre-existing diabetes (29). Therefore, lanreotide was stopped, and pegvisomant at 10 mg/d was started. After 1 month, fasting blood glucose slightly decreased (164 mg/dL), with normal serum hepatic enzymes. Because pegvisomant can cross-react with routine GH assays (34), we biochemically followed acromegaly only with IGF-I assay (31). After 3 months, IGF-I (315 ng/mL) and HbA$_{1c}$ (7%) were decreased. Pegvisomant dose was increased to 15 mg/d, and after 6 months, IGF-I was controlled (228 ng/mL). Blood glucose control was further improved (HbA$_{1c}$, 6.6%), and repaglinide was stopped.

Question 3
Which parameters should be monitored during pegvisomant therapy?
   A. Pituitary MRI
   B. Liver enzymes
   C. Comorbidities
   D. Creatine kinase

Answers A, B, and C
Efficacy of pegvisomant may be relatively limited in clinical practice (17) by intolerance, adverse effects, and reluctance to increase doses (36). One possible concern regarding pegvisomant use is tumor remnant enlargement, although this according to most recent observational studies (37) occurs rarely and prevalently because of the natural history of the disease. Moreover, in a small proportion of treated patients, an increase in liver enzymes has been reported, which has rarely been relevant enough to lead to stopping treatment (37).

Finally, pegvisomant has been shown to improve several complications of acromegaly, particularly ventricular hypertrophy and sleep apnea (36), which may be linked to an increased risk of death.

In our patient, subcutaneous injections of pegvisomant were well tolerated. Pituitary MRI and hepatic enzymes were persistently negative, and sleep apnea was in remission.

Case 3
S.D. was a 74-year-old woman who was referred to a private practice endocrinologist by the bone unit of a regional orthopedic and traumatologic hospital, where the patient was followed for a postmenopausal osteopenia. Multiple morphometric vertebral fractures were found at dual energy x-ray absorptiometry (DXA), with a bone density T score of −2.6 DS at lumbar spine and −0.9 DS at total hip. The patient had undergone in the same hospital bilateral carpal tunnel syndrome surgery and underwent surgery 7 years ago for an *in situ* breast cancer. She had acromegalic facies and enlarged hands. She had normal weight (BMI, 23 kg/m^2) and had diabetes mellitus, for which she was receiving insulin treatment. Oral glucose tolerance test was not performed because of the baseline diabetic status (30).

Pituitary function was slightly reduced, and supplementation with low doses of L-thyroxine and cortisone acetate was started. Pituitary MRI reported a pituitary macroadenoma (maximal diameter, 2.5 cm) with upper growth and contact with the optic chiasm in the presence of modest alterations at campimetric evaluations (quadrantopsia).

S.D. was sent to the PTCOE of the regional hospital.

Question 1
What was the therapeutic decision of the MDT?
   A. Surgery
   B. Medical treatment with SRLs
   C. Medical treatment with pegvisomant
   D. Radiosurgery

Answer A
The patient underwent pituitary surgery, which was not successful in entirely removing the adenoma, but remission of the campimetric alterations was achieved. GH at discharge was 7.7 ng/mL. Three months after surgery, GH levels were stable, and IGF-I was 898 ng/mL. MRI showed a reduced pituitary mass with modest extrasellar extension with no contact with the optic chiasm (maximal diameter, 1.4 cm). The patient was started on octreotide LAR at 30 mg every 28 days. After 6 months, GH was 3.3 ng/mL and IGF-I was 420 ng/mL. Serum HbA$_{1c}$ was worse (8.8%). Further reduction in pituitary tumor size was observed (maximal diameter, 1.2 cm). The case was reassessed by the MDT.

Question 2
What was the next step decided by the MDT?
   A. No change of treatment
   B. Reoperation

C. Add pegvisomant

D. Switch to pasireotide

Answer C

A recently published consensus article (19) advised continuing conventional SRL treatment when the tumor represents a clinical concern, because SRLs have a consistent shrinkage effect on the residual mass (38) without generally serious negative effects on glucose metabolism (39), and adding pegvisomant, which does not have any effect at the pituitary tumor level but may allow better biochemical control (17, 19). Therefore, octreotide was continued, and pegvisomant at 10 mg/d was added. After 1 month, fasting blood glucose had slightly decreased (204 mg/dL), with normal serum hepatic enzymes. Subcutaneous injections were well tolerated. Because pegvisomant can cross-react with routine GH assays (34), we biochemically followed acromegaly only with IGF-I assay. After 3 months, IGF-I (190 ng/mL) was normalized and HbA$_{1c}$ decreased (7.2%). Insulin dose was reduced, and pituitary MRI was stable. At this point, the MDT decided to send the patient back for consultation with the bone expert of the PTCOE.

Question 3

What type of follow-up will be recommended to the patient for optimal management of skeletal complications?

A. DXA bone mineral density (BMD) measurement

B. Bone markers

C. DXA vertebral morphometry

D. No need for specific follow-up

Answers A and C

Bone metabolic alterations in acromegaly are frequent and often observed at diagnosis of the disease (40), even in the presence of not very low BMD (41). During follow-up of acromegaly, the bone profile may improve in those patients with controlled disease (42), but incident fractures may often occur in well-controlled patients as well (43). In acromegaly, changes in BMD may predict the risk of incident fractures (43). Moreover, because vertebral fractures often occur asymptomatically, proactive follow-up with vertebral morphometry should be put into practice (42). In the patient, BMD on DXA scan performed at the bone unit of the PTCOE had slightly improved at lumbar spine (T score, −2.4 DS), with no evidence of worsening of previous morphometric fractures and no appearance of new vertebral fractures. Therefore, as shown in clinical trials, pegvisomant added to conventional SRLs can improve control of acromegaly patients (36) without risks of tumor growth resulting from the growth control obtained by both octreotide (38) and lanreotide (44).

CONCLUSIONS

New consensus guidelines published in August 2018 (19) are the first available guidelines that integrate the use of the new SRL pasireotide and use of pegvisomant into the second-line medical treatment of acromegaly. Presence of a clinically significant tumor remnant and diabetes mellitus are the two situations that mainly inform the pharmacological choice. New guidelines also recommend that acromegaly patients are optimally managed in PTCOEs, and holistic evaluation of the clinical condition, possibly through ad hoc tools [*i.e.*, SAGIT (Symptoms Associated Comorbidities Growth Hormone IGF-I Tumor)] (45), is recommended to optimize clinical management of acromegaly. Finally, novel tumor biomarkers, such as sparsely vs densely granulated pathologic subtypes, as well as tumor differential somatostatin receptor subtype expression, although not yet included in the guidelines as predictors to response to therapy (46), will probably help in the future refinement of the management of acromegaly, with better personalization of treatment.

Acknowledgments

I thank Prof. Pietro Mortini, neurosurgeon, and Dr. Anna Maria Formenti and Dr. Stefano Frara, endocrinologists, as the members of the MDT in our PTCOE who coauthored this contribution.

References

1. Melmed S. Acromegaly pathogenesis and treatment. *J Clin Invest.* 2009;**119**(11):3189–3202.
2. Lavrentaki A, Paluzzi A, Wass JA, Karavitaki N. Epidemiology of acromegaly: review of population studies. *Pituitary.* 2017;**20**(1):4–9.
3. Melmed S, Casanueva FF, Klibanski A, Bronstein MD, Chanson P, Lamberts SW, Strasburger CJ, Wass JA, Giustina A. A consensus on the diagnosis and treatment of acromegaly complications. *Pituitary.* 2013;**16**(3):294–302.
4. Mazziotti G, Maffezzoni F, Frara S, Giustina A. Acromegalic osteopathy. *Pituitary.* 2017;**20**(1):63–69.
5. Davì MV, Dalle Carbonare L, Giustina A, Ferrari M, Frigo A, Lo Cascio V, Francia G. Sleep apnoea syndrome is highly prevalent in acromegaly and only partially reversible after biochemical control of the disease. *Eur J Endocrinol.* 2008;**159**(5):533–540.
6. Frara S, Maffezzoni F, Mazziotti G, Giustina A. Current and emerging aspects of diabetes mellitus in acromegaly. *Trends Endocrinol Metab.* 2016;**27**(7):470–483.
7. Gadelha MR, Kasuki L, Lim DS, Fleseriu M. Systemic complications of acromegaly and the impact of the current treatment landscape: an update. *Endocr Rev.* 2019;**40**(1):268–322.
8. Melmed S. Medical progress: acromegaly. *N Engl J Med.* 2006; **355**(24):2558–2573.
9. Webb SM, Crespo I, Santos A, Resmini E, Aulinas A, Valassi E. Management of endocrine disease: quality of life tools for the management of pituitary disease. *Eur J Endocrinol.* 2017;**177**(1):R13–R26.
10. Holdaway IM, Bolland MJ, Gamble GD. A meta-analysis of the effect of lowering serum levels of GH and IGF-I on mortality in acromegaly. *Eur J Endocrinol.* 2008;**159**(2):89–95.
11. Melmed S, Colao A, Barkan A, Molitch M, Grossman AB, Kleinberg D, Clemmons D, Chanson P, Laws E, Schlechte J, Vance ML, Ho K, Giustina A; Acromegaly Consensus Group. Guidelines for acromegaly management: an update. *J Clin Endocrinol Metab.* 2009;**94**(5):1509–1517.
12. Abu Dabrh AM, Mohammed K, Asi N, Farah WH, Wang Z, Farah MH, Prokop LJ, Katznelson L, Murad MH. Surgical interventions and medical treatments in treatment-naive patients with acromegaly: systematic review and meta-analysis. *J Clin Endocrinol Metab.* 2014;**99**(11):4003–4014.
13. Mortini P, Barzaghi LR, Albano L, Panni P, Losa M. Microsurgical therapy of pituitary adenomas. *Endocrine.* 2018;**59**(1):72–81.
14. Babu H, Ortega A, Nuno M, Dehghan A, Schweitzer A, Bonert HV, Carmichael JD, Cooper O, Melmed S, Mamelak AN. Long-term endocrine outcomes following endoscopic endonasal transsphenoidal surgery for acromegaly and associated prognostic factors. *Neurosurgery.* 2017;**81**(2):357–366.

15. Maffezzoni F, Formenti AM, Mazziotti G, Frara S, Giustina A. Current and future medical treatments for patients with acromegaly. *Expert Opin Pharmacother.* 2016;**17**(12):1631–1642.

16. Giustina A, Chanson P, Kleinberg D, Bronstein MD, Clemmons DR, Klibanski A, van der Lely AJ, Strasburger CJ, Lamberts SW, Ho KK, Casanueva FF, Melmed S; Acromegaly Consensus Group. Expert consensus document: a consensus on the medical treatment of acromegaly. *Nat Rev Endocrinol.* 2014;**10**(4):243–248.

17. Giustina A. Optimal use of pegvisomant in acromegaly: are we getting there? *Endocrine.* 2015;**48**(1):3–8.

18. Giustina A, Mazziotti G, Maffezzoni F, Amoroso V, Berruti A. Investigational drugs targeting somatostatin receptors for treatment of acromegaly and neuroendocrine tumors. *Expert Opin Investig Drugs.* 2014;**23**(12):1619–1635.

19. Melmed S, Bronstein MD, Chanson P, Klibanski A, Casanueva FF, Wass JAH, Strasburger CJ, Luger A, Clemmons DR, Giustina A. A consensus statement on acromegaly therapeutic outcomes. *Nat Rev Endocrinol.* 2018;**14**(9):552–561.

20. Casanueva FF, Barkan AL, Buchfelder M, Klibanski A, Laws ER, Loeffler JS, Melmed S, Mortini P, Wass J, Giustina A; Pituitary Society, Expert Group on Pituitary Tumors. Criteria for the definition of Pituitary Tumor Centers of Excellence (PTCOE): a Pituitary Society statement [published correction appears in *Pituitary.* 2018;**21**(6): 663]. *Pituitary.* 2017;**20**(5):489–498.

21. Caron PJ, Bevan JS, Petersenn S, Flanagan D, Tabarin A, Prévost G, Maisonobe P, Clermont A; PRIMARYS Investigators. Tumor shrinkage with lanreotide 120mg as primary therapy in acromegaly: results of a prospective multicenter clinical trial. *J Clin Endocrinol Metab.* 2014;**99**(4):1282–1290.

22. Carlsen SM, Lund-Johansen M, Schreiner T, Aanderud S, Johannesen O, Svartberg J, Cooper JG, Hald JK, Fougner SL, Bollerslev J; Preoperative Octreotide Treatment of Acromegaly study group. Preoperative octreotide treatment in newly diagnosed acromegalic patients with macroadenomas increases cure short-term postoperative rates: a prospective, randomized trial. *J Clin Endocrinol Metab.* 2008;**93**(8):2984–2990.

23. Colao A, Auriemma RS, Galdiero M, Cappabianca P, Cavallo LM, Esposito F, Grasso LF, Lombardi G, Pivonello R. Impact of somatostatin analogs versus surgery on glucose metabolism in acromegaly: results of a 5-year observational, open, prospective study. *J Clin Endocrinol Metab.* 2009;**94**(2):528–537.

24. Giustina A, Bonadonna S, Bugari G, Colao A, Cozzi R, Cannavò S, de Marinis L, Degli Uberti E, Bogazzi F, Mazziotti G, Minuto F, Montini M, Ghigo E. High-dose intramuscular octreotide in patients with acromegaly inadequately controlled on conventional somatostatin analogue therapy: a randomised controlled trial. *Eur J Endocrinol.* 2009;**161**(2):331–338.

25. Petersenn S, Bollerslev J, Arafat AM, Schopohl J, Serri O, Katznelson L, Lasher J, Hughes G, Hu K, Shen G, Reséndiz KH, Giannone V, Beckers A. Pharmacokinetics, pharmacodynamics, and safety of pasireotide LAR in patients with acromegaly: a randomized, multicenter, open-label, phase I study. *J Clin Pharmacol.* 2014;**54**(11):1308–1317.

26. Colao A, Bronstein MD, Freda P, Gu F, Shen CC, Gadelha M, Fleseriu M, van der Lely AJ, Farrall AJ, Hermosillo Reséndiz K, Ruffin M, Chen Y, Sheppard M; Pasireotide C2305 Study Group. Pasireotide versus octreotide in acromegaly: a head-to-head superiority study. *J Clin Endocrinol Metab.* 2014;**99**(3):791–799.

27. Gadelha MR, Bronstein MD, Brue T, Coculescu M, Fleseriu M, Guitelman M, Pronin V, Raverot G, Shimon I, Lievre KK, Fleck J, Aout M, Pedroncelli AM, Colao A; Pasireotide C2402 Study Group. Pasireotide versus continued treatment with octreotide or lanreotide in patients with inadequately controlled acromegaly (PAOLA): a randomized, phase 3 trial. *Lancet Diabetes Endocrinol.* 2014;**2**(11):875–884.

28. Breitschaft A, Hu K, Hermosillo Reséndiz K, Darstein C, Golor G. Management of hyperglycemia associated with pasireotide (SOM230): healthy volunteer study. *Diabetes Res Clin Pract.* 2014;**103**(3):458–465.

29. Schmid HA, Brue T, Colao A, Gadelha MR, Shimon I, Kapur K, Pedroncelli AM, Fleseriu M. Effect of pasireotide on glucose- and growth-hormone-related biomarkers in patients with inadequately controlled acromegaly. *Endocrine.* 2016;**53**(1):210–219.

30. Mazziotti G, Bonadonna S, Doga M, Patelli I, Gazzaruso C, Solerte SB, De Menis E, Giustina A. Biochemical evaluation of patients with active acromegaly and type 2 diabetes mellitus: efficacy and safety of the galanin test. *Neuroendocrinology.* 2008;**88**(4):299–304.

31. Giustina A, Mazziotti G, Cannavò S, Castello R, Arnaldi G, Bugari G, Cozzi R, Ferone D, Formenti AM, Gatti E, Grottoli S, Maffei P, Maffezzoni F, Montini M, Terzolo M, Ghigo E. High-dose and high-frequency autogel in acromegaly: a randomized, multicenter study. *J Clin Endocrinol Metab.* 2017;**102**(7):2454–2464.

32. Trainer PJ, Drake WM, Katznelson L, Freda PU, Herman-Bonert V, van der Lely AJ, Dimaraki EV, Stewart PM, Friend KE, Vance ML, Besser GM, Scarlett JA, Thorner MO, Parkinson C, Klibanski A, Powell JS, Barkan AL, Sheppard MC, Malsonado M, Rose DR, Clemmons DR, Johannsson G, Bengtsson BA, Stavrou S, Kleinberg DL, Cook DM, Phillips LS, Bidlingmaier M, Strasburger CJ, Hackett S, Zib K, Bennett WF, Davis RJ. Treatment of acromegaly with the growth hormone-receptor antagonist pegvisomant. *N Engl J Med.* 2000;**342**(16): 1171–1177.

33. Frara S, Maffezzoni F, Mazziotti G, Giustina A. The modern criteria for medical management of acromegaly. *Prog Mol Biol Transl Sci.* 2016; **138**:63–83.

34. Giustina A, Chanson P, Bronstein MD, Klibanski A, Lamberts S, Casanueva FF, Trainer P, Ghigo E, Ho K, Melmed S; Acromegaly Consensus Group. A consensus on criteria for cure of acromegaly. *J Clin Endocrinol Metab.* 2010;**95**(7):3141–3148.

35. Schreiber I, Buchfelder M, Droste M, Forssmann K, Mann K, Saller B, Strasburger CJ; German Pegvisomant Investigators. Treatment of acromegaly with the GH receptor antagonist pegvisomant in clinical practice: safety and efficacy evaluation from the German Pegvisomant Observational Study. *Eur J Endocrinol.* 2007;**156**(1):75–82.

36. Giustina A, Arnaldi G, Bogazzi F, Cannavò S, Colao A, De Marinis L, De Menis E, Degli Uberti E, Giorgino F, Grottoli S, Lania AG, Maffei P, Pivonello R, Ghigo E. Pegvisomant in acromegaly: an update [published correction appears in *J Endocrinol Invest.* 2018;**41**(2):267]. *J Endocrinol Invest.* 2017;**40**(6):577–589.

37. van der Lely AJ, Biller BM, Brue T, Buchfelder M, Ghigo E, Gomez R, Hey-Hadavi J, Lundgren F, Rajicic N, Strasburger CJ, Webb SM, Koltowska-Häggström M. Long-term safety of pegvisomant in patients with acromegaly: comprehensive review of 1288 subjects in ACROSTUDY. *J Clin Endocrinol Metab.* 2012;**97**(5):1589–1597.

38. Giustina A, Mazziotti G, Torri V, Spinello M, Floriani I, Melmed S. Meta-analysis on the effects of octreotide on tumor mass in acromegaly. *PLoS One.* 2012;**7**(5):e36411.

39. Mazziotti G, Floriani I, Bonadonna S, Torri V, Chanson P, Giustina A. Effects of somatostatin analogs on glucose homeostasis: a metaanalysis of acromegaly studies. *J Clin Endocrinol Metab.* 2009;**94**(5):1500–1508.

40. Bonadonna S, Mazziotti G, Nuzzo M, Bianchi A, Fusco A, De Marinis L, Giustina A. Increased prevalence of radiological spinal deformities in active acromegaly: a cross-sectional study in postmenopausal women. *J Bone Miner Res.* 2005;**20**(10):1837–1844.

41. Mazziotti G, Frara S, Giustina A. Pituitary diseases and bone. *Endocr Rev.* 2018;**39**(4):440–488.

42. Chiloiro S, Mazziotti G, Giampietro A, Bianchi A, Frara S, Mormando M, Pontecorvi A, Giustina A, De Marinis L. Effects of pegvisomant and somatostatin receptor ligands on incidence of vertebral fractures in patients with acromegaly [published correction appears in *Pituitary.* 2018;**21**(3):309]. *Pituitary.* 2018;**21**(3):302–308.

43. Mazziotti G, Bianchi A, Porcelli T, Mormando M, Maffezzoni F, Cristiano A, Giampietro A, De Marinis L, Giustina A. Vertebral fractures in patients with acromegaly: a 3-year prospective study. *J Clin Endocrinol Metab.* 2013;**98**(8):3402–3410.

44. Mazziotti G, Giustina A. Effects of lanreotide SR and autogel on tumor mass in patients with acromegaly: a systematic review. *Pituitary.* 2010;**13**(1):60–67.

45. Giustina A, Bevan JS, Bronstein MD, Casanueva FF, Chanson P, Petersenn S, Thanh XM, Sert C, Houchard A, Guillemin I, Melmed S; SAGIT Investigator Group. SAGIT®: clinician-reported outcome instrument for managing acromegaly in clinical practice-development and results from a pilot study. *Pituitary.* 2016;**19**(1):39–49.

46. Kasuki L, Wildemberg LE, Gadelha MR. Management of endocrine disease: personalized medicine in the treatment of acromegaly. *Eur J Endocrinol.* 2018;**178**:R89-R100.

Perioperative Management and Complications of Pituitary Neurosurgery: DI and SIADH

M47
Presented, March 23–26, 2019

Janice M. Kerr, MD. University of Colorado Denver, Anschutz Medical Center, Aurora, Colorado 80045, E-mail: janice.kerr@ucdenver.edu

SIGNIFICANCE OF THE CLINICAL PROBLEM

Transient diabetes insipidus (DI) and hyponatremia from isolated syndrome of inappropriate antidiuretic hormone (SIADH) excess are the most common fluid and electrolyte abnormalities in neurosurgery patients. SIADH occurs in upward of 25% of patients after transsphenoidal surgery (TSS) and accounts for the majority of 30-day rehospitalizations (1, 2). In addition, untreated adrenal insufficiency and hypothyroidism may cause perioperative hyponatremia. Most cases of post-TSS hyponatremia are mild and can be prevented or managed in the outpatient setting. Less commonly, hyponatremia is severe (Na ≤120 to 125 mmol/L) and requires hospitalization. Long term, a small subset of pituitary patients have chronic DI, including the very challenging cases of DI with impaired thirst sensation [hypodipsic DI, adipsic DI (ADI)]. Endocrinologists who routinely care for surgical patients with pituitary conditions should be familiar with the management of these conditions.

BARRIERS TO OPTIMAL PRACTICE

The major barriers to optimal management of patients with pituitary conditions in the perioperative period include the following:

- An understanding of the basic physiology that contributes to water balance disturbances
- The implementation of proven strategies to prevent postoperative hyponatremia in the outpatient setting
- Optimal evaluation and treatment of SIADH-related hyponatremia after pituitary surgery
- Challenges in the optimal management of patients with DI, including ADI

LEARNING OBJECTIVES

As a result of participating in this session, learners should be able to:

- Describe the normal physiology of sodium and water balance and understand abnormalities related to pituitary diseases and neurosurgery
- Describe strategies to prevent hyponatremia after pituitary surgery
- Understand the evaluation and management of postoperative DI and SIADH
- Detail long-term strategies for managing chronic DI, including ADI

STRATEGIES FOR DIAGNOSIS, THERAPY, AND/OR MANAGEMENT
Physiology of Sodium/Water Balance

Under normal conditions, plasma sodium and osmolality levels are maintained within narrow ranges, despite marked variations in water and salt intake. Plasma sodium concentration and osmolality are determined mainly by the plasma water content and vary according to water intake, urinary losses, and insensible losses (*e.g.*, sweat, gastrointestinal, respiration). Normal water balance is maintained primarily by two osmoregulated mechanisms: thirst and arginine vasopressin (AVP)/antidiuretic hormone (ADH) release.

Thirst, a major driver of water intake, is mediated by specialized osmoreceptors in the anterior hypothalamus. These neurons are juxtaposed to the hypothalamic neurons of the paraventricular and supraoptic nuclei that synthesize ADH. Physiologic mediators of ADH release include primarily osmotic stimuli, specifically serum osmolality >282 to 285 mOsm/kg water, and serum Na >145 mmol/L (145 mEq/L). In addition, less-potent nonosmotic stimuli cause ADH release, specifically hypovolemia, hypotension, and various physiologic factors (*e.g.*, pain, nausea, infection). ADH acts on the kidney to increase aquaporin channel expression and water reabsorption (3).

Hypothalamic abnormalities of osmoreceptors that regulate thirst are an uncommon manifestation of sellar lesions and/or their treatment. Most patients with pituitary conditions with DI maintain normal thirst sensation, which allows for hydration in response to hyperosmolality. In contrast, patients with DI and concomitant defective thirst centers (hypodipsic DI, ADI) are at increased risk for hypernatremia (4).

Endocrinopathies That Contribute to Perioperative Hyponatremia in Patients With Pituitary Conditions

Glucocorticoids play an important role in free water excretion, and euvolemic hyponatremia from ACTH deficiency may be the initial presentation of a pituitary tumor. The putative mechanism of hyponatremia is loss of tonic inhibition of cortisol on ADH secretion (5). In addition, glucocorticoids may affect aquaporin channel expression either directly or indirectly. The clinical and biochemical pictures of these adrenally insufficient patients are often indistinguishable from SIADH, although the hallmark is that the serum sodium levels usually normalize only after glucocorticoid replacement.

Hypothyroidism is also a well-recognized cause of hyponatremia, although it is a less important factor than glucocorticoid deficiency. Impaired free water excretion from hypothyroidism usually only is associated with severe hypothyroidism. The putative mechanism of hyponatremia is through decreased glomerular filtration rates from hypothyroid-related increased peripheral vascular resistance and decreased cardiac output. In more severe cases of hypothyroidism, ADH release is also stimulated nonosmotically (6).

Based on the potential contribution of pituitary hormone deficiencies to perioperative complications, adrenal and thyroid hormonal levels routinely are assessed preoperatively, and these hormones are replaced as indicated. In addition, patients who develop postoperative hyponatremia, if not already on hormone replacement, may be reevaluated for these deficiencies.

Evaluation and Treatment of Perioperative DI in Patients With Pituitary Conditions

DI is such a rare presentation for pituitary adenomas that it should prompt consideration of other sellar lesions, most notably craniopharyngiomas, inflammatory hypophysitis, and metastatic diseases. In contrast, transient DI is common after pituitary surgeries, occurring in upward of 25% to 30% of patients. Exclusion of other causes of polyuria should be performed before establishing the diagnosis of central DI, including osmotic diuresis, diuresis from high intraoperative fluid administration, and GH tumor resection–related diuresis (7).

DI is characterized clinically and biochemically by the abrupt onset of hypotonic polyuria and thirst within 24 to 48 hours of surgery (Table 1). As such, postoperative patients routinely are monitored closely for fluid intake, urinary output, and serial sodium levels with or without urine specific gravity and urine osmolality. Most DI cases spontaneously resolve before hospital discharge. More commonly, an isolated SIADH phase occurs on postoperative days 5 to 10 from the release of prestored ADH. Rarely, a triphasic ADH response occurs, which is characterized by an initial DI phase, followed by SIADH, and then by a final permanent DI phase (7). Fortunately, permanent DI is noted in <5% of TSS cases, most notably in patients with either proximal pituitary stalk resection or extensive pituitary surgeries.

In anticipation of spontaneous recovery, most postoperative DI cases are managed expectantly in the hospital and without medications. Patients are allowed to drink to thirst, and serum sodium levels are followed closely (*i.e.*, every 4 to 6 hours). For persistent polyuria >24 to 48 hours after TSS, however, and particularly if associated with hypernatremia or disruptive nocturia, patients are given

Table 1. Diagnosis of Postoperative DI in Adults

Diagnostic Criteria for DI in Adults
1. Dilute urine (osmolality <200 mOsm/kg water or urine specific gravity <1.005)
2. Polyuria/nocturia (≥3 L/d or >250 mL/h urine output for 2–3 consecutive hours)
3. Polydipsia
4. Exclusion of other etiologies for postoperative polyuria

limited antidiuretic hormones parenterally as desmopressin/1-desamino 8-D-arginine vasopressin (DDAVP) 0.5 to 2.0 μg (subcutaneously or IV) or, less commonly, as ADH/vasopressin. The duration of DDAVP action is ~6 to 12 hours, although there are important individual variations in response, with some patients having a prolonged effect. Desmopressin should be prescribed rarely and judiciously for postsurgical patients at the time of discharge. It is mostly limited to patients with high-risk features such as antecedent DI, prolonged postoperative DI, craniopharyngiomas, or known pituitary stalk resection.

Regarding outpatient desmopressin formulations, patients typically are started on a low nighttime DDAVP dose, either nasal spray (10 μg) or oral tablets (0.10 mg), and only as needed to prevent nocturia. The intranasal form is provided as an aqueous formula that can be delivered in 10-μg metered doses (preferred by most adults) or through a calibrated rhinal tube (if smaller doses are needed). Dosing desmopressin on an as-needed basis instead of on a fixed schedule allows for detection of normalized ADH secretion or the start of the second/SIADH phase of a triple-phase response. With more severe DI, higher nighttime doses or additional morning doses may be needed. Patients should be questioned at each clinic visit about polyuria and their DDAVP use, and the desmopressin dose should be adjusted or discontinued accordingly. Recovery from DI usually is observed in the first few weeks postoperatively and, less commonly, in the months after TSS.

Strategies to Prevent Hyponatremia From SIADH After TSS

Hyponatremia after TSS is primarily attributable to isolated SIADH from pituitary stalk manipulation. Predictors of postoperative hyponatremia remain controversial. Some studies have suggested that postoperative hyponatremia risks include female sex, Cushing disease, larger tumors, cerebral spinal fluid leak, hypopituitarism, or craniopharyngiomas, whereas other investigators have not found these associations (8–10).

Nadir sodium levels occur most commonly between postoperative days 5 and 9 when patients typically are at home. Symptoms vary depending on the degree of hyponatremia and the rate of its development but generally include headaches, irritability, anorexia, lethargy, and nausea in mild hyponatremia (125 < Na < 134 mmol/L) to more severe, potentially life-threatening complications in marked hyponatremia (Na ≤ 120 mmol/L), such as altered mental status, vomiting, neurogenic pulmonary edema, seizure, coma, brain herniation, and death.

Based on the high prevalence of postoperative hyponatremia, the American Association of Clinical Endocrinologists guidelines recommend a routine serum sodium check at ~1 week postoperatively (11). A growing body of literature now supports early fluid restriction in addition to a routine sodium test after TSS to prevent hyponatremia (12, 13). With the use of a modest fluid restriction (1.5 L or 50 fl oz for 2 weeks), we reported a 70% reduction in 30-day readmissions for symptomatic hyponatremia after TSS for pituitary adenomas (14). We recommend the following general guidelines (or a similarly published, ideally nurse-driven protocol) to assist endocrinologists who routinely care for patients after TSS (Fig. 1). All fluid intake must be included in the fluid restriction. Salt and protein intake are not limited unless clinically indicated (*e.g.*, congestive heart failure). Importantly, as an exclusionary criterion, patients who have DI and/or are prescribed DDAVP at the time of hospital discharge are not placed on fluid restriction until there is evidence for resolution of DI.

A recognized small subset of post-TSS patients experience a rapid decrease in serum sodium levels, and it is postulated that additional factors beyond SIADH, such as natriuresis and/or low oral salt intake, may be culprits (1). The role of liberal salt intake to mitigate further against such rapid sodium declines in such post-TSS patients has yet to be investigated.

Management of Hyponatremia in Hospitalized, Postoperative Patients With Pituitary Conditions

Patients with symptomatic, severe hyponatremia (generally defined as Na $\leq$ 120 to 125 mmol/L) typically require an emergency department visit and/or hospitalization. The laboratory evaluation of hyponatremia should include a serum osmolality measurement to confirm true hypo-osmolality (15). A clinical assessment of extracellular volume status also should be made from among hypovolemic, euvolemic, and hypervolemic states. Studies have shown, however, that the sensitivity and specificity for clinically distinguishing euvolemic from hypovolemic hyponatremic conditions are low at ~50%, particularly in mild cases (16). In contrast, a spot urinary sodium level of <30 mmol/L has a high positive predictive value for identifying patients whose sodium levels

will increase in response to isotonic/0.9% normal saline (*i.e.*, saline-responsive hyponatremia) (16). An important caveat is that patients with renal causes of salt wasting (*i.e.*, diuretic use, primary adrenal insufficiency), may also have high urinary sodium levels and saline responsiveness. Furthermore, because normal saline may worsen SIADH-related hyponatremia, particularly if patients are volume replete and have a urinary osmolality >500 mOsm/kg water, it is best to initiate a diagnostic SIADH work-up before starting therapy whenever possible (17) (Table 2). As such, all patients should be tested initially for serum sodium, serum osmolality, spot urine sodium, and spot urine osmolality levels. A spot urine potassium level also will allow for the calculation of the electrolyte-free water clearance. Additional retesting may be indicated during the hospitalization, particularly if there is concern about a mixed etiology of hyponatremia (*e.g.*, hypovolemia and SIADH). Finally, although new-onset adrenal insufficiency and hypothyroidism are uncommon after an uncomplicated TSS, these pituitary hormones are typically reassessed at the time of hospitalization, with baseline laboratories including free T_4 and morning cortisol levels, as indicated.

Severe symptomatic hyponatremia (usually Na $\leq$ 120 to 125 mmol/L), particularly if acute and/or complicated by altered mental status, delirium, nausea/vomiting, neurogenic pulmonary edema, seizure, coma, or impending brain herniation, is best treated with hypertonic (3%) saline. The US hyponatremia guidelines recommend an initial rise in serum sodium of 4 to 6 mmol/L over 4 hours using either IV boluses (100 mL over 10 minutes × 3 maximum) or hypertonic (3%) saline infusions (~1 mL/kg per hour for a few hours) (15). For severe chronic hyponatremia (>48 hours or unknown duration), hypertonic saline also is used, although the subsequent sodium correction rate should be stratified according to the risk for osmotic demyelination syndrome (ODS) and limited to $\leq$10 to 12 mmol in the first 24 hours and $\leq$18 mmol in the

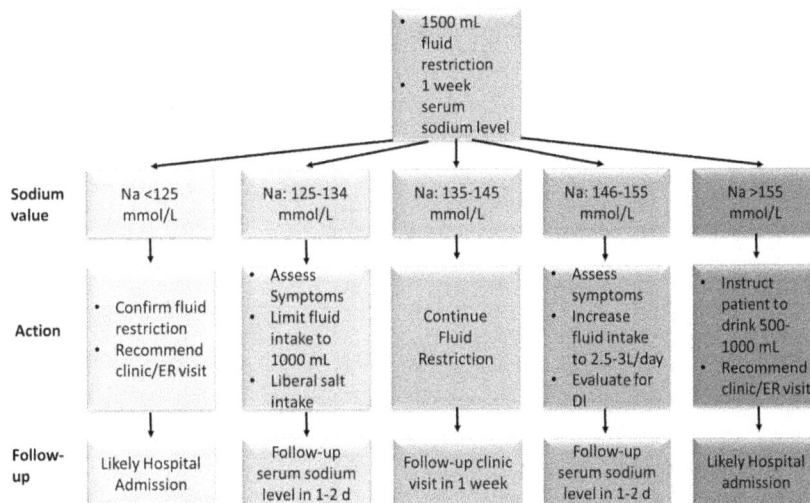

Figure 1. Outpatient strategy to prevent hyponatremia in post-TSS patients. ER, emergency room.

Table 2. Diagnostic Criteria for SIADH

1. Decreased effective osmolality (<275 mOsm/kg water)
2. Urinary osmolality >100 mOsm/kg water
3. Clinical euvolemia
4. Urinary sodium >40 mmol/L and normal dietary salt intake
5. Normal renal function and absence of diuretic use
6. Normal thyroid and adrenal function

first 48 hours for most post-TSS patients. For patients with higher ODS risk factors, specifically an initial sodium <105 mmol/L, hypokalemia, advanced liver disease, alcoholism, or poor nutritional status, an even lower rate of sodium correction is recommended, ≤8 mmol/24 h (15). Of note, ODS rarely has been reported as a complication of pituitary surgery. Currently, <30 case reports exist in the literature possibly because of the relatively shorter duration of hyponatremia. In addition, most of the patients with pituitary-related ODS had profound hyponatremia (serum sodium levels <115 mmol/L), which is uncommon in closely monitored neurosurgical patients (18).

Several factors have been identified that predict the likelihood of fluid restriction failure, including (i) a high urinary osmolality (>500 mOsm/kg water), (ii) an electrolyte-free water clearance >1.0 (defined as urine sodium + urine potassium levels / serum sodium concentration), (iii) a 24-hour urinary volume <1500 mL/d, and (iv) a slow increase in serum sodium concentration (<2 mmol/L/d) on a ≤1 L/d fluid restriction (15). For refractory hyponatremia, consideration could be given to additional treatments, such as salt tablets (as tolerated), a loop diuretic, urea (although limited availability in the United States), or a V2 receptor antagonist (vaptans). Vaptans have the advantage of addressing the underlying pathophysiology in SIADH and cause a pure aquaresis. Some small, retrospective studies have supported vaptan use in

postsurgical patients with pituitary conditions, although most endocrinologists have limited experience with these medications (10).

Chronic DI: Management Considerations, Including Patients With ADI

The goal of chronic DI therapy is control of nocturia and partial control of daytime polyuria. A number of ADH analogs/desmopressin formulations are available, with intranasal preparations and oral tablets being the preferred therapies in the United States. Comparison of the various DDAVP formulations, their relative dosages, and treatment considerations (19) are shown in Table 3. In patients with complete DI and for intranasal formulas, 10- to 20-μg doses twice daily usually are required. Intranasal formulations have a quicker onset of action compared with the oral tablets and are therefore generally preferred by adult patients. Most spray formulations require refrigeration, however, which may limit their utility for some patients. For oral desmopressin tablets, because of proteolytic degradation, much higher doses (10- to 20-fold) are needed. Both intranasal and tablet formulations have comparable durations of action (between 6 and 12 hours), although marked individual differences exist in response to any DDAVP formulation, and empiric dosing is required. Higher doses are associated with comparable urinary concentrating abilities but slightly longer durations of actions. Finally, sometimes a third afternoon desmopressin dose is required for adequate daytime DI control and to maintain normal sodium levels.

ADI is an uncommon manifestation of sellar masses and rarely has been reported as a pituitary surgery complication. It is most commonly associated with large/invasive tumors, such as craniopharyngiomas, germinomas, and germ cell tumors (20). Informally, ADI can be assumed if hypernatremia develops without complaint of thirst in an awake person with

Table 3. Characteristics of Antidiuretic Hormones

	ADH Injectable	DDAVP Injectable	DDAVP Tablets	DDAVP Spray	DDAVP Melt Sublingual
Dose comparison	5–10 units subcutaneously or lower infusion doses	NA	100 mg	2.5–5 μg	60 μg
		<0.5 μg	200 mg	5–10 μg	120 μg
		<1 μg	400 mg	10–20 μg	240 μg
Issues	Very short half-life of 20 min	All DDAVP formulations: individual variability in duration	Reduced absorption with food (40%)	Refrigerated and nonrefrigerated formulations	NA in the United States
	AVP V1 actions/side effects at higher dose	Higher dose = greater duration of effect		Rhinal tubes for lowest doses	
		Prolonged effect with CRI		Absorption may be affected by mucosal congestion, allergic rhinitis, surgical packing, *etc.*	

Adapted with permission from Oiso Y, Robertson GL, Norgaard JP, Vinter Juul K. Treatment of neurohypophyseal aiabetes insipidus. *J Clin Endocrinol Metab.* 2013;98:3958–3967.

Abbreviations: CRI, chronic renal insufficiency; NA, not available; V1, vasopressin 1 receptor.

hypotonic polyuria and unlimited access to water. The management of ADI is complex and often confounded by the patient's cognitive impairment from the tumor and/or its treatment.

The general principles of outpatient management of ADI, as first published by Ball *et al.* (4), include the following:

1. Regularly scheduled desmopressin and given at least twice daily.
2. A goal fluid intake of ~1.5 to 2 L/d, with additional adjustments for obligate losses on the basis of daily weights, exercise, temperature, or intercurrent illness.
3. Daily weights should be performed and compared with the patient's optimal weight as determined in the normonatremic and euvolemic states. Potential daily adjustments in fluid intake should be made on a 1:1 kilogram-to-liter basis. For example, a patient ~1.0 lb (0.5 kg) below his/her normonatremia body weight should consume an extra 0.5 L of water that day and vice versa if he/she is above their optimal body weight.
4. Patients should be followed regularly with plasma sodium levels. Substantial weight changes (>3%) or symptoms of sodium abnormalities should prompt an earlier reassessment.

In the inpatient hospital setting, the management of DI/ADI is similar and, importantly, should include continued desmopressin use that controls DI and close monitoring of fluid balances and serum sodium levels.

1. Hypernatremia management in patients with ADI: Water deficit due to pure water loss (as in DI) can be estimated using the following equation: water deficit = total body water (TBW) × [(Na concentration/140) – 1] (3). TBW = weight (kg) × 0.6 (male) or 0.5 (female). Patients with mild biochemical hypernatremia (145 ≥ Na ≥ 148 mmol/L) usually can be managed safely by oral free water supplementation. Patients with more severe hypernatremia (Na ≥149 mmol/L), particularly if associated with altered mental status, should be maintained with subcutaneous/IV desmopressin and parenteral dextrose/hypotonic infusions. For acute hypernatremia (<48-hour duration), a goal ~2 mmol/L/h decrease in plasma sodium concentration is recommended until the serum sodium concentration is ~145 mmol/L. For chronic cases of severe hypernatremia, slower rates of sodium corrections (≤10 to 12 mmol/L per day) are recommended to avoid iatrogenic cerebral injury, although this is a less-well-described problem in hypernatremia than for hyponatremia overcorrection (3). Finally, endocrinologists should be aware to avoid the frequent mistakes of withholding desmopressin during procedures and/or giving isotonic saline to correct hypernatremia in patients with DI.
2. Hyponatremia management in patients with ADI: For mild hyponatremia (125 ≤ Na ≤ 135 mmol/L) with minimal symptoms, this can be managed by decreasing

fluid intake or delaying the next DDAVP dosing by 2 to 4 hours. Conversely, more severe and symptomatic hyponatremia (≤120 to 125 mmol/L) should be managed by temporarily withholding DDAVP and possibly administering 3% saline, depending on the clinical severity and as previously detailed (15). For chronic hyponatremia (>48-hour duration), sodium adjustments should be limited to the maximum sodium correction needed to prevent ODS, as previously detailed.

Even with regimented desmopressin and fluid administrations, abnormal serum sodium levels are common in patients with ADI. Unfortunately, ADI is usually a lifelong condition, although a limited recovery of defective thirst mechanisms occurs in a small subset of patients (4, 20).

MAIN CONCLUSIONS
Transient DI and SIADH are common after pituitary surgery and require close monitoring during the perioperative period. Newer postoperative strategies that include a mild fluid restriction, in addition to a routine sodium level test, have been shown to minimize hospital readmissions for hyponatremia. Desmopressin should be started judiciously in post-TSS patients after hospital discharge, as inappropriate desmopressin use in transient DI may result in hyponatremia. Conversely, patients with chronic DI, especially if associated with hypernatremia or impaired thirst, should be placed on scheduled desmopressin and free water replacement.

CASES
Case 1. Pituitary Hormone Deficiencies and Hyponatremia
A 44-year-old Hispanic male presented with headaches, weakness, nausea, and hyponatremia (Na 124 mmol/L). Clinically, he appeared euvolemic, and the initial laboratories were consistent with SIADH. His pituitary laboratories showed panhypopituitarism, and a pituitary MRI revealed a 1.8- × 1.4- × 2.4-cm, T1-hyperintense mass consistent with acute hemorrhage. The patient was started on thyroid and glucocorticoid replacement therapy, and the follow-up serum sodium level normalized.

Question 1
Regarding the relative contribution of central hormone deficiencies to hyponatremia in pituitary patients, the following is generally true:
- A. Hypocortisolism > hypothyroidism
- B. Hypothyroidism > hypocortisolism
- C. Hypocortisolism = hypothyroidism
- D. Isolated secondary adrenal insufficiency > primary adrenal insufficiency
- E. Isolated secondary hypothyroidism > primary hypothyroidism

Answer

A. Both central glucocorticoid and thyroid hormone deficiencies can cause hyponatremia, and hyponatremia may be a presenting feature for a pituitary adenoma. Glucocorticoids, however, assume a greater physiologic role on free water excretion, presumably through tonic inhibition on ADH secretion. Hyponatremia is generally greater in primary adrenal insufficiency compared with isolated secondary adrenal insufficiency because of the concomitant mineralocorticoid deficiency. Finally, hyponatremia in isolated secondary hypothyroidism is not greater than in primary hypothyroidism.

Case 2. Outpatient Management of Post-TSS Patients

A 55-year-old white female with normal pituitary hormones was noted incidentally to have a 1.3-cm pituitary adenoma. She underwent an uncomplicated TSS for a gonadotroph adenoma. On postoperative day 1, she had a brief episode of DI (urinary output ~310 mL/h for 3 consecutive hours), which was treated with a single 0.5-µg DDAVP injection. Her high urinary output subsequently improved over the next 24 to 48 hours, the serum sodium remained normal, and she was ready for hospital discharge on postoperative day 3.

Question 2

For optimal postoperative TSS management, this patient should now be instructed to:

    A. Use nighttime desmopressin as needed and return to the clinic in ~2 weeks

    B. Intake fluid *ad libitum* and return to the clinic in ~2 weeks

    C. Undergo mild fluid restriction and check serum sodium level on postoperative day 7

    D. Intake fluid *ad libitum* and check serum sodium level on postoperative day 7

    E. Undergo mild fluid restriction and return to the clinic in ~2 weeks

Answer

C. Delayed hyponatremia from SIADH is the leading cause of 30-day hospital readmission after TSS. Strategies to address this problem include a routine serum sodium level on postoperative day 7 as recommended by American Association of Clinical Endocrinologists guidelines. In recent years, a number of studies also have demonstrated the added benefit of a mild to moderate fluid restriction to reduce hospital readmissions in properly selected patients.

Case 3. Hospital Management of Hyponatremia After TSS

The patient in case 2 was discharged from the hospital but presented to the emergency department the evening of postoperative day 9 with complaints of generalized headaches, anorexia, and fatigue. Because of recent travel, she did not obtain a 7-day postoperative serum sodium level or limit her fluid intake as recommended. Per the emergency department physician's evaluation, the patient appeared tired, borderline hypovolemic, but alert and oriented. Her blood pressure was 131/79 mm Hg and pulse 78 beats/min. Her physical and neurologic examinations were normal, and her serum sodium level was low at 124 mmol/L (normal 135 to 145 mmol/L).

Question 3

The following is the next best step now:

    A. Start 0.9% saline infusion

    B. Check spot urinary sodium/osmolality levels

    C. Start 3% saline infusion

    D. Check orthostatic blood pressures

    E. Check serum cortisol level

Answer

B. The clinical assessment of extracellular fluid volume status and orthostatic blood pressure measurements are generally inaccurate in mild cases of hypovolemia. In contrast, the kidneys are the most sensitive indicator of hydration status, and a spot urinary sodium level of <30 mEq/L (in patients not on a diuretic) has a high positive predictive value for identifying saline-responsive hyponatremia and is the next best step. Consideration could be given to infusing 1 L of 0.9% saline in cases of mild hyponatremia and diagnostic uncertainty but ideally, if supported by a low urine osmolality (<500 mOsm/kg water). Infusion of hypertonic (3%) saline infusion is not clinically warranted in this case. Finally, new-onset adrenal insufficiency in a patient who had normal adrenal function preoperatively and an uncomplicated TSS is unlikely, although a serum cortisol could be checked the following morning in this noncritically ill patient.

Case 4. Management of Chronic DI

A 25-year-old Hispanic male with a history of childhood germinoma, status post-TSS and radiation therapy, is being seen for management of his DI and panhypopituitarism. He has been on long-standing stable doses of glucocorticoids, levothyroxine, testosterone, and desmopressin. His pituitary hormone levels and tests were at goal, with the exception of mild hypernatremia (Na 148 mmol/L). The patient reported that the hypernatremia was chronic, despite good compliance with desmopressin 20 µg nasal spray twice a day and a robust fluid intake of ~3.2 L/d (108 fl oz/d). He denied thirst or nocturia but endorsed a mildly disruptive, daytime polyuria.

Question 4

You now recommend the following:

    A. Increase the morning DDAVP dose

    B. Switch desmopressin to oral tablets, starting with 200 mg twice a day

    C. Undergo an empiric trial of carbamazepine (renal ADH sensitizer)

D. Increase nighttime fluids

E. Add an afternoon DDAVP dose

Answer

E. The goal of chronic DI therapy is to control nocturia and partially control daytime polyuria. Because this patient has daytime polyuria and associated hypernatremia despite high fluid intake, additional therapy is recommended. Higher DDAVP doses are associated with increased duration of action, although this patient is already on the maximum intranasal DDAVP dose, and switching to a comparable oral DDAVP dose is unlikely to be helpful. The best option for this patient is the addition of an afternoon DDAVP dose; usually one half the morning dose is sufficient. Additional agents to increase renal ADH responsiveness have been studied in patients with DI (*e.g.*, carbamazepine, chlorpropamide) or a thiazide diuretic with low-sodium diet, although none of these therapies are superior to desmopressin.

References

1. Olson BR, Gumowski J, Rubino D, Oldfield EH. Pathophysiology of hyponatremia after transsphenoidal pituitary surgery. *J Neurosurg*. 1997;**87**(4):499–507.
2. Bohl MA, Ahmad S, Jahnke H, Shepherd D, Knecht L, White WL, Little AS. Delayed hyponatremia is the most common cause of 30-day unplanned readmission after transsphenoidal surgery for pituitary tumors. *Neurosurgery*. 2016;**78**(1):84–90.
3. Sterns RH. Disorders of plasma sodium—causes, consequences, and correction. *N Engl J Med*. 2015;**372**(1):55–65.
4. Ball SG, Vaidja B, Baylis PH. Hypothalamic adipsic syndrome: diagnosis and management. *Clin Endocrinol (Oxf)*. 1997;**47**(4): 405–409.
5. Raff H. Glucocorticoid inhibition of neurohypophysial vasopressin secretion. *Am J Physiol*. 1987;**252**(4 Pt 2):R635–R644.
6. Derubertis FR Jr, Michelis MF, Bloom ME, Mintz DH, Field JB, Davis BB. Impaired water excretion in myxedema. *Am J Med*. 1971;**51**(1):41–53.
7. Loh JA, Verbalis JG. Disorders of water and salt metabolism associated with pituitary disease. *Endocrinol Metab Clin North Am*. 2008;**37**(1): 213–234.
8. Hensen J, Henig A, Fahlbusch R, Meyer M, Boehnert M, Buchfelder M. Prevalence, predictors and patterns of postoperative polyuria and hyponatraemia in the immediate course after transsphenoidal surgery for pituitary adenomas. *Clin Endocrinol (Oxf)*. 1999;**50**(4): 431–439.
9. Cote DJ, Dasenbrock HH, Muskens IS, Broekman MLD, Zaidi HA, Dunn IF, Smith TR, Laws ER Jr. Readmission and other adverse events after transsphenoidal surgery: prevalence, timing, and predictive factors. *J Am Coll Surg*. 2017;**224**(5):971–979.
10. Jahangiri A, Wagner J, Tran MT, Miller LM, Tom MW, Kunwar S, Blevins L Jr, Aghi MK. Factors predicting postoperative hyponatremia and efficacy of hyponatremia management strategies after more than 1000 pituitary operations. *J Neurosurg*. 2013;**119**(6):1478–1483.
11. Woodmansee WW, Carmichael J, Kelly D, Katznelson L for the AACE Neuroendocrine and Pituitary Scientific Committee. American Association of Clinical Endocrinologists and American College of Endocrinology Disease state clinical review: postoperative management following pituitary surgery. *Endocr Pract*. 2015;**21**(7):832–838.
12. Bohl MA, Ahmad S, White WL, Little AS. Implementation of a postoperative outpatient care pathway for delayed hyponatremia following transsphenoidal surgery. *Neurosurgery*. 2018;**82**(1):110–117.
13. Burke WT, Cote DJ, Iuliano SI, Zaidi HA, Laws ER. A practical method for prevention of readmission for symptomatic hyponatremia following transsphenoidal surgery. *Pituitary*. 2018;**21**(1):25–31.
14. Deaver KE, Catel CP, Lillehei KO, Wierman ME, Kerr JM. Strategies to reduce readmissions for hyponatremia after transsphenoidal surgery for pituitary adenomas. *Endocrine*. 2018;**62**(2):333–339.
15. Verbalis JG, Goldsmith SR, Greenberg A, Korzelius C, Schrier RW, Sterns RH, Thompson CJ. Diagnosis, evaluation, and treatment of hyponatremia: expert panel recommendations. *Am J Med*. 2013; **126**(10, Suppl 1):S1–S42.
16. Chung HM, Kluge R, Schrier RW, Anderson RJ. Clinical assessment of extracellular fluid volume in hyponatremia. *Am J Med*. 1987;**83**(5): 905–908.
17. Ellison DH, Berl T. The syndrome of inappropriate antidiuresis. *N Engl J Med*. 2007;**356**:2064–2072.
18. Perikal PJ, Jagannatha AT, Khanapure KS, Furtado SV, Joshi KC, Hegde AS. Extrapontine myelinolysis and reversible parkinsonism after hyponatremia correction in a case of pituitary adenoma: hypopituitarism as a predisposition for osmotic demyelination. *World Neurosurg*. 2018;**118**:304–310.
19. Oiso Y, Robertson GL, Nørgaard JP, Juul KV. Clinical review: treatment of neurophyseal diabetes insipidus. *J Clin Endocrinol Metab*. 2013; **98**(10):3958–3967.
20. Cuesta M, Hannon MJ, Thompson CJ. Adipsic diabetes insipidus in adult patients. *Pituitary*. 2017;**20**(3):372–380.

"New" Types of Hypophysitis: Current Knowledge in Diagnosis and Management

M55
Presented, March 23–26, 2019

Elena Varlamov, MD. Northwest Pituitary Center, Departments of Medicine and Neurologic Surgery, Oregon Health & Science University, Portland, Oregon 97239, E-mail: varlamoe@ohsu.edu

Maria Fleseriu, MD. Northwest Pituitary Center, Departments of Medicine and Neurologic Surgery, Oregon Health & Science University, Portland, Oregon 97239, E-mail: fleseriu@ohsu.edu

SIGNIFICANCE OF THE CLINICAL PROBLEM

Hypophysitis (Hy) is an inflammatory "state" of the pituitary gland and/or pituitary stalk. It can occur as a primary disorder [e.g., autoimmune lymphocytic Hy (LyHy)] or as a result of secondary involvement in systemic diseases [e.g., Langerhans cell histiocytosis, sarcoidosis, IgG4-related disease (IgG4-RD)], infection (e.g., tuberculosis), tumors (e.g., germinoma), or immune therapy (immune checkpoint inhibitor–induced Hy) and other drugs. Histologically, Hy is classified as lymphocytic, xanthomatous, IgG4-related, or necrotizing type (1).

Immune checkpoint inhibitors have become the mainstay of treatment of a variety of cancers, but their use is associated with a number of serious immune-related adverse events. Hy is one of the most severe endocrine complications, and although increasingly recognized by physicians, there is no standardized treatment approach.

IgG4-related Hy is a relatively new classified form of Hy, which can present alone or as part of systemic IgG4-RD. Little is known about its natural history, and diagnosis may be challenging due to a lack of sensitive laboratory markers and clear-cut pathologic criteria.

BARRIERS TO OPTIMAL PRACTICE

Due to overall Hy rarity and absence of randomized controlled trials evaluating treatment of Hy types, optimal management is still up for debate. Although high-dose (HD) glucocorticoids (GCs) frequently are used in treatment of both immune checkpoint inhibitor–induced Hy and IgG4-related Hy, some reports suggest that physiologic GC replacement therapy may be appropriate in most cases.

LEARNING OBJECTIVES

As a result of participating in this session, learners should be able to:
- Understand the pathophysiology of immune checkpoint inhibitor–induced Hy
- Illustrate new evidence on treatment and outcomes of immune checkpoint inhibitor–induced Hy
- Recognize the clinical spectrum of IgG4-related Hy
- Assess management options for IgG4-related Hy

STRATEGIES FOR DIAGNOSIS AND MANAGEMENT
Immune Checkpoint Inhibitor–Induced Hy
Pathophysiology

Cytotoxic T-lymphocyte–associated antigen 4 (CTLA-4) and programmed cell death receptor 1 (PD-1) and its associated ligand PD-L1 are T-cell proteins that serve as immune checkpoints by downregulating T-cell activation and proliferation. This mechanism is necessary to maintain immune tolerance against self-antigens. However, it may allow cancer cells to escape immune surveillance (2, 3). Anti-CTLA-4, anti-PD-1, and anti-PD-L1 agents block these proteins, leading to an enhanced immune response against tumor cells (Figs. 1 and 2; Table 1). At the same time, this also leads to nonspecific activation of autoimmune and inflammatory processes, which can affect nearly every organ system. Within the endocrine system, immune checkpoint inhibitors can cause Hy, thyroid gland dysfunction, primary adrenal insufficiency (AI), and type 1 diabetes mellitus.

Precise pathogenesis of immune therapy–induced Hy is unknown. Some possible mechanisms are T-cell cytotoxicity, antibody-directed destruction of pituitary cells, and tissue damage due to inflammation (3). Furthermore, the CTLA-4 receptor is expressed by the pituitary cells; however, its function is unknown. Stronger expression of CTLA-4 has been found in patients with more severe Hy. It has been proposed

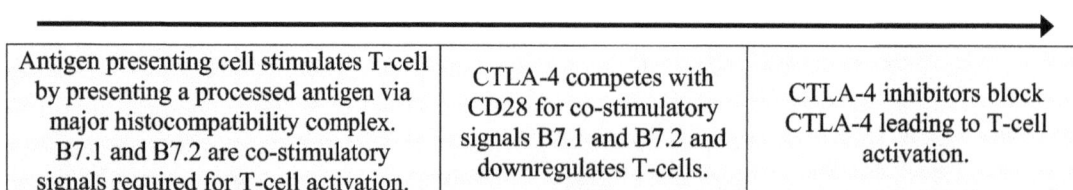

Antigen presenting cell stimulates T-cell by presenting a processed antigen via major histocompatibility complex. B7.1 and B7.2 are co-stimulatory signals required for T-cell activation.	CTLA-4 competes with CD28 for co-stimulatory signals B7.1 and B7.2 and downregulates T-cells.	CTLA-4 inhibitors block CTLA-4 leading to T-cell activation.

Figure 1. Summary of CTLA-4 role in T-cell activation and suppression.

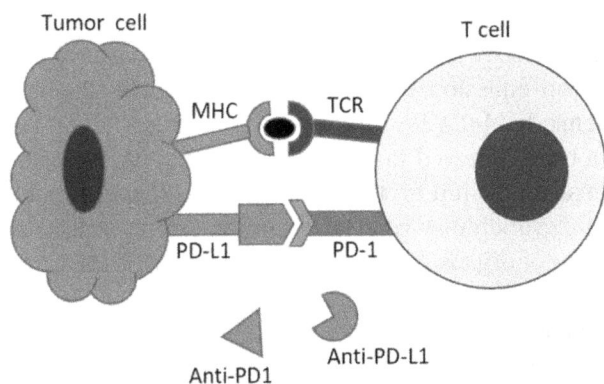

Figure 2. Role of PD-1 and PD-L1 in T-cell function. PD-L1 expressed on tumor cells binds to PD-1 receptor on T cells and inactivates them. PD-1 inhibitors and PD-L1 inhibitors block this interaction and allow T cells to become active. MHC, major histocompatibility complex; TCR, T-cell receptor.

that blocking of pituitary CTLA-4 by anti-CTLA agents triggers activation of type 2 (complement) and type 4 (autoreactive T cells) hypersensitivity reactions (4). Expression of PD-1 or PD-L1 by the pituitary has not yet been demonstrated, which is consistent with the clinical observation that Hy is observed less frequently with PD-1 or PD-L1 than with CTLA-4 inhibitors (3).

Incidence

Reported Hy incidence varies, with higher rates observed in CTLA-4 inhibitor–treated patients (up to 17.4%), which seems to correlate with high doses (5). A recent meta-analysis reported a 6.4% incidence with combination therapy followed by 3.2% with CTLA-4 inhibitors, 0.4% with PD-1 inhibitors, and <0.1% with PD-L1 inhibitors (6). Some investigators observed a higher frequency of CTLA-4–induced Hy in males; however, this may be due to a higher proportion of males in those clinical trials (7, 8).

Clinical Presentation and Diagnosis

Hy typically develops early in the course of check point inhibitor treatment, usually within 4 months or during the first four doses, especially with CTLA-4 inhibitors (9, 10). The most common presenting symptoms are headache, fatigue, nausea, hypotension, amenorrhea, and sexual dysfunction. Visual disturbances are rare (5, 11).

Anterior pituitary hormones are classically affected [thyrotropin (TSH) and follicle-stimulating hormone (FSH)/luteinizing

Table 1.   Classification of Immune Checkpoint Inhibitors

Class	Drug
CTLA-4 inhibitors	Ipilimumab
PD-1 inhibitors	Pembrolizumab, nivolumab
PD-L1 inhibitors	Atezolizumab, durvalumab, avelumab

hormone (LH) ~85%, adrenocorticotropic hormone (ACTH) ~73%, growth hormone, and prolactin (PRL) ~25%], whereas diabetes insipidus (DI) is much rarer compared with LyHy. Therefore, if a patient with cancer presents with DI, brain metastases should be higher in the differential diagnosis (5, 11).

MRI demonstrates some degree of pituitary enlargement (usually mild to moderate), stalk thickening (2, 3, 11), heterogeneous enhancement of the pituitary gland, or even normal findings (5). Optic chiasm compression is rare. MRI changes may precede clinical manifestations of Hy. Upon resolution of Hy, reduced pituitary volume or empty sella commonly are observed (12).

Other checkpoint inhibitor–induced endocrine disorders may occur concurrently or prior to Hy. Additionally, there are no known predictors of development of endocrinopathies (13, 14); therefore, increased awareness and close monitoring are important.

Management

Systemic HD GCs have been used to treat LyHy, although effectiveness of pituitary deficiency reversal has not been demonstrated consistently (15). Likewise, administration of HD GCs and discontinuation of immune therapy were recommended initially to treat immune therapy–induced Hy (3, 8). However, subsequent evidence has suggested that HD GCs do not improve Hy outcomes. Retrospective studies found no difference in the frequency or time of resolution of pituitary deficiencies and pituitary enlargement between patients who were and were not treated with systemic HD GCs for ipilimumab-induced Hy (8, 12). Pituitary enlargement resolved quickly (typically within 3 months), and corticotroph deficiency persisted long term in the majority of patients, irrespective of GC dose (2, 3). Recovery of other pituitary functions was variable, with thyroid and gonadal axes having a more favorable prognosis (7, 8, 11, 12).

Furthermore, GCs might reduce effectiveness of immune checkpoint inhibitors. A new retrospective study showed that patients with melanoma (n = 98) with ipilimumab-induced Hy had a better survival rate if they were treated with low-dose (LD) (replacement) rather than HD GCs (7), suggesting a possible negative effect on the efficacy of immune therapy. In this study, hypopituitarism resolved in a small fraction of patients treated with either HD or LD GCs, without a significant difference between the two groups. Radiologic resolution occurred in all but one patient, independent of the GC dose. Therefore, replacement doses of GCs and continuation of immune therapy have been recommended unless the patient is experiencing compressive symptoms (intractable headache, vision changes due to mass effect on optic chiasm) or if HD GCs are indicated for treatment of other concurrent toxicities (dermatologic, rheumatologic, gastrointestinal/hepatic, and pneumonitis) (7, 12, 15). A typical HD GC regimen is prednisone 1 mg/kg/d or equivalent but may vary slightly followed by a gradual taper to a physiologic replacement dose. Additionally, patients presenting with adrenal crisis or severe hyponatremia should be treated with an HD (*i.e.*, stress dose) GC (intravenous hydrocortisone is preferred) and fluids per current Endocrine Society guidelines (16, 17). Other pituitary deficiencies should be replaced as appropriate (16, 17). Management guidelines of the American Society of Clinical Oncology are based on the severity of endocrine toxicity and therefore are less specific but are still in line with the above recommendations. In addition, withholding immune therapy for more advanced (grades 3 to 4) Hy until the patient is clinically stable on replacement hormones is recommended (18). Testing for recovery of pituitary function or development of new hormone deficiencies can be performed at 3- to 6-month intervals or as clinically indicated.

IgG4-Related Hy
Pathophysiology
IgG4-RD is a systemic disorder characterized by inflammation and infiltration of the affected organs by lymphocytes, IgG4-positive plasma cells, and some degree of fibrosis. IgG4-related Hy is a rare manifestation, occurring as an isolated entity or as part of multiple organ involvement. Like other types of IgG4-RD, IgG4-related Hy occurs more commonly in middle-aged and older men (19, 20).

Pathophysiology of IgG4-RD is not completely understood but possibly is driven by an autoimmune, allergic, or infectious process. IgG4 antibody elevation could be a secondary event rather than a primary immune process, and IgG4 antibodies are not considered pathogenic by themselves.

Clinical Presentation and Diagnosis
Patients present with headache, visual defects, and anterior and/or posterior pituitary hormone deficiencies. Panhypopituitarism develops in 44%, with DI being the most common deficiency, followed by gonadal, corticotroph, somatotroph, and thyroid deficiency (19). Some authors reported no pituitary deficiencies or mild hypopituitarism (21, 22).

MRI demonstrates pituitary enlargement and stalk thickening. Additional body imaging, such as CT and fluorodeoxyglucose-positron emission tomography, is helpful in diagnosing systemic IgG4-RD. Variable levels of serum IgG4 antibodies have been observed in IgG4-RD, including often completely normal values (up to 40%), which limits diagnostic utility. IgG4 elevation may correlate with the extent of disease or number of organs involved (23). Decreasing levels are seen during treatment with GCs.

A pituitary biopsy can confirm IgG4-related Hy and rule out other types of inflammatory or neoplastic sellar masses. However, when pituitary tissue diagnosis is not available, the diagnosis of IgG4-related Hy can be established using criteria proposed by Leporati *et al.* (24) (Table 2). Occasionally, pathology may be atypical, lacking IgG4 plasma cell infiltration, whereas clinical presentation is consistent with IgG4-RD (systemic organ involvement with elevated serum IgG4). Previous use of GCs is believed to affect the biopsy results (25, 26).

Management
GCs are effective at decreasing pituitary size, which reportedly occurs rapidly within 1 to 2 months. Although moderate dose to HD GCs often are used to treat IgG4-related Hy, several groups have documented normalization of pituitary size and symptoms with physiologic doses (21). Little is known about the natural history of IgG4-related Hy, and one cannot exclude that it is a self-limiting disease prone to spontaneous resolution independent of GC use (27). At the same time, relapses and refractory cases have been reported, necessitating use of rituximab and other immunosuppressive therapies. Surgery may be necessary for prompt decompression of the optic chiasm. Recovery of pituitary function has been observed infrequently (20).

MAIN CONCLUSIONS
Immune therapy–related Hy likely will remain a clinical problem given more widespread use of checkpoint inhibitors. More studies

Table 2.   Diagnostic Criteria for IgG4-Related Hy

Diagnostic Criteria	Clinical Features	
Criterion 1: pituitary histopathology	Mononuclear infiltration of the pituitary gland, rich in lymphocytes and plasma cells, with >10 IgG4-positive cells per high-power field	
Criterion 2: pituitary MRI	Sellar mass and/or thickened pituitary stalk	
Criterion 3: biopsy-proven involvement in other organs	Association with IgG4-positive lesions in other organs	
Criterion 4: serology	Increased serum IgG4 (>140 mg/dL)	
Criterion 5: response to GCs	Shrinkage of the pituitary mass and symptom improvement with steroids	
Diagnosis of IgG4-related Hy is established when any of the following is fulfilled	Criterion 1	
	Criteria 2 and 3	
	Criteria 2, 4, and 5	

Reproduced with permission from Leporati P, Landek-Salgado MA, Lupi I, et al. IgG4-related hypophysitis: a new addition to the hypophysitis spectrum. *J Clin Endocrinol Metab.* 2011;96(7):1971–1980.

are needed to determine prognostic factors for patients who are at a higher risk and optimal individualized management. Currently, physiologic hormone replacement is recommended for a majority of patients unless they develop compressive neurologic symptoms or require HD GCs for other concurrent toxicities.

IgG4-related Hy has a broad clinical spectrum but should be suspected in middle-aged men with DI and anterior pituitary dysfunction. GCs are the mainstay of therapy and are effective in decreasing pituitary size but not at recovery of pituitary function. Further studies are needed to identify and develop diagnostic markers and determine appropriate treatment.

DISCUSSION OF CASES AND ANSWERS
Case 1
A 67-year-old male treated in a clinical trial with ipilimumab for prostate cancer presented with headache, fatigue, and anorexia. He denied visual changes, nausea, abdominal pain, increased thirst, or increased urination. He had a blood pressure of 122/75 mm Hg, pulse of 89 beats/min, temperature of 98.6°F, TSH of <0.01 mIU/L (0.46 to 5.56 mIU/L), free T_4 of 0.4 ng/dL (0.6 to 1.2 ng/dL), cortisol of <1 µg/dL (5.3 to 22.50 µg/dL); ACTH of <5 pg/mL (0 to 45 pg/mL), PRL of 3 ng/mL (2.1 to 17.7 ng/mL), IGF-1 of 103 ng/mL (34 to 240 ng/mL), FSH of <1 mIU/mL (0 to 19 mIU/mL), and LH of 1 mIU/mL (0 to 10 mIU/mL). MRI showed mild enlargement of the pituitary gland with pituitary stalk thickening.

1. How Would You Treat This Patient?
The patient presented with ipilimumab-induced Hy and multiple anterior pituitary deficiencies. There were no clinical symptoms of adrenal crisis and no evidence of optic chiasm compression clinically or on imaging. Therefore, HD GCs usually are not necessary, and the patient can be treated with replacement doses of GCs. The patient was started on hydrocortisone 30 mg daily, and after that, levothyroxine 125 µg/d was added. Symptoms quickly resolved with treatment. Ipilimumab treatment was continued.

2. A Few Weeks Later, a New Temporal Visual Field Defect Was Noted. How Would You Proceed?
HD GCs are indicated due to visual impairment. There is no universal protocol; however, prednisone 1 mg/kg/d or equivalent generally is recommended. The patient was started on prednisone 60 mg/d with subsequent taper and eventually switched to a physiologic dose of hydrocortisone. Ipilimumab treatment was stopped. Vision recovered, and 3 months later, MRI showed complete resolution of pituitary enlargement; the thyroid axis recovered, but secondary AI persisted.

Case 2
A 64-year-old male with metastatic small cell lung cancer treated with nivolumab/ipilimumab in a clinical trial was admitted with weakness, nausea, abdominal pain, and frequent bowel movements after a fourth nivolumab/ipilimumab injection. Vital signs were normal. Laboratory results on admission showed a TSH of <0.01 mIU/L (0.46 to 5.56 mIU/L), free T_4 of 3.5 ng/dL (0.6 to 1.2 ng/dL), sodium of 138 mmol/L (136 to 145 mmol/L), potassium of 3.0 mmol/L (3.4 to 5.0 mmol/L), and creatine of 1.2 mg/dL (0.70 to 1.30 mg/dL). Standard cortisol stimulation test results were 8.4 µg/dL at baseline (6 AM), 26.6 µg/dL at 30 minutes, and 25.9 µg/dL at 60 minutes. ACTH was not measured. TSH receptor antibody was normal. Thyroglobulin was 319 ng/mL (1.4 to 29 ng/mL). Brain MRI 4 weeks prior to presentation was normal.

1. What Is the Diagnosis?
Checkpoint inhibitor–induced thyroiditis. Additionally, symptomology suggests a possibility of AI. A normal ACTH stimulation test result does not rule out secondary AI during the acute phase of Hy (before adrenal atrophy has occurred). Therefore, it should be suspected particularly in the setting of hypotension, hyponatremia, and hypoglycemia, even with a normal ACTH stimulation test.

2. How Would You Manage This Patient?
GCs have been used for treatment of checkpoint inhibitor–induced thyroiditis; however, it is unknown whether GCs can alter disease course. In most cases, a hyperthyroid phase resolves quickly without treatment and is followed by a hypothyroid phase requiring thyroid hormone replacement. Therefore, experts have recommended only supportive measures and β-blockers for symptomatic management of mild to moderate thyroiditis (18, 28). In severe cases or if thyroid storm is suspected, prednisone 1 mg/kg/d over 1 to 2 weeks may be considered (18).

An accurate determination of whether this patient has secondary AI cannot be made. Baseline cortisol levels were low, and Endocrine Society guidelines recommend ruling out AI in patients with a morning cortisol <15 µg/dL (16, 17). However, absence of hypotension, hyponatremia, and hypoglycemia are reassuring, but in the presence of hyperthyroidism, replacement GCs should be administered until a clear diagnosis is made. HD/stress dose GCs are needed if the clinical situation deteriorates.

This patient was treated for thyroiditis with 40 mg oral prednisone daily for 7 days, followed by a taper over the next 3 weeks and transition to 20 mg hydrocortisone daily. Free T_4 normalized within 2 weeks; the patient then entered a hypothyroid phase and was started on levothyroxine 125 µg/d. Checkpoint inhibitor treatment was resumed after the hyperthyroidism resolved. Repeat ACTH stimulation test results were normal, and GCs were discontinued. However, 2 months later, the patient was readmitted with nausea, vomiting, weight loss, and hypoglycemic episodes. Empiric stress-dose GCs and fluids were administered with an excellent response.

3. What Is the Next Step in Diagnosis and Management?

Repeat morning cortisol and ACTH (or ACTH stimulation test). Repeat thyroid function tests to ensure appropriate thyroid replacement dose. Check FSH/LH, testosterone, PRL, and IGF-1 to assess for other pituitary deficiencies. If headache or vision changes are present, obtain a pituitary MRI.

This patient's ACTH stimulation test results showed a cortisol level of 7.9 µg/dL at baseline, 7.7 µg/dL at 30 minutes, and 10 µg/dL at 60 minutes and an ACTH level of 1 pg/mL, confirming secondary AI. He was treated with 20 mg of hydrocortisone daily. The patient denied headache or vision changes, thus an MRI was not performed. He remained in the clinical trial without evidence of cancer progression.

Case 3

A 69-year-old man presented with 4 months of fatigue, weakness, weight loss, polyuria, and polydipsia. Laboratory results revealed glucose of 120 mg/dL (70 to 99 mg/dL), creatine of 1.8 mg/dL (0.70 to 1.30 mg/dL), cortisol of 2.9 µg/dL (5.3 to 22.50 µg/dL), ACTH of 6 pg/mL (0 to 45 pg/mL), TSH of 0.8 mIU/L, free T_4 of 0.5 ng/dL (0.6 to 1.2 ng/dL), FSH of <1 mIU/mL, LH of <1 mIU/mL, PRL of 16 ng/mL (2.1 to 17.7 ng/mL), IGF-1 of 50 ng/mL (34 to 240 ng/mL), urine osmolality of 190 mOsm/kg H_2O, and serum osmolality of 300 mOsm/kg H_2O (275 to 295 mOsm/kg H_2O). MRI showed a normal-sized pituitary gland and thickened pituitary stalk.

1. Which Pituitary Disorder Do You Suspect and Why?

Although the differential diagnosis is broad (sarcoidosis, histiocytosis, tumor, lymphoma, infection, *etc.*), IgG4-related Hy should be suspected in this instance. Clinical features that are common in IgG4-related Hy include older age, male sex, and presence of DI.

2. What Additional Studies Would You Perform?

Although only a pituitary biopsy would provide a definitive diagnosis, clinicians often obtain a variety of noninvasive studies to try to establish an etiology. These tests may include chest x-ray or a CT of the chest/abdomen, angiotensin-converting enzyme, tuberculosis, antineutrophil cytoplasmic antibody, serum IgG4, and sometimes lumbar puncture. This patient's IgG4 level was elevated. CT scan showed bilateral low-attenuation lesions in the kidneys. Biopsy of the kidney nodules confirmed IgG4-RD.

3. How Would You Treat This Patient?

IgG4-RD responds well to GCs; however, an optimal regimen is not well established. International consensus guidance recommends that active IgG4-RD be treated with moderate doses of GCs (prednisone 30 to 40 mg/d) as initial treatment for 2 to 4 weeks followed by gradual taper with a goal to discontinue treatment in 3 to 6 months. Some experts recommend maintenance

therapy with LD prednisone (5 mg/d) for up to 3 years (29). With treatment, this patient's serum IgG4 level normalized, renal lesions improved, and the pituitary stalk was thinner on a 6-month follow-up scan. However, pituitary deficiencies persisted, as in most cases of Hy.

References

1. Joshi MN, Whitelaw BC, Carroll PV. Mechanisms in endocrinology: hypophysitis: diagnosis and treatment. *Eur J Endocrinol.* 2018; **179**(3):R151–R163.
2. Dillard T, Yedinak CG, Alumkal J, Fleseriu M. Anti-CTLA-4 antibody therapy associated autoimmune hypophysitis: serious immune related adverse events across a spectrum of cancer subtypes. *Pituitary.* 2010;**13**(1):29–38.
3. Joshi MN, Whitelaw BC, Palomar MT, Wu Y, Carroll PV. Immune checkpoint inhibitor-related hypophysitis and endocrine dysfunction: clinical review. *Clin Endocrinol (Oxf).* 2016;**85**(3):331–339.
4. Caturegli P, Di Dalmazi G, Lombardi M, Grosso F, Larman HB, Larman T, Taverna G, Cosottini M, Lupi I. Hypophysitis secondary to cytotoxic T-lymphocyte-associated protein 4 blockade: insights into pathogenesis from an autopsy series. *Am J Pathol.* 2016;**186**(12):3225–3235.
5. González-Rodríguez E, Rodríguez-Abreu D for the Spanish Group for Cancer Immuno-Biotherapy (GETICA). Immune checkpoint inhibitors: review and management of endocrine adverse events. *Oncologist.* 2016;**21**(7):804–816.
6. Barroso-Sousa R, Barry WT, Garrido-Castro AC, Hodi FS, Min L, Krop IE, Tolaney SM. Incidence of endocrine dysfunction following the use of different immune checkpoint inhibitor regimens: a systematic review and meta-analysis. *JAMA Oncol.* 2018;**4**(2):173–182.
7. Faje AT, Lawrence D, Flaherty K, Freedman C, Fadden R, Rubin K, Cohen J, Sullivan RJ. High-dose glucocorticoids for the treatment of ipilimumab-induced hypophysitis is associated with reduced survival in patients with melanoma. *Cancer.* 2018;**124**(18):3706–3714.
8. Min L, Hodi FS, Giobbie-Hurder A, Ott PA, Luke JJ, Donahue H, Davis M, Carroll RS, Kaiser UB. Systemic high-dose corticosteroid treatment does not improve the outcome of ipilimumab-related hypophysitis: a retrospective cohort study. *Clin Cancer Res.* 2015;**21**(4):749–755.
9. Johnson DB. Toxicities and outcomes: do steroids matter? *Cancer.* 2018;**124**(18):3638–3640.
10. Sznol M, Postow MA, Davies MJ, Pavlick AC, Plimack ER, Shaheen M, Veloski C, Robert C. Endocrine-related adverse events associated with immune checkpoint blockade and expert insights on their management. *Cancer Treat Rev.* 2017;**58**:70–76.
11. Faje AT, Sullivan R, Lawrence D, Tritos NA, Fadden R, Klibanski A, Nachtigall L. Ipilimumab-induced hypophysitis: a detailed longitudinal analysis in a large cohort of patients with metastatic melanoma. *J Clin Endocrinol Metab.* 2014;**99**(11):4078–4085.
12. Albarel F, Gaudy C, Castinetti F, Carré T, Morange I, Conte-Devolx B, Grob JJ, Brue T. Long-term follow-up of ipilimumab-induced hypophysitis, a common adverse event of the anti-CTLA-4 antibody in melanoma. *Eur J Endocrinol.* 2015;**172**(2):195–204.
13. Sum M, Garcia FV. Immunotherapy-induced autoimmune diabetes and concomitant hypophysitis. *Pituitary.* 2018;**21**(5):556–557.
14. Zeng MF, Chen LL, Ye HY, Gong W, Zhou LN, Li YM, Zhao XL. Primary hypothyroidism and isolated ACTH deficiency induced by nivolumab therapy: case report and review. *Medicine (Baltimore).* 2017;**96**(44): e8426.
15. Johnston PC, Chew LS, Hamrahian AH, Kennedy L. Lymphocytic infundibulo-neurohypophysitis: a clinical overview. *Endocrine.* 2015; **50**(3):531–536.
16. Chang LS, Barroso-Sousa R, Tolaney SM, Hodi FS, Kaiser UB, Min L. Endocrine toxicity of cancer immunotherapy targeting immune checkpoints. *Endocr Rev.* 2019;**40**(1):17–65.
17. Fleseriu M, Hashim IA, Karavitaki N, Melmed S, Murad MH, Salvatori R, Samuels MH. Hormonal replacement in hypopituitarism in adults:

an Endocrine Society clinical practice guideline. *J Clin Endocrinol Metab.* 2016;**101**(11):3888–3921.

18. Brahmer JR, Lacchetti C, Schneider BJ, Atkins MB, Brassil KJ, Caterino JM, Chau I, Ernstoff MS, Gardner JM, Ginex P, Hallmeyer S, Holter Chakrabarty J, Leighl NB, Mammen JS, McDermott DF, Naing A, Nastoupil LJ, Phillips T, Porter LD, Puzanov I, Reichner CA, Santomasso BD, Seigel C, Spira A, Suarez-Almazor ME, Wang Y, Weber JS, Wolchok JD, Thompson JA for the National Comprehensive Cancer Network. Management of immune-related adverse events in patients treated with immune checkpoint inhibitor therapy: American Society of Clinical Oncology clinical practice guideline. *J Clin Oncol.* 2018; **36**(17):1714–1768.

19. Shikuma J, Kan K, Ito R, Hara K, Sakai H, Miwa T, Kanazawa A, Odawara M. Critical review of IgG4-related hypophysitis. *Pituitary.* 2017;**20**(2): 282–291.

20. Liu Y, Wang L, Zhang W, Pan H, Yang H, Deng K, Lu L, Yao Y, Chen S, Chai X, Feng F, You H, Jin Z, Zhu H. Hypophyseal involvement in immunoglobulin G4-related disease: a retrospective study from a single tertiary center. *Int J Endocrinol.* 2018;**2018**:7637435.

21. Harano Y, Honda K, Akiyama Y, Kotajima L, Arioka H. A case of IgG4-related hypophysitis presented with hypopituitarism and diabetes insipidus. *Clin Med Insights Case Rep.* 2015;**8**:23–26.

22. Hattori Y, Tahara S, Ishii Y, Kitamura T, Inomoto C, Osamura RY, Teramoto A, Morita A. A case of IgG4-related hypophysitis without pituitary insufficiency. *J Clin Endocrinol Metab.* 2013;**98**(5):1808–1811.

23. Takano K, Yamamoto M, Takahashi H, Himi T. Recent advances in knowledge regarding the head and neck manifestations of IgG4-related disease. *Auris Nasus Larynx.* 2017;**44**(1):7–17.

24. Leporati P, Landek-Salgado MA, Lupi I, Chiovato L, Caturegli P. IgG4-related hypophysitis: a new addition to the hypophysitis spectrum. *J Clin Endocrinol Metab.* 2011;**96**(7):1971–1980.

25. Yuen KCJ, Moloney KJ, Mercado JU, Rostad S, McCullough BJ, Litvack ZN, Delashaw JB, Mayberg MR. A case series of atypical features of patients with biopsy-proven isolated IgG4-related hypophysitis and normal serum IgG4 levels. *Pituitary.* 2018;**21**(3):238–246.

26. Bernreuther C, Illies C, Flitsch J, Buchfelder M, Buslei R, Glatzel M, Saeger W. IgG4-related hypophysitis is highly prevalent among cases of histologically confirmed hypophysitis. *Brain Pathol.* 2017;**27**(6):839–845.

27. Anno T, Kawasaki F, Takai M, Shigemoto R, Kan Y, Kaneto H, Mune T, Kaku K, Okimoto N. Clinical course of pituitary function and image in IgG4-related hypophysitis. *Endocrinol Diabetes Metab Case Rep.* 2017;**2017**:16–0148.

28. Iyer PC, Cabanillas M, Waguespack SG, Hu MI, Thosani SN, Lavis VR, Busaidy NL, Subudhi SK, Diab A, Dadu R. Immune-related thyroiditis with immune checkpoint inhibitors. *Thyroid.* 2018;**28**(10):1243–1251.

29. Khosroshahi A, Wallace ZS, Crowe JL, Akamizu T, Azumi A, Carruthers MN, Chari ST, Della-Torre E, Frulloni L, Goto H, Hart PA, Kamisawa T, Kawa S, Kawano M, Kim MH, Kodama Y, Kubota K, Lerch MM, Löhr M, Masaki Y, Matsui S, Mimori T, Nakamura S, Nakazawa T, Ohara H, Okazaki K, Ryu JH, Saeki T, Schleinitz N, Shimatsu A, Shimosegawa T, Takahashi H, Takahira M, Tanaka A, Topazian M, Umehara H, Webster GJ, Witzig TE, Yamamoto M, Zhang W, Chiba T, Stone JH for the Second International Symposium on IgG4-Related Disease. International consensus guidance statement on the management and treatment of IgG4-related disease. *Arthritis Rheumatol.* 2015;**67**(7): 1688–1699.

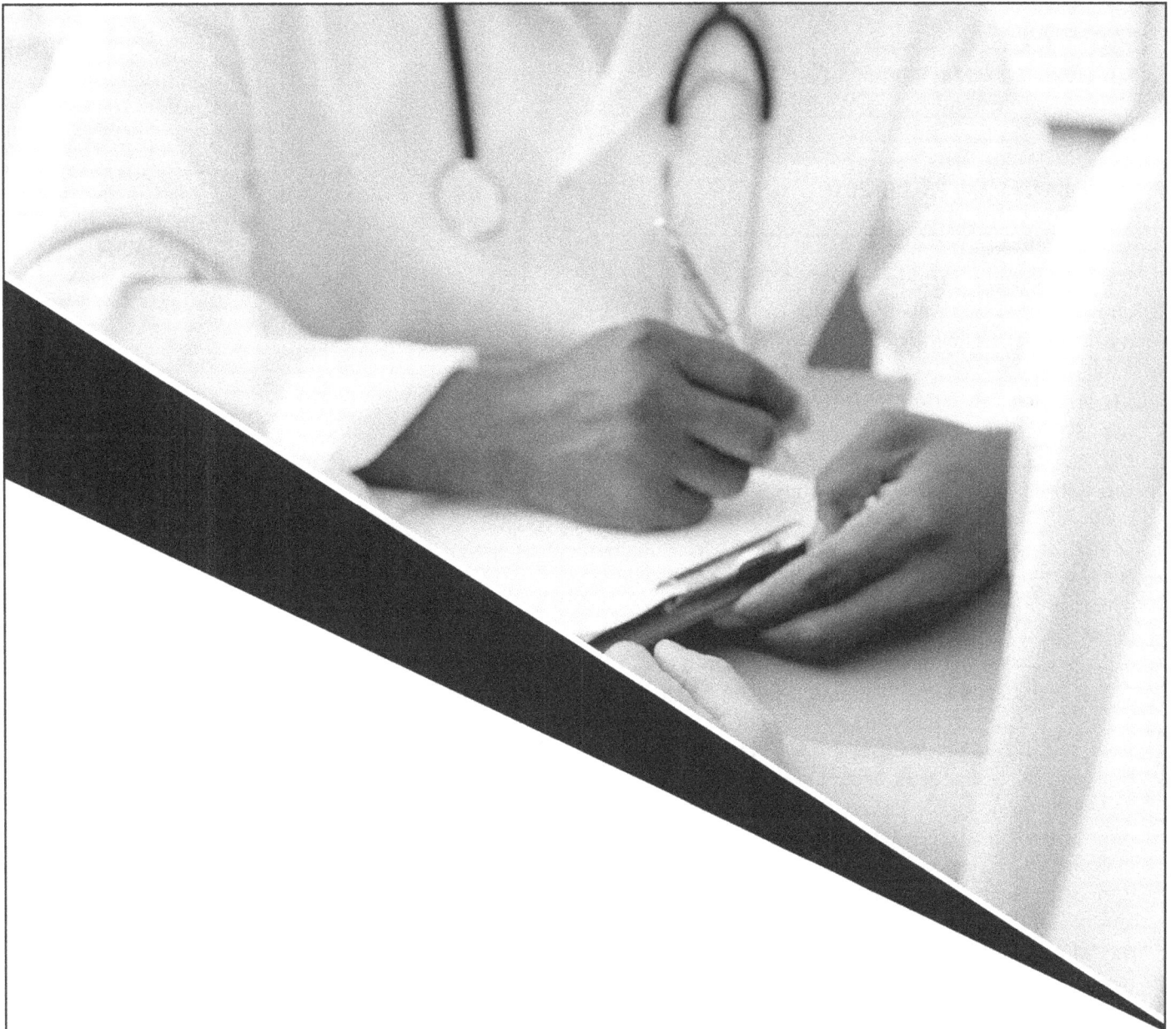

PEDIATRIC ENDOCRINOLOGY

Growth Hormone Transition

M08
Presented, March 23–26, 2019

Jens Otto Lunde Jørgensen, DMSci. Department of Endocrinology and Diabetes, Aarhus University Hospital, Aarhus 8400, Denmark, E-mail: joj@clin.au.dk

SIGNIFICANCE OF THE PROBLEM

Growth-promoting activity of anterior pituitary extracts was discovered almost 100 years ago, and growth hormone (GH) was isolated in 1944 (1). Subsequently, GH extracted from human cadaveric pituitary glands was used therapeutically to promote longitudinal growth in children with hypopituitarism and severe growth retardation. The scarce supply demanded a restrictive use, and treatment was terminated when a certain target height was reached. This scenario changed completely with the advent and approval of biosynthetic human GH (2).

The first extension of clinical practice became GH substitution in adults with verified pituitary disease and GH deficiency (GHD). The pivotal trial in 1989 was a collaboration between adult and pediatric endocrinologists and included patients with a mean age of ~24 years with reconfirmed childhood-onset GHD who had received childhood GH replacement that was discontinued ~6 years before the trial (3). A substantial increase in muscle volume and a substantial reduction in fat volume together with improved exercise capacity were recorded. The second trial comprised patients with adult-onset GHD with a mean age of ~39 years and confirmed beneficial effects on body composition (4). These observations were replicated in numerous trials, which led to the approval of adult GHD as an indication for GH replacement in 1994 (5).

However, neither trial captured patients in transition from childhood to adulthood, which is noteworthy for several reasons. First, peripuberty is characterized by continued growth and very high serum insulin-like growth factor I (IGF-I) levels, which suggests a particular role for ongoing GH activity (Fig. 1). Second, uncritical continuation of GH replacement in all children does not take into account that a proportion of the patients respond normally to a GH stimulation retest after completion of longitudinal growth (6). Third, the etiology of hypopituitarism developing in peripubertal children is different from adult-onset GHD, which may have therapeutic implications. Finally, the patients in this age-group may require particular attention to ensure treatment adherence, which is particularly critical as their care transitions from pediatricians to adult endocrinologists.

BARRIERS TO OPTIMAL PRACTICE

- Nonformalized collaboration between pediatricians and adult endocrinologists

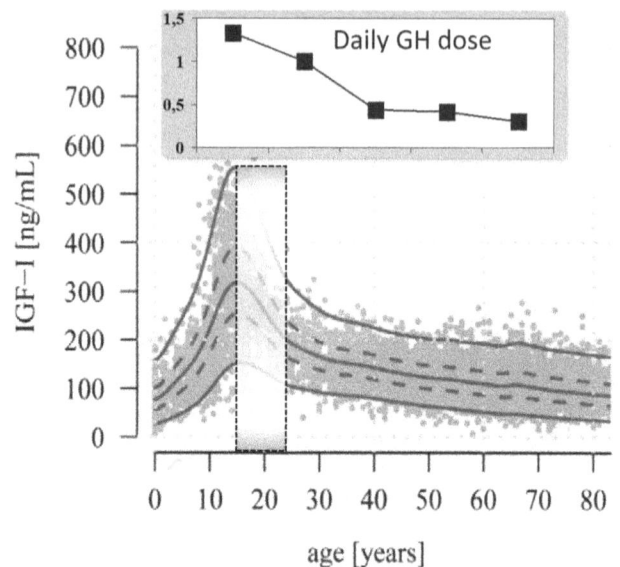

Figure 1. Serum IGF-I levels as a function of age. Inset shows daily GH dose tailored to maintain serum IGF-I within the upper limit of normal. The transition period is indicated. Adapted with permission from Bidlingmaier M, Friedrich N, Emeny RT, et al. Reference intervals for insulin-like growth factor-1 (IGF-1) from birth to senescence: results from amulticenter study using a new automated chemiluminescence IGF-1 immunoassay conforming to recent international recommendations. *J Clin Endocrinol Metab.* 2014;99(5):1712–1721.

- Incomplete knowledge of diagnosis and treatment
- Failure to ensure patient adherence

LEARNING OBJECTIVES

As a result of participating in this session, learners should be able to:

- Understand the history of GH replacement before and after the availability of biosynthetic GH
- Define and describe the transition phase with emphasis on GH status
- Understand specific challenges in the management of transition phase patients

STRATEGIES FOR DIAGNOSIS, TREATMENT, AND MANAGEMENT

Puberty is the transition from childhood to adulthood and represents a period with marked physical changes, including a pubertal growth spurt and the development of secondary sexual characteristics. Muscle and bone mass increase markedly during this period, leading to the adult phenotype. These important physical changes depend on amplified GH secretion and action, resulting in very high, and even acromegalic, IGF-I levels (Fig. 1).

Serum IGF-I levels remain elevated 2 to 5 years after peak height velocity, suggesting additional physiological actions of GH on muscle and bone mass accrual in this period. The transition phase starts in late puberty when final adult height is attained (mean age, ~15 to 17 years) and terminates in early adulthood when peak bone mass is reached (mean age, ~20 to 23 years) (Fig. 1).

As mentioned previously, the early adult GH replacement trials did not recruit patients within this critical age-group, but a prospective study reported that discontinuation of GH replacement in patients with childhood-onset GHD at the time of transition induced unfavorable changes in lipid profile and body composition (7). Subsequently, a double-blind, placebo-controlled parallel study evaluated the effects of continuation versus discontinuation of GH replacement after cessation of linear growth (8, 9). It showed that GH discontinuation resulted in decreased IGF-I as well as increased body fat and insulin sensitivity. After resumption of GH, lean body mass and IGF-I increased. Comparable results were reported from an open study of 12-month continuation versus discontinuation of GH replacement (10).

Guidelines regarding the management of patients with GHD during the transition are available, of which certain points merit mention here (11). First, a large proportion of children with GHD exhibit normal stimulated GH secretion when retested after completion of GH treatment (6). Therefore, GH status and the indication for continued GH replacement in adulthood must be evaluated on an individual basis, which requires retesting unless there is strong evidence of either organic panhypopituitarism or a genetic cause of GHD. Second, GH dosing is no longer based on longitudinal growth response but relies predominantly on serum IGF-I measurements. Finally, the proper management of transition patients includes patient involvement and a close collaboration between pediatric and adult endocrinologists.

CASES WITH QUESTIONS AND ANSWERS
Case 1
An 18-year-old female was diagnosed with a craniopharyngeoma at age 5 years. The presenting symptoms were headache and impaired visual function. The patient underwent transcranial surgery and was left with panhypopituitarism and central diabetes insipidus. The substitution therapy included hydrocortisone, levothyroxine, estradiol, GH, and desmopressin.

Question
What are next steps with regard to GH substitution?
  A. Discontinue GH substitution if an acceptable linear height is achieved.
  B. Discontinue GH substitution for 1 month and perform a GH stimulation test.
  C. Continue GH substitution without any retesting.
  D. Perform pituitary imaging and continue GH substitution if no tumor is remnant.

  E. Measure IGF-I after 1-month GH discontinuation, and restart GH if IGF-I is <-2 standard deviations.

Answer
As a rule, a diagnosis of GHD requires an appropriate clinical context in addition to a GH stimulation test (12). Exceptions to the rule exist, one of which is a transition patient with multiple (three or more) pituitary deficiencies (11, 12). However, the jury is out about whether C or E is correct. The Pediatric Endocrine Society favors C (12), whereas the Growth Hormone Research Society (GRS) recommends E (11). With today's experience, I favor C, but the patient was retested with an insulin tolerance test without any evidence of residual GH secretory capacity.

It is important to emphasize that the majority of patients treated with GH in childhood have idiopathic GHD, and most of these patients exhibit a normal GH response when retested after attainment of their target height (6).

Question
How would you dose and monitor GH substitution?
  A. Continue weight-based dosing and monitor according to serum IGF-I.
  B. Continue weight-based dosing and monitor according to body composition.
  C. Switch to a fixed dose of 0.2 to 0.5 mg/d and adjust on the basis of serum IGF-I.
  D. Same as C plus structured quality-of-life assessments.
  E. Use the nomogram developed by GRS that takes into account age, sex, and body composition.

Answer
A non–weight-based regimen is recommended with the dose adjusted according to IGF-I; thus, answer C is correct (11). Also recommended is to avoid serum IGF-I levels above the upper limit of normal and to check HbA_{1c} levels and evidence of fluid retention. Although GH affects body composition at all ages, it is not recommended to monitor treatment according to this in the transition patient. Quality-of-life assessments are mandatory in some countries (United Kingdom) to reimburse and guide GH replacement in adults, but they are not in the guidelines for transition patients. Moreover, it remains unproven whether GH replacement improves quality of life compared with placebo (5). Unfortunately, no nomogram was available.

Question
Which is correct with regard to management of underlying disease and additional hormone replacement?
  A. The patient may develop impaired quality of life and psychosocial problems related to GHD and/or the underlying chronic disease for which she may need counseling.
  B. The following minimum observations are recommended: height, weight, body mass index, and waist and hip

circumference yearly; blood pressure, heart rate, and quality-of-life assessment yearly; duel-energy x-ray absorptiometry (DXA) and lipid profiles at baseline and at 2- to 5-year intervals.

C. Patients with treated intracranial malignancy require an annual MRI for at least 3 years after primary tumor therapy and subsequently as appropriate. Patients with treated craniopharyngioma should be reimaged at a frequency determined by the perceived risk of tumor regrowth.

D. The patient on hydrocortisone replacement should continue this treatment with a daily dose of 8 to 12 mg/m^2 three times daily (early morning, lunch, and evening). GH replacement may accelerate cortisol metabolism, which may increase the risk of cortisol insufficiency in those with untreated subtle degrees of adrenocorticotropic hormone or those on suboptimal hydrocortisone replacement.

E. As part of the transition management, fertility issues should be discussed in collaboration with a reproductive specialist.

Answer

All statements are correct according to the GRS guideline (11). With regard to DXA measurements, however, the more recent Pediatric Endocrine Society guidelines argue against DXA scanning as obligatory during follow-up of GH treatment in transition patients (12), and it has been challenged whether there is a true increased risk of osteopenia in adolescents with GHD to justify bone densitometry measurements (13).

The patient did encounter psychosocial problems, which also caused her to express ambivalence about adherence to her substitution therapy apart from hydrocortisone. However, after counseling, she resumed all substitution therapy and has since lived a successful life.

Case 2

A 17-year-old female is referred to the outpatient clinic with a pituitary mass lesion. She was first seen by a private gynecologist because of secondary amenorrhea for 2 years. Serum prolactin was 83 µg/L (~1600 mU/L).

Question

What is the most likely diagnosis?
A. Prolactinoma
B. Nonfunctioning pituitary adenoma
C. Craniopharyngeoma
D. Germinoma
E. Pilocytic astrocytoma

Answer

Pituitary adenomas are rare in this age-group, wherefore other causes must be considered first. A craniopharyngeoma is a relatively frequent intracranial tumor in this age-group, and a computed tomography scan may be considered to visualize calcifications.

Astrocytomas account for ~50% of childhood intracranial tumors and may be located in the optic chiasm or the hypothalamus. Intracranial germinomas also occur in this age-group, and tandem lesions affecting both the suprasellar region and the pineal body are pathognomonic. Thus, the correct answer is D.

Panhypopituitarism, including central diabetes insipidus, developed, and the patient was given replacements of hydrocortisone, levothyroxine, estradiol, and desmopressin. The patient was treated with cranial irradiation (40 Gy) and responded well without notable adverse effects. She was a former elite swimmer, her father was a physician, and her mother was a nurse. The family asked specifically about GH testing and treatment.

Question

Which statement is correct regarding GHD in this context?
A. GHD should not be considered because GH replacement is contraindicated at any time in this patient.
B. It is recommended to assess for GHD in all survivors treated for tumors in the region of the hypothalamic pituitary axis, including radiation (≥18 Gy).
C. Annual serum IGF-I measurements are recommended to monitor GH status.
D. The preferred GH stimulation test is GHRH in combination with arginine.
E. It is not necessary to test for GHD if there are more than three other anterior pituitary deficits.

Answer

Although intracranial germinoma has a very good prognosis, it is a malignant disease, so the decision to test for and treat GHD is not trivial. However, there is overwhelming consensus that GHD should be tested for. Serum IGF-I is not useful in this regard, and a GHRH stimulation test may elicit a falsely normal response if the lesion is predominantly hypothalamic (14). Thus, the correct answer is E. The patient underwent an insulin tolerance test that showed severe GHD and opted for GH replacement.

Question

Which statement is correct with regard to GH substitution in childhood cancer survivors?
A. It is suggested to wait until the patient has been at least 2 years disease free.
B. The GH dose should be reduced compared with that in patients with GHD from the noncancer population.
C. GH replacement generally is recommended.
D. Although GH replacement generally is recommended, the risk of recurrence of the original tumor is slightly increased.
E. All of the above are correct.

Answer

GH replacement generally is recommended when the patient is 1 year disease free and treatment dose and monitoring should be done according to standard guidelines (14). According to a recent meta-analysis, the risk of tumor recurrence is not increased (15). Thus, the correct answer is C.

DISCUSSION

The transition period refers to a broad set of physical and psychosocial changes, arbitrarily defined as starting in late puberty and ending with full adult maturation (11). It is a challenging phase for the patient with hypopituitarism and their caregivers because a transition takes place simultaneously between pediatricians and adult endocrinologists. Moreover, it is necessary to reevaluate frequently the disease and its treatment. Not the least, treatment adherence is not always optimal in this age-group and demands close collaboration among all parties. At the same time, it is essential to offer continued care to ensure optimal lifelong health and quality of life. GH replacement is only one piece of the puzzle. The two case reports illustrate the veracity of the guidelines and the good prognosis with regard to quality of health if proper treatment and care are provided.

References

1. Beck JC, McGarry EE, Dyrenfurth I, Venning EH. Metabolic effects of human and monkey growth hormone in man. *Science.* 1957;**125**(3253):884–885.
2. Kaplan SL, Underwood LE, August GP, Bell JJ, Blethen SL, Blizzard RM, Brown DR, Foley TP, Hintz RL, Hopwood NJ, et al. Clinical studies with recombinant-DNA-derived methionyl human growth hormone in growth hormone deficient children. *Lancet.* 1986;**327**(8483):697–700.
3. Jørgensen JO, Pedersen SA, Thuesen L, Jørgensen J, Ingemann-Hansen T, Skakkebaek NE, Christiansen JS. Beneficial effects of growth hormone treatment in GH-deficient adults. *Lancet.* 1989;**333**(8649):1221–1225.
4. Salomon F, Cuneo RC, Hesp R, Sönksen PH. The effects of treatment with recombinant human growth hormone on body composition and metabolism in adults with growth hormone deficiency. *N Engl J Med.* 1989;**321**(26):1797–1803.
5. Jørgensen JOL, Juul A. Therapy of endocrine disease: growth hormone replacement therapy in adults: 30 years of personal clinical experience. *Eur J Endocrinol.* 2018;**179**(1):R47–R56.
6. Tauber M, Moulin P, Pienkowski C, Jouret B, Rochiccioli P. Growth hormone (GH) retesting and auxological data in 131 GH-deficient patients after completion of treatment. *J Clin Endocrinol Metab.* 1997;**82**(2):352–356.
7. Johannsson G, Albertsson-Wikland K, Bengtsson BA; Swedish Study Group for Growth Hormone Treatment in Children. Discontinuation of growth hormone (GH) treatment: metabolic effects in GH-deficient and GH-sufficient adolescent patients compared with control subjects. *J Clin Endocrinol Metab.* 1999;**84**(12):4516–4524.
8. Vahl N, Juul A, Jørgensen JO, Orskov H, Skakkebaek NE, Christiansen JS. Continuation of growth hormone (GH) replacement in GH-deficient patients during transition from childhood to adulthood: a two-year placebo-controlled study. *J Clin Endocrinol Metab.* 2000;**85**(5):1874–1881.
9. Nørrelund H, Vahl N, Juul A, Møller N, Alberti KG, Skakkebaek NE, Christiansen JS, Jørgensen JO. Continuation of growth hormone (GH) therapy in GH-deficient patients during transition from childhood to adulthood: impact on insulin sensitivity and substrate metabolism. *J Clin Endocrinol Metab.* 2000;**85**(5):1912–1917.
10. Carroll PV, Drake WM, Maher KT, Metcalfe K, Shaw NJ, Dunger DB, Cheetham TD, Camacho-Hübner C, Savage MO, Monson JP. Comparison of continuation or cessation of growth hormone (GH) therapy on body composition and metabolic status in adolescents with severe GH deficiency at completion of linear growth. *J Clin Endocrinol Metab.* 2004;**89**(8):3890–3895.
11. Clayton PE, Cuneo RC, Juul A, Monson JP, Shalet SM, Tauber M; European Society of Paediatric Endocrinology. Consensus statement on the management of the GH-treated adolescent in the transition to adult care. *Eur J Endocrinol.* 2005;**152**(2):165–170.
12. Grimberg A, DiVall SA, Polychronakos C, Allen DB, Cohen LE, Quintos JB, Rossi WC, Feudtner C, Murad MH; Drug and Therapeutics Committee and Ethics Committee of the Pediatric Endocrine Society. Guidelines for growth hormone and insulin-like growth factor-I treatment in children and adolescents: growth hormone deficiency, idiopathic short stature, and primary insulin-like growth factor-I deficiency. *Horm Res Paediatr.* 2016;**86**(6):361–397.
13. Högler W, Shaw N. Childhood growth hormone deficiency, bone density, structures and fractures: scrutinizing the evidence. *Clin Endocrinol (Oxf).* 2010;**72**(3):281–289.
14. Sklar CA, Antal Z, Chemaitilly W, Cohen LE, Follin C, Meacham LR, Murad MH. Hypothalamic-pituitary and growth disorders in survivors of childhood cancer: an Endocrine Society Clinical practice guideline. *J Clin Endocrinol Metab.* 2018;**103**(8):2761–2784.
15. Tamhane S, Sfeir JG, Kittah NEN, Jasim S, Chemaitilly W, Cohen LE, Murad MH. GH therapy in childhood cancer survivors: a systematic review and meta-analysis. *J Clin Endocrinol Metab.* 2018;**103**(8):2794–2801.

Adolescent Bariatric Surgery

M30
Presented, March 23–26, 2019

Ellen Lancon Connor, MD. Division of Pediatric Endocrinology and Diabetes, University of Wisconsin–Madison, Madison, Wisconsin 53706, E-mail: elconnor@wisc.edu

Dennis Styne, MD. Department of Pediatrics, Division of Pediatric Endocrinolgy, University of California Davis Health, Sacramento, California 95817; E-mail: dmstyne@ucdavis.edu

SIGNIFICANCE OF THE CLINICAL PROBLEM

Adolescent obesity is prevelent and places many American youth at risk of severe metabolic and cardiovascular comorbidities, even during the teen years. The risk of obesity and comorbidities for an adult who was an adolescent with obesity is significant. The condition is often refractory to lifestyle modifications and there are no effective approved pharmaceutical agents available so that bariatric surgery becomes an appropriate choice for the most severely affected individuals.

BARRIERS TO OPTIMAL PRACTICE

Barriers to optimal practice include a lack of availability of adolescent bariatric surgery centers of excellence to accommodate adolescents in all regions of the country. Previously there was a reluctance to refer adolescents for this type of surgery over concerns over impaired growth. Lower socioeconomic status or ethnic minority status are also associated with lower likelihood of referral to bariatric surgery centers. Additionally, families often face lack of insurance coverage for the procedure. Last, lack of family support may impair the essential follow-up care.

LEARNING OBJECTIVES

As a result of participating in this session, learners should be able to:
- Recognize who is a candidate for adolescent bariatric surgery
- Identify the various procedures and their efficacy in adolescents
- Understand the monitoring needed after bariatric surgery

STRATEGIES FOR DIAGNOSIS, THERAPY, AND/OR MANAGEMENT

In the United States between 2014 and 2016, 5% to 7% of youth had a body mass index (BMI) ≥ 35 kg/m^2 or a BMI $\geq 120\%$ of the 95th percentile for age and sex (1). Youth with severe obesity are at high risk for current and future cardiovascular and metabolic disease. Long-term weight loss programs fail to demonstrate enduring substantial loss of weight or BMI values in pediatric obesity (2–4). However, adolescent bariatric surgery in bariatric surgery centers of excellence is proven to be a meaningful tool in reducing BMI and metabolic and cardiovascular complications, although there are no long-term studies in this age group (5). Candidates for surgery must be carefully selected and require close monitoring for many years after surgery to prevent and address surgical and other complications. Three-year studies of weight loss indicate that patients can maintain a decrease in BMI of 15 to 20 kg/m^2 or over 5 years, a weight loss of 20%, but weight regain from years 1 to 5 has been noted (5, 6).

Guidelines for the choice of a candidate for adolescent bariatric surgery were developed mainly by bariatric surgery centers of excellence for this age group (7–9). A summary includes the following (10):

1. The patient has attained Tanner stage 4 or 5 pubertal development and final or near-final adult height.
2. The patient has a BMI of 40 kg/m^2 or has a BMI of 35 kg/m^2 and substantial, extreme comorbidities.
3. Extreme obesity and comorbidities persist despite compliance with a formal program of lifestyle modification with or without pharmacotherapy.
4. Psychological evaluation confirms the stability and competence of the family unit. Psychological distress due to impaired quality of life from obesity may be present, but the patient does not have an underlying untreated psychiatric illness.
5. The patient demonstrates the ability to adhere to the principles of healthy dietary and activity habits.
6. The patient has access to an experienced surgeon in a pediatric bariatric surgery center of excellence that provides the necessary infrastructure for patient care, including a team capable of long-term follow-up of the metabolic and psychosocial needs of the patient and family.

Adolescents chosen for bariatric surgery traditionally have been at or near full skeletal maturation, but some evidence suggests that those who have not reached skeletal maturation may not have adverse effects from surgery on adult height (5). Because of potential risks to the fetus, girls who are pregnant or planning to become pregnant in the next 2 years should not undergo bariatric surgery procedures.

Psychological illness that is untreated is a contraindication, but psychopathology that is being treated and/or related to obesity itself does not preclude surgery and may be a comorbidity to include in screening. Untreated substance abuse or eating disorders are contraindications to surgery.

Before surgery, patients must have attempted lifestyle modification with dietary and exercise prescriptions for weight loss for at least 6 months. Patients must have family or guardian support and an understanding that bariatric surgery may not make them thin but will decrease their BMI and its consequences.

Some studies of patients with cognitive impairment have been reported. Gibbons *et al.* (11) reported a summary of 16 studies in 49 patients with intellectual disabilities. The most frequently performed surgeries were biliopancreatic diversion and Roux-en-Y-gastric bypass (RYGB). Weight loss varied from 12% to 86% of excess weight. Improved quality of life and resolved sleep apnea, hypertension, and type 2 diabetes were reported.

Patients and/or their guardians must be able to understand and comply with the dietary changes and follow-up essential to the surgery. Although initially, surgery was offered only to those with a BMI ≥ 40 kg/m^2 or to those ≥ 35 kg/m^2 with severe comorbidities, experience now suggests that surgery may be even more beneficial at a lower BMI before comorbidities occur (9). Presurgical comorbidities must be addressed before surgery.

CASE 1

A 17-year-old male is admitted to the intensive care unit with altered mental status. He is combative and confused. Pulse is 120 beats/min, respiration is 20 breaths/min, and blood pressure in the right arm is 158/94 mm Hg. BMI is 61 mg/m^2. Serum sodium is 152 mEq/L, potassium is 3.9 mEq/L, carbon dioxide is 22 mEq/L, glucose is 1350 mg/dL, alanine aminotransferase is 62 U/L, and γ-glutamyltransferase is 105 U/L. HbA$_{1c}$ is 12%. Serum ammonia is normal.

Appropriate management for diabetes and weight loss after initial intravenous (IV) insulin drip would be:

A. Metformin after weaning from insulin
B. Insulin subcutaneously and referral for bariatric surgery
C. Institution of lifestyle modification while weaning from insulin to pioglitazone
D. Lifestyle modification, insulin, and liraglutide with referral to bariatric surgery
E. Leptin plus referral for bariatric surgery

Various procedures first developed in adults have been adapted for adolescent bariatric surgery. Although laparoscopic gastric banding achieved some popularity, the results were inferior to RYGB and gastric sleeve procedures, which are used presently with greater frequency (6).

The Surgical Procedures
The following describe the various bariatric surgical procedures performed commonly in adolescents who undergo bariatric surgery, which are illustrated in Figure 1:
- Adjustable gastric banding: a restrictive procedure that isolates the upper stomach. It is associated with higher reoperation and complication rates.
- Roux-en-Y gastric bypass or RYGB: a procedure that is both malabsorptive and restrictive. A small stomach pouch is isolated and connected to a portion of jejunum;

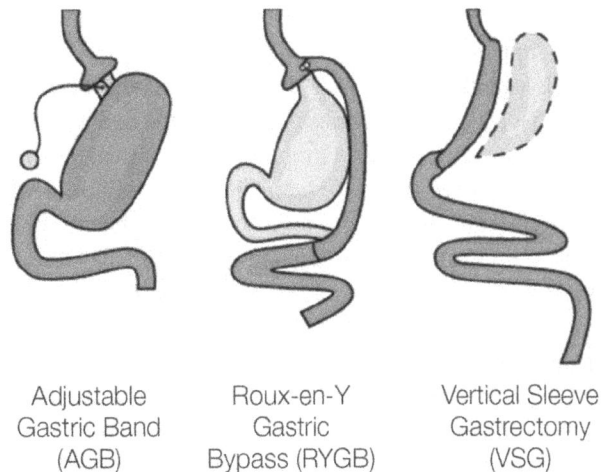

Adjustable Gastric Band (AGB) — Roux-en-Y Gastric Bypass (RYGB) — Vertical Sleeve Gastrectomy (VSG)

Figure 1. Illustration of the various bariatric surgical procedures. Reproduced from Weight Control Information Network and National Institute of Diabetes and Digestive and Kidney Diseases. ©University of North Carolina.

the rest of the jejunum drains the remainder of the stomach and duodenum. Dumping syndrome and decreases in ghrelin and increases in glucagon-like peptide-1 and peptide YY occur.
- Vertical sleeve gastrectomy: the larger portion of the fundus of the stomach is separated from a small portion of remaining stomach that links the esophagus and duodenum. Decreases in ghrelin and increases glucagon-like peptide-1 and peptide YY occur.

Positive effects of bariatric surgery in adolescents include remission of type 2 diabetes; improved insulin sensitivity and glucose metabolism; resolution of obstructive sleep apnea; and improvements in hepatic steatosis, hyperlipidemia, arthropathy, hypertension, and inflammatory markers. Laboratory profiles favorably affected include HbA$_{1c}$, adiponectin, IL-1, IL-8, C-reactive protein, and TNF-α.

Monitoring After Bariatric Surgery
Adolescent bariatric surgery should occur in pediatric bariatric surgery centers of excellence, and monitoring for immediate and long-term complications and comorbidities should occur. The team following the youth should include pediatric surgeons, pediatric endocrinologists, pediatric obesity specialists, psychologists, social workers, dieticians, specialty nurses, gastroenterologists, and other health care providers as indicated by comorbidities.

CASE 2
The patient is a 16-year-old girl, formerly with a BMI of 41 kg/m^2, type 2 diabetes mellitus, and hepatic steatosis. She is now 1-year post-RYGB surgery with a BMI of 40 kg/m^2 and returns to the bariatric surgery clinic. She complains of some

leg tingling and fatigue. She has not been taking her prescribed vitamin supplements.

Which vitamin and mineral deficiencies should be considered? What are possible causes of her paresthesia and fatigue?

Monitoring after bariatric surgery in an adolescent includes evaluation for perioperative complications in the first month after surgery and in the long term. In the first postoperative month, complications include gastrointestinal leaks, suicidal ideation, and pulmonary embolus, as well as the more common finding of abdominal pain, diarrhea, nausea, and dehydration. Less common are stricture with RYGB and wound infection with vertical sleeve gastrectomy. Screening for dumping syndrome symptoms and treatment of dumping are necessary. Late complications in 10% to 15% of adolescents include incisional hernia, cholelithiasis, small bowel obstruction, stomal stenosis, protein-calorie malnutrition, weight regain, and vitamin and mineral deficiencies. Psychological complications must be considered and addressed. Overall complication rates are quite low: Thirty days of data from a comparative efficacy study in 554 adolescents by Inge *et al.* (6) showed no deaths; a 4% incidence of venous thromboembolism; 3.3% percutaneous, endoscopic, or operative intervention after the procedure; and 0.7% failure to be discharged by postoperative day 30.

Causes of vitamin and mineral deficiencies include nutrient restriction; decreased gastric acid, intrinsic factor, and digestive enzyme production; and food intolerance with dumping. Mineral deficiencies can include iron (most common), calcium and phosphate, copper, selenium, zinc, and magnesium. Vitamin deficiencies include B12, B1, folate, and D. Hair loss, anemia, osteopenia, fatigue, and neurologic complications also may occur.

References

1. Ogden CL, Fryar CD, Hales CM, Carroll MD, Aoki Y, Freedman DS. Differences in obesity prevalence by demographics and urbanization in US children and adolescents, 2013-2016. *JAMA.* 2018;**319**(23): 2410-2418.

2. O'Connor EA, Evans CV, Burda BU, Walsh ES, Eder M, Lozano P. Screening for obesity and intervention for weight management in children and adolescents: evidence report and systematic review for the US Preventive Services Task Force. *JAMA.* 2017;**317**(23): 2427-2444.

3. Mead E, Brown T, Rees K, Azevedo LB, Whittaker V, Jones D, Olajide J, Mainardi GM, Corpeleijn E, O'Malley C, Beardsmore E, Al-Khudairy L, Baur L, Metzendorf MI, Demaio A, Ells LJ. Diet, physical activity and behavioural interventions for the treatment of overweight or obese children from the age of 6 to 11 years. *Cochrane Database Syst Rev.* 2017;**6**:CD012651.

4. Al-Khudairy L, Loveman E, Colquitt JL, Mead E, Johnson RE, Fraser H, Olajide J, Murphy M, Velho RM, O'Malley C, Azevedo LB, Ells LJ, Metzendorf MI, Rees K. Diet, physical activity and behavioural interventions for the treatment of overweight or obese adolescents aged 12 to 17 years. *Cochrane Database Syst Rev.* 2017;**6**: CD012691.

5. Pedroso FE, Angriman F, Endo A, Dasenbrock H, Storino A, Castillo R, Watkins AA, Castillo-Angeles M, Goodman JE, Zitsman JL. Weight loss after bariatric surgery in obese adolescents: a systematic review and meta-analysis. *Surg Obes Relat Dis.* 2018;**14**(3):413-422.

6. Inge TH, Coley RY, Bazzano LA, Xanthakos SA, McTigue K, Arterburn D, Arterburn D, Williams N, Wellman R, Coleman KJ, Courcoulas A, Desai NK, Anau J, Pardee R, Toh S, Janning C, Cook A, Sturtevant J, Horgan C, Zebrick AJ, Michalsky M for the PCORnet Bariatric Study Collaborative. Comparative effectiveness of bariatric procedures among adolescents: the PCORnet bariatric study. *Surg Obes Relat Dis.* 2018;**14**(9):1374-1386.

7. Childerhose JE, Alsamawi A, Mehta T, Smith JE, Woolford S, Tarini BA. Adolescent bariatric surgery: a systematic review of recommendation documents. *Surg Obes Relat Dis.* 2017;**13**(10):1768-1779.

8. Desai NK, Wulkan ML, Inge TH. Update on adolescent bariatric surgery. *Endocrinol Metab Clin North Am.* 2016;**45**(3):667-676.

9. Pratt JSA, Browne A, Browne NT, Bruzoni M, Cohen M, Desai A, Inge T, Linden BC, Mattar SG, Michalsky M, Podkameni D, Reichard KW, Stanford FC, Zeller MH, Zitsman J. ASMBS pediatric metabolic and bariatric surgery guidelines, 2018. *Surg Obes Relat Dis.* 2018;**14**(7): 882-901.

10. Styne DM, Arslanian SA, Connor EL, Farooqi IS, Murad MH, Silverstein JH, Yanovski JA. pediatric obesity-assessment, treatment, and prevention: an Endocrine Society Clinical practice guideline. *J Clin Endocrinol Metab.* 2017;**102**(3):709-757.

11. Gibbons E, Casey AF, Brewster KZ. Bariatric surgery and intellectual disability: furthering evidence-based practice. *Disabil Health J.* 2017; **10**(1):3-10.

Youth-Onset Type 2 Diabetes

M36
Presented, March 23–26, 2019

Philip Zeitler, MD, PhD. Section of Endocrinology, Department of Pediatrics, University of Colorado School of Medicine, Aurora, Colorado 80045, E-mail: philip.zeitler@ childrenscolorado.org

Petter Bjornstad, MD. Section of Endocrinology, Department of Pediatrics, University of Colorado School of Medicine, Aurora, Colorado 80045, E-mail: petter. bjornstad@childrenscolorado.org

SIGNIFICANCE OF THE CLINICAL PROBLEM

Youth-onset type 2 diabetes (T2D) is an emerging disorder in children, adolescents, and young adults with unique clinical challenges. The incidence of T2D in youths has increased dramatically over the last 20 years, although it remains a rare disorder. In the United States, the best estimates are that the incidence is as high as 5000 new cases per year, with total prevalence of <50,000 (1, 2). T2D in youths resembles the pathophysiology in adults: insulin resistance and nonautoimmune β-cell injury. However, studies indicate that youth-onset T2D has a number of unique aspects. For example, there is an important association of T2D with pubertal development—the median age of onset of T2D in youths is ~14 years old. This is likely related to the transient reduction in insulin sensitivity that occurs in children as they enter puberty (3) and the need for compensation in insulin secretion, which may lead to hyperglycemia in youths with limited β-cell capacity. Furthermore, diabetes onset during puberty may be reversible in some youths due to the dynamic nature of the underlying insulin resistance. Also, although rates in adult men and women are similar, adolescent girls have a 60% higher prevalence rate than boys (2). In addition, although decline in β-cell function also occurs in adults with T2D, β-cell failure seems to be more rapid in youths than in adults, leading to loss of glycemic control on oral therapy that is more rapid than in adults (4–9). Finally, there is evidence of microvascular complications and risk markers for macrovascular complications at the time of diagnosis along with rapid progression of these complications (10–13).

T2D has a disproportionate impact on youths from ethnic/racial minorities and disadvantaged backgrounds and occurs in complex psychosocial and cultural environments that make durable lifestyle change elusive and adherence to medical recommendations a struggle. Furthermore, these complexities hinder successful recruitment into and completion of research programs, leaving large gaps in knowledge on pathophysiology and treatment optimization (2, 14–16).

BARRIERS TO OPTIMAL PRACTICE
- Complex social milieu
- Knowledge gaps in understanding underlying pathophysiology
- Rapidly progressive course with frequent oral treatment failure
- High risk of vascular complications
- Limited clinical experience
- Restricted access to diabetes medications
- No evidence-based treatment guidelines

LEARNING OBJECTIVES
As a result of participating in this session, learners should be able to
- Know the initial approach to evaluation and management of new-onset diabetes in the obese adolescent
- Understand how to select and modify pharmacologic agents for treatment of youths with T2D
- Develop an approach to management of complications and cardiovascular risk in youths with T2D

STRATEGIES FOR DIAGNOSIS, THERAPY, AND MANAGEMENT
The diagnosis of T2D in youths requires two steps: confirmation of the presence of diabetes mellitus followed by determination of diabetes type. The criteria and classification of diabetes mellitus are provided in the American Diabetes Association (ADA) annual guidelines and the International Society for Pediatric and Adolescent Diabetes (ISPAD) Clinical Practice Consensus Guidelines (17, 18). However, there are a couple of important points. First, although the ADA has added hemoglobin A_{1c} (HbA$_{1c}$) as a diagnostic criterion, this assumes laboratory-measured, the Diabetes Control and Complications Trial (DCCT)-aligned assay, not point of care testing, and it has not been specifically validated in youth. Second, in the absence of symptoms, hyperglycemia detected incidentally or under conditions of acute physiologic stress may be transitory and should not be regarded as diagnostic of diabetes. Accordingly, a second test on a different day is required.

After the diagnosis of diabetes is established, consideration should be given to determining diabetes type. There are features of presentation and phenotype that may be useful in developing a presumption of T2D, although there is substantial overlap between characteristics of T2D and type 1 diabetes (T1D) in the obese adolescent, making these features of limited value. The degree of pubertal development may be the most useful, although in a negative fashion; youths with T2D are almost always in puberty, with a mean age of diagnosis of 13 or 14 years old and Tanner stage 4 or 5, and rarely, prepubertal (10, 19). Most importantly, diabetes autoantibody testing should be done in all youths with the clinical diagnosis of T2D because of the high frequency of islet cell autoimmunity in patients with otherwise "typical" T2D (20); the presence of antibodies predicts rapid development of insulin requirement as well as risk for development of other autoimmune disorders. Diabetes autoantibody testing should also be considered in overweight/obese pubertal children with a clinical picture of T1D (weight loss, ketosis/ketoacidosis), some of whom may have T2D and may be able to be weaned off of insulin for extended periods of time (21, 22). Finally, single-gene mutation forms of diabetes, such as maturity-onset diabetes of the young should be considered in individuals who have a presentation and course that is not characteristic of either T1D or T2D.

Initial treatment of the obese adolescent with diabetes must take into account that diabetes type is often not certain in the first few weeks of treatment, that 10% to 15% of obese adolescents will have T1D and that a substantial percentage of adolescents with T2D will present with clinically important ketoacidosis (19, 23). Therefore, initial treatment should be based on the clinical presentation while an open mind regarding both the diabetes type and eventual therapy is maintained (17).

Obese adolescents presenting with acidosis require initiation of intravenous insulin. However, after acidosis is resolved, subsequent therapy depends on the provisional clinical diagnosis. In those patients with a clinical impression of T2D, basal insulin at a dose of 0.2 to 0.4 U/kg once a day is started and titrated based on finger stick glucose measurements. Insulin is administered at whatever time of day is the most likely to promote good adherence. At the same time, metformin is initiated at 500 mg once a day and titrated weekly to a maximally tolerated dose, with a target of 2000 mg/d. Insulin can generally be discontinued within a few weeks after antibody negativity has been confirmed.

Asymptomatic patients with an initial HbA_{1c} >9% to 10% may also require initiation of once daily basal insulin therapy to allow for sufficient recovery of β-cell function for successful monotherapy with an oral medication. However, results from the Treatment Options for Type 2 Diabetes in Adolescents and Youth (TODAY) study suggest that initiation of metformin and basic dietary intervention will result in an HbA_{1c} in the nondiabetic range with or without insulin (22). Obese asymptomatic adolescents presenting with less decompensation can be started on metformin alone, with a high likelihood of initial success. Patients not on insulin are asked to check their finger stick glucose twice a day a few days a week and whenever the patient feels ill. This frequency of blood glucose monitoring represents a sustainable balance between providing adequate safety to identify gradual deterioration and avoiding excessive burden on this generally poorly adherent population, particularly as the adolescents quickly recognize that daily glucose readings are not used for medication adjustment.

Lifestyle change is critical to treatment of T2D, and clinicians should initiate a lifestyle modification program, including nutrition and physical activity, for children and adolescents at the time of diagnosis of T2D (24). The interventions include promoting a healthy lifestyle through behavior change, including nutrition, exercise training, weight management, and smoking cessation. However, the challenges in implementing lifestyle modifications in adolescents are greater than in adult patients, because adolescents typically come from families where overeating and a sedentary lifestyle are considered the norm. Thus, many adolescents with T2D will not maintain the recommended lifestyle changes and will remain overweight with poor diabetes control (25).

The target of therapy is to attain and maintain HbA_{1c} <6.5. In most cases, this target can be successfully achieved and maintained for extended periods with metformin monotherapy combined with focused lifestyle counseling and support. The approach to the adolescent with T2D who fails to attain and/or maintain target HbA_{1c} has not been studied systematically. In most cases, pediatric endocrinologists will add basal insulin as a second agent and titrate to achieve the target HbA_{1c} (17). This combination of basal insulin and metformin is often effective and may provide reliable glycemic control for extended periods. Failure to achieve the target at an insulin dose of 1 U/kg or evidence for poor control of postprandial glycemia may prompt consideration of the addition of rapid-acting insulin, but the known challenges with adherence in this population should be kept in mind. Premixed insulins may offer some benefits in ease of administration over rapid-acting insulin, but they require a degree of attention to meal times and snacks that is not always achievable.

Other than metformin, no oral hypoglycemic agent is approved for use in adolescents, and few studies have been reported to date, although a number of clinical trials of newer agents are in various stages of design and execution (25). Many of these agents offer promise for improving insulin resistance (thiazolidinediones), reducing weight [glucagon-like peptide-1 (GLP-1) agonists, sodium-glucose cotransporter-2 (SGLT2) inhibitors], and/or improving β-cell survival [GLP-1 agonists, dipeptidyl peptidase-4 (DPP-4) inhibitors], but at this time, there is no evidence base for their use in youth.

CASES

Case 1: The Obese Minority Youth With New Diabetes

DW is a 16-year-old Hispanic girl who was diagnosed with diabetes 3 years ago by her primary doctor. At that time, diabetes type was determined based on clinical presentation and family history of T2D. She was started on metformin 2000 mg/d but reports that she took this for only a few months. Since that time, she has been off all medications and reports no symptoms of diabetes, including polyuria, polydipsia, or weight loss. One month ago, DW was admitted to the hospital after a suicide attempt. During that admission, she was noted to have a glucose of 550 ng/dL and glucosuria, with small ketonuria and normal venous pH. HbA_{1c} was 12.5%. She was treated by the inpatient team with subcutaneous basal and bolus insulin and restarted on metformin. She was referred to the diabetes center for additional evaluation. At that visit, body mass index (BMI) was 28 kg/m^2, and blood pressure (BP) was 125/72 mm Hg.

Given the length of time since original diagnosis, obtaining which of the following is the most important next step in the evaluation of this patient?

A. Fasting lipid panel
B. Fasting and stimulated C-peptide
C. Home glucose measurements
D. Liver enzymes
E. Pancreatic autoantibodies

The answer is E (pancreatic autoantibodies).

Although this patient has had diabetes for 3 years without severe metabolic decompensation off treatment, there is no clinical characteristic with 100% sensitivity in excluding T1D. Because T1D remains more common than T2D at all ages and in most ethnicities, the *a priori* risk for type 1 is higher than type 2, despite "typical" characteristics. Furthermore, even among those race/ethnicity groups (black, American Indian) where type 2 is more common in adolescents, T1D still occurs. Furthermore, a substantial percentage of adolescents with type 1 in the United States are obese, and obesity does not protect from autoimmunity. Therefore, even in this setting, the most important step in the evaluation of an adolescent with diabetes is rigorous determination of diabetes type. The presence of positive antibodies, no matter what the phenotype, is associated with more rapid progression to insulin requirement, and patients with positive antibodies should be treated with insulin irrespective of how they are doing on oral therapy. Measurement of fasting C-peptide may be helpful in determining degree of insulin resistance, and stimulated C-peptide may be a reasonable measure of insulin secretory capacity, potentially contributing to the distinction of T2D from T1D. However, this is only true in the setting of stable metabolic status. During acute decompensation, insulin and C-peptide secretion are transiently decreased. Measurement of C-peptide may be more useful in the asymptomatic patient, the patient who has recovered from decompensation, or the evaluation of the patient with presumed T2D who has a persistent insulin requirement. The remaining options would be important to obtain at diagnosis in an obese individual with diabetes, irrespective of diabetes type, but would be unlikely to make an immediate difference in therapeutic decisions. However, the specific screening done would depend on whether the individual has positive antibodies (thyrotropin, celiac antibodies, lipids) or negative antibodies (lipids, aspartate aminotransferase/alanine aminotransferase, urine albumin, creatinine clearance).

Case 2: The Adolescent With New-Onset T2D

AJ is a 15-year-old Hispanic boy with a long history of being overweight who was recently found to have a fasting glucose of 289 mg/dL during a yearly examination for school. He had no complaints initially, but on questioning, he recalls some polyuria, polydipsia, and fatigue for the last few months. His mother had noted increased thirst but thought it was due to the hot summer. AJ has previously been healthy and is on no medications. On examination, he has a BMI of 32 kg/m^2 and a BP of 120/58 mm Hg. He is Tanner stage 5, and the remainder of his examination is unremarkable. His HbA$_{1c}$ is 8.7%, and antibodies (glutamic acid decarboxylase, islet antigen 2, zinc transporter 8, microinsulin auto-antibody) are negative. You start him on metformin and titrate to 2000 mg/d. He returns in 3 months and reports that he has been taking his metformin every day; his mother confirms that she has been watching him. His HbA$_{1c}$ is 7.1%.

Of the following, the best next step in management is
A. Measure fasting C-peptide level
B. Measure stimulated C-peptide level
C. Start canagliflozin 100 mg once daily
D. Start basal insulin once a day
E. Start multiple daily injections with glargine and glulisine (apidra)

The answer is D (start basal insulin once a day).

The patient is nearly at the ADA and the ISPAD targets for glycemia (17, 18), and a common response would be that no changes are needed. However, recently published results from the TODAY study (9) indicate that HbA$_{1c}$ >6.3% after a few months of metformin monotherapy is associated with a 4- to 10-fold increased risk for loss of glycemic control depending on sex and race/ethnicity, with a median time to loss of control of ~11 months. Although it may be premature to start basal insulin at this initial visit, failure to get to an HbA$_{1c}$ in the nondiabetic range on metformin monotherapy suggests that the provider taking care of this patient should initiate a discussion with the family, informing them that response to metformin has not been sufficient to date and that add-on therapy may be necessary soon. Initiation of basal insulin is the standard approach to add-on therapy in the absence of evidence for oral or injected agents other than metformin and insulin (17, 25). Starting multiple daily injections will help with glycemia, but adherence among youths with T2D is generally poor, and it is preferable to use the simplest regimen possible. Measurement of fasting C-peptide will provide information on insulin sensitivity, and stimulated C-peptide will provide information on β-cell reserve, but these factors are already incorporated into the HbA$_{1c}$ and will not affect management. Additional agents, including GLP-1RA, SGLT-2i, and DPP-4, are likely useful but not yet Food and Drug Administration approved in pediatrics; therefore, they cannot be formally recommended.

Case 3: The Adolescent With T2D and Dyslipidemia

AA is a 15-year-old Hispanic girl who was recently diagnosed with T2D at the time of a routine physical examination. She was started on metformin by her primary care provider and referred to the diabetes center. She has been healthy and was not on medications. Her review of systems is negative. On examination, her BMI is 35 kg/m^2, and her HbA$_{1c}$ is 7.8%.

Of the following, which is the most important next step in management?

A. Start atorvastatin 10 mg/d for low-density lipoprotein of 160 mg/dL
B. Start fenofibrate 67 mg/d for triglycerides of 745 mg/dL
C. Start lisinopril 10 mg/d for BP of 145/82 mm Hg
D. Start lisinopril 20 mg/d for urine albumin to creatinine of 48 mg/g
E. Start vitamin E 600 IU/d for alanine aminotransferase of 87 U/L

The answer is B (start fenofibrate 67 mg/d for triglycerides of 745 mg/dL).

T2D generally occurs in the setting of other insulin-resistant abnormalities, including lipid abnormalities, endothelial and cardiac dysfunction, increased procoagulant and inflammatory markers, increased hepatic and muscle lipid deposition, mitochondrial dysfunction, increased plasma uric acid, ovarian hyperandrogenism, and sleep disorders, all of which increase cardiovascular risk. Given the prevalence of comorbidities at the time of diagnosis (26, 27), evaluation should occur either at the time of initial diagnosis or on re-establishment of metabolic stability (17, 24).

BP should be measured at every clinic visit and normalized for sex, height, and age. Initial treatment of BP above the 95th percentile consists of weight loss, limitation of dietary salt, and increased physical activity. After 6 months, if BP is still above the 95th percentile, an angiotensin-converting enzyme (ACE) inhibitor is started to achieve BP values that are <90th percentile. If the ACE inhibitor is not tolerated due to adverse effects (mainly cough), an angiotensin receptor blocker may be used. Combination therapy may be required if hypertension does not normalize on single-agent therapy. Workup of hypertension not responsive to initial medication should also include a renal ultrasound and an echocardiogram.

Urine albumin excretion should be assessed at diagnosis and annually. Microalbuminuria is defined as albumin to creatinine ratio 30 to 299 mg/g on a spot urine sample. Because an elevated value can be secondary to exercise, smoking, menstruation, and orthostasis, the diagnosis of persistent abnormal microalbumin excretion requires documentation of two of three consecutive abnormal values obtained on different days, preferably on rising, because benign orthostatic proteinuria is common in adolescents. ACE inhibitors are the agents of choice due to proven renal protection, even if BP is normal. Albumin excretion should be repeated at 3- to 6-month intervals, and therapy should be titrated to achieve a normal albumin to creatinine ratio. Nondiabetes-related causes of renal disease should be excluded, and consultation should be obtained if an albumin to creatinine ratio >300 mg/g is present.

Testing for dyslipidemia should be performed soon after diagnosis when blood glucose control has been achieved and annually thereafter. Goals for lipids are low-density lipoprotein cholesterol (LDL-C) <100 mg/dL and triglycerides <150 mg/dL along with high-density lipoprotein cholesterol >40 mg/dL. If LDL-C is above goal, blood glucose control should be maximized, and dietary counseling should be provided (dietary cholesterol <200 mg/d, saturated fat <7% of total calories, and <30% calories from fat). If LDL-C remains >130 mg/dL after 6 months, statin therapy should be started with a target of <100 mg/dL. The use of statins in sexually active adolescent females must be carefully considered, and the risks should be explicitly discussed. Elevated triglycerides are not treated for cardiovascular disease prevention. However, if fasting triglycerides are >500 mg/dL, a fibric acid is started due to substantially increased risk for acute pancreatitis, with a treatment goal of <150 mg/dL.

Hepatic steatosis is present in 25% to 50% of adolescents with T2D, and more advanced forms of fatty liver disease are increasingly common and associated with progression to cirrhosis, portal hypertension, and liver failure. Fatty liver is now the most frequent cause of chronic liver disorders among obese youth, and it is the most common reason for liver transplantation in adults in the United States. T2D therapies that improve insulin resistance seem to improve fatty liver. However, due to the potential for progression to steatohepatitis, fibrosis, and cirrhosis, ongoing monitoring of liver enzymes is recommended in youths with T2D, with referral for biopsy if enzymes remain markedly elevated.

In addition, the clinician should explore the presence of polycystic ovary syndrome, depression, eating disorders, and sleep disturbance and address these as appropriate.

References

1. Lawrence JM, Imperatore G, Dabelea D, Mayer-Davis EJ, Linder B, Saydah S, Klingensmith GJ, Dolan L, Standiford DA, Pihoker C, Pettitt DJ, Talton JW, Thomas J, Bell RA, D'Agostino RB, Jr; Search for Diabetes in Youth Study Group. Trends in incidence of type 1 diabetes among non-Hispanic white youth in the U.S., 2002-2009. *Diabetes.* 2014;**63**(11):3938–3945.
2. Dabelea D, Mayer-Davis EJ, Saydah S, Imperatore G, Linder B, Divers J, Bell R, Badaru A, Talton JW, Crume T, Liese AD, Merchant AT, Lawrence JM, Reynolds K, Dolan L, Liu LL, Hamman RF; SEARCH for Diabetes in Youth Study. Prevalence of type 1 and type 2 diabetes among children and adolescents from 2001 to 2009. *JAMA.* 2014; **311**(17):1778–1786.
3. Hannon TS, Janosky J, Arslanian SA. Longitudinal study of physiologic insulin resistance and metabolic changes of puberty. *Pediatr Res.* 2006;**60**(6):759–763.
4. TODAY Study Group; Zeitler P, Hirst K, Pyle L, Linder B, Copeland K, Arslanian S, Cuttler L, Nathan DM, Tollefsen S, Wilfley D, Kaufman F. A clinical trial to maintain glycemic control in youth with type 2 diabetes. *N Engl J Med.* 2012;**366**(24):2247–2256.
5. Rascati K, Richards K, Lopez D, Cheng LI, Wilson J. Progression to insulin for patients with diabetes mellitus on dual oral antidiabetic therapy using the US Department of Defense Database. *Diabetes Obes Metab.* 2013;**15**(10):901–905.
6. Kahn SE. Clinical review 135: the importance of β-cell failure in the development and progression of type 2 diabetes. *J Clin Endocrinol Metab.* 2001;**86**(9):4047–4058.
7. Kahn SE, Lachin JM, Zinman B, Haffner SM, Aftring RP, Paul G, Kravitz BG, Herman WH, Viberti G, Holman RR; ADOPT Study Group. Effects of rosiglitazone, glyburide, and metformin on β-cell function and insulin sensitivity in ADOPT. *Diabetes.* 2011;**60**(5):1552–1560.
8. TODAY Study Group. Effects of metformin, metformin plus rosiglitazone, and metformin plus lifestyle on insulin sensitivity and β-cell function in TODAY. *Diabetes Care.* 2013;**36**(6):1749–1757.

9. Zeitler P, Hirst K, Copeland KC, El Ghormli L, Levitt Katz L, Levitsky LL, Linder B, McGuigan P, White NH, Wilfley D; TODAY Study Group. HbA1c after a short period of monotherapy with metformin identifies durable glycemic control among adolescents with type 2 diabetes. *Diabetes Care.* 2015;**38**(12):2285–2292.

10. Copeland KC, Zeitler P, Geffner M, Guandalini C, Higgins J, Hirst K, Kaufman FR, Linder B, Marcovina S, McGuigan P, Pyle L, Tamborlane W, Willi S; TODAY Study Group. Characteristics of adolescents and youth with recent-onset type 2 diabetes: the TODAY cohort at baseline. *J Clin Endocrinol Metab.* 2011;**96**(1):159–167.

11. Sellers EAC, Yung G, Dean HJ. Dyslipidemia and other cardiovascular risk factors in a Canadian First Nation pediatric population with type 2 diabetes mellitus. *Pediatr Diabetes.* 2007;**8**(6):384–390.

12. Hannon TS, Arslanian SA. The changing face of diabetes in youth: lessons learned from studies of type 2 diabetes. *Ann N Y Acad Sci.* 2015;**1353**(1):113–137.

13. Dart AB, Martens PJ, Rigatto C, Brownell MD, Dean HJ, Sellers EA. Earlier onset of complications in youth with type 2 diabetes. *Diabetes Care.* 2014;**37**(2):436–443.

14. Zeitler P, Chou HS, Copeland KC, Geffner M. Clinical trials in youth-onset type 2 diabetes: needs, barriers, and options. *Curr Diab Rep.* 2015;**15**(5):28.

15. Fazeli Farsani S, van der Aa MP, van der Vorst MMJ, Knibbe CA, de Boer A. Global trends in the incidence and prevalence of type 2 diabetes in children and adolescents: a systematic review and evaluation of methodological approaches. *Diabetologia.* 2013;**56**(7): 1471–1488.

16. Petitti DB, Klingensmith GJ, Bell RA, Andrews JS, Dabelea D, Imperatore G, Marcovina S, Pihoker C, Standiford D, Waitzfelder B, Mayer-Davis E; SEARCH for Diabetes in Youth Study Group. Glycemic control in youth with diabetes: the SEARCH for diabetes in Youth Study. *J Pediatr.* 2009;**155**(5):668–72.e1–3.

17. Zeitler P, Fu J, Tandon N, Nadeau K, Urakami T, Barrett T, Maahs D; International Society for Pediatric and Adolescent Diabetes. ISPAD Clinical Practice Consensus Guidelines 2014. Type 2 diabetes in the child and adolescent. *Pediatr Diabetes.* 2014;**15**(Suppl 20):26–46.

18. American Diabetes Association. Standards of medical care in diabetes—2018. *Diabetes Care.* 2018;**41**(Suppl 1):S1–S2.

19. Fagot-Campagna A, Pettitt DJ, Engelgau MM, Burrows NR, Geiss LS, Valdez R, Beckles GL, Saaddine J, Gregg EW, Williamson DF, Narayan KM. Type 2 diabetes among North American children and adolescents: an epidemiologic review and a public health perspective. *J Pediatr.* 2000;**136**(5):664–672.

20. Klingensmith GJ, Pyle L, Arslanian S, Copeland KC, Cuttler L, Kaufman F, Laffel L, Marcovina S, Tollefsen SE, Weinstock RS, Linder B; TODAY Study Group. The presence of GAD and IA-2 antibodies in youth with a type 2 diabetes phenotype: results from the TODAY study. *Diabetes Care.* 2010;**33**(9):1970–1975.

21. Laffel L, Chang N, Grey M, Hale D, Higgins L, Hirst K, Izquierdo R, Larkin M, Macha C, Pham T, Wauters A, Weinstock RS; TODAY Study Group. Metformin monotherapy in youth with recent onset type 2 diabetes: experience from the prerandomization run-in phase of the TODAY study. *Pediatr Diabetes.* 2012;**13**(5):369–375.

22. Kelsey MM, Geffner ME, Guandalini C, Pyle L, Tamborlane WV, Zeitler PS, White NH; Treatment Options for Type 2 Diabetes in Adolescents and Youth Study Group. Presentation and effectiveness of early treatment of type 2 diabetes in youth: lessons from the TODAY study. *Pediatr Diabetes.* 2016;**17**(3):212–221.

23. Pinhas-Hamiel O, Dolan LM, Zeitler PS. Diabetic ketoacidosis among obese African-American adolescents with NIDDM. *Diabetes Care.* 1997;**20**(4):484–486.

24. Copeland KC, Silverstein J, Moore KR, Prazar GE, Raymer T, Shiffman RN, Springer SC, Thaker VV, Anderson M, Spann SJ, Flinn SK; American Academy of Pediatrics. Management of newly diagnosed type 2 Diabetes Mellitus (T2DM) in children and adolescents. *Pediatrics.* 2013;**131**(2):364–382.

25. Nadeau KJ, Anderson BJ, Berg EG, Chiang JL, Chou H, Copeland KC, Hannon TS, Huang TT, Lynch JL, Powell J, Sellers E, Tamborlane WV, Zeitler P. Youth-onset Type 2 diabetes consensus report: current status, challenges, and priorities. *Diabetes Care.* 2016;**39**(9):1635–1642.

26. West NA, Hamman RF, Mayer-Davis EJ, D'Agostino RB, Jr, Marcovina SM, Liese AD, Zeitler PS, Daniels SR, Dabelea D. Cardiovascular risk factors among youth with and without type 2 diabetes: differences and possible mechanisms. *Diabetes Care.* 2009;**32**(1):175–180.

27. Pinhas-Hamiel O, Zeitler P. Acute and chronic complications of type 2 diabetes mellitus in children and adolescents. *Lancet.* 2007;**369**(9575):1823–1831.

Pediatric Endocrine Tumors: Hereditary Syndromes and Prospective Monitoring

M43
Presented, March 23–26, 2019

Steven G. Waguespack, MD. Department of Endocrine Neoplasia and Hormonal Disorders and the Children's Cancer Hospital, The University of Texas MD Anderson Cancer Center, Houston, Texas 77230, E-mail: swagues@ mdanderson.org

SIGNIFICANCE OF THE CLINICAL PROBLEM

Endocrine tumors comprise a variety of neoplasms that arise from the endocrine glands or other neuroendocrine tissues such as the paraganglia. Most childhood endocrine tumors, typified by papillary thyroid carcinoma, are sporadic without an identifiable mutation in the germline DNA. However, other endocrine neoplasms, especially when neuroendocrine in nature, are familial and occur as part of one of the well-recognized hereditary tumor syndromes (Table 1). Pediatric endocrine tumors are rare, but when encountered, the clinician should have a high index of suspicion that the clinical presentation could be a manifestation of a hereditary tumor syndrome, primarily given the early age of disease onset. Additional clues to a familial endocrine tumor syndrome include a positive family history (*i.e.*, a family history of other endocrine tumors/cancers), abnormalities on the physical examination [*e.g.*, oral mucosal neuromas in multiple endocrine neoplasia 2B (MEN2B)], and other aspects of clinical presentation (*e.g.*, multifocal/bilateral disease). When a hereditary tumor syndrome is suspected, the patient should be referred for formal genetic counseling and testing. Identification of a germline tumor-predisposing mutation will inform decisions about treatment, alert first-degree relatives that they are at risk, and lead to prospective clinical monitoring of the child for other manifestations of the specific tumor syndrome.

BARRIERS TO OPTIMAL PRACTICE

- The incidence of pediatric endocrine tumors is low, such that few providers are proficient in the diagnosis and management of these rare neoplasms.
- Knowledge regarding the genetic causes of endocrine tumors continues to rapidly expand, which makes it challenging for endocrine providers to remain updated.
- The rarity of hereditary endocrine tumors and the lack of large-scale prospective studies create uncertainty as relates to the optimal strategy for the management of asymptomatic individuals who have a germline mutation that predisposes them to the development of one or more endocrine tumors.

LEARNING OBJECTIVES

As a result of participating in this session, learners should be able to
- Provide an overview of the major hereditary endocrine tumor syndromes occurring in childhood
- Understand the genetics of the hereditary endocrine tumors and how to pursue a genetic diagnosis
- Discuss current recommendations for prospective clinical screening in patients with a tumor-predisposing germline mutation

STRATEGIES FOR DIAGNOSIS, THERAPY, AND/OR MANAGEMENT
Introduction

Endocrine tumors comprise a variety of benign and malignant neoplasms that arise from the endocrine glands or other neuroendocrine tissues. A subset of these tumors is hereditary and secondary to mutations in one of many known tumor-predisposing genes, which are primarily tumor suppressor genes that require a "second hit"/loss of heterozygosity at the tissue level for tumor development to occur. Heritable endocrine neoplasms typically occur in the context of a larger hereditary tumor syndrome and are inherited in an autosomal-dominant manner.

Advances in genetic testing and ongoing research have led to the ongoing discovery of novel tumor-susceptibility genes in addition to a better understanding of the underlying pathophysiology of these disorders. Knowledge regarding genotype-phenotype relationships continues to evolve, as has clinical practice regarding the age of predictive genetic testing, screening for endocrine tumors in an asymptomatic carrier, and the timing of therapeutic intervention. A diagnosis of an endocrine tumor in a child, especially one that is neuroendocrine in nature, should always raise concern for the possibility of an underlying genetic predisposition, which can subsequently have medical, reproductive, psychological, and/or social consequences for the patient and family.

Genetic Counseling and Testing

Genetic counseling is a critical component of the care of children with a heritable endocrine tumor and one that should be incorporated into all stages of care, both at diagnosis and during long-term follow-up. Genetic testing, nicely exemplified in MEN2 (1), is a multistep process that should always begin with a patient who already has clinical manifestations of disease. In most cases, such as in MEN1 and MEN2A, this is likely to be a parent or another blood relative, but in other hereditable disorders with low disease penetrance, such as the familial paraganglioma syndromes, genetic testing of the

Table 1.   Hereditary Endocrine Tumor Syndromes[a]

Syndrome	Gene (Chromosome)	Associated Endocrine Neoplasms	Other
APC-associated polyposis [familial adenomatous polyposis (FAP), attenuated FAP, Gardner syndrome, and Turcot syndrome]	*APC* (5q22.2)	• ACT • PTC (Cribriform-morular variant)	• Colorectal polyps/colorectal carcinoma • Osteomas • Desmoid tumors • Pancreas adenocarcinomas • Medulloblastoma • Hepatoblastoma

Carney complex	*PRKAR1A* (17q24.2) and unknown gene at chromosome locus 2p16	• Mammosomatotroph hyperplasia/GH-secreting PA
		• Primary pigmented nodular adrenocortical disease/ACT
		• Thyroid neoplasia
		  • Follicular adenomas
		  • Thyroid carcinoma (PTC and FTC)
		• Large-cell calcifying Sertoli cell tumors
			• GH excess and hyperprolactinemia
			• Spotty skin pigmentation
			• Blue nevus
			• Cardiac, cutaneous, or breast myxomas
			• Psammomatous melanotic schwannoma

DICER1 syndrome	*DICER1* (14q32.13)	• MNG • PTC • Pituitary blastoma	• Pleuropulmonary blastoma • Ovarian Sertoli-Leydig cell tumor • Cystic nephroma • Cervical embryonal rhabdomyosarcoma • Ciliary body medulloepithelioma • Pineoblastoma

Familial PGL syndromes
  PGL1
  PGL2
  PGL3
  PGL4
  PGL5
	SDHD (11q23.1)
	SDHAF2 (11q12.2)
	SDHC (1q23.3)
	SDHB (1p36.13)
	SDHA (5p15.33)
		• PHEO/PGL
		• PA
			• GIST
			• RCC
			• High rate of malignancy with *SDHB* mutations
			• Parent of origin effects in *SDHD* and *SDHAF2* genes (clinical disease inherited from father only)

MEN1	*MEN1* (11q13.1)	• Parathyroid adenomas/hyperplasia • PA • Bronchopulmonary and GEP-NET • ACT • PHEO (rare)	• Lipomas/angiofibromas/collagenomas • Meningiomas • Ependymomas • Leiomyomas • ? Breast cancer
MEN2A	*RET* (10q11.21)	• MTC • PHEO/PGL • Parathyroid adenoma/hyperplasia	• Codon-specific risk of MTC • Variants with cutaneous lichen amyloidosis and Hirschsprung disease • Adrenal ganglioneuroma in rare cases

(Table Continues)

TABLE 1. Hereditary Endocrine Tumor Syndromes[a] **(Continued)**

Syndrome	Gene (Chromosome)	Associated Endocrine Neoplasms	Other
MEN2B	*RET* (10q11.21)	• MTC • PHEO/PGL	• Very high risk for early onset and metastasis of MTC • Mucosal neuromas of the lips, tongue, and eyelids • Medullated corneal nerve fibers • Distinctive facies with enlarged lips • Megacolon/ganglioneuromatosis of the gastrointestinal tract • "Marfanoid" body habitus • Absent tears in infancy • Feeding difficulties and constipation in infancy • Adrenal ganglioneuroma in rare cases
MEN4	*CDKN1B* (12p13.1)	• PA • Parathyroid adenoma/hyperplasia • Bronchopulmonary and GEP-NET • ? ACT (case report) • ? PTC (case report)	• Neuroendocrine cervical cancer
NF1	*NF1* (17q11.2)	• PHEO/PGL • GEP-NET • Primarily peri-ampullary duodenal somatostatinomas but also insulinomas, gastrinomas, and nonfunctioning tumors • ? Parathyroid tumors (case reports) • ? ACT (case reports)	• Café-au-lait macules with smooth borders • Axillary and inguinal freckling • Dermal and plexiform neurofibromas • Lisch nodules of the iris • Learning disabilities • Scoliosis, vertebral dysplasia, pseudarthrosis, and bony overgrowth • Optic and other central nervous system gliomas • Malignant peripheral nerve sheath tumors • Vasculopathy • Macrocephaly
VHL	*VHL* (3p25.3)	• PHEO/PGL • Nonfunctioning PETs • Ovarian steroid cell tumor (case reports)	• Hemangioblastomas of the central nervous system and retina • Renal cysts and clear cell RCC • Pancreatic cysts and cystadenomas • Endolymphatic sac tumors • Papillary cystadenomas of the epididymis (males) and round ligament (females)

Abbreviations: ACT, adrenocortical tumor; FTC, follicular thyroid carcinoma; GEP-NET, gastroenteropancreatic neuroendocrine tumor; GH, growth hormone; GIST, gastrointestinal stromal tumor; MNG, multinodular goiter; PA, pituitary adenoma; PET, pancreatic endocrine tumor; PGL, familial paraganglioma syndrome or paraganglioma; PHEO, pheochromocytoma; PTC, papillary thyroid carcinoma; RCC, renal cell carcinoma; VHL, von Hippel-Lindau disease.
[a] Showing only those hereditary tumor syndromes that are clearly associated with two or more endocrine tumors.

family may actually begin with the child who is clinically affected.

Genetic testing serves multiple purposes, including the confirmation of the genetic cause of an endocrine tumor, the identification of asymptomatic patients who are at risk for disease, family planning, and guidance regarding management (2). When ordering predictive genetic testing, it is important to understand how the results will be used in patient management. In some cases, such as in MEN2, knowledge of the genotype will lead to a disease-preventing intervention (early thyroidectomy), whereas in other hereditary syndromes, it only will lead to an earlier diagnosis of disease but not disease that can be prevented by an early intervention. When multiple family members require testing, it is best to separate the testing temporally (*i.e.*, obtain the samples for testing on different days, starting with the oldest patient) to minimize the unlikely but potentially devastating consequences from an accidental sample switch.

The process of genetic testing in children is engrained with various ethical, legal, and psychosocial implications (3). Despite the clear medical benefits afforded from an early diagnosis, genetic testing in children has the potential for psychosocial harm, such as alteration of the child's self-image and of the parents' perception of the child, modification of the patient's outlook on life and worry about the potential for genetic discrimination, changes in family relationships, early "medicalization" of an otherwise healthy child, and concerns regarding future reproductive issues. Timely medical benefit to the child should be the primary justification for genetic testing. In all cases where the risks versus benefits of genetic testing are unclear, *e.g.*, testing at a very early age in MEN1 and MEN2A, the provider should respect the decision of the family.

Other important concepts surrounding genetic testing that are important for the clinician to understand include (i) the age at which genetic testing should be pursued for predictive genetic testing, which can vary based upon the familial mutation and the desires of the patient/parents; (ii) the limitations of sequencing, which will not identify large gene insertions or deletions and which may not look at the entire gene and thus miss a mutation outside of the known mutation "hot spots;" (iii) the differences between multigene next generation sequencing panels and single gene or single-site testing; and (iv) a DNA variant of unknown significance (VUS) is not synonymous with a disease-causing mutation and may represent a rare polymorphism (2). There are several online resources regarding genetic counseling and testing, including the National Society of Genetic Counselors (www.nsgc.org), the National Cancer Institute "The Genetics of Cancer" website (www.cancer.gov/cancertopics/genetics), and the internet site GeneReviews® (https://www.ncbi.nlm.nih.gov/books/NBK1116/).

Hereditary Endocrine Tumor Syndromes

Hereditary endocrine tumors can arise from any component of the endocrine system and can be isolated to one gland, such as seen in familial isolated pituitary adenoma, or include multiple endocrine tissues, exemplified by MEN1. Over time, the phenotypes of the heritable endocrine tumor syndromes continue to evolve and newer genes are implicated in the development of endocrine tumors. A thorough discussion of the various hereditary endocrine tumor syndromes is beyond the scope of the current handout, and the reader is referred elsewhere for a contemporary overview of these varied disorders (1, 4–16).

Prospective Clinical Screening

After a child has been identified to carry a pathogenic mutation, a plan for prospective clinical monitoring should be developed. Various recommendations for the monitoring of the asymptomatic patient who has been diagnosed with a hereditary endocrine tumor syndrome have been published (1, 4, 6, 9–11, 14, 15, 17–20). In some settings, optimal screening strategies have yet to be established. It should be acknowledged that screening guidelines primarily rely on retrospective studies and expert opinion and thus are not based upon the highest levels of evidence. In general, the age at which to begin clinical screening is linked to the earliest reported onset of disease. Although this approach may offer the best chance at diagnosing disease early in almost all at-risk patients, it also likely leads to overscreening of the youngest patients, who as a whole are less likely to develop overt clinical manifestations at a young age. Some other issues to consider regarding prospective screening include the psychological and physical risks to the patient, the medical costs, and the induction of "screening fatigue" in those subjected to very frequent monitoring. Certainly, the screening plan can be adjusted based upon the family history, recognizing that genotype-phenotype correlations are imperfect and that family members who share a common mutation do not all follow the same clinical course. Finally, given the concern that ionizing radiation may increase the risk of tumor development, the use of computerized tomography for screening should be limited and reserved for specific circumstances such as surgical planning.

MAIN CONCLUSIONS

- Endocrine tumors, especially when neuroendocrine in origin, are commonly familial and occur as a component of one of the well-recognized hereditary tumor syndromes.
- The possibility of hereditary disease should be considered in any child presenting with an endocrine neoplasm.
- Genetic counseling and testing should be pursued based upon the type of endocrine tumor, the clinical presentation (multifocal/bilateral disease), and the family history. For apparently sporadic disease, the decision to pursue genetic testing is based upon the tumor type (*e.g.*, genetic testing is rarely needed for differentiated thyroid cancer but is always recommended for pheochromocytoma/paraganglioma).

- Once a germline mutation has been identified, prospective monitoring is undertaken to diagnosis early the clinical manifestations of disease and, in the case of MEN2, to determine the age of early thyroidectomy. In many cases, optimal screening procedures have yet to be determined based upon a high level of evidence.

CASES/DISCUSSION OF CASES AND ANSWERS

Case 1

You are called by the genetic counselor regarding a 33-year-old man with clinical MEN1 (primary hyperparathyroidism, hyperprolactinemia, lipomas, and angiofibromas) who has been found to have a VUS in the MEN1 gene. He has four children, ages 8 months to 8 years.

Question

What would you recommend?
  A. Check an annual calcium level in his children.
  B. Recommend no further testing in his children because he has a VUS.
  C. Test for the VUS in all of his children.
  D. Pursue further genetic counseling/family studies and get parents' input regarding testing of the children.

Answer: D

In this case, the father has a clinical diagnosis of MEN1 and has been found to have a VUS in the *MEN1* gene. This conclusion by the testing laboratory implies that there is not enough information available to call this DNA variant a pathogenic, disease-causing mutation. This typically is because a particular DNA variant has not yet been reported to be associated with disease. The frequency of the DNA variant in the general population and the predicted effects of the variant on gene function can help to understand the likelihood that it is a mutation. Performing a functional assay of the "mutated" versus wild-type protein would also help to confirm the pathogenic nature of the DNA change, but this is usually not feasible due to the lack of access to a basic science laboratory to perform such studies. Additionally, identifying segregation of clinical disease with the VUS in other family members can lead to the conclusion that a given DNA change is likely a pathogenic mutation, and VUS clarification services are available from the major genetic testing laboratories. In the case presented, the next best step would be to pursue further genetic counseling and testing of the family, with a decision to test the children based upon additional data derived from family studies and the preference of the children's parents. In the case presented, the children's paternal grandmother also had clinical MEN1 and the same *MEN1* VUS, and so it was eventually concluded that this was in fact a likely pathogenic mutation. Answer A is not appropriate because genetic testing for MEN1 is preferred over clinical screening alone, understanding that primary hyperparathyroidism is not always

the first clinical manifestation of MEN1, and thus calcium screening alone could miss another clinically relevant MEN1 manifestation. Answer B is not the preferred answer because it ignores the fact that the VUS may in fact be a pathogenic mutation, and answer C is not the optimal answer, because, as discussed above, it is best to pursue additional counseling/family testing before embarking on testing of the children for a DNA variant that may or may not be pathogenic.

Case 2

You are seeing four children (ages 5 to 9 years) for predictive genetic testing for MEN2A. The maternal grandfather had locally metastatic medullary thyroid carcinoma (MTC) diagnosed at age 24 years, and the mother had an intrathyroidal microscopic MTC diagnosed at age 39 years when she presented with symptomatic bilateral pheochromocytomas. The familial RET mutation is the C618S mutation [American Thyroid Association (ATA) level moderate risk]. You recommend genetic testing for all of the children.

Question

If an RET mutation is confirmed, when would you recommend that early thyroidectomy be pursued?
  A. Now; >5 years of age
  B. By the age of 10 years
  C. When the basal calcitonin becomes abnormal and based on parent preference
  D. By the age of 24 years, which is the earliest age of MTC diagnosis in the family

Answer: C

There is widespread agreement that the therapeutic goal in a child with MEN2 is to remove the at-risk thyroid before incurable MTC metastasis occurs while minimizing potential medical and surgical morbidity. In experienced surgeons' hands, children who have a total thyroidectomy performed prior to the onset of metastatic disease have an excellent chance of remaining disease-free. After the identification of *RET* as the gene responsible for MEN2 in 1993, recommendations regarding the appropriate age for surgery were made on the basis of the specific *RET* mutation and the earliest age at which clinically relevant disease had been described for that particular mutation. In 2009, in the inaugural ATA MTC guidelines (21), the concept of safely delaying thyroidectomy while offering expectant monitoring of the neck ultrasound and basal calcitonin level in children with lower-risk *RET* mutations was introduced. In 2015, this approach was perpetuated in the revised ATA guidelines (18). The familial mutation in the presented case is currently considered a moderate-risk mutation, and early thyroidectomy could be delayed until the basal calcitonin becomes abnormal. The timing of thyroidectomy also depends on the preference of the parents. Thus, answer C is the most appropriate answer.

Answer D is incorrect because, as demonstrated in the vignette, family history does not necessary predict the disease course in other affected family members. Answer A would be appropriate if this family had a high-risk *RET* codon 634 mutation. Although answer B is historically correct, early thyroidectomy by age 10 years for this mutation is no longer universally recommended.

Case 3

A 14-year-old boy has a history of constipation, episodic abdominal pain with headaches, declining school performance, and behavioral issues. Due to abdominal pain, an ultrasound is ordered and a 4.1-cm left suprarenal mass is identified. Family history is unremarkable. He is admitted to his local hospital, where he was also found to have hypertension. A diagnosis of pheochromocytoma is made after additional evaluation confirmed a metaiodobenzylguanidine-avid left adrenal mass associated with significantly elevated normetanephrine levels.

Question

A mutation in which of the following genes is most suspected?

  A. *RET*
  B. *VHL*
  C. *SDHD*
  D. *NF1*

Answer: B

There are now many genes that have been associated with the development of pheochromocytomas and paragangliomas (PPGL), as reviewed elsewhere (14–16, 20). In general, of the known susceptibility genes, the one most likely to be mutated in a child presenting with a PPGL is *VHL*, followed by *SDHB*. Answer A is not the correct answer because it is extraordinarily rare for PPGL to be the initial presentation of MEN2 in childhood. In addition, *RET*-associated PPGL are adrenergic tumors, producing both epinephrine and metanephrine, whereas the tumor in the clinical vignette is a noradrenergic tumor, producing only norepinephrine and its metabolite normetanephrine. Noradrenergic tumors are highly indicative of a mutation in the *VHL* or the *SDHx* genes. Answer C is not correct because *SDHD*-related disease is primarily located in the neck and is not associated with catecholamine hypersecretion, and answer D is not correct because the patient does not have a clinical diagnosis of neurofibromatosis 1 (NF1) and because NF1-related tumors are adrenergic, not noradrenergic, neoplasms. After a germline mutation in one of the PPGL-susceptibility genes is identified, annual biochemical screening is undertaken to identify a functional tumor. In the case of *VHL* and *SDHx* mutations, imaging is also incorporated into prospective monitoring. In VHL, this is primarily done in the context of concomitant screening for pancreatic and renal manifestations, but in the case of the familial paraganglioma

syndromes (*SDHx*), it is done because of the possibility of nonfunctional tumors and, in the case of *SDHB*, a high risk of malignant PPGL.

Other questions for discussion will be covered during the session.

References

1. Waguespack SG, Rich TA, Perrier ND, Jimenez C, Cote GJ. Management of medullary thyroid carcinoma and MEN2 syndromes in childhood. *Nat Rev Endocrinol.* 2011;**7**(10):596–607.
2. De Sousa SM, Hardy TS, Scott HS, Torpy DJ. Genetic testing in endocrinology. *Clin Biochem Rev.* 2018;**39**(1):17–28.
3. Botkin JR, Belmont JW, Berg JS, Berkman BE, Bombard Y, Holm IA, Levy HP, Ormond KE, Saal HM, Spinner NB, Wilfond BS, McInerney JD. Points to consider: ethical, legal, and psychosocial implications of genetic testing in children and adolescents [published correction appears in *Am J Hum Genet.* 2015;97(3):501]. *Am J Hum Genet.* 2015;**97**(1):6–21.
4. Petr EJ, Else T. Genetic predisposition to endocrine tumors: diagnosis, surveillance and challenges in care. *Semin Oncol.* 2016; **43**(5):582–590.
5. Goudie C, Hannah-Shmouni F, Kavak M, Stratakis CA, Foulkes WD. 65 years of the double helix: endocrine tumour syndromes in children and adolescents. *Endocr Relat Cancer.* 2018;**25**(8):T221–T244.
6. Schultz KAP, Rednam SP, Kamihara J, Doros L, Achatz MI, Wasserman JD, Diller LR, Brugières L, Druker H, Schneider KA, McGee RB, Foulkes WD. *PTEN, DICER1, FH*, and their associated tumor susceptibility syndromes: clinical features, genetics, and surveillance recommendations in childhood. *Clin Cancer Res.* 2017;**23**(12):e76–e82.
7. Guilmette J, Nosé V. Hereditary and familial thyroid tumours. *Histopathology.* 2018;**72**(1):70–81.
8. Castinetti F, Moley J, Mulligan L, Waguespack SG. A comprehensive review on MEN2B. *Endocr Relat Cancer.* 2018;**25**(2):T29–T39.
9. Wasserman JD, Tomlinson GE, Druker H, Kamihara J, Kohlmann WK, Kratz CP, Nathanson KL, Pajtler KW, Parareda A, Rednam SP, States LJ, Villani A, Walsh MF, Zelley K, Schiffman JD. Multiple endocrine neoplasia and hyperparathyroid-jaw tumor syndromes: clinical features, genetics, and surveillance recommendations in childhood. *Clin Cancer Res.* 2017;**23**(13):e123–e132.
10. Hyde SM, Cote GJ, Grubbs EG. Genetics of multiple endocrine neoplasia type 1/multiple endocrine neoplasia type 2 syndromes. *Endocrinol Metab Clin North Am.* 2017;**46**(2):491–502.
11. van Leeuwaarde RS, de Laat JM, Pieterman CRC, Dreijerink K, Vriens MR, Valk GD. The future: medical advances in MEN1 therapeutic approaches and management strategies. *Endocr Relat Cancer.* 2017; **24**(10):T179–T193.
12. Pepe S, Korbonits M, Iacovazzo D. Germline and mosaic mutations causing pituitary tumours: genetic and molecular aspects. *J Endocrinol.* 2019;**240**(2):R21–R45.
13. Bonnet-Serrano F, Bertherat J. Genetics of tumors of the adrenal cortex. *Endocr Relat Cancer.* 2018;**25**(3):R131–R152.
14. Rednam SP, Erez A, Druker H, Janeway KA, Kamihara J, Kohlmann WK, Nathanson KL, States LJ, Tomlinson GE, Villani A, Voss SD, Schiffman JD, Wasserman JD. Von Hippel-Lindau and hereditary pheochromocytoma/paraganglioma syndromes: clinical features, genetics, and surveillance recommendations in childhood. *Clin Cancer Res.* 2017;**23**(12):e68–e75.
15. Muth A, Crona J, Gimm O, Elmgren A, Filipsson K, Stenmark Askmalm M, Sandstedt J, Tengvar M, Tham E. Genetic testing and surveillance guidelines in hereditary pheochromocytoma and paraganglioma [published online ahead of print 8 December 2018]. *J Intern Med.* doi:10.1111/joim.12869.
16. Neumann HP, Young WF, Jr, Krauss T, Bayley JP, Schiavi F, Opocher G, Boedeker CC, Tirosh A, Castinetti F, Ruf J, Beltsevich D, Walz M, Groeben HT, von Dobschuetz E, Gimm O, Wohllk N, Pfeifer M, Lourenço DM, Jr, Peczkowska M, Patocs A, Ngeow J, Makay O, Shah NS, Tischler A, Leijon H, Pennelli G, Villar Gómez de Las Heras K, Links

TP, Bausch B, Eng C. 65 years of the double helix: genetics informs precision practice in the diagnosis and management of pheochromocytoma. *Endocr Relat Cancer.* 2018;**25**(8):T201–T219.

17. Thakker RV, Newey PJ, Walls GV, Bilezikian J, Dralle H, Ebeling PR, Melmed S, Sakurai A, Tonelli F, Brandi ML; Endocrine Society. Clinical practice guidelines for multiple endocrine neoplasia type 1 (MEN1). *J Clin Endocrinol Metab.* 2012;**97**(9):2990–3011.

18. Wells SA, Jr, Asa SL, Dralle H, Elisei R, Evans DB, Gagel RF, Lee N, Machens A, Moley JF, Pacini F, Raue F, Frank-Raue K, Robinson B, Rosenthal MS, Santoro M, Schlumberger M, Shah M, Waguespack SG; American Thyroid Association Guidelines Task Force on Medullary Thyroid Carcinoma. Revised American Thyroid Association guidelines for the management of medullary thyroid carcinoma. *Thyroid.* 2015;**25**(6):567–610.

19. Manoharan J, Albers MB, Bartsch DK. The future: diagnostic and imaging advances in MEN1 therapeutic approaches and management strategies. *Endocr Relat Cancer.* 2017;**24**(10):T209–T225.

20. Eisenhofer G, Klink B, Richter S, Lenders JW, Robledo M. Metabologenomics of phaeochromocytoma and paraganglioma: an integrated approach for personalised biochemical and genetic testing. *Clin Biochem Rev.* 2017;**38**(2):69–100.

21. Kloos RT, Eng C, Evans DB, Francis GL, Gagel RF, Gharib H, Moley JF, Pacini F, Ringel MD, Schlumberger M, Wells SA, Jr; American Thyroid Association Guidelines Task Force. Medullary thyroid cancer: management guidelines of the American Thyroid Association [published correction appears in *Thyroid.* 2009;**19**(11):1295]. *Thyroid.* 2009;**19**(6):565–612.

Turner Syndrome: Growth, Puberty, and Fertility

M48
Presented, March 23–26, 2019

Patricia Y. Fechner, MD. Seattle Children's Hospital, Seattle, Washington 98105; and Department of Pediatrics, Division of Endocrinology, University of Washington, Seattle, Washington 98195, E-mail: patricia. fechner@seattlechildrens.org

SIGNIFICANCE OF THE CLINICAL PROBLEM

Turner syndrome (TS), a condition in which one of the sex chromosomes is missing in an individual with a female phenotype, occurs 1 in 2000 live female births, yet only ~50% of females with TS are diagnosed (1). The age of diagnosis depends on the severity of the phenotype, with the most severe presenting at younger ages. Typically, infants present with a webbed neck or pedal edema, or they may have been identified *in utero* secondary to ultrasound findings or an amniocentesis due to advanced maternal age or cell-free DNA. Other girls are identified during childhood when they present with short stature. Another subset of girls are diagnosed when they fail to initiate puberty or have premature ovarian failure. Some women are not recognized as having TS until they develop menstrual irregularities or premature ovarian failure. Thus, the spectrum of phenotype for girls with TS is broad and more diverse than what was originally believed. If diagnosed in childhood, many of these girls are followed by pediatric endocrinologists for issues of growth and puberty. However once these girls are discharged from pediatric endocrinology, the question arises about whom should follow these girls. Endocrinologists, gynecologists, and internists may not be familiar with caring for a woman with TS. The most recent set of clinical practice guidelines (2) is an outstanding resource for anyone caring for a girl or woman with TS.

Women with TS have a multitude of unique issues that need to be addressed. They may have cardiac anomalies, and all are at risk for dilation and rupture of the aorta. They usually have primary ovarian failure and thus need estrogen and progesterone replacement for induction of puberty, maintenance of healthy bone mineral density, maintenance of their uterus, and cardiovascular health. They are at increased risk for metabolic syndrome with lipid disorders, abnormal glucose tolerance or insulin resistance, hypertension, and obesity. Women with TS have an increased incidence of sensorineural hearing loss and require regularly scheduled audiology evaluations. Some may contemplate pregnancy with donor oocytes.

BARRIERS TO OPTIMAL PRACTICE

- There is no one specialty provider who is ideally suited to care for women with TS; instead, a multidisciplinary team approach may be needed.
- Most providers do not have experience with caring for a woman with TS, which makes it difficult for them to be aware of all of the areas of health that need to be screened.
- Patient adherence with estrogen replacement may be suboptimal.

LEARNING OBJECTIVES

As a result of participating in this session, learners should be able to:
- Recognize the features of TS
- Apply the clinical practice guidelines for TS
- Discuss the risks of pregnancy in a woman with TS

STRATEGIES FOR DIAGNOSIS, THERAPY, AND/OR MANAGEMENT

To make the diagnosis of TS, one first needs to consider the diagnosis. In childhood, girls with TS are usually shorter than expected based on parental heights. If an adolescent fails to go through puberty or has amenorrhea or irregular periods, an elevated follicle-stimulating hormone (FSH) will establish primary gonadal failure and lead to obtaining a karyotype. But in other females, the features of TS may be more subtle, especially in girls or women who have mosaicism with a 46,XX cell line. Table 1 lists the most common features of TS and the criteria for obtaining a karyotype for the diagnosis of TS.

The gold standard for diagnosing TS is a karyotype with at least 20 cells but preferably 30 cells. A 20-cell count will detect a level of 10% mosaicism with 95% confidence. If a 45,X karyotype is identified without mosaicism, an additional 200 cells can be studied using fluorescence *in situ* hybridization for the X and Y centromere because the absent chromosome could be an X or a Y. Both males and females may present with the 45,X/46,XY karyotype. The key is that the phenotype must be female for the diagnosis of TS. Females with the 45,X/46, XY karyotype have an increased risk for germ cell tumors; thus, a gonadectomy currently is recommended. If a female has the 46,XX karyotype with no 45,X cell line but TS is highly suspected, then karyotyping can be done on a second tissue, such as skin fibroblasts, buccal mucosa cells, or bladder epithelial cells, to look for the 45,X cell line. Structural abnormalities of the X chromosome may predispose it to be lost, as in the mosaic karyotype 45,X/46,X,isoXq.

Females diagnosed with TS are at risk for cardiac and renal congenital malformations, which need to be screened for with an echocardiogram and renal ultrasound. In addition, she is at risk for hearing loss (conductive and sensorineural), autoimmune disease, and metabolic syndrome. The most recent

Table 1. Indications for Obtaining a Karyotype to Diagnose TS

If one of the following
Fetal cystic hygroma or hydrops
Short stature
Heart defects: bicuspid aortic valve, coarctation, aortic stenosis, mitral valve abnormalities, hypoplastic left heart
Delayed puberty/onset of menarche due to primary ovarian failure
Short, broad neck with or without webbing, narrow palate, micrognathia, low-set abnormal pinnae, downslanted palpebral fissures, epicanthal folds
If two of the following
Kidney: horseshoe, absent, or hypoplastic
Madelung deformity
Neuropsychological/psychiatric issues
Multiple nevi
Dysplastic or hyperconvex nails
Congenital heart defects: partial anomalous pulmonary venous return, atrial septal defect, ventricular septal defects
Hearing impairment at <40 years and short stature
Adapted with permission from Gravholt CH, Andersen NH, Conway GS, et al. Clinical practice guidelines for the care of girls and women with Turner syndrome: proceedings from the 2016 Cincinnati International Turner Syndrome Meeting. *Eur J Endocrinol.* 2017;177:G1–G70.

clinical practice guidelines for TS (2) is an excellent source for determining which studies are required at diagnosis and for follow-up based on the age of the female to promote good health and prevent comorbidities.

Most girls with TS end up as adults shorter than expected based on midparental height. Growth hormone (GH) therapy has been shown to make up some, but not all, of the 8-in (20-cm) deficit. Current recommendations are to initiate GH at 4 to 6 years of age or as soon as TS is diagnosed if after 6 years of age, and the girl is short, has a strong chance of being short, or has a height velocity <50% for 6 months. GH stimulation testing does not need to be done. GH is initiated at 45 to 50 µg/kg per day in the United States or 4.0 to 4.5 IU/m^2 per day in Europe. Insulin-like growth factor-1 should be checked at least once a year and should be <2 SD above the mean for age. GH is discontinued once growth velocity is <2 cm/y or if growth plates are closed or bone age ≥14 years.

Approximately one-third of girls with TS have spontaneous breast development, and some have onset of menarche. Most of the girls who have thelarche have mosaicism with a 46,XX cell line (3). For those girls who do not have spontaneous thelarche, estrogen replacement therapy is initiated. The goal is to begin estrogen therapy if luteinizing hormone (LH) and FSH are elevated or anti-Müllerian hormone is low at 11 to 12 years of age (4). In this way, the girl can go through puberty at the same time as her peers. Estrogen therapy is initiated at a very low dose to promote breast development without compromising bone age advancement and ultimate height. If diagnosis of TS is late and height is quite short, then estrogen therapy can be initiated at a very low dose with a longer time to adult dosing to maximize height potential but with the risk of decreased bone mass

accrual, lack of uterine growth, and possible decreased self-esteem. Transdermal estradiol is the preferred method of therapy to induce puberty. The dose is increased gradually every 6 months from 3 to 4 µg for 12 hours at night to the adult dose of 25 to 100 µg/d over a 2- to 3-year period. If transdermal estrogen is unavailable or not approved by insurance, micronized oral 17β-estradiol can be started at 0.25 mg/d and increased to 1 to 4 mg/d. The transdermal form is preferred because it avoids the first pass through the liver that is necessary for the oral form. A progesterone needs to be added once there is vaginal bleeding or after 2 years of estrogen therapy to decrease the risk of endometrial cancer due to unopposed estrogen. Progesterone can be given as micronized crystalline progesterone 100 to 200 mg/d or medroxyprogesterone 5 to 10 mg/d for 10 days to cause withdrawal bleeding. Estrogen and progesterone therapy should be continued for bone and uterine health until the usual age of menopause, unless the risks outweigh the benefits.

Infertility is a major factor affecting the quality of life in a woman with TS (5). At the time of diagnosis, it is important to let the girl and her family know that there are many ways to have children and that carrying one's biologic child is just one way. Adoption is a possibility, as is surrogacy and pregnancy using a donor oocyte. Infertility is due to the premature loss of oocytes in the ovary beginning at 20 weeks gestation. Thus, at birth, many girls with TS already have ovarian failure. A few women with TS have spontaneous pregnancies, but the majority achieve pregnancies through the use of donor oocytes. If a girl and her family are interested in fertility preservation, oocyte cryopreservation has moved from being available only through research to now being a clinical procedure. Oocyte cryopreservation is not recommended in a girl <12 years of age. Individuals with TS need to be informed that if fertility is present, it decreases rapidly with age. They also need to know that the risk of miscarriage is high and that only 58% of conceptions result in a live birth, with 34% of the infants having aneuploidy or other fetal malformation when spontaneous pregnancy occurs (6). Women with TS who are pregnant are at higher risk than the general population for complications. They have a higher incidence of preeclampsia, infants born prematurely with a lower median birth weight, and higher rate of cesarean section.

Any woman with TS contemplating a pregnancy with her own oocytes or a donor oocyte needs to undergo careful screening for cardiac disease. Women with TS have increased cardiovascular risk during pregnancy over the general population. They should be evaluated by a multidisciplinary team that includes a cardiologist. A transthoracic echocardiogram and computed tomography/magnetic resonance imaging must be done within 2 years before becoming pregnant (7). If the ascending aortic size index (ASI) is >2.5 cm/m^2 or an ascending ASI is 2.0 to 2.5 cm/m^2 with a risk factor for aortic dissection such as bicuspid aortic valve, elongation of the transverse aorta, coarctation of the aorta, or hypertension, pregnancy is contraindicated. Pregnancy should be monitored closely in specialized centers by a multidisciplinary team. Women with TS have a higher incidence of hypertension and preeclampsia. Follow-up transthoracic echocardiogram should be done at least at 20 weeks of gestation and more frequently if indicated. Follow-up during the postpartum period is also critical because the cardiovascular risk does not end when the baby is delivered. It is estimated that risk of aortic dissection during pregnancy is 2% in a woman with TS, and this risk increases fivefold with a multiple gestation pregnancy. There is also a higher risk of hypertension and preeclampsia with a multiple gestation pregnancy. Therefore, only one embryo should be transferred in an *in vitro* fertilization cycle to decrease the maternal risk for complications associated with a multiple gestation.

MAIN CONCLUSIONS

TS is more common than expected, with 1 in 2000 females affected. The phenotypic range is extensive from normal female to a female with short stature, primary ovarian failure, webbed neck, and congenital heart disease. As genetic testing has become more frequent and physicians are aware of the broad spectrum of TS, more females are diagnosed with this condition. Advances in assisted reproductive technology provide women with TS the opportunity to become pregnant. Women with TS need life-long screening for aortic dilation, hypertension, hyperlipidemia, elevated transaminase levels, autoimmune disease, bone mineral density, and sensorineural hearing loss.

CASE 1

Anne is a 9-year-old female who has always been short and is referred for short stature. Her parents and primary care provider had not been concerned because the mom is only 4 ft, 10 in. However, in the past year, Anne's younger sister surpassed Anne in height. Anne has always been well except for frequent otitis media. She has had pressure equalization tubes in the past. On examination, her height is below the first percentile. She has bilateral ptosis with posterior rotation and cupping of her pinnae. She has a high arched palate with a short neck but no webbing. Anne is prepubertal on physical examination. She has an increased carrying angle and shortened fourth metacarpals bilaterally.

Question 1
What is the next best test to order?
   A. Echocardiogram
   B. FSH and LH
   C. Thirty-cell karyotype
   D. Thyroid function tests
   E. GH stimulation test

Discussion
The answer is C. TS is high on the differential with the findings of short stature, history of frequent otitis media, physical features of ptosis, posterior rotation and cupping of pinnae, high-arched palate, short neck, increased carrying angle, and shortened fourth metacarpals. After the diagnosis of TS is made, an echocardiogram and ECG should be done to look for cardiac anomalies. Girls with TS are also at risk for autoimmune disease, so Anne should be screened for thyroid and celiac disease. GH stimulation testing is not needed prior to starting GH for the indication of TS.

CASE 2

Barbara is a 9-year-old female who has been consistently growing along the 5th percentile for height. She was just diagnosed with compensated hypothyroidism and is referred for thyroid hormone replacement therapy. She has always been in good health. Family history is noteworthy for midparental height at the 90th percentile. Physical examination is normal except for a small goiter and increased nevi. You are concerned about the fact that Barbara is so much shorter than expected based on midparental height and do not believe that the degree of hypothyroidism explains this height discrepancy. A karyotype is ordered and returns with a 45,X/46,XX result. An echocardiogram is performed and is normal. Renal ultrasound reveals a horseshoe kidney. Barbara is initiated on GH therapy and continues with levothyroxine replacement therapy.

Question 2
Barbara's mother would like to know whether Barbara will be able to have children. What would you say to her?
   A. Women with TS are unable to be mothers.
   B. Pregnancy is possible if approved by her cardiologist.
   C. Barbara's pregnancy is at no higher risk than any other woman's pregnancy.

D. Barbara does not have a uterus, so she cannot become pregnant.

Discussion

The answer is B. All women with TS can be mothers, but most will not have a biologic child. Adoption is one way to have children, and the concept of different ways to have a family should be introduced to Barbara. Pregnancy is contraindicated in women who have an ASI >2.5 cm/m^2 and no cardiovascular risk factors and in those with an ASI of 2 to 2.5 cm/m^2 and one risk factor, such as aortic dissection (*e.g.*, bicuspid aortic valve), elongation of the transverse aorta, coarctation of the aorta, or hypertension. Barbara currently has no contraindication to pregnancy but most likely will require a donor oocyte to achieve a pregnancy. It is critical that she undergo cardiac evaluation just before undergoing pregnancy to ensure that she has no contraindications to pregnancy. She needs to be followed closely by a cardiologist during the pregnancy as well as by a high-risk obstetrician. Barbara is at higher risk during her pregnancy than other pregnant women for aortic dissection, hypertension and preeclampsia, preterm delivery, and a lower-birth-weight infant. If she has a spontaneous pregnancy with her own oocyte, then her baby has a one in three chance of aneuploidy or other congenital malformation. If she has had spontaneous puberty or received sufficient estrogen and progesterone replacement therapy, her uterus will grow large enough to support implantation and pregnancy.

Question 3

How and when should puberty be induced?

A. Barbara should be started on an oral contraceptive, which has both estrogen and progesterone, when she is 12 years old.

B. Barbara should wait until she is 14 years old to see whether she has spontaneous puberty before initiating puberty with estrogen.

C. Barbara should complete her growth before starting puberty with estrogen.

D. Gonadotropins should be checked beginning at age 11 years, and if increased, Barbara should start on low-dose estrogen therapy at 11 to 12 years of age.

Discussion

The answer is D. Starting at age 11 years, LH and FSH can be checked. If they are not elevated, then Barbara can continue to wait for the onset of spontaneous puberty. If she has no pubertal signs but elevated LH and FSH, then low-dose estrogen therapy, preferably using a transdermal patch, can be initiated. The dose of estrogen is increased gradually every 6 months over a 2- to 3-year period to adult doses. Once she has vaginal bleeding or has been on unopposed estrogen for 2 years, progesterone can be added to the regimen to induce withdrawal bleeding. If Barbara's height is still short and she is growing well, the increase in estrogen dosing can be slower to allow her more time to grow.

References

1. Stochholm K, Juul S, Juel K, Naeraa RW, Gravholt CH. Prevalence, incidence, diagnostic delay, and mortality in Turner syndrome. *J Clin Endocrinol Metab.* 2006;**91**(10):3897–3902.

2. Gravholt CH, Andersen NH, Conway GS, Dekkers OM, Geffner ME, Klein KO, Lin AE, Mauras N, Quigley CA, Rubin K, Sandberg DE, Sas TCJ, Silberbach M, Söderström-Anttila V, Stochholm K, van Alfen-van derVelden JA, Woelfle J, Backeljauw PF for the International Turner Syndrome Consensus Group. Clinical practice guidelines for the care of girls and women with Turner syndrome: proceedings from the 2016 Cincinnati International Turner Syndrome Meeting. *Eur J Endocrinol.* 2017;**177**(3):G1–G70.

3. Pasquino AM, Passeri F, Pucarelli I, Segni M, Municchi G. Spontaneous pubertal development in Turner's syndrome. Italian Study Group for Turner's Syndrome. *J Clin Endocrinol Metab.* 1997;**82**:1810–1813.

4. Klein KO, Rosenfield RL, Santen RJ, Gawlik AM, Backeljauw PF, Gravholt CH, Sas TCJ, Mauras N. Estrogen replacement in Turner syndrome: literature review and practical considerations. *J Clin Endocrinol Metab.* 2018;**103**(5):1790–1803.

5. Sutton EJ, McInerney-Leo A, Bondy CA, Gollust SE, King D, Biesecker B. Turner syndrome: four challenges across the lifespan. *Am J Med Genet A.* 2005;**139A**(2):57–66.

6. Tarani L, Lampariello S, Raguso G, Colloridi F, Pucarelli I, Pasquino AM, Bruni LA. Pregnancy in patients with Turner's syndrome: six new cases and review of literature. *Gynecol Endocrinol.* 1998;**12**(2):83–87.

7. Silberbach M, Roos-Hesselink JW, Andersen NH, Braverman AC, Brown N, Collins RT, De Backer J, Eagle KA, Hiratzka LF, Johnson WH Jr, Kadian-Dodov D, Lopez L, Mortensen KH, Prakash SK, Ratchford EV, Saidi A, van Hagen I, Young LT for the American Heart Association Council on Cardiovascular Disease in the Young; Council on Genomic and Precision Medicine; and Council on Peripheral Vascular Disease. Cardiovascular health in Turner syndrome: a scientific statement from the American Heart Association. *Circ Genom Precis Med.* 2018;**11**(10):e000048.

Interesting Cases in Pediatric DXA Interpretation

M51
Presented, March 23–26, 2019

Melissa S. Putman, MD. Bone Health Program, Division of Endocrinology, Boston Children's Hospital, Boston, Massachusetts 02115; and Harvard Medical School, Boston, Massachusetts 02115, E-mail: melissa.putman@ childrens.harvard.edu

SIGNIFICANCE OF THE CLINICAL PROBLEM

As with most aspects of pediatrics, children are not just little adults when it comes to bone densitometry, and the principles that guide how dual energy x-ray absorptiometry (DXA) is applied and interpreted in pediatric patients are very different than those used for adults. The International Society for Clinical Densitometry (ISCD) developed guidelines initially in 2007 (1) and revised them in 2013 (2) that provide official recommendations for the use and interpretation of DXA in pediatrics.

BARRIERS TO OPTIMAL PRACTICE

The purpose of this presentation is to use interesting DXA cases to illustrate some of the unique challenges in interpreting bone density in growing children and adolescents and in managing bone disorders in pediatrics.

LEARNING OBJECTIVES

As a result of participating in this session, participants should be able to:

- Appreciate the unique challenges in pediatric DXA interpretation
- Understand the role for DXA in children and adolescents and how to interpret pediatric DXA results on the basis of the most recent International Society for Clinical Densitometry (ISCD) Position Statement
- Identify strategies to account for short stature and pubertal status in interpreting DXA results

STRATEGIES, DIAGNOSIS, THERAPY, AND/OR MANAGEMENT

The clinical pearls listed below are based on the 2013 ISCD Pediatric Position Statement to keep in mind when discussing the clinical cases.

DXA Is Useful in Pediatric Patients With Primary Bone Disease and Those at Risk for Secondary Bone Disease or Fracture in Whom Knowing Bone Mineral Density (BMD) and/or Changes in BMD Over Time Would Affect Their Management

Studies suggest that there is a direct association between DXA results and fracture risk in pediatric patients with primary bone disease as well as in those with medical conditions that place them at risk for secondary bone disease (3, 4). For patients with primary bone disease, DXA scans are important for providing a baseline evaluation of bone health, to monitor disease status over time, and to gauge the effects of interventions. For patients with medical conditions that put them at risk for skeletal fragility, DXA scans can provide important information by which to identify patients who are at the highest risk for fracture as well as to inform decision making for both their primary condition and their bone health.

Recommended Imaging Sites in Children and Adolescents Are the Posterior-Anterior Spine and Total Body Less Head

In adults, the posterior-anterior spine, total hip, and femoral neck are the standard sites for determining BMD and predicting fracture. In children and adolescents, the hip is not a preferred skeletal site because of the variability and changes in skeletal anatomy with growth. Alternative sites for pediatric patients in whom standard sites cannot be imaged include the distal radius and lateral distal femur, although there are less reference data available for these sites and positioning can be tricky.

T-Scores Have No Role in Pediatrics

T-scores compare BMD with a young adult standard, but children and adolescents have not yet reached their adult height or peak bone mass. Although using T-scores for fracture prediction is helpful in postmenopausal women and older men, a child will have a low T-score as a result of his or her small size, despite having perfectly normal BMD for his or her age. For this reason, T-scores should never be reported on pediatric DXA interpretations. Rather, BMD Z-scores are used to compare the child's BMD with reference data that match the child's own age, race, and gender. According to the ISCD Official Positions, a BMD Z-score of −2.0 or below qualifies as low bone density or low bone mass.

In Pediatrics, Osteoporosis Cannot Be Diagnosed on the Basis of DXA Alone

World Health Organization criteria for the diagnosis of osteopenia and osteoporosis in adults do not apply to children and adolescents. In postmenopausal women and older men, osteoporosis can be diagnosed in patients with a T-score −2.5 or lower, nor osteopenia in patients with a T-score of −1.0 to −2.4. However, the diagnosis of osteoporosis in pediatrics requires both low bone density—a BMD Z-score of −2.0 or lower—and a significant fracture history, defined as two or more long bone fractures at age < 10 years or three or more fractures at age < 19 years. Similar to adults, diagnosis of osteoporosis can also be made in children with one or more vertebral fracture regardless of BMD. In addition, there is no place for the term osteopenia in pediatric DXA interpretation.

Pediatric DXA Scans Are Best Interpreted in the Context of Growth and Pubertal Status

Areal BMD measurements are two dimensional and are therefore affected by bone size such that smaller bones seem to be less dense on DXA imaging. Children with short stature will therefore appear to have lower BMD compared with their age-matched peers regardless of whether they have inherent bone disease or skeletal fragility. In addition, dramatic growth and gains in BMD occur during puberty; thus, pubertal status can have a profound impact on BMD measures. There are several potential approaches to addressing variations in height and puberty on DXA interpretation. ISCD recommends adjusting pediatric BMD Z-scores for height Z-score to account for short stature, which can be done using the Web site: https://zscore. research.chop.edu/bmdCalculator.php. Bone mineral apparent density provides a volumetric estimate of BMD on the basis of bone size of the spine. A bone age X-ray of the hand can identify an underlying delay or advancement in growth and development, and this bone age can be substituted for chronologic age to account for any variation in the patient's development. Even without specific BMD Z-score adjustments, knowing the patient's pubertal status, particularly if advanced or delayed, can help the clinician to interpret BMD Z-scores in the appropriate context.

Bone Loss in Growing Children Is Never Normal

Children are constantly growing, on average 5 to 7 cm/y in childhood and 8 to 11 cm/y during puberty. This growth is accompanied by significant gains in BMD. If serial DXA scans in a child show bone loss instead of gain, this is always a cause for concern and should be investigated.

Z-Score Change Captures Whether (or Not) Gains in BMD Are Appropriate for Age

Given the growth and gains in BMD that occur in childhood, knowing that there has been an increase in absolute BMD over time is not enough. These changes must be put in the context of what would be expected given the interval growth that has occurred. A positive Z-score change indicates that greater than expected changes in BMD have occurred during the interval between DXA scans, and a negative Z-score change suggests that gains in BMD have been less than what would be expected. A Z-score change that approximates zero suggests that interval changes in BMD have been appropriate for age.

CASES
Case 1

A 14-year-old girl was referred to the Boston Children's Hospital Bone Health Program for low bone density and fractures. She was otherwise healthy with no significant medical problems and took no medications. She participated in competitive ice skating on a national level, which involved skating 2 to 3 h/d, 7 d/wk. She fractured her right wrist after being dropped on the ice by her skating partner while lifted in the air during a competition. Her second fracture was of the

left distal fibula, which was sustained after twisting and falling on the ice. Her third fracture was a stress fracture of the right third metatarsal. Family history was remarkable for osteoporosis in the maternal grandmother, and midparental target height was 62 inches. Anthropometric measures showed a height of 146 cm (Z-score, −2.2), weight of 36 kg (Z-score, −2.0), and body mass index (BMI) of 16.9 mg/kg^2 (Z-score, −1.0). Physical examination was remarkable for normal sclera, normal dentition, no joint laxity, normal skin exam, and Tanner II breast and pubic hair development. Laboratory assessment included normal calcium, phosphorus, renal function, parathyroid hormone (PTH), and first morning urine calcium-creatinine ratio. 25-Hydroxyvitamin D was 26 ng/mL. DXA scan was obtained and showed Z-scores of −2.2 at the total body, less head (TBLH) and −2.6 at the spine.

Questions
1. Does this child have osteoporosis?
2. What additional testing would you recommend?
3. How would you treat this patient?

Discussion

There are several interesting points about this case that illustrate the challenges in pediatric bone health evaluation. First, to make the diagnosis of osteoporosis in this adolescent, she should have a clinically significant fracture history. Although she does have three fractures before age 19 years, two of her fractures were quite traumatic and whether these fractures should be included as clinically significant is not readily clear. Data to determine exactly what degree of trauma would warrant consideration for skeletal fragility are lacking, and often the clinician must use his or her best judgment in making these decisions. In this case, one could argue that a child with normal bone strength could sustain these fractures in similar circumstances. In addition, stress fractures are usually related to overuse and are not necessarily associated with skeletal fragility; therefore, this patient's metatarsal stress fracture would not typically be considered a clinically significant fracture. Second, this patient is short with a height Z-score < −2.0, and she is only Tanner II for sexual development at an age when most girls would be postmenarchal. Both her short stature and delayed puberty affect how we should interpret her DXA results. If we adjust her DXA results for her height Z-score, her TBLH Z-score becomes −0.8 and spine Z-score −1.5, which suggests that her bone density is not nearly as low as her unadjusted BMD Z-scores would imply. It might also be helpful to obtain a bone age, which could also be used to adjust her DXA results. Other additional testing to consider in this particular patient could include additional evaluation of the cause of her short stature and delayed puberty. Assuming this evaluation is normal, one could surmise that her excessive exercise may be contributing to her pubertal delay, and reducing the amount of her exercise may be of benefit. Treatment would include starting vitamin D to optimize her 25-hydroxyvitamin D level, ensuring adequate calcium intake, and optimizing nutritional status. Bisphosphonate therapy would not be indicated in this patient.

Case 2

A 15-year-old male with cystic fibrosis (CF) with mutation F508del/F508del and pancreatic insufficiency was referred for bone health evaluation. He underwent a bilateral lung transplantation 1 year before presentation that was complicated by two episodes of acute rejection that required high-dose IV glucocorticoid treatment. He suffered a left humerus fracture last month after falling while playing basketball outside his home but has had no other fractures. Current medications include prednisone 10 mg/d, mycophenolate, tacrolimus, pancreatic enzymes, inhaled antibiotics, and vitamin D_3 50,000 IU/wk. Anthropometric measures include height of 168 cm (Z-score, -0.3), weight of 48 kg (Z-score, -1.0), and BMI of 17.0 (Z-score, -1.4). Physical examination was remarkable for a thin male, rounded facies, proximal muscle wasting, nontender spine, and Tanner IV pubic hair with testicular size 18 mL bilaterally. Recent laboratory tests included normal calcium, phosphorus, renal function, and PTH. 25-Hydroxyvitamin D was 32 ng/mL. Prior testing also included negative celiac antibodies and thyroid function tests. DXA scan shortly before his lung transplantation showed BMD Z-scores of -2.0 at the TBLH and -1.6 at the spine. A DXA scan 1 year later showed BMD Z-scores of -3.1 at the TBLH and -2.2 at the spine, with a 5% to 7% decline in absolute BMD compared with the preceding year.

Questions

1. Does this patient have osteoporosis?
2. How would you treat this patient?

Discussion

Children and adults with CF are at risk for skeletal fragility for multiple reasons, including vitamin D deficiency, pancreatic insufficiency, malnutrition, chronic inflammation, reduced physical activity, glucocorticoid use, diabetes, and delayed puberty/hypogonadism. Lung transplantation is also associated with significant bone loss and a high fracture rate in adults, although data are limited in children and adolescents. According to ISCD guidelines, this patient technically may not meet criteria for the diagnosis of osteoporosis as he has had only a single long bone fracture; however, a humerus fracture sustained under these circumstances in a patient with this clinical history is concerning for underlying skeletal fragility. In addition, the bone loss that has occurred in the interval year between DXA scans is worrisome. According to a consensus statement from the Cystic Fibrosis Foundation (5), bisphosphonates should be considered in adult and pediatric patients with CF who have low BMD Z-scores, a decline in BMD by 3% to 5% or more per year, a prior fragility fracture, and/or undergoing lung

transplantation. Given this patient's constellation of clinical findings, including the fracture, low bone density, recent lung transplantation, ongoing glucocorticoid and calcineurin inhibitor treatment, and significant bone loss, this patient was treated with zoledronic acid along with counseling on lifestyle interventions to optimize bone health.

Case 3

A 15-year-old male with a history of Duchenne's muscular dystrophy (DMD) presented in consultation for low bone density. Although previously ambulatory, he had been wheelchair bound for the past year. He received regular physical and occupational therapy, but weightbearing activities were limited. He recently suffered a distal femur fracture that was sustained during a difficult transfer from his motorized wheelchair. He had been treated with prednisone 20 mg/d for many years and his neurologist had no plans to reduce this dose. Other medications included vitamin D_3 2000 IU/d. His family history was notable for delayed puberty in his mother, who reported menarche at age 16 years. Anthropometric measures included height of 153 cm (Z-score, -2.4), weight of 68 kg (Z-score, $+0.7$), and BMI of 28.6 kg/m^2 (Z-score, $+1.82$). Physical examination was notable for an overweight male, round facies, normal visual fields, intact sense of smell, nontender spine with no scoliosis or kyphosis, and Tanner III pubic hair with testicular size 3 mL bilaterally. Laboratory results were notable for normal calcium, phosphorus, PTH, prolactin, thyrotropin, and free T_4. Creatine was 0.2 mg/dL, and 25-hydroxyvitamin D was 36 ng/mL. Morning follicle-stimulating hormone and luteinizing hormone were in the prepubertal range and testosterone was undetectable. Bone age was within 1 year of chronologic age. DXA scan results were as follows:

Age 13 years
    Spine: BMD, 0.698 g/cm^2
              BMD Z-score, -0.5
              Height Z-score–adjusted BMD Z-score, $+1.6$

    TBLH: BMD, 0.560 g/cm^2
              BMD Z-score, -4.4
              Height Z-score–adjusted BMD Z-score, -3.4

Age 15 years
    Spine: BMD, 0.704 g/cm^2
              BMD Z-score, -1.9
              Height Z-score–adjusted BMD Z-score, -0.3

    TBLH: BMD, 0.611 g/cm^2
              BMD Z-score, -6.5
              Height Z-score–adjusted BMD Z-score, -4.9

Questions

1. What additional evaluation would you recommend?
2. How would you treat this patient?

Discussion

Patients with DMD are at high risk of low bone density and fractures as a result of progressive muscle weakness, immobilization, and glucocorticoid use. Vertebral fractures occur frequently and may not be initially clinically apparent. Given this patient's clinical history and BMD, a lateral thoracolumbar spine X-ray was obtained to evaluate for an asymptomatic vertebral fracture, which was negative. Recently published guidelines (6) recommend IV bisphosphonate treatment in patients with DMD who have evidence of clinically significant fragility, which is defined as one or more low-trauma long bone or vertebral fracture. However, this patient's case is also complicated by significantly delayed puberty, which certainly contributes to his low BMD, declining BMD Z-scores, and skeletal fragility. At age 15 years, without signs of puberty and particularly in the setting of psychosocial concerns expressed by the patient, hormonal therapy with testosterone is indicated and would likely help to improve his skeletal health and BMD. This patient started testosterone 50 mg IM monthly for a planned 6-month course followed by re-evaluation of pubertal progression and testicular size. After a long discussion with the patient and his family about the benefits and risks of bisphosphonate treatment, they preferred to avoid starting two treatments at the same time and the decision was made to delay bisphosphonate therapy for the time being while focusing on optimizing calcium intake, vitamin D, and physical therapy with ongoing annual DXA monitoring and annual lateral spine X-rays.

References

1. Gordon CM, Bachrach LK, Carpenter TO, Crabtree N, El-Hajj Fuleihan G, Kutilek S, Lorenc RS, Tosi LL, Ward KA, Ward LM, Kalkwarf HJ. Dual energy X-ray absorptiometry interpretation and reporting in children and adolescents: The 2007 ISCD Pediatric Official Positions. *J Clin Densitom.* 2008;**11**(1):43–58.
2. Gordon CM, Leonard MB, Zemel BS, for the International Society for Clinical Densitometry. 2013 Pediatric Position Development Conference: Executive summary and reflections [published correction appears in *J Clin Densitom.* 2014;17(4):517]. *J Clin Densitom.* 2014; **17**(2):219–224.
3. Bianchi ML, Leonard MB, Bechtold S, Högler W, Mughal MZ, Schönau E, Sylvester FA, Vogiatzi M, van den Heuvel-Eibrink MM, Ward L, for the International Society for Clinical Densitometry. Bone health in children and adolescents with chronic diseases that may affect the skeleton: The 2013 ISCD Pediatric Official Positions. *J Clin Densitom.* 2014;**17**(2):281–294.
4. Bishop N, Arundel P, Clark E, Dimitri P, Farr J, Jones G, Makitie O, Munns CF, Shaw N, for the International Society of Clinical Densitometry. Fracture prediction and the definition of osteoporosis in children and adolescents: The ISCD 2013 Pediatric Official Positions. *J Clin Densitom.* 2014;**17**(2):275–280.
5. Aris RM, Merkel PA, Bachrach LK, Borowitz DS, Boyle MP, Elkin SL, Guise TA, Hardin DS, Haworth CS, Holick MF, Joseph PM, O'Brien K, Tullis E, Watts NB, White TB. Guide to bone health and disease in cystic fibrosis. *J Clin Endocrinol Metab.* 2005;**90**(3):1888–1896.
6. Ward LM, Hadjiyannakis S, McMillan HJ, Noritz G, Weber DR. Bone health and osteoporosis management of the patient with Duchenne muscular dystrophy. *Pediatrics.* 2018;**142**(Suppl 2): S34–S42.

Congenital Adrenal Hyperplasia: Transition, New Insights Into Etiology, and Prescriptions

M56
Presented, March 23–26, 2019

Deborah P. Merke, MD, MS. National Institutes of Health Clinical Center, Bethesda, Maryland 20892, E-mail: dmerke@nih.gov

Wiebke Arlt, MD, DSc. University of Birmingham, Birmingham B15 2TT, United Kingdom, E-mail: w.arlt@bham.ac.uk

SIGNIFICANCE OF THE CLINICAL PROBLEM

Congenital adrenal hyperplasia (CAH) due to 21-hydroxylase deficiency is an autosomal recessive disorder of steroidogenesis and the cause of disease in the overwhelming majority of patients with CAH. In the "classic" form of CAH, the adrenal does not produce adequate amounts of cortisol, there is variable effect on aldosterone production, and accumulation of cortisol precursors is diverted to sex hormone biosynthesis, resulting in androgen excess. Classic CAH has an estimated worldwide prevalence of one in 16,000 births, and it is part of the neonatal screen in over 40 countries (1). The majority of patients with classic CAH are salt wasters (*i.e.*, suffer from both glucocorticoid and mineralocorticoid deficiency and if not treated soon after birth, would present with a life-threatening adrenal crisis at 7 to 21 days of life). About 25% of patients with classic CAH make small amounts of aldosterone sufficient to escape a neonatal salt-wasting adrenal crisis and if not identified by neonatal screening, would present as toddlers with signs and symptoms of androgen excess.

The clinical management of CAH involves treatment of adrenal insufficiency and suppression of adrenal androgen production. Current glucocorticoid formulations mostly fail to mimic the pattern of physiologic diurnal glucocorticoid production, resulting in intermittent upregulation of ACTH and the frequent requirement for supraphysiologic doses of glucocorticoid to control excess adrenal androgen production. However, iatrogenic glucocorticoid excess can result in obesity, growth suppression in children, decreased bone mineral density, cardiovascular risk, and adverse psychosocial outcomes. However, inadequate androgen suppression can result in precocious puberty, virilization of females, infertility in both sexes, and adverse psychosocial outcomes. Patient management strives to control excess androgen production while avoiding signs and symptoms of glucocorticoid excess. Suboptimal outcomes are common (2).

During childhood, disease management focuses on optimization of growth and development and the prevention and treatment of adrenal crises. Treatment goals during the transition from childhood to adulthood are particularly challenging (3); in adolescence, the general psychosocial challenges of puberty are combined with the need for the affected patient to take control of the management of their disease, a role usually taken by the parents during childhood. Management in adulthood aims to prevent comorbidities, such as infertility, metabolic syndrome, and poor quality of life (4, 5).

BARRIERS TO OPTIMAL PRACTICE

- The clinical management of CAH involves suppression of adrenal androgen production in addition to the treatment of primary adrenal insufficiency. Control of upregulated adrenal androgen production is often difficult to achieve without supraphysiological glucocorticoid doses. Current therapy requires individual fine tuning.
- Classic CAH is a rare disease; therefore, there are few centers with expertise in the management of CAH. This is especially true for adults, who are often lost to follow-up. The prevalence of CAH is similar to that of primary adrenal insufficiency due to autoimmune adrenalitis, but many endocrine centers look after more patients with Addison disease than patients with CAH. This points to the importance of the handover between pediatric and adult care at the point of transition for ensuring that patients with CAH are under specialist care throughout their life.

LEARNING OBJECTIVES

As a result of participating in this session, learners should be able to

- Explain the challenges in managing and treating patients with classic CAH during childhood and into adulthood and understand the role of both glucocorticoid and mineralocorticoid therapy
- Identify the long-term comorbidities associated with classic CAH, including infertility and poor quality of life in both men and women
- Develop strategies for transitioning patients from pediatric to adult care

STRATEGIES FOR MANAGEMENT

With the advent of neonatal screening, the majority of patients with classic CAH are now diagnosed during infancy, making the distinction between "salt-wasting" and "simple-virilizing" CAH unclear. However, this distinction is not an essential aspect of the management. All patients with classic CAH benefit from fludrocortisone therapy throughout childhood and adequate dietary sodium during infancy. Subclinical aldosterone deficiency is present in all classic patients (1).

Maintaining sodium balance and euvolemia is important in reducing vasopressin and ACTH, leading to decreased adrenal androgen production, and allowing for reduced glucocorticoid doses, leading to improved growth (6).

The glucocorticoid of choice for treatment of CAH is the short-acting hydrocortisone (1). Compounded forms of hydrocortisone should be used with caution due to risk of variable dose accuracy (7). In childhood, long-acting glucocorticoid preparations, such as prednisone, prednisolone, and dexamethasone, are discouraged because of potential growth suppression (1). In adulthood, prednisolone can be considered if disease control cannot be reliably achieved with hydrocortisone (8); dexamethasone should be avoided or restricted to short, targeted treatment periods, because it is long acting and frequently results in adverse metabolic side effects (9, 10). Hydrocortisone is best given three to four times a day, with the first dose given in the early morning on awakening and the last dose given at bedtime. The timing of the midday dose is less important, because physiologic cortisol and ACTH are low at this time. Fludrocortisone is given once or twice daily.

Laboratory evaluation helps guide the management. Serum 17-hydroxyprogesterone and androstenedione are the traditional biomarkers of CAH disease control; they help guide hydrocortisone treatment, whereas plasma renin should be maintained in the mid- to upper normal range to help guide fludrocortisone therapy. In general, 17-hydroxyprogesterone levels should not be suppressed to within the normal reference range; this would indicate excessive glucocorticoid therapy. However, androstenedione should be maintained within a normal range for sex and tanner stage. Tandem mass spectrometry is the gold standard for measurement of blood or saliva samples for treatment monitoring, because immunoassay results may not be accurate due to cross-reactivity by steroid precursors that accumulate in CAH. Consistently timed hormone measurements are important for treatment monitoring; levels are influenced by time of day and relationship to ingestion of medication (11). Disease markers that are highly likely to play a major role in the monitoring of CAH are the 11-oxygenated androgens, which are generated from conversion of androstenedione to 11-hydroxyandrostenedione and 11-ketotestosterone, the latter binding and activating the androgen receptor with similar potency to testosterone (12). Recent work has shown that 11-oxygenated androgens are major markers of disease activity and the predominant androgens in CAH (13–15).

Adjustments to medication should be made in the context of the overall clinical picture (1, 2). Pertinent aspects of the clinical status include signs and symptoms of hyperandrogenism (accelerated growth velocity; increased pubic hair, apocrine odor, or phallic size) or hypercortisolism (decreased growth velocity, weight gain, striae). Bone age, blood pressure, and symptoms of salt craving are also important and help guide management. Bone age is a lagging indicator of

inadequate adrenal suppression. Blood pressure should be maintained in the normal range, and hypertension may occur with excess fludrocortisone dosing. Hypertension in children with CAH has been associated with higher fludrocortisone doses and lack of plasma renin activity monitoring (16). Doses of hydrocortisone >20 mg/m^2 per day in infancy or 17 mg/m^2 per day in adolescents have been found to be associated with decreased adult height (1, 9). Attention should be given to these important periods of growth during childhood.

Close monitoring early in life is recommended, especially in the first 3 to 6 months. Mineralocorticoid sensitivity increases in the first year, and therefore, monitoring blood pressure and plasma renin activity is especially important. Often, fludrocortisone dose can be decreased around 6 months of age. After 18 months, evaluation should occur every 4 months.

Adolescence is a particularly challenging time. Pubertal activation of the hypothalamic-pituitary-gonadal axis may indirectly affect management; changes in the clearance of cortisol during puberty have been shown and may influence glucocorticoid effectiveness in suppressing adrenal androgens. During adolescence, psychosocial pressures often affect adherence to medical therapy. Inconsistent compliance can result in underreplacement of cortisol. Educating patients about their disease is an important aspect of the transition to adulthood. Goals include understanding that CAH is a genetic disease, learning self-administration of stress dosing, comprehending long-term risks, and open discussion of sexual issues. After growth is complete, the glucocorticoid regimen should be reassessed. The goal is to use the lowest possible glucocorticoid dose to adequately suppress adrenal androgens and optimize compliance based on lifestyle. Mineralocorticoid receptor sensitivity changes throughout childhood and adolescence and settles into a steady state after completion of puberty. Therefore, the need for mineralocorticoid replacement should be reassessed at transitional age (16 to 20 years old) to ensure the appropriate choice of treatment; both regular under- and overreplacement with fludrocortisone were found in a large cross-sectional study of adults with CAH, with increased plasma renin in 53% of adults on fludrocortisone therapy but also, in 36% of adults not on fludrocortisone due to being wrongly assumed to have a normal mineralocorticoid reserve (17).

All patients with classic CAH require increased glucocorticoid dosing (stress dosing) for febrile illnesses, gastroenteritis, major surgery, or major trauma (18, 19). Children, especially young children, are at risk for hypoglycemia during illness episodes, and ingestion of simple and complex sugars in addition to fluids is recommended (18). Adrenal crisis prevention should include equipping every patient with a glucocorticoid injection kit for emergency use as well as a steroid emergency card or alternatively, an emergency bracelet or necklace as per general guidelines for primary adrenal insufficiency (19). In children, parents/guardians should be taught parenteral administration; patients should be trained in hydrocortisone self-administration at transitional age, and emergency treatment education sessions may also be offered to friends and partners as appropriate to an individual's living situation.

An important issue, in particular in early to midadulthood, is fertility, and this can be compromised in both men and women with CAH. In female adolescents and adult women with CAH, cycle irregularity is a common finding; in the majority of cases, it is driven by excess production of progesterone, which creates a functional chronic luteal phase, and this can disrupt both the menstrual cycle and implantation of a fertilized egg. For women with CAH who attempt to conceive, glucocorticoid therapy should be tailored to maintain a serum progesterone of <0.6 ng/mL (<2 nmol/L). Women with CAH wishing to conceive should be jointly managed by an expert endocrinologist and expert gynecologist, and the latter should evaluate whether a vaginal birth may be possible. Vaginal delivery is usually not recommended in women with CAH who underwent two or more genital corrective surgeries, but this requires individualized assessment in all cases.

In men with CAH, adrenal androgen excess can lead to downregulation of gonadal function. Physiologic androgen production in men arises mainly from gonadal testosterone production, and healthy men have a serum androstenedione over testosterone (A/T) ratio of <0.2. In men with CAH, an A/T ratio > 0.5 indicates that a substantial fraction of circulating testosterone is of adrenal origin. If A/T is more than one with concurrent suppression of serum LH and FSH, most of circulating testosterone in the affected man with CAH is of adrenal origin. Another problem that regularly affects male patients with CAH is testicular adrenal rest tumor (TART). These are thought to arise from the urogenital ridge during fetal development, with cells of adrenal origin migrating with the emerging gonad. However, the term "TART" might need revision for three reasons. First, the word "tumor" can be misunderstood as "cancer" by both patients and urologists. Second, TARTs have now also been described in women with CAH, and thus, they are not strictly of "testicular" origin. Third, recent work has shown that the cells are not of adrenal origin but actually harbor features that characterize both adrenal and gonadal cells (i.e., may represent a more stem cell–like urogenital ridge precursor cell) (20). TARTs are found in a large number of male patients with CAH (21, 22) and can best be assessed by ultrasound, because in particular, smaller lesions are not palpable. However, TARTs can be detected even in boys with CAH under the age of 10 years old (23); therefore, a monitoring strategy has to also include children and adolescents as appropriate. At transition, all young men with CAH should be offered testicular ultrasound and if TARTs are found, a sperm count and motility assessment with the opportunity for sperm banking, because TARTs substantially impact sperm quality and production. Although testis-sparing surgery of TARTs does not restore fertility (24), time-limited,

individually tailored administration of long-acting glucocorticoids can, in some cases, reverse azoospermia and facilitate fertility (25).

CASE 1

A 2.5-year-old male presents with pubic hair and increased growth velocity. Bone age is 8 years. The diagnosis of classic simple-virilizing CAH is made based on a serum 17-hydroxyprogesterone level of 5300 ng/dL. He is started on hydrocortisone 5 mg three times a day (37.5 mg/m^2 per day) and subsequently weaned to 20 mg/m^2 per day. Follow-up laboratory results measured in the early morning (around 0800 hours) show 17-hydroxyprogesterone levels ranging from undetectable (while receiving 37.5 mg/m^2 per day) to 8200 ng/dL (while receiving 20 mg/m^2 per day). One year later, he has gained 10 kg, grown 5 cm, and developed abdominal striae, and his bone age is 10 years. Pubic hair is tanner 3, and testes are 2 mL bilateral on physical examination.

Question

What is the next best step in the management?
  A. Measure gonadotropin levels and start treatment with an luteinizing hormone-releasing hormone analog
  B. Measure plasma renin activity and start treatment with fludrocortisone
  C. Discuss barriers to compliance with the family; no change in therapy
  D. Consider starting an aromatase inhibitor

CASE 2

A 17-year-old female has classic CAH. She was born with ambiguous genitalia and diagnosed at 4 days old based on 17-hydroxyprogesterone (17OHP) of 19,000 ng/dL (574 nmol/L). She was treated with hydrocortisone, fludrocortisone, and salt during the first 2 years of life. Genital surgery was at 6 months of age. Menarche started at 14 years old, and she now has regular menses. She has reached adult height. She will be starting college soon. On physical examination, height is at the 10th percentile, weight is at the 50th percentile, and body mass index is 23.3 kg/m^2. There is no hirsutism, acne, or striae. She is receiving hydrocortisone 10 mg (awakening), 5 mg (midday), and 10 mg (bedtime) = 15.5 mg/m^2 per day and fludrocortisone 100 μg (awakening). Laboratory evaluation indicates 17OHP 1150 ng/dL (35 nmol/L), androstenedione 170 ng/dL (5.7 nmol/L; normal range: 30 to 200 ng/dL), and plasma renin activity 2.1 ng/mL per hour (0.2 to 4.5 ng/mL per hour).

Question

What is the best plan for treatment as she transitions from adolescence to adulthood?

A. Continue hydrocortisone; this patient has done well on hydrocortisone
B. Switch to dexamethasone once daily to optimize compliance
C. Switch to dexamethasone and an oral contraceptive pill
D. Switch to prednisone twice daily to optimize compliance

DISCUSSION OF CASES AND ANSWERS
Case 1
This patient is receiving high doses of hydrocortisone. Although noncompliance (or intermittent compliance) is a possibility and this needs to be reviewed with the family, a 2-year-old child should not be receiving 20 mg/m^2 per day of hydrocortisone. Clinically, he is showing signs and symptoms of both hypercortisolism and hyperandrogenism, supporting the fact that he is receiving the prescribed high doses of hydrocortisone. This patient is at risk for central precocious puberty, but this is not his immediate concern. His testicular size is prepubertal. The correct answer is B. Mild salt wasting can stimulate vasopressin and ACTH, leading to increased adrenal androgen production and an apparent need for high glucocorticoid doses. All patients with classic CAH, even those who fall into the simple-virilizing subgroup, benefit from daily fludrocortisone therapy. Starting fludrocortisone will allow for lower hydrocortisone dosing. Plasma renin activity should be measured routinely. Review of other medications should also be checked. Medications that increase the metabolism of hydrocortisone (Cytochrome P450 3A1 inducers) might increase glucocorticoid requirement. An aromatase inhibitor would be considered experimental therapy for this patient.

Case 2
This patient is doing well on hydrocortisone. There is no need to change her medication. The correct answer is A. However, if she has concerns about compliance with her midday dose, then prednisone or prednisilone could be considered (answer D). Dexamethasone should not be used in heterosexually active women, because it is not inactivated by placental 11-β-hydroxysteroid dehydrogenase type 2 and would, therefore, result in fetal exposure should a pregnancy occur (1). The glucocorticoid dose is individualized, aiming to use the lowest glucocorticoid dose possible that adequately suppresses adrenal androgens and optimizes compliance based on lifestyle.

MAIN CONCLUSIONS
Children, adolescents, and adults with classic CAH require lifelong treatment and care, and they should be regularly reviewed and educated regarding their condition by an endocrine specialist with patient age–appropriate input of members of a multidisciplinary specialist team, including geneticists, urological surgeons, gynecologists, psychologists mand specialist nurses.

References
1. Speiser PW, Arlt W, Auchus RJ, Baskin LS, Conway GS, Merke DP, Meyer-Bahlburg HFL, Miller WL, Murad MH, Oberfield SE, White PC. Congenital adrenal hyperplasia due to steroid 21-hydroxylase deficiency: an Endocrine Society clinical practice guideline. *J Clin Endocrinol Metab.* 2018;**103**(11):4043–4088.
2. El-Maouche D, Arlt W, Merke DP. Congenital adrenal hyperplasia. *Lancet.* 2017;**390**(10108):2194–2210.
3. Merke DP, Poppas DP. Management of adolescents with congenital adrenal hyperplasia. *Lancet Diabetes Endocrinol.* 2013;**1**(4):341–352.
4. Han TS, Walker BR, Arlt W, Ross RJ. Treatment and health outcomes in adults with congenital adrenal hyperplasia. *Nat Rev Endocrinol.* 2014;**10**(2):115–124.
5. Arlt W, Willis DS, Wild SH, Krone N, Doherty EJ, Hahner S, Han TS, Carrol PV, Conway GS, Rees DA, Stimson RH, Walker BR, Connell JM, Ross RJ; United Kingdom Congenital adrenal Hyperplasia Adult Study Executive (CaHASE). Health status of adults with congenital adrenal hyperplasia: a cohort study of 203 patients. *J Clin Endocrinol Metab.* 2010;**95**(11):5110–5121.
6. Muthusamy K, Elamin MB, Smushkin G, Murad MH, Lampropulos JF, Elamin KB, Abu Elnour NO, Gallegos-Orozco JF, Fatourechi MM, Agrwal N, Lane MA, Albuquerque FN, Erwin PJ, Montori VM. Clinical review: adult height in patients with congenital adrenal hyperplasia: a systematic review and metaanalysis. *J Clin Endocrinol Metab.* 2010;**95**(9):4161–4172.
7. Neumann U, Burau D, Spielmann S, Whitaker MJ, Ross RJ, Kloft C, Blankenstein O. Quality of compounded hydrocortisone capsules used in the treatment of children. *Eur J Endocrinol.* 2017;**177**(2):239–242.
8. Auchus RJ, Arlt W. Approach to the patient: the adult with congenital adrenal hyperplasia. *J Clin Endocrinol Metab.* 2013;**98**(7):2645–2655.
9. Han TS, Stimson RH, Rees DA, Krone N, Willis DS, Conway GS, Arlt W, Walker BR, Ross RJ; United Kingdom Congenital adrenal Hyperplasia Adult Study Executive (CaHASE). Glucocorticoid treatment regimen and health outcomes in adults with congenital adrenal hyperplasia. *Clin Endocrinol (Oxf).* 2013;**78**(2):197–203.
10. Han TS, Krone N, Willis DS, Conway GS, Hahner S, Rees DA, Stimson RH, Walker BR, Arlt W, Ross RJ; United Kingdom Congenital adrenal Hyperplasia Adult Study Executive (CaHASE). Quality of life in adults with congenital adrenal hyperplasia relates to glucocorticoid treatment, adiposity and insulin resistance: United Kingdom Congenital adrenal Hyperplasia Adult Study Executive (CaHASE). *Eur J Endocrinol.* 2013;**168**(6):887–893.
11. Debono M, Mallappa A, Gounden V, Nella AA, Harrison RF, Crutchfield CA, Backlund PS, Soldin SJ, Ross RJ, Merke DP. Hormonal circadian rhythms in patients with congenital adrenal hyperplasia: identifying optimal monitoring times and novel disease biomarkers. *Eur J Endocrinol.* 2015;**173**(6):727–737.
12. Storbeck KH, Bloem LM, Africander D, Schloms L, Swart P, Swart AC. 11β-Hydroxydihydrotestosterone and 11-ketodihydrotestosterone, novel C19 steroids with androgenic activity: a putative role in castration resistant prostate cancer? *Mol Cell Endocrinol.* 2013;**377**(1-2):135–146.
13. Turcu AF, Nanba AT, Chomic R, Upadhyay SK, Giordano TJ, Shields JJ, Merke DP, Rainey WE, Auchus RJ. Adrenal-derived 11-oxygenated 19-carbon steroids are the dominant androgens in classic 21-hydroxylase deficiency. *Eur J Endocrinol.* 2016;**174**(5):601–609.
14. Jones CM, Mallappa A, Reisch N, Nikolaou N, Krone N, Hughes BA, O'Neil DM, Whitaker MJ, Tomlinson JW, Storbeck KH, Merke DP, Ross RJ, Arlt W. Modified-release and conventional glucocorticoids and diurnal androgen excretion in congenital adrenal hyperplasia. *J Clin Endocrinol Metab.* 2017;**102**(6):1797–1806.
15. Turcu AF, Mallappa A, Elman MS, Avila NA, Marko J, Rao H, Tsodikov A, Auchus RJ, Merke DP. 11-Oxygenated androgens are biomarkers of adrenal volume and testicular adrenal rest tumors in 21-hydroxylase deficiency. *J Clin Endocrinol Metab.* 2017;**102**(8):2701–2710.
16. Bonfig W, Roehl FW, Riedl S, Dörr HG, Bettendorf M, Brämswig J, Schönau E, Riepe F, Hauffa B, Holl RW, Mohnike K; AQUAPE CAH

Study Group. Blood pressure in a large cohort of children and adolescents with classic adrenal hyperplasia (CAH) due to 21-hydroxylase deficiency. *Am J Hypertens.* 2016;**29**(2):266–272.

17. Bonfig W, Pozza SB, Schmidt H, Pagel P, Knorr D, Schwarz HP. Hydrocortisone dosing during puberty in patients with classical congenital adrenal hyperplasia: an evidence-based recommendation. *J Clin Endocrinol Metab.* 2009;**94**(10):3882–3888.

18. El-Maouche D, Hargreaves CJ, Sinaii N, Mallappa A, Veeraraghavan P, Merke DP. Longitudinal assessment of illnesses, stress dosing, and illness sequelae in patients with congenital adrenal hyperplasia. *J Clin Endocrinol Metab.* 2018;**103**(6):2336–2345.

19. Bornstein SR, Allolio B, Arlt W, Barthel A, Don-Wauchope A, Hammer GD, Husebye ES, Merke DP, Murad MH, Stratakis CA, Torpy DJ. Diagnosis and treatment of primary adrenal insufficiency: an Endocrine Society clinical practice guideline. *J Clin Endocrinol Metab.* 2016;**101**(2):364–389.

20. Smeets EE, Span PN, van Herwaarden AE, Wevers RA, Hermus AR, Sweep FC, Claahsen-van der Grinten HL. Molecular characterization of testicular adrenal rest tumors in congenital adrenal hyperplasia: lesions with both adrenocortical and Leydig cell features. *J Clin Endocrinol Metab.* 2015;**100**(3):E524–E530.

21. Reisch N, Flade L, Scherr M, Rottenkolber M, Pedrosa Gil F, Bidlingmaier M, Wolff H, Schwarz HP, Quinkler M, Beuschlein F, Reincke M. High prevalence of reduced fecundity in men with congenital adrenal hyperplasia. *J Clin Endocrinol Metab.* 2009;**94**(5):1665–1670.

22. Engels M, Gehrmann K, Falhammar H, Webb EA, Nordenstrom A, Sweep FC, Span PN, van Heerwaarden AE, Rohayem J, Richter-Unruh A, Bouvattier C, Kohler B, Kormann BB, Arlt W, Roeleveld N, Reisch N, Stikkelbroeck NMML, Claahsen-van der Grinten HL; dsd-LIFE group. Gonadal function in adult male patients with congenital adrenal hyperplasia. *Eur J Endocrinol.* 2018;**178**(3):285–294.

23. Claahsen-van der Grinten HL, Sweep FC, Blickman JG, Hermus AR, Otten BJ. Prevalence of testicular adrenal rest tumours in male children with congenital adrenal hyperplasia due to 21-hydroxylase deficiency. *Eur J Endocrinol.* 2007;**157**(3):339–344.

24. Claahsen-van der Grinten HL, Otten BJ, Takahashi S, Meuleman EJ, Hulsbergen-van de Kaa C, Sweep FC, Hermus AR. Testicular adrenal rest tumors in adult males with congenital adrenal hyperplasia: evaluation of pituitary-gonadal function before and after successful testis-sparing surgery in eight patients. *J Clin Endocrinol Metab.* 2007;**92**(2):612–615.

25. Claahsen-van der Grinten HL, Otten BJ, Sweep FC, Hermus AR. Repeated successful induction of fertility after replacing hydrocortisone with dexamethasone in a patient with congenital adrenal hyperplasia and testicular adrenal rest tumors. *Fertil Steril.* 2007;**88**(3):705.e5–705.e8.

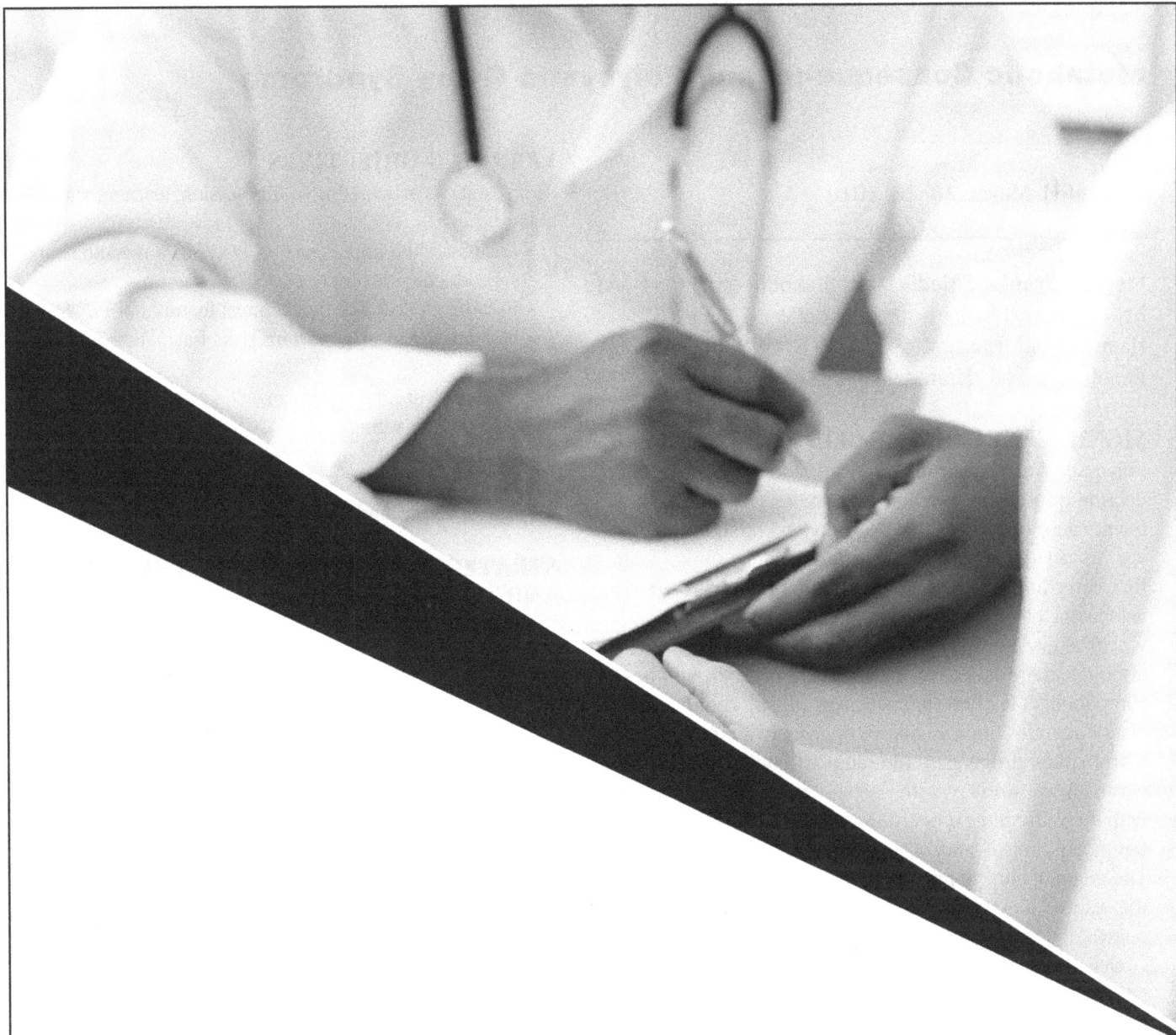

REPRODUCTIVE
ENDOCRINOLOGY

Metabolic Consequences of Polycystic Ovary Syndrome

M09
Presented, March 23–26, 2019

Stephen Franks, FMedSci. Institute of Reproductive and Developmental Biology, Imperial College London, Hammersmith Hospital, London W12 0NN, United Kingdom, E-mail: s.franks@imperial.ac.uk

SIGNIFICANCE OF THE CLINICAL PROBLEM

Polycystic ovary syndrome (PCOS) is the most common endocrine disorder in women. Not only is PCOS the most frequent cause of anovulatory infertility and hirsutism, but it is also associated with characteristic metabolic abnormalities that carry an increased risk in the longer term for the development of type 2 diabetes mellitus (T2DM) and cardiovascular disease (CVD). The etiology remains uncertain, although there is increasing evidence of a strong genetic component. It is a heterogeneous disorder and, although the classic manifestation is that of oligo/anovulation, together with hyperandrogenism, the range of clinical presentation varies from women with infrequent or absent menses without androgen excess to those who have regular cycles but have clinical and/or biochemical hyperandrogenism. The mode of clinical presentation of PCOS has a bearing on the risk of metabolic consequences, as will be discussed below.

Obesity is more prevalent in women with PCOS than in the general population and there is no doubt that there is an important interaction of obesity and PCOS that has a significant impact on metabolic dysfunction and the risk of both T2DM and CVD. The risk of obstructive sleep apnea may also be increased in obese women with the syndrome. The recent publication of the International Guideline for Management of PCOS (1) recognizes the importance of this interaction and informs recommendations on the management of PCOS, as will be discussed below.

BARRIERS TO OPTIMAL PRACTICE

- There is a need for consideration of ethnic variations in the risk of T2DM and CVD in women with PCOS and how that knowledge could—and should—affects strategies for investigation and management.
- Lack of long-term follow-up and longitudinal data for cardiovascular events in women with PCOS limits the effectiveness of screening, monitoring, and possible interventions.
- There are difficulties in implementing and sustaining effective measures for diet and lifestyle changes in overweight and obese women.

LEARNING OBJECTIVES

As a result of participating in this session, learners should be able to:

- Recognize the importance of PCOS as a metabolic and reproductive disorder
- Identify clinical and biochemical features of PCOS that indicate the most important risks for metabolic dysfunction
- Have a clear strategy for investigating metabolic disorders in women with PCOS
- Have a clear strategy for long-term monitoring of at-risk patients and, when appropriate, intervene to reduce the risk of T2DM and CVD

STRATEGIES FOR DIAGNOSIS, THERAPY, AND/OR MANAGEMENT

With the increasing prevalence of obesity in the population, there is concern over the negative effects of PCOS on metabolic and cardiovascular health. Of course, it is well known that obesity alone increases the risk of diabetes and CVD, but overweight and obesity have a more profound negative impact in women with PCOS—who are more likely to be insulin resistant—than in those without. Cross-sectional, clinic-based studies of women with PCOS suggest that 30% to 40% of young women with the disorder have impaired glucose tolerance (IGT) and an additional 5% to 10% have frank T2DM. Epidemiologic studies are likely to provide a more accurate reflection of the risk of IGT and T2DM in women with PCOS, and results suggest that there is an up to twofold increased risk in lean women with PCOS, but an alarming threefold to fivefold increased risk in obese women with PCOS compared with the appropriate reference population (2–5). Not surprisingly, the risk of gestational diabetes (GDM) is also increased (5). A recent prospective study of pregnancies in women with PCOS in The Netherlands reported a prevalence of GDM of 22% (6) against an expected background rate of <5% in the general population. The new international, evidence-based guideline for the assessment and management of PCOS (7) includes a clinical consensus recommendation that "Health professionals and women with PCOS should be aware that, regardless of age, the prevalence of gestational diabetes, impaired glucose tolerance and type 2 diabetes (fivefold in Asia, fourfold in the Americas, and threefold in Europe) are significantly increased in PCOS, with risk independent of, yet exacerbated by, obesity" (7). In terms of monitoring and management, it is recommended that glycemic status be assessed at diagnosis in all women with PCOS and thereafter every 1 to 3 years, depending the presence of other risk factors for GDM or T2DM. An oral glucose tolerance test is recommended if such risk factors exist—for example, family history, obesity, or previous GDM—and for all women planning a pregnancy.

Effects of PCOS on cardiovascular health are less clear cut. Biochemical risk factors for heart disease, including dyslipidemia (8) and elevated concentrations of inflammatory markers (2, 9), have been widely reported. In addition, other surrogate markers of cardiovascular dysfunction, such as impaired indices of endothelial function (10, 11), are abnormal and point to an increased risk of coronary heart disease and stroke. Even so, no study to date has convincingly demonstrated that there is a greater risk of cardiovascular events in women with PCOS, even in obese patients. This may simply reflect the fact that CVD in young or middle-aged women is uncommon and that we lack longitudinal studies of women with PCOS into the postmenopausal years. It is also possible that there are as-yet-unidentified protective factors that compensate for the apparently adverse cardiovascular risk profile. Nevertheless, it seems wise to counsel strategies for intervention in women with PCOS and additional risk factors, such as obesity and abnormal lipid profile—in particular, lower-than-normal serum levels of high-density lipoprotein cholesterol. Indeed, the new guideline recommends that body mass index should be monitored at each clinic visit—or a minimum of every 12 months—and that the presence of other important risk factors for CVD, including lack of exercise, cigarette smoking, dyslipidemia, hypertension, IGT, and ethnicity, should be considered in the determination of the frequency and intensity of follow-up.

It is helpful to consider which patients with PCOS are at an increased risk of metabolic disease and CVD. Among the varied phenotypes defined by the Rotterdam diagnostic criteria, it is those women with the classic presentation of PCOS as defined by the experts' meeting at the National Institutes of Health in 1990—that is, those with both oligomenorrhea and hyperandrogenism—who are most at risk. Insulin resistance and other metabolic abnormalities seem to be fewer in those women with androgen excess and regular cycles or those with anovulation and normal androgens (12, 13); however, it is important to bear in mind that the clinical presentation may change within an individual. For example, weight gain in a woman with hyperandrogenism but regular menses may then lead to irregular periods and, at the same time, an increase in metabolic risk factors.

What then should be the optimum management of women with PCOS for the prevention of or reduction of T2DM and CVD risk (14)? First, it is important to identify those who are most at risk—that is, those with both menstrual disorders and hyperandrogenism (clinical and/or biochemical) who are overweight or obese. A positive family history of T2DM adds to the risk. As stated in the recent guideline, screening should include an oral glucose tolerance test or at least fasting glucose measurement together with HbA$_{1c}$. There is no firm evidence to inform how often an oral glucose tolerance test should be repeated, but assessment every 6 to 12 months for those who are at highest risk of IGT—that is, obese with a positive family history—seems to be sensible and is in line with the guideline's recommendations. For those at risk but

without overt IGT or T2DM, diet and lifestyle changes have been shown not only to reduce metabolic risk factors but also to improve rates of ovulation and fertility. The international guideline includes important clinical practice points for patient-centered advice on lifestyle and emphasizing that a healthy lifestyle can contribute positively to health and wellbeing even in the absence of weight loss. There is no evidence that any specific, energy-equivalent, calorie-restricted diet is better than another (7).

In women who already have IGT or T2DM, lifestyle changes may also be effective, but there is an increased likelihood of the requirement for medication. Metformin has been used extensively in women with PCOS and often as a first-line treatment of symptoms of anovulation or androgen excess. However, although metformin may have a minor benefit in improving menstrual regularity, it is neither an effective fertility drug, nor a useful treatment of hirsutism. It does, however, have proven efficacy in reducing the rate of conversion from IGT to T2DM (15) and is therefore important in women with PCOS and IGT who have not responded well to modulation of diet and lifestyle. Orlistat is the only drug in the United Kingdom to be licensed for weight loss, but there are promising studies in progress to examine the efficacy of GLP-1 agonists as weight loss therapy. There is emerging evidence that bariatric surgery is an effective treatment for both fertility and metabolic improvement in women with PCOS and morbid obesity, but this treatment is not universally available, is expensive, and is not without significant adverse effects that may themselves affect long-term health.

MAIN CONCLUSIONS

In summary, PCOS is a common endocrine disorder with a well-known impact on ovarian function, but it is not just a reproductive disorder. Women with PCOS are at an increased risk of diabetes and, potentially, heart disease. Therefore, it is important to recognize as early as possible—and that may be in the teenage years—those who are particularly prone to problems with long-term health. It is also important to recognize those patients who are most at risk and institute an individualized program of regular monitoring, lifestyle advice, and, when necessary, therapeutic intervention to prevent complications or treat established disease.

CASES
Case 1
A patient (J.D.), age 32 years and of European ancestry, was diagnosed with PCOS at age 17 when she presented with irregular menses and bad acne. The patient had a body mass index (BMI) of 24, LH of 15 U/L (4–13), an FSH of 6 U/L (4–11), and total testosterone of 3.5 nmol/L (0.5 to 3.0). Pelvic ultrasound (transabdominal) demonstrated enlarged ovaries and multiple follicles. The patient has a family history of T2DM (paternal grandfather). The patient was treated with combined oral contraceptive (COC) with good control of symptoms. She re-presented at age 26, hoping to conceive. Symptoms remain well controlled on COC, and her BMI is 32.

1. Was the original diagnosis correct?
2. What tests should she undergo?
3. How should she be managed in the short term and for long-term health?

Discussion

The original diagnosis was probably correct because although irregular menses, acne, and multiple ovarian follicles are commonplace—and not diagnostic—in teenagers, the abnormal endocrine profile and consequent development of symptoms support the diagnosis. The patient should undergo repeat endocrine and metabolic testing and will need careful monitoring during pregnancy and beyond because of PCOS and additional risk factors (obesity and a family history of T2DM).

A1. Yes.

A2. Repeat endocrine tests as well as oral glucose tolerance test and that for lipids and lipoproteins.

A3. Observe the patient's menstrual pattern after stopping COC, provide diet and lifestyle advice, consider the induction of ovulation if not ovulating, and carefully monitor pregnancy. Consider the long-term risk of T2DM and CVD, and provide regular assessment.

Case 2

A patient (A.R.), age 40 years and of South Asian ancestry, was diagnosed with PCOS at age 27 when she presented with a delay in conceiving and oligomenorrhea but no symptoms or biochemical evidence of androgen excess. Her BMI was 23. A pelvic ultrasound showed multiple follicles and enlarged ovaries. Her LH was 16 and FSH was 5 U/L. The patient achieved successful induction of ovulation and normal singleton pregnancy after clomiphene treatment. She has a family history of premature CVD (her father had coronary heart disease at age 50), and her lipid profile showed slightly raised serum cholesterol and slightly low high-density lipoprotein 2C.

The patient re-presented at age 38. She had another child (age 5 years) after spontaneous ovulation and her family is completed. The patient now complains of oligomenorrhea but also facial hirsutism. She has gained weight gain since her last pregnancy. Her BMI is 28, LH is 18 U/L, FSH is 5 U/L, and testosterone is 3.5 nmol/L. The patient has been referred for dietary advice.

1. Is she at risk for metabolic dysfunction and long term-health problems?
2. What additional tests should be considered?
3. Is it reasonable to prescribe combined oral contraceptive to control her symptoms?
4. How would you monitor her progress?

Discussion

Weight gain, high BMI (South Asian origin puts her at a greater relative risk of metabolic dysfunction), dyslipidemia (although originally mild), and family history of CVD put her at high risk of long-term complications. COC is not ideal treatment but not contraindicated. There is no clear evidence that any one particular type of COC is better than another. Metabolic tests, dietary advice, and long-term monitoring should be implemented.

A1. Yes, she is at risk for both—overweight, family history of heart disease, South Asian origin, abnormal lipid profile

A2. Fasting lipids and lipoproteins, fasting glucose/ HbA_{1c} or oral glucose tolerance test

A3. COC is not ideal but would provide control of symptoms and is relatively safe if the patient is nonsmoker with no history of thromboembolic episodes; there is little evidence that COC would significantly worsen an adverse metabolic profile

A4. Regular measurement of (6 to 12 months) weight, blood pressure, fasting glucose, and lipids

References

1. Monash University. PCOS program: guideline. Available at: https://www.monash.edu/__data/assets/pdf_file/0004/1412644/PCOS_Evidence-Based-Guidelines_20181009.pdf. Accessed September 2018.
2. Ollila MM, West S, Keinänen-Kiukaanniemi S, Jokelainen J, Auvinen J, Puukka K, Ruokonen A, Järvelin MR, Tapanainen JS, Franks S, Piltonen TT, Morin-Papunen LC. Overweight and obese but not normal weight women with PCOS are at increased risk of type 2 diabetes mellitus-a prospective, population-based cohort study. *Hum Reprod.* 2017; **32**(2):423–431.
3. Wild S, Pierpoint T, McKeigue P, Jacobs H. Cardiovascular disease in women with polycystic ovary syndrome at long-term follow-up: a retrospective cohort study. *Clin Endocrinol (Oxf).* 2000;**52**(5): 595–600.
4. Solomon CG, Hu FB, Dunaif A, Rich-Edwards JE, Stampfer MJ, Willett WC, Speizer FE, Manson JE. Menstrual cycle irregularity and risk for future cardiovascular disease. *J Clin Endocrinol Metab.* 2002;**87**(5): 2013–2017.
5. Joham AE, Ranasinha S, Zoungas S, Moran L, Teede HJ. Gestational diabetes and type 2 diabetes in reproductive-aged women with polycystic ovary syndrome. *J Clin Endocrinol Metab.* 2014;**99**(3):E447–E452.
6. de Wilde MA, Veltman-Verhulst SM, Goverde AJ, Lambalk CB, Laven JS, Franx A, Koster MP, Eijkemans MJ, Fauser BC. Preconception predictors of gestational diabetes: a multicentre prospective cohort study on the predominant complication of pregnancy in polycystic ovary syndrome. *Hum Reprod.* 2014;**29**(6):1327–1336.
7. Teede HJ, Misso ML, Costello MF, Dokras A, Laven J, Moran L, Piltonen T, Norman RJ, for the International PCOS Network. Recommendations from the international evidence-based guideline for the assessment and management of polycystic ovary syndrome. *Clin Endocrinol (Oxf).* 2018;**89**(3):251–268.
8. Couto Alves A, Valcarcel B, Mäkinen VP, Morin-Papunen L, Sebert S, Kangas AJ, Soininen P, Das S, De Iorio M, Coin L, Ala-Korpela M, Järvelin MR, Franks S. Metabolic profiling of polycystic ovary syndrome reveals interactions with abdominal obesity. *Int J Obes.* 2017; **41**(9):1331–1340.
9. Escobar-Morreale HF, Luque-Ramirez M, Gonzalez F. Circulating inflammatory markers in polycystic ovary syndrome: a systematic review and metaanalysis. *Fertil Steril.* 2011;**95**(3):1048-1058.e1-2.
10. Talbott EO, Zborowski JV, Boudreaux MY, McHugh-Pemu KP, Sutton-Tyrrell K, Guzick DS. The relationship between C-reactive protein and carotid intima-media wall thickness in middle-aged women with polycystic ovary syndrome. *J Clin Endocrinol Metab.* 2004;**89**(12): 6061–6067.
11. Sorensen MB, Franks S, Robertson C, Pennell DJ, Collins P. Severe endothelial dysfunction in young women with polycystic ovary syndrome is only partially explained by known cardiovascular risk factors. *Clin Endocrinol (Oxf).* 2006;**65**(5):655–659.

12. Barber TM, Wass JA, McCarthy MI, Franks S. Metabolic characteristics of women with polycystic ovaries and oligo-amenorrhoea but normal androgen levels: implications for the management of polycystic ovary syndrome. *Clin Endocrinol (Oxf)*. 2007;**66**(4):513–517.

13. Moghetti P, Tosi F, Bonin C, Di Sarra D, Fiers T, Kaufman JM, Giagulli VA, Signori C, Zambotti F, Dall'Alda M, Spiazzi G, Zanolin ME, Bonora E. Divergences in insulin resistance between the different phenotypes of the polycystic ovary syndrome. *J Clin Endocrinol Metab*. 2013;**98**(4): E628–E637.

14. Moran LJ, Norman RJ, Teede HJ. Metabolic risk in PCOS: phenotype and adiposity impact. *Trends Endocrinol Metab*. 2015;**26**(3):136–143.

15. Diabetes Prevention Program Research Group. Reduction in the incidence of type 2 diabetes with lifestyle intervention or metformin. *N Engl J Med*. 2002;**346**:393–403.

What Endocrinologists Really Need to Know About Polycystic Ovary Syndrome

M12
Presented, March 23–26, 2019

Andrea Dunaif, MD. Division of Endocrinology, Diabetes and Bone Disease, Mount Sinai Hospital System, New York, New York 10029, E-mail: andrea.dunaif@mssm.edu

SIGNIFICANCE OF THE CLINICAL PROBLEM

Polycystic ovary syndrome (PCOS) is an exceptionally common disorder that affects 5% to 15% of reproductive-age women worldwide, depending on the diagnostic criteria applied (1). It is the leading cause of hirsutism, oligoamenorrhea, and anovulatory infertility (2–4). PCOS is also a major metabolic disorder due to its frequent association with insulin resistance (1). Affected women have an approximately fourfold increased risk for type 2 diabetes (T2D) as well as for other disorders associated with insulin resistance, such as metabolic syndrome and nonalcoholic fatty liver disease (1, 5, 6). There is an increased prevalence of obesity in PCOS that exacerbates both the metabolic and the reproductive morbidities of the syndrome (1). Finally, anxiety and depression are increased in women with PCOS (7).

The specific etiologies of PCOS remain unknown; however, it is a highly heritable, complex genetic disease (8). The three major diagnostic criteria—National Institutes of Health (NIH) (9), Rotterdam (10, 11), and Androgen Excess Society (AES) (12)—are based on expert opinion rather than on pathophysiologic understanding. The original NIH diagnostic criteria require the presence of hyperandrogenism (HA) and ovulatory dysfunction (OD). The Rotterdam criteria added polycystic ovarian morphology (PCOM) and require the presence of at least two of the three key reproductive traits resulting in three affected phenotypes: HA and OD with or without PCOM (also known as NIH PCOS) and non-NIH Rotterdam phenotypes HA and PCOM and OD and PCOM. The AES criteria require the presence of HA, reducing the number of phenotypes to two (HA and OD with or without PCOM and HA and PCOM) (12).

Almost 20 genetic susceptibility loci have been reproducibly mapped for PCOS in genome-wide association studies in European and Han Chinese case-control cohorts, many of which are shared between these ethnic groups (8). Biologic pathways implicated include gonadotropin secretion and action, androgen biosynthesis, and metabolic homeostasis (13–16). Male as well as female relatives have reproductive and metabolic features of the syndrome consistent with genetic susceptibility to these phenotypes (1). However, a recent meta-analysis (16) found that only one of 14 PCOS susceptibility loci was significantly more strongly associated with the NIH compared with the Rotterdam diagnostic criteria or self-reported PCOS. There

was no difference in the association between the other 13 PCOS susceptibility loci and the NIH PCOS, non-NIH Rotterdam PCOS, or self-reported PCOS. These findings suggest that the genetic architecture of the phenotypes defined by the various PCOS diagnostic criteria is generally similar (16).

BARRIERS TO OPTIMAL PRACTICE

Women with PCOS see on average four physicians before diagnosis and are highly dissatisfied with their medical care (17, 18). The difficulty in physician diagnosis of PCOS implies that diagnostic criteria are poorly disseminated, difficult to use, and/or poorly understood (19). Survey findings suggest that endocrinologists use the NIH diagnostic criteria more frequently than the Rotterdam diagnostic criteria (20). The syndrome itself is incorrectly named because the structures in the ovary are follicles and not cysts. The expert panel from the 2012 NIH evidence-based methodology workshop on PCOS noted that the name PCOS "is a distraction and an impediment to progress" (21).

There are evidence-based guidelines for the diagnosis and management of PCOS, such as those published in 2013 by the Endocrine Society (3) and the 2018 international evidence-based guideline (22, 23). However, the quality of the evidence upon which these guidelines are based is predominantly low due to a paucity of randomized clinical trials. Of the 34 recommendations in the Endocrine Society clinical practice guideline (3), the evidence supporting 24 of these was rated as low or very low. There were almost 175 recommendations in the international guideline (22, 23) of which only 31 were ranked as evidence based; the remainder were clinical consensus recommendations or clinical practice points.

LEARNING OBJECTIVES

As a result of participating in this session, learners should be able to:
- Describe the endocrine pathophysiology of PCOS
- Assess critically the diagnostic criteria for PCOS
- Review management of endocrine and metabolic features of PCOS

STRATEGIES FOR DIAGNOSIS, THERAPY, AND/OR MANAGEMENT

Monitoring of ovarian morphology is an essential component of assisted reproductive technologies. However, there is no evidence that the presence or absence of PCOM has any implications with regard to endocrine or metabolic features of PCOS (3, 24). Furthermore, there is no evidence to support the addition of assessment of PCOM to the diagnosis of NIH phenotype PCOS (22, 23). Indeed, the international evidence-based guidelines (22, 23) state that ovarian ultrasound is not needed for the diagnosis of PCOS in women with HA and OD (*i.e.*, NIH PCOS). Similarly, the recently updated Endocrine Society guideline on hirsutism (4) states that demonstrating PCOM to diagnose ovulatory PCOS is unlikely to affect management of hirsutism. Of note, there is expert consensus that the NIH criteria define the phenotype that is at greatest metabolic risk (25). In summary, the management of the endocrine and metabolic features of PCOS does not require the assessment of ovarian morphology. The PCOS genome-wide association study meta-analysis (16) supports this conclusion because no differences in genetic architecture, except for one locus more strongly associated with NIH PCOS, were present when the NIH PCOS, non-NIH Rotterdam PCOS, and PCOS by self-report cohorts were compared (16).

MAIN CONCLUSIONS

Characterization of chronic oligoanovulation, HA, and metabolic status are sufficient for the endocrine and metabolic management of PCOS. There is no need to assess ovarian morphology to diagnose PCOS when HA and chronic anovulation are present (22, 23). Similarly, assessment of ovarian morphology is not needed to managed HA symptoms such as hirsutism (4). The most recent genetic evidence supports this approach (16). Specific therapies are directed at patient concerns because there is no therapeutic intervention to reverse PCOS.

CASE 1

G.B. is a 23-year-old graduate student who presents for the evaluation of oligomenorrhea and inability to lose weight. She experienced menarche at age 14 years and subsequently has had two to three menstrual bleeds annually. She has a few terminal hairs on her chin that she removes with waxing every 2 weeks. She began to gain weight around the time of menarche and her weight increased by 50 lb during her first year of college. She takes three aerobics classes per week and follows the Weight Watchers® diet. Nevertheless, the patient reports that she is unable to lose weight. She denies binging and purging. She was evaluated by her gynecologist for these problems several years ago and was told that she should lose weight. No further evaluation was performed. She has no signs or symptoms of other endocrinopathies.

G.B. is of Dutch and Irish ancestry. Her mother is 50 years old with no known medical problems, but she had difficulty conceiving. Her father is 60 years old, is overweight, and has T2D. There is a 15-year-old sister who experienced menarche at age 13 years and currently has about six menstrual periods per year. She is obese and also has difficulty losing weight. The patient has a 25-year-old brother who is overweight but otherwise healthy.

Physical Examination

G.B.'s blood pressure (BP) was 130/85 mm Hg; pulse, 82/min; body mass index, 33.8 kg/m^2; and waist circumference, 90 cm.

She has normal habitus. There is stubble on her chin from waxing and moderate acanthosis nigricans with skin tags on her neck and in her axillae. Her examination is otherwise normal.

Laboratory Evaluation

The patient's urine pregnancy test was negative. Her other laboratory test findings were as follows: testosterone, 56 ng/dL (<58 ng/dL) [1.93 nmol/L (<2.01)]; sex hormone–binding globulin, 40.1 nmol/L (24.6 to 122.0 nmol/L); bioavailable testosterone, 21 ng/dL (<16 ng/dL) [0.73 nmol/L (<0.56 nmol/L)]; dehydroepiandrosterone sulfate (DHEAS), 350 µg/dL (<263 µg/dL) [9.49 µmol/L (<7.13 µmol/L)]; 17-hydroxy-progesterone (17-OHP), 175 ng/dL (<200 ng/dL) [5.30 nmol/L (<6.06 nmol/L)] at 0800 hours; prolactin, 20 ng/mL (<25 ng/mL) [0.87 nmol/L (<1.09 nmol/L)]; thyrotropin (TSH) 2.0 mIU/L (0.4 to 4.5 mIU/L); and follicle-stimulating hormone (FSH), 3.0 mIU/mL (<40 mIU/mL).

1. What additional testing would you perform to determine her diagnosis?
   A. Androstenedione level
   B. Ovarian ultrasound
   C. Luteinizing hormone (LH) level
   D. None

Answer

D is correct. The patient fulfills all three diagnostic criteria for PCOS, NIH, Rotterdam, and AES, because of the presence of HA, both clinical, hirsutism, and biochemical, elevated bioavailable testosterone and DHEAS levels, as well as chronic anovulation indicated by oligomenorrhea. Other disorders have been excluded with normal TSH, prolactin, and 17-OHP levels. There is no need for additional androgen testing [*e.g.*, androstenedione (A)]. An ovarian ultrasound (B) is not needed for the diagnosis. In the United States, these studies often are not interpreted according to criteria for PCOM. Although increased LH levels relative to FSH levels are a common feature of PCOS, LH levels are not part of any diagnostic criteria for PCOS. FSH levels can be measured to assess for primary ovarian damage.

2. A hemoglobin A$_{1c}$ level is 5.4% (35.5 mmol/mol) and a fasting glucose 95 mg/dL (<100 mg/dL) [5.83 mmol/L (<5.55 mmol/L)]. Would you perform additional metabolic testing?
   A. Yes
   B. No

Answer

A is correct. Women with PCOS have an ~40% decrease in insulin-mediated glucose uptake independent of obesity, whereas increased hepatic glucose production is seen only in affected obese women (1). As a consequence, impaired glucose tolerance rather than fasting dysglycemia is the major defect in glucose homeostasis in PCOS (26, 27). In the United

States, ~40% of women have PCOS glucose intolerance (30% with impaired glucose tolerance and ~10% T2D). Prevalence rates of glucose tolerance are lower in Europe. Obesity and a family history of diabetes, both of which G.B. has, increase the risk for T2D. Lipid and lipoprotein levels also should be assessed in PCOS because low high-density lipoprotein (HDL) and elevated triglyceride levels are common, as are modestly elevated low-density lipoprotein (LDL) levels (5). Finally, elevated aspartate aminotransferase and alanine aminotransferase, which suggest the presence of nonalcoholic fatty liver disease, can be a feature of PCOS, although the utility of routine screening has not been established (28).

Additional Test Results

The patient's 2-hour post–75-g oral glucose challenge level was 180 mg/dL (<140 mg/dL) [9.99 mmol/L (<7.77 mmol/L)]. Other test results were as follows: cholesterol, 210 mg/dL (<200 mg/dL) [5.44 mmol/L (<5.18 mmol/L)]; LDL, 110 mg/dL (<100 mg/dL) [2.85 mmol/L (<2.59 mmol/L)]; HDL, 40 mg/dL (≥50 mg/dL) [1.04 mmol/L (<1.30 mmol/L)]; triglycerides, 500 mg/dL (<150 mg/dL) [2.26 mmol/L (<1.70 mmol/L)]; aspartate aminotransferase, 76 IU/L (<40 IU/L); and alanine aminotransferase, 88 IU/L (<32 IU/L).

3. What therapy or therapies would you recommend?
A. Combined oral contraceptive pill (COCP)
B. Metformin
C. Lifestyle and moderate exercise
D. Pioglitazone

Answer

B and C are correct. As little as a 5% reduction of body weight can result in improvements in testosterone levels and resumption of ovulatory menses in women with PCOS (29). The patient has impaired glucose tolerance and fulfills criteria for metabolic syndrome (30). There are no studies of diabetes prevention in women with PCOS; however, the Diabetes Prevention Program lifestyle intervention produced the greatest decrease in risk of progression to T2D (58%) as well as substantial reversal of metabolic syndrome in individuals with prediabetes (31). Metformin also reduced the incidence of T2D (31%) and metabolic syndrome in the Diabetes Prevention Program (31). Meta-analyses have indicated that metformin improves menstrual frequency and slightly decreases fasting glucose, LDL levels, and systolic BP in PCOS (32, 33).

The patient has relative contraindications to COCP because she is obese, has impaired glucose tolerance, and has elevated triglyceride levels. Pioglitazone is a possibility, but there are concerns about using thiazolidinediones in reproductive-age women because of weight gain, potential effects on bone density, and safety during pregnancy.

4. What additional therapy is needed if the patient does not have regular menses with your therapeutic intervention?
A. Intermittent progestin-induced withdrawal bleeding
B. Progestin intrauterine device (IUD)

C. COCP
D. Any of the above

Answer

D is correct. The patient has chronic anovulation and is at risk for endometrial hyperplasia/neoplasia (22, 23). Endometrial protection can be achieved with intermittent progestin-induced withdrawal bleeding, progestin IUDs, or COCP. As discussed in question 3, COCP is relatively contraindicated in this patient.

CASE 2

D.D. is a 26-year-old fashion magazine editor who presents for evaluation of hirsutism, acne, and alopecia. She has had irregular menses since menarche at age 14 years, with cycle lengths of 3 to 6 months. She had severe acne as an adolescent and had a course of Accutane (Roche, Basel, Switzerland) at that time. She began to note increasing terminal hair growth on her chin and sideburn area during college and progressive hair thinning of the frontal and vertex scalp. She also has had recurrent acne lesions. Her dermatologist started her on oral spironolactone 50 mg once daily. She has never had hormonal testing, but her gynecologist sent her for an ovarian ultrasound examination.

She has always been slender. She is Italian ancestry. Her mother and maternal aunt have hair thinning; a maternal cousin has hirsutism and was diagnosed recently with PCOS.

Physical Examination

D.D.'s BP was 115/70 mm Hg; pulse, 84/min, body mass index, 22.6 kg/m², and waist circumference, 80 cm. She had normal habitus. There is frontal and vertex hair thinning with the hairline preserved. Increased terminal hair exists in the sideburn, chin, and presacral areas, there are moderately severe acne lesions on her face and upper back. There is no acanthosis nigricans. The rest of the examination was normal.

Laboratory Evaluation

The patient's laboratory findings were as follows: testosterone, 72 ng/dL (<58 ng/dL) [2.50 nmol/L (<2.01 nmol/L)]; sex hormone-binding globulin, 71.3 nmol/L (24.6 to 122.0 nmol/L); bioavailable testosterone, 18 ng/dL (<16 ng/dL) [0.62 nmol/L (<0.56 nmol/L)]; DHEAS, 245 μg/dL (<263 μg/dL) [6.64 μmol/L (<7.13 μmol/L)]; 17-OHP, 175 ng/dL (<200 ng/dL) at 0800 hours; prolactin, 20 ng/mL (<25 ng/mL) [0.87 nmol/L (<1.09 nmol/L)]; and TSH, 2.0 mIU/L (0.4 to 4.5 mIU/L).

1. What additional testing would you perform to determine her diagnosis?
A. Androstenedione level
B. Ovarian ultrasound
C. LH level
D. None

Answer

D is correct. Analogous to case 2, the diagnosis of PCOS can be made in this patient by NIH, Rotterdam, and AES criteria by the presence of HA, both clinical, hirsutism, acne and alopecia, and biochemical, elevated total and bioavailable testosterone levels, as well as chronic anovulation indicated by oligomenorrhea.

2. A fasting glucose is 80 mg/dL ($<$100 mg/dL) [4.44 mmol/L ($<$5.56 mmol/L)]. Would you perform additional metabolic testing?
   A. Yes
   B. No

Answer

Either A or B is reasonable. Although nonobese women with PCOS can be insulin resistant and at increased risk for T2D, the prevalence rates of glucose tolerance are low (26, 27). Similarly, the risk for dyslipidemia is low in the absence of obesity.

Additional Test Results

The patient's 2-hour post–75-g oral glucose challenge glucose level was 120 mg/dL ($<$140 mg/dL) [6.66 mmol/L ($<$7.77)]. Other test results were as follows: cholesterol, 180 mg/dL ($<$200 mg/dL) [4.66 mmol/L ($<$5.18 mmol/L)]; LDL, 95 mg/dL ($<$100 mg/dL) [2.46 mmol/L ($<$2.59 mmol/L)]; HDL, 60 mg/dL ($\geq$50 mg/dL) [1.55 mmol/L ($<$1.30 mmol/L]; and triglycerides, 88 mg/dL ($<$150 mg/dL) [0.99 mmol/L ($<$1.70 mmol/L)].

3. What therapy or therapies would you recommend?
   A. COCP
   B. Metformin
   C. COCP with antiandrogen
   D. Topical minoxidil

Answer

A, C, and D are correct. COCP alone or in combination with an antiandrogen is an appropriate first-line therapy for androgenic symptoms. If symptoms are severe, it is reasonable to begin with the combination of COCP and antiandrogen. In the United States, the antiandrogen of choice is spironolactone; there are no Food and Drug Administration–approved antiandrogens for the treatment of hirsutism, acne, or alopecia in women. Adequate contraception during antiandrogen treatment is preferred, usually with COCP, because antiandrogens cross the placenta and interfere with the virilization of a male fetus. There is also additive beneficial effects of COCP and antiandrogens. Minoxidil alone or in combination with hormonal therapies is an appropriate therapy for androgenetic alopecia.

4. Would your therapy change if she was a 37-year-old smoker?
   A. Yes
   B. No

Answer

A is correct. COCPs are contraindicated in women 35 years of age and older who are also smokers. In this setting, contraception can be provided with an IUD, and antiandrogen therapy can be continued. The additive beneficial effect of COCP on androgenic symptoms will be lost.

References

1. Diamanti-Kandarakis E, Dunaif A. Insulin resistance and the polycystic ovary syndrome revisited: an update on mechanisms and implications. *Endocr Rev.* 2012;**33**(6):981–1030.
2. Paparodis R, Dunaif A. The Hirsute woman: challenges in evaluation and management. *Endocr Pract.* 2011;**17**(5):807–818.
3. Legro RS, Arslanian SA, Ehrmann DA, Hoeger KM, Murad MH, Pasquali R, Welt CK, for the Endocrine Society. Diagnosis and treatment of polycystic ovary syndrome: an Endocrine Society clinical practice guideline. *J Clin Endocrinol Metab.* 2013;**98**(12):4565–4592.
4. Martin KA, Anderson RR, Chang RJ, Ehrmann DA, Lobo RA, Murad MH, Pugeat MM, Rosenfield RL. Evaluation and treatment of hirsutism in premenopausal women: an Endocrine Society Clinical Practice Guideline. *J Clin Endocrinol Metab.* 2018;**103**(4):1233–1257.
5. Randeva HS, Tan BK, Weickert MO, Lois K, Nestler JE, Sattar N, Lehnert H. Cardiometabolic aspects of the polycystic ovary syndrome. *Endocr Rev.* 2012;**33**(5):812–841.
6. Rubin KH, Glintborg D, Nybo M, Abrahamsen B, Andersen M. Development and risk factors of type 2 diabetes in a nationwide population of women with polycystic ovary syndrome. *J Clin Endocrinol Metab.* 2017;**102**(10):3848–3857.
7. Dokras A. Mood and anxiety disorders in women with PCOS. *Steroids.* 2012;**77**(4):338–341.
8. Dunaif A. Perspectives in polycystic ovary syndrome: from hair to eternity. *J Clin Endocrinol Metab.* 2016;**101**(3):759–768.
9. Zawadzki JK, Dunaif A. Diagnostic criteria for polycystic ovary syndrome; towards a rational approach. In: Dunaif A, Givens JR, Haseltine F, Merriam G, eds. *Polycystic Ovary Syndrome.* Boston, MA: Blackwell Scientific; 1992:377–384.
10. Rotterdam ESHRE/ASRM-Sponsored PCOS Consensus Workshop Group. Revised 2003 consensus on diagnostic criteria and long-term health risks related to polycystic ovary syndrome (PCOS). *Hum Reprod.* 2004;**19**(1):41–47.
11. Rotterdam ESHRE ASRM-Sponsored PCOS Consensus Workshop Group. Revised 2003 consensus on diagnostic criteria and long-term health risks related to polycystic ovary syndrome. *Fertil Steril.* 2004;**81**(1):19–25.
12. Azziz R, Carmina E, Dewailly D, Diamanti-Kandarakis E, Escobar-Morreale HF, Futterweit W, Janssen OE, Legro RS, Norman RJ, Taylor AE, Witchel SF, for the Androgen Excess Society. Positions statement: criteria for defining polycystic ovary syndrome as a predominantly hyperandrogenic syndrome: an Androgen Excess Society guideline. *J Clin Endocrinol Metab.* 2006;**91**(11):4237–4245.
13. Shi Y, Zhao H, Shi Y, Cao Y, Yang D, Li Z, Zhang B, Liang X, Li T, Chen J, Shen J, Zhao J, You L, Gao X, Zhu D, Zhao X, Yan Y, Qin Y, Li W, Yan J, Wang Q, Zhao J, Geng L, Ma J, Zhao Y, He G, Zhang A, Zou S, Yang A, Liu J, Li W, Li B, Wan C, Qin Y, Shi J, Yang J, Jiang H, Xu JE, Qi X, Sun Y, Zhang Y, Hao C, Ju X, Zhao D, Ren CE, Li X, Zhang W, Zhang Y, Zhang J, Wu D, Zhang C, He L, Chen ZJ. Genome-wide association study identifies eight new risk loci for polycystic ovary syndrome. *Nat Genet.* 2012;**44**(9):1020–1025.
14. Hayes MG, Urbanek M, Ehrmann DA, Armstrong LL, Lee JY, Sisk R, Karaderi T, Barber TM, McCarthy MI, Franks S, Lindgren CM, Welt CK, Diamanti-Kandarakis E, Panidis D, Goodarzi MO, Azziz R, Zhang Y, James RG, Olivier M, Kissebah AH, Stener-Victorin E, Legro RS, Dunaif A, for the Reproductive Medicine Network. Genome-wide association of polycystic ovary syndrome implicates alterations in gonadotropin secretion in European ancestry populations [published correction appears in *Nat Commun.* 2016;**7**:10762]. *Nat Commun.* 2015;**6**(1):7502.

15. Day FR, Hinds DA, Tung JY, Stolk L, Styrkarsdottir U, Saxena R, Bjonnes A, Broer L, Dunger DB, Halldorsson BV, Lawlor DA, Laval G, Mathieson I, McCardle WL, Louwers Y, Meun C, Ring S, Scott RA, Sulem P, Uitterlinden AG, Wareham NJ, Thorsteinsdottir U, Welt C, Stefansson K, Laven JS, Ong KK, Perry JR. Causal mechanisms and balancing selection inferred from genetic associations with polycystic ovary syndrome. *Nat Commun.* 2015;**6**(1):8464.

16. Day F, Karaderi T, Jones MR, Meun C, He C, Drong A, Kraft P, Lin N, Huang H, Broer L, Magi R, Saxena R, Laisk-Podar T, Urbanek M, Hayes GM, Thorleifsson G, Fernandez-Tajes J, Mahajan A, Mullin BH, Stuckey BGA, Spector TD, Wilson SG, Goodarzi MO, Davis L, Obermeyer-Pietsch B, Uitterlinden AG, Anttila V, Neale BM, Jarvelin M-R, Fauser B, Kowalska I, Visser JA, Anderson M, Ong K, Stener-Victorin E, Ehrmann D, Legro RS, Salumets A, McCarthy MI, Morin-Papunen L, Thorsteinsdottir U, Stefansson K, Styrkarsdottir U, Perry J, Dunaif A, Laven JSE, Franks S, Lindgren CM, Welt CK. Large-scale genome-wide meta-analysis of polycystic ovary syndrome suggests shared genetic architecture for different diagnosis criteria. *PLoS Genet.* 2018;**14**(12): e1007813.

17. Gibson-Helm M, Teede H, Dunaif A, Dokras A. Delayed diagnosis and a lack of information associated with dissatisfaction in women with polycystic ovary syndrome. *J Clin Endocrinol Metab.* 2017;**102**(2): 604–612.

18. Lin AW, Bergomi EJ, Dollahite JS, Sobal J, Hoeger KM, Lujan ME. Trust in physicians and medical experience beliefs differ between women with and without polycystic ovary syndrome. *J Endocr Soc.* 2018;**2**(9): 1001–1009.

19. March WA, Moore VM, Willson KJ, Phillips DIW, Norman RJ, Davies MJ. The prevalence of polycystic ovary syndrome in a community sample assessed under contrasting diagnostic criteria. *Hum Reprod.* 2010;**25**(2):544–551.

20. Conway G, Dewailly D, Diamanti-Kandarakis E, Escobar-Morreale HF, Franks S, Gambineri A, Kelestimur F, Macut D, Micic D, Pasquali R, Pfeifer M, Pignatelli D, Pugeat M, Yildiz B, for the ESE PCOS Special Interest Group. European survey of diagnosis and management of the polycystic ovary syndrome: results of the ESE PCOS Special Interest Group's questionnaire. *Eur J Endocrinol.* 2014;**171**(4):489–498.

21. National Institutes of Health. *Evidence-Based Methodology Workshop on Polycystic Ovary Syndrome: Final Report.* Bethesda, MD: National Institutes of Health; 2012.

22. Teede HJ, Misso ML, Costello MF, Dokras A, Laven J, Moran L, Piltonen T, Norman RJ for the International PCOS Network. Recommendations from the international evidence-based guideline for the assessment and management of polycystic ovary syndrome. *Fertil Steril.* 2018; **110**(3):364–379.

23. Teede HJ, Misso ML, Costello MF, Dokras A, Laven J, Moran L, Piltonen T, Norman RJ for the International PCOS Network. Recommendations from the international evidence-based guideline for the assessment and management of polycystic ovary syndrome. *Clin Endocrinol (Oxf).* 2018;**89**(3):251–268.

24. Johnstone EB, Rosen MP, Neril R, Trevithick D, Sternfeld B, Murphy R, Addauan-Andersen C, McConnell D, Pera RR, Cedars MI. The polycystic ovary post-Rotterdam: a common, age-dependent finding in ovulatory women without metabolic significance. *J Clin Endocrinol Metab.* 2010;**95**(11):4965–4972.

25. Fauser BC, Tarlatzis BC, Rebar RW, Legro RS, Balen AH, Lobo R, Carmina E, Chang J, Yildiz BO, Laven JS, Boivin J, Petraglia F, Wijeyeratne CN, Norman RJ, Dunaif A, Franks S, Wild RA, Dumesic D, Barnhart K. Consensus on women's health aspects of polycystic ovary syndrome (PCOS): the Amsterdam ESHRE/ASRM-Sponsored 3rd PCOS Consensus Workshop Group. *Fertil Steril.* 2012;**97**(1):28–38.

26. Legro RS, Kunselman AR, Dodson WC, Dunaif A. Prevalence and predictors of risk for type 2 diabetes mellitus and impaired glucose tolerance in polycystic ovary syndrome: a prospective, controlled study in 254 affected women. *J Clin Endocrinol Metab.* 1999;**84**(1): 165–169.

27. Ehrmann DA, Barnes RB, Rosenfield RL, Cavaghan MK, Imperial J. Prevalence of impaired glucose tolerance and diabetes in women with polycystic ovary syndrome. *Diabetes Care.* 1999;**22**(1):141–146.

28. Kumarendran B, O'Reilly MW, Manolopoulos KN, Toulis KA, Gokhale KM, Sitch AJ, Wijeyaratne CN, Coomarasamy A, Arlt W, Nirantharakumar K. Polycystic ovary syndrome, androgen excess, and the risk of nonalcoholic fatty liver disease in women: a longitudinal study based on a United Kingdom primary care database. *PLoS Med.* 2018; **15**(3):e1002542.

29. Kiddy DS, Hamilton-Fairley D, Bush A, Short F, Anyaoku V, Reed MJ, Franks S. Improvement in endocrine and ovarian function during dietary treatment of obese women with polycystic ovary syndrome. *Clin Endocrinol (Oxf).* 1992;**36**(1):105–111.

30. Alberti KG, Eckel RH, Grundy SM, Zimmet PZ, Cleeman JI, Donato KA, Fruchart JC, James WP, Loria CM, Smith SC Jr for the International Diabetes Federation Task Force on Epidemiology and Prevention; National Heart, Lung, and Blood Institute; American Heart Association; World Heart Federation; International Atherosclerosis Society; International Association for the Study of Obesity. Harmonizing the metabolic syndrome: a joint interim statement of the International Diabetes Federation Task Force on Epidemiology and Prevention; National Heart, Lung, and Blood Institute; American Heart Association; World Heart Federation; International Atherosclerosis Society; and International Association for the Study of Obesity. *Circulation.* 2009;**120**(16):1640–1645.

31. Knowler WC, Barrett-Connor E, Fowler SE, Hamman RF, Lachin JM, Walker EA, Nathan DM for the Diabetes Prevention Program Research Group. Reduction in the incidence of type 2 diabetes with lifestyle intervention or metformin. *N Engl J Med.* 2002;**346**(6):393–403.

32. Tang T, Lord JM, Norman RJ, Yasmin E, Balen AH. Insulin-sensitising drugs (metformin, rosiglitazone, pioglitazone, D-chiro-inositol) for women with polycystic ovary syndrome, oligo amenorrhoea and subfertility. *Cochrane Database Syst Rev.* 2012;(5):CD003053.

33. Morley LC, Tang T, Yasmin E, Norman RJ, Balen AH. Insulin-sensitising drugs (metformin, rosiglitazone, pioglitazone, D-chiro-inositol) for women with polycystic ovary syndrome, oligo amenorrhoea and subfertility. *Cochrane Database Syst Rev.* 2017;**11**:CD003053.

Hirsutism: Practical Approaches to Diagnosis and Treatment

M19
Presented, March 23–26, 2019

Ricardo Azziz, MD, MBA, MPH. Department of Health Policy, Management & Behavior, School of Public Health, University at Albany, State University of New York, Albany, New York 12222; Department of Obstetrics & Gynecology, Albany Medical College, Albany, New York 12222; and Department of Obstetrics & Gynecology, David Geffen School of Medicine, University of California, Los Angeles, California 90095, E-mail: ricardo.azziz@suny.edu

Daria Lizneva, MD, PhD. Division of Endocrinology, Diabetes and Bone Disease, Icahn School of Medicine at Mount Sinai, New York, New York 10029, E-mail: daria.lizneva@mssm.edu

SIGNIFICANCE OF THE CLINICAL PROBLEM

Hirsutism or the presence of male pattern terminal hair growth in women is the most common and recognizable sign of female androgen excess, and it is present in 5% to 10% of women (1). One-half of the women with mild hirsutism and the majority of those with moderate to severe hirsutism have elevated plasma total and free testosterone (T) levels. Hirsutism can be a clinical sign of polycystic ovary syndrome (PCOS), 21-hydroxylase (21-OH)–deficient nonclassic adrenal hyperplasia (NC-CAH), hyperandrogenic insulin-resistant acanthosis nigricans (HAIRAN) syndrome, idiopathic hirsutism (IH), and androgen-secreting neoplasms (ASNs). More rare causes include acromegaly iatrogenic/drug-induced hyperandrogenism, and chronic skin irritation. In general terms, the most common clinical sign of androgen excess is, in fact, hirsutism.

BARRIERS TO OPTIMAL PRACTICE

- The need for better definitions of clinically detected hirsutism
- The lack of well-designed studies to evaluate the best medical therapy for hirsutism
- The lack of well-designed studies to compare the effects of different hormonal contraceptives (HC) formulations
- The lack of data on the optimal duration of medical treatment of androgen excess
- The lack of long-term data on cosmetic treatments for hirsutism, including electrology, laser, and intense pulsed light (IPL)

LEARNING OBJECTIVES

As a result of participating in this session, learners should be able to:
- Evaluate the patient with the modified Ferriman–Gallwey scoring system (mFG)
- Refer the patient with hirsutism for specific laboratory evaluation
- Formulate the treatment plan for the hirsute patient
- Recognize the limitations of current diagnostic and treatment strategies

STRATEGIES FOR DIAGNOSIS, THERAPY, AND MANAGEMENT

We should first note that, although in general terms, the authors agree with the recent Endocrine Society guidelines on the diagnosis and treatment of hirsutism (1) and commend them a useful guideline, some of the specific recommendations have been modified based on the authors' experience or interpretation of the standing literature. When possible, these areas of discrepancy will be highlighted and explained.

Diagnosis of Hirsutism

Objective and subjective methods are available for the diagnosis of hirsutism. Objective methods of evaluation (*i.e.*, photographic evaluations and weighing of extracted hairs) are generally time consuming, and they are mainly used for research purposes. More applicable to the clinical setting is the visual, albeit more subjective, scoring system widely used for the evaluation of hair growth. Several scales have been proposed; however, the mFG scoring system is currently considered the gold standard for the clinical evaluation of hirsutism. To improve the quality of assessment, patients should be advised to avoid use of electrolysis or lasers for at least 3 months and depilation or waxing for 4 weeks, and they should be cautioned not to shave at least 5 days before evaluation.

Establishing the cutoff for determining an abnormal score (*i.e.*, one indicating hirsutism) has generally relied on establishing the 95th percentile of a "normal" or "control" population, with mFG cutoff scores ranging from 3 to 8 and even as high as 10 (2–4). However, a better method of defining the degree of hirsutism and that of any other continuous parameter in a population that one suspects detects an "abnormal" subset is to use cluster analysis or similar approaches to identify natural breaks in the data that would suggest the presence of these distinctive populations. Using this approach in a large population of unselected women seeking an employment physical assessment consisting of black (n = 350) and white (n = 283) women, we found that a cutoff of three or more clearly detected a population that was abnormal or different (3). A similarly designed study in Chinese women determined that the cutoff level in that population was five (5).

Overall, the cutoff mFG score value indicating abnormal seems to be closer to three to five, less than the higher values reported previously. Thus, although an mFG score of six to eight may be used as evidence of pathologic hirsutism, this definition is much stricter than how patients perceive their hair growth. Finally, current data suggest relatively little difference in the cutoff mFG scores between Asians, whites, and blacks, although additional studies are needed.

Differential Diagnosis of Hirsutism
PCOS

Approximately 80% or more of hirsute women will suffer from PCOS, the most frequent cause of hirsutism, which affects 10% to 15% of all women. PCOS is diagnosed today using Rotterdam 2003/National Institutes of Health 2012 criteria (6) by the presence of (i) androgen excess (either biochemical or clinical), (ii) ovulatory dysfunction/oligoamenorrhea, and/or (iii) polycystic ovarian morphology (PCOM) after the exclusion of similar/mimicking disorders. Some similar/mimicking disorders are screened for by laboratory tests (including thyroid dysfunction, hyperprolactinemia, and NC-CAH), and others are screened for (not diagnosed) clinically (ASNs, HAIRAN syndrome, iatrogenic causes, *etc.*). Key to the contemporary diagnosis of PCOS is the need for clinicians to specify the phenotype of PCOS diagnosed (phenotypes A to D) (Table 1).

NC-CAH

21-OH–deficient NC-CAH affects between 1% and 10% of hirsute women depending on ethnicity. NC-CAH is clinically indistinguishable from PCOS (7) and requires assessment of 17-hydroxyprogesterone (17-HP) levels and response to ACTH stimulation for screening and diagnosis (see below).

HAIRAN Syndrome

The HAIRAN syndrome affects 3% to 5% of clinically seen hirsute women, although the diagnostic criteria for this syndrome remain unclear. HAIRAN syndrome can be suspected when patients show acanthosis nigricans (AN) in association with extraordinarily high insulin levels, generally >300 miU/mL during an oral glucose tolerance test (OGTT). Clinically, the degree of AN and hirsutism in patients with HAIRAN syndrome is usually severe.

Table 1. PCOS Diagnostic Criteria

Clinical Feature	PCOS Phenotype[a]			
	A	B	C	D
Clinical and/or biochemical hyperandrogenism	X	X	X	
Oligoanovulation (OA)	X	X		X
PCOM	X		X	X

Based on Rotterdam 2003/National Institutes of Health 2012 criteria.
[a] After the exclusion of similar/mimicking disorders.

ASNs

ASNs are suspected clinically based on the progression and/or severity of symptoms or the presence of concomitant signs (*e.g.*, cachexia or Cushingoid features). ASNs are evident in 1:500 to 1:1000 hirsute women: mostly ovarian (*e.g.*, Sertoli-Leydig cell/androblastoma; granulosa-theca cell; adrenal like, including lipoid cell; and hilar tumors, including thecal, leydig, and metastases) and less frequently, adrenal (*e.g.*, adenoma and carcinomas).

IH

IH is a diagnosis of exclusion after all other causers of hirsutism have been assessed for. IH affects between 5% and 8% of hirsute women depending on the degree and sensitivity of the testing undertaken (8–10). It is likely that the prevalence of IH in hirsute women is decreasing as the diagnostic criteria of PCOS have expanded and the quality of androgen assays, the resolution of ultrasonographic equipment, and the completeness of the evaluation have improved.

Evaluation of the Hirsute Patient

The evaluation of the hirsute patient rests on three factors: (i) determination of ovulatory status and ovarian morphology; (ii) confirmation, if necessary, of androgen excess; and (iii) exclusion of specific disorders (*e.g.*, causes of ovulatory dysfunction, NC-CAH, HAIRAN syndrome, ASNs, or iatrogenic etiologies). We will detail these as follows.

Determination Ovulatory Status and Ovarian Morphology

In many cases, OA is clearly evident by the presence of overt menstrual dysfunction (oligoamenorrhea or polymenorrhea). However, up to 40% of hirsute women with apparently regular menstrual cycles are actually oligo-ovulatory (8), and in these women, measurement of a luteal (days 22 to 24) progesterone level is required to exclude OA. Ovarian morphology, including PCOM, is detected by ultrasonography, preferably transvaginal.

Confirmation of Androgen Excess

Although hirsutism itself is the most common clinical evidence of hyperandrogenism, it is recommended that androgen levels be measured in all women with hirsutism, including total and free T.

A few caveats should be considered. Total and free T should be measured using the highest-quality assays possible. The measurement of dehydroepiandrosterone sulfate (DHEAS) and/or androstenedione adds only a small increase to the detection of hyperandrogenemia. The total T may be useful for determining the severity of androgen excess, although it has limited usefulness for the screening of hirsute patients for an ASN. The DHEAS measurement may rarely suggest an adrenal ASN. The clinical presentation and history are generally the best tests to screen for ASNs.

Finally, we should note that, because hirsutism itself is a sign of androgen excess, the measurement of circulating androgens generally adds little to the evaluation of the patient who is already hirsute other than to help identify women with IH (if normal). Androgen levels are of greatest value in the evaluation of women with equivocal or absent signs of hyperandrogenism: for example, to diagnose PCOS in the minimally hirsute or nonhirsute patient.

Exclusion of Specific Disorders
As noted above, many specific disorders can be suspected by the history and physical examination (*e.g.*, ASNs, HAIRAN syndrome, drug-induced androgen excess, *etc.*). However, laboratory testing is necessary to screen for others, most notably 21-OH–deficient NC-CAH, thyroid dysfunction, and hyperprolactinemia.

A 17-HP level, obtained in the follicular phase and preferably in the morning, is required to screen for 21-OH–deficient NC-CAH. A basal 17-HP level should be obtained in all women with signs of androgen excess, regardless of androgen-level results. If the basal follicular 17-HP level is >2 ng/mL (200 ng/dL), the patient should undergo an acute adrenal stimulation testing with 250 μg of 1-24 ACTH (*e.g.*, Cortrsoyn®). If the 17-HP level 60 minutes after ACTH administration is >10 ng/mL (or 1000 ng/dL) and more frequently, 15 ng/mL (1500 ng/dL), the diagnosis of 21-OH–deficient NC-CAH is established.

In hirsutism women with OA, thyrotropin (TSH) and prolactin (PRL) levels should be assessed. An OGTT assessing both glucose and insulin may be necessary to diagnosis HAIRAN syndrome. Ovarian ultrasonography is performed to detect PCOM (see above) but should also be used to exclude ovarian ASNs when clinically indicated. A computed tomography scan/magnetic resonance imaging of the adrenal should be performed only when adrenal ASNs are suspected.

THERAPY AND MANAGEMENT
Initiation of the treatment should be based on the patient's perception of the problem rather than quantitative characteristics of hirsutism. As noted above, ~70% of patients with hirsutism defined by an mFG score of more than three complain of being hirsute (3), and about one-half of women with minimal hair growth (mFG score of 3 to 5) have PCOS (4). The hirsutism score correlates poorly with serum androgens (11); therefore, monitoring of T and other androgens is generally not needed. The choice of specific intervention depends on the patient's plan for pregnancy and the severity of hirsutism.

Hirsutism is a sign and is not a disease in and of itself; therefore, the underlying cause should be considered. PCOS is the most common etiology, and it is found in 72% to 82% of patients with hyperandrogenism (9, 10). Treatment of clinical signs of hyperandrogenism primarily centers on the suppression of androgen production and/or action. The most useful medical treatment includes oral contraceptive pills

(OCPs) and antiandrogen therapy, preferably in combination. Finally, treatment of these hyperandrogenic signs necessities understanding and incorporating cosmetic means of treatment, including shaving, depilating, hair bleaching, electrology, laser hair removal, hair transplantation, and others. Smoking cessation is strongly recommended for hirsute patients, because many of the undesirable side effects of the medications prescribed to treat hirsutism are exacerbated when patients indulge in this habit. Suppression of androgen biosynthesis may be achieved by the use of hormonal contraceptives, GnRH analogs, glucocorticoids, or insulin sensitizers as well as lifestyle modification.

OCPs
Progestins in OCPs cause suppression of LH levels and inhibition of LH-mediated ovarian androgen synthesis. The contained ethinylestradiol leads to a substantial increase in SHBG, thus contributing to a reduction of free testosterone. Moreover, OCPs modestly affect adrenal steroidogenesis by decreasing the synthesis and release of androgens. Several progestins have antiandrogenic properties that can antagonize the AR and/or inhibit the activity of 5α-reductase (5α-RA), although the amount found in OCPs alone is generally insufficient to mount a robust therapeutic response. OCPs are more effective than no treatment of hirsutism. Between 60% and 100% of hirsute women show improvement with OCPs alone. Consistent with the Endocrine Society guidelines (1), for most women, we do not suggest one oral contraceptive over another as initial therapy, because all oral contraceptives seem to be equally effective for hirsutism, and the risk of side effects is low.

However, differing from the guidelines, we prefer not to initiate treatment of hirsutism solely with an oral contraceptive other than in women with very mild degrees of hirsutism, but rather, we begin therapy in most women with clinically substantial hirsutism with combination therapy (*e.g.*, an OCP plus an antiandrogen). Four randomized, controlled trials (RCTs) show that antiandrogens in combination with OCPs were more effective than monotherapy with HCs (12). Furthermore, our published long-term clinical experience (13) suggests that this approach provides an effective long-term treatment of hirsute women who otherwise may become frustrated with the slow rate of the response when using OCPs alone.

Androgen Blockade
Antiandrogens generally include two androgen receptor (AR) blockers, spironolactone and flutamide, and one 5α-RA inhibitor, finasteride. Although there are other AR blockers and 5α-RA inhibitors available, these have not been used with any regularity in women. The side effects of antiandrogens vary some, although there are two side effects and risks that are common to all. First, all antiandrogens are teratogenic in that they may cause feminization of the genitalia in a male fetus. This is why antiandrogens alone are generally

discouraged unless they are used in a patient with very secure contraception.

Second, they all have the potential to cause side effects related to their antiandrogenic properties, including some muscle weakness and decreased libido, although this varies greatly from patient to patient. In general, because efficacy is generally higher when using a combination of OCPs and antiandrogens (see above) and because OCPs minimize the risk of teratogenicity, we generally begin therapy with a combination of OCPs and antiandrogens.

Third, there are legitimate concerns about the use of flutamide for the treatment of hirsutism in view of rare but serious and even fatal cases of associated hepatotoxicity. Although the Endocrine Society guidelines (1) advocate against using flutamide, we and others (14, 15) have found it clinically useful in patients who cannot tolerate other antiandrogens. However, administration of flutamide must be closely supervised, with frequent periodic monitoring of liver function tests.

Eflornithine Hydrochloride

Depending on accessibility and availability, in some countries, the topical use of 13.9% eflornithine hydrochloride (HCL) is available for the treatment of facial hirsutism. This medication acts as permanent inhibitor of enzyme ornithine decarboxylase, which is required for the growth and differentiation of cells in the hair follicle. Topical administration of eflornithine HCL was shown to slow facial hair growth (16). This action is reversible, and hirsutism relapsed after 8 weeks of cessation of treatment. Percutaneous absorption of eflornithine is <1%. The general use of eflornithine HCL is not approved for large surface areas of the skin due to systemic effects; therefore, its use should be restricted to the removal of facial hair only. Two RCTs showed that eflornithine promotes a more rapid response to therapy when combined with laser treatment (17, 18).

Lifestyle Modification and Weight Loss

The prevalence and degree of hirsutism are higher among obese women with PCOS. Some evidence suggests that obesity itself may negatively impact the effects of pharmacologic treatments for hirsutism. In a systematic review of nine small RCTs enrolling 583 women with a high loss to follow-up rate, lack of blinding, and short follow-up, the effect of lifestyle modification on hirsutism was unclear (19).

Cosmetic Approaches

Cosmetic methods are widely used and can be categorized as short or long term. Short-term mechanical methods include shaving, chemical depilation, plucking (threading), waxing, and bleaching; long-term mechanical methods include electrolysis, laser therapy, and IPL therapy.

Short-Term Mechanical Methods of Hair Removal

Depilation is the removal of the hair shaft from the skin's surface and includes shaving and chemical depilation. Conversely, epilation is the extraction of hair above the bulb (e.g., plucking or waxing). Between these two methods, epilation provides the most long-lasting action on hair regrowth, with hair absent for 6 to 8 weeks. If epilation is performed during the anagen phase, it could possibly destroy the dermal papilla.

Long-Term Mechanical Methods of Hair Removal
Electrology

Electrolysis has been commonly used for the treatment of unwanted hair since 1875. Galvanic electrolysis facilitates chemical destruction of the dermal papilla, resulting in the long-term reduction of hirsutism. Thermolytic electrolysis induces heat injury of the hair follicle in the treated area. Currently available blended electrolysis includes the synergetic application of both energies. Data on the clinical effectiveness of electrolysis are limited. Side effects associated with electrolysis include discomfort, erythema, skin discoloration, and scarring. Application of local anesthetics has been shown to be effective in reducing the discomfort associated with this procedure.

Laser Therapy

Laser therapy is based on selective photothermolysis, wherein melanin of hair follicles accumulates the light energy, which in turn, destroys the hair bulb. Several lasers with varying wavelengths are available for hair removal: ruby, alexandrite, diode, and the neodymium: yttrium-aluminum-garnet (Nd:YAG). Darker skin types are usually more difficult to treat using photoepilation. In this case, light energy is absorbed by the surrounding epidermis beside the hair follicle, which makes the procedure less effective and could be associated with skin discoloration and burns. Therefore, the Nd-YAG laser, which has a longer wavelength, is the preferred treatment of patients with darker skin. A Cochrane systematic review showed almost 50% hair reduction in a period of 6 months after treatment with alexandrite and diode lasers and limited evidence of effectiveness with other lasers (20). Maintenance therapy is recommended every 6 to 12 months.

IPL

Data regarding IPL efficacy are limited. It is shown to be superior to the ruby laser, similar to the Nd:YAG laser, and less effective compared with diode laser therapy. IPLs with radiofrequency can be used for women with blond hair and light skin when lasers are not effective. For darker skin, in an assessor-blinded comparison, the Nd:YAG laser was more effective than the IPL (21).

MAIN CONCLUSIONS

Hirsutism excess is a common disorder of reproductive-age women. The mFG scoring system is currently considered the gold standard for the clinical evaluation of hirsutism. Treatment of hirsutism includes topical eflornithine HCL for mild facial hirsutism, electrolysis for localized hirsutism as a monotherapy or in combination with pharmacological approaches, use of lasers for generalized hirsutism in mild cases or in combination with medical therapy in patients with moderate to severe causes, and low-dose neutral or antiandrogenic HCs as first-line monotherapy for women with mild hirsutism or in combination with antiandrogens for women with moderate or severe hirsutism. The use of metformin or other insulin sensitizers, glucocorticoids, or GnRH is not routinely recommended.

CLINICAL CASES

Case 1

A 24-year-old female presents with complaints of excess and unwanted hair growth and increased scalp hair shedding. On questioning, she states that she has "always" had more hair than her friends but that it has been getting worse over the past 4 years. The excess hair appears to be on her upper lip, chin and neck, chest, and lower abdomen, with an mFG score of six. She now shaves her face twice weekly. Her cycles are relatively irregular at about every 40 to 60 days. Her mother and sister also have excess hair growth on their face and abdomen but less than she does. A clinical evaluation reveals a black woman who is moderately obese with extensive terminal hair growth on the abdomen and face, moderate acanthosis, normal thyroid on palpation, and no galactorrhea. The next best option is

   A. OGTT for insulin and glucose
   B. 17-HP, TSH, and PRL
   C. Total and free T and DHEAS
   D. Ovarian ultrasonography

Case 1 Discussion

In patients presenting with long-term gradually worsening hirsutism and oligoamenorrhea, the most common cause is PCOS, a diagnosis of exclusion. The next best step is to exclude hyperprolactinemia and thyroid dysfunction as causes of the ovulatory dysfunction and 21-OH NC-CAH as the cause of the androgen excess by measuring PRL, TSH, and 17-HP, respectively. An OGTT should be performed after the diagnosis of PCOS is made to exclude glucose intolerance and if also measuring insulin, hyperinsulinemia. Total and free T and DHEAS are most helpful in patients with equivocal clinical signs of androgen excess. Ovarian ultrasonography will help show the presence of PCOM and establish the exact PCOS phenotype, although in this case, it will not add to the diagnosis.

Case 2

A 56-year-old white female presents with complaints of excess hair growth; she states that she feels that is more than her husband's hair growth. Also, we find that she had vasomotor flushing 6 to 7 years ago, but they have since stopped, and her unwanted hair growth started developing 2 years ago and has progressively worsened. Family history reveals a cousin with excess unwanted hair and "Stein–Leventhal." On evaluation, we document an mFG score of 18, an estrogenic vaginal mucosa, a normal thyroid on palpation, and no galactorrhea. The next best option is

   A. OGTT for insulin and glucose
   B. 17-HP, TSH, and PRL
   C. Total and free T and DHEAS
   D. Ovarian ultrasonography

Case 2 Discussion

In this patient, the advanced age of onset and the rapidity of progression of the hirsutism should suggest an ASN. Because the most frequent ASN is an ovarian tumor, an ovarian ultrasound using a high-resolution transducer would be the next best step. The measurement of 17-HP, TSH, and PRL would be useful if an ASN is not detected and if PCOS is suspected. An OGTT is useful to exclude metabolic dysfunction and glucose intolerance if PCOS is eventually diagnosed. total and free T and DHEAS are most helpful in patients with equivocal clinical signs of androgen excess, which is not the case in this patient. Furthermore, although androgen measures can be very elevated in ASNs, this is not always a consistent finding, and it can be misleading.

References

1. Martin KA, Anderson RR, Chang RJ, Ehrmann DA, Lobo RA, Murad MH, Pugeat MM, Rosenfield RL. Evaluation and treatment of hirsutism in premenopausal women: an Endocrine Society clinical practice guideline. *J Clin Endocrinol Metab.* 2018;**103**(4):1233–1257.
2. Yildiz BO, Bolour S, Woods K, Moore A, Azziz R. Visually scoring hirsutism. *Hum Reprod Update.* 2010;**16**(1):51–64.
3. DeUgarte CM, Woods KS, Bartolucci AA, Azziz R. Degree of facial and body terminal hair growth in unselected black and white women: toward a populational definition of hirsutism. *J Clin Endocrinol Metab.* 2006;**91**(4):1345–1350.
4. Souter I, Sanchez LA, Perez M, Bartolucci AA, Azziz R. The prevalence of androgen excess among patients with minimal unwanted hair growth. *Am J Obstet Gynecol.* 2004;**191**(6):1914–1920.
5. Zhao X, Ni R, Li L, Mo Y, Huang J, Huang M, Azziz R, Yang D. Defining hirsutism in Chinese women: a cross-sectional study. *Fertil Steril.* 2011;**96**(3):792–796.
6. Lizneva D, Suturina L, Walker W, Brakta S, Gavrilova-Jordan L, Azziz R. Criteria, prevalence, and phenotypes of polycystic ovary syndrome. *Fertil Steril.* 2016;**106**(1):6–15.
7. Azziz R, Waggoner WT, Ochoa T, Knochenhauer ES, Boots LR. Idiopathic hirsutism: an uncommon cause of hirsutism in Alabama. *Fertil Steril.* 1998;**70**(2):274–278.
8. Pall M, Azziz R, Beires J, Pignatelli D. The phenotype of hirsute women: a comparison of polycystic ovary syndrome and 21-hydroxylase-deficient nonclassic adrenal hyperplasia. *Fertil Steril.* 2010;**94**(2):684–689.
9. Azziz R, Sanchez LA, Knochenhauer ES, Moran C, Lazenby J, Stephens KC, Taylor K, Boots LR. Androgen excess in women: experience with over 1000 consecutive patients. *J Clin Endocrinol Metab.* 2004;**89**(2):453–462.
10. Carmina E, Rosato F, Jannì A, Rizzo M, Longo RA. Extensive clinical experience: relative prevalence of different androgen excess

disorders in 950 women referred because of clinical hyperandrogenism. *J Clin Endocrinol Metab.* 2006;**91**(1):2–6.

11. Landay M, Huang A, Azziz R. Degree of hyperinsulinemia, independent of androgen levels, is an important determinant of the severity of hirsutism in PCOS. *Fertil Steril.* 2009;**92**(2):643–647.

12. Swiglo BA, Cosma M, Flynn DN, Kurtz DM, Labella ML, Mullan RJ, Erwin PJ, Montori VM. Clinical review: antiandrogens for the treatment of hirsutism: a systematic review and metaanalyses of randomized controlled trials. *J Clin Endocrinol Metab.* 2008;**93**(4):1153–1160.

13. Ezeh U, Huang A, Landay M, Azziz R. Long-term response of hirsutism and other hyperandrogenic symptoms to combination therapy in polycystic ovary syndrome. *J Womens Health (Larchmt).* 2018;**27**(7):892–902.

14. Castelo-Branco C, Hernández-Angeles C, Alvarez-Olivares L, Balasch J. Long-term satisfaction and tolerability with low-dose flutamide: a 20-year surveillance study on 120 hyperandrogenic women. *Gynecol Endocrinol.* 2016;**32**(9):723–727.

15. Fulghesu AM, Melis F, Murru G, Canu E, Melis GB. Very low dose of flutamide in the treatment of hyperandrogenism [published correction appears in *Gynecol Endocrinol.* 2018;34(5):i]. *Gynecol Endocrinol.* 2018;**34**(5):394–398.

16. Wolf JE Jr, Shander D, Huber F, Jackson J, Lin CS, Mathes BM, Schrode K; Eflornithine HCl Study Group. Randomized, double-blind clinical evaluation of the efficacy and safety of topical eflornithine HCl 13.9% cream in the treatment of women with facial hair. *Int J Dermatol.* 2007;**46**(1):94–98.

17. Smith SR, Piacquadio DJ, Beger B, Littler C. Eflornithine cream combined with laser therapy in the management of unwanted facial hair growth in women: a randomized trial. *Dermatol Surg.* 2006;**32**(10):1237–1243.

18. Hamzavi I, Tan E, Shapiro J, Lui H. A randomized bilateral vehicle-controlled study of eflornithine cream combined with laser treatment versus laser treatment alone for facial hirsutism in women. *J Am Acad Dermatol.* 2007;**57**(1):54–59.

19. Domecq JP, Prutsky G, Mullan RJ, Hazem A, Sundaresh V, Elamin MB, Phung OJ, Wang A, Hoeger K, Pasquali R, Erwin P, Bodde A, Montori VM, Murad MH. Lifestyle modification programs in polycystic ovary syndrome: systematic review and meta-analysis. *J Clin Endocrinol Metab.* 2013;**98**(12):4655–4663.

20. Haedersdal M, Gøtzsche PC. Laser and photoepilation for unwanted hair growth. *Cochrane Database Syst Rev.* 2006;**2006**(4):CD004684.

21. Ismail SA. Long-pulsed Nd:YAG laser vs. intense pulsed light for hair removal in dark skin: a randomized controlled trial. *Br J Dermatol.* 2012;**166**(2):317–321.

Testosterone Therapy: Maximizing the Benefits, Minimizing the Risks

M20
Presented, March 23–26, 2019

Margaret E. Wierman, MD. University of Colorado Anschutz Medical Campus, Rocky Mountain Regional Veterans Affairs Medical Center, Aurora, Colorado 80045, E-mail: margaret.wierman@ucdenver.edu

SIGNIFICANCE OF THE PROBLEM

Testosterone (T) therapy is indicated for the treatment of male hypogonadism, a disorder of the reproductive axis with signs and symptoms that are due to lack of T and usually with decreased spermatogenesis (1–3). Many of the signs and symptoms are nonspecific, including fatigue, in addition to the more specific signs of decrease in sexual function, loss of virilization, and muscle mass. In addition to classic disorders of the male reproductive axis (with defects in the hypothalamus, pituitary, or testes), over recent years, T preparations have been marketed for their anabolic properties such as antiaging, antifrailty, or antifatigue (3, 4). Changes in the measurement of T levels with imperfect and imprecise platform assays compared with sensitive radioimmunoassays or mass spectrometry measurements have resulted in difficulty in interpreting results, changes in normative data ranges, and confusion for providers and patients alike (5). Effects of obesity that alter total T levels because of effects on sex hormone binding globulin (SHBG) need to be considered. Careful evaluation for age-related hypogonadism suggests that the disorder is not common, but rare, and is usually associated with morbid obesity (6, 7). Risks of T therapy (including cardiovascular risk) and somewhat modest beneficial effects of physiologic dosing in prospective studies have created controversy and confusion about who should receive T treatment, in what formulation, and to what benefit or risk—especially in older men (8). As the prescriptions for T have dramatically increased over the last 8 years (often without evidence of a T measurement or diagnosis of hypogonadism and with lack of appropriate follow-up), guidelines from various endocrine societies internationally have tried to give guidance and put individual risk/benefit into perspective (1–3).

BARRIERS TO OPTIMAL PRACTICE

- Changes in the T assay and definitions of what is normal or abnormal to allow the clinician to make a diagnosis of hypogonadism
- Pressure from lay press and marketing to patients with direct-to-consumer advertising to administer T for reasons other than real hypogonadism
- Controversy about the benefit/risk of physiologic vs pharmacologic T therapy in different populations

LEARNING OBJECTIVES

- Summarize the physiology of the male reproductive axis and the common causes of hypogonadism
- Identify the common causes of transient reversible causes of low T measurements
- Outline the risks of T therapy in different patient populations and with different preparations

STRATEGIES FOR DIAGNOSIS, THERAPY, AND MANAGEMENT

Diagnosis

Diagnosis of hypogonadism should be made with signs and symptoms as well as evidence of low morning T levels measured at least twice (1). With obesity, changes in SHBG often result in changes in total T levels, and measurement of SHBG and calculation of free T levels should be performed (1, 2, 9). In these men, diet, weight loss, and lifestyle intervention are indicated, rather than administration of T therapy.

Treatment

Exclusion of causes of transient (or reversible) causes of low T (including dietary supplements, anabolic steroids, glucocorticoid injections, illness or stress, and obstructive sleep apnea) should be assessed before considering T therapy. There are many formulations of T therapy available (10–12). T gel and patches result in physiologic levels when applied to dry skin without lotion in soap or on skin. Depot T injections usually result in high followed by low levels, depending on dose and timing of administration. The pharmacologic peaks may be decreased by more frequent dosing with lower amounts of the drug (*i.e.*, 75 to 100 mg testosterone cypionate injection weekly vs 200 mg every 2 weeks IM). The use of T pellets (implants) or testosterone undecanoate always results in pharmacologic T levels for at least several weeks to months. Although these preparations may increase compliance in patients, their risk in older men or in those with coronary artery disease (CAD) is of concern (13, 14).

CASES WITH QUESTIONS AND ANSWERS

Case 1

A 20-year-old man presented with complaints of decreased muscle mass and fatigue. He related a normal puberty with normal virilization during adolescence and normal sexual function. Over the last year, he has experienced fatigue and inability to keep up with a rigorous exercise regimen. Following a training injury, he has had three trigger-point injections in the last 6 months. He takes vitamin supplements and protein powders to increase his muscle mass, without effect. His physical examination was normal. Testes were 12 mL bilaterally. A random T level was just below the normal range in a platform radioimmunoassay.

What are the best laboratory tests to obtain for evaluation of his symptoms?
   A. Morning fasting glucose, T, and complete blood count
   B. Morning prolactin, luteinizing hormone (LH), follicle-stimulating hormone (FSH), and T
   C. Morning cortisol, LH, FSH, and T
   D. Afternoon cortisol, LH, FSH, and T

Answer: C (morning cortisol, LH, FSH, and T)

Discussion (Case 1)

To confirm hypogonadism, repeat early morning laboratory results are required. The patient described a normal pubertal development and sexual maturation. Therefore, the differential diagnosis switches from a genetic disorder (*e.g.*, normosmic hypogonadotropic hypogonadism) to an acquired process. Before considering any therapy with T, it is critical to exclude causes of acquired reversible hypogonadism. In this scenario, both supplements and glucocorticoid injections could be the culprit. Although there is published literature about the effects of glucocorticoid injections to cause secondary adrenal insufficiency, especially when given repeatedly and with higher doses or multiple injection sites (15–17); however, data about the risk of secondary hypogonadism are not as well documented. Other supplements often are contaminated with prohormones that are converted into androgens and suppress the hypothalamic pituitary testisticular axis. Waiting 4 to 6 weeks for supplements, but much longer for anabolic steroid use, will be necessary. Repeating laboratory testing after the steroid injection and withholding supplements will allow assessment of whether these are the causes of the symptoms and signs, and the laboratory results should normalize. If not, further work-up would be indicated (*e.g.*, evaluation of prolactin, other disorders of the pituitary such as hemochromatosis, *etc.*). Other causes of reversible hypogonadism include higher-dose use of opioids, especially morphine, methadone, oxycontin, and fentanyl (18). A primary goal would be to taper the narcotics. However, some patients using chronic narcotics who are unable to lower their doses may be candidates for short- or longer-term T therapy.

Case 2

A 38-year-old man presented to the clinic with a history of delayed puberty. He had normal sexual function. He and his wife were trying to start a family, and he complained of infertility. His examination was notable for mild gynecomastia, testes 8 mL bilaterally (normal, >10 mL).

Laboratory results revealed T 240 ng/dL (normal range, 240 to 840 ng/dL), FSH 18 mIU/mL, LH 9 mIU/mL, and prolactin 10 ng/mL. Upon semen analysis, no sperm were detected.

What is the most probable diagnosis for this patient's symptoms and clinical picture?
   A. Gonadotrope pituitary tumor
   B. Germ cell testicular tumor
   C. Exogenous androgen use
   D. Klinefelter syndrome

Answer: D (Klinefelter syndrome)

Discussion (Case 2)

This patient has signs and symptoms that suggest a disorder of the pubertal process and normal sexual maturation. He has normal sexual function, low-normal T level, but no sperm and gynecomastia. A karyotype is indicated to evaluate for XXY or mosaic XY/XXY. Other causes of primary testicular failure associated with a primary spermatic defect can be considered if the karyotype is normal (1). Intracytoplasmic semen injection can sometimes be used for fertility in men with Klinefelter syndrome, understanding that the genetic defect can be transmitted unless genetic testing of the embryos is performed (19). Long-term issues in these patients include an ultimate need for T therapy at physiologic dosing, some increased risk of venous insufficiency, possible increased risk of deep venous thrombosis on therapy, and need for monitoring of breast tissue for tumors (20, 21). Topical T therapy is optimal for these patients.

Case 3

A 54-year-old man with diabetes and hypertension (HTN) complained of fatigue and erectile dysfunction. He has diabetes type 2, hyperlipidemia, and hypertension, and for 5 years has been treated with metformin, a statin, and lisinopril. He had normal pubertal development and fathered three children. After being an athlete in high school and in college, he has been more inactive and has had progressive weight gain, with a current body mass index (BMI) of 38 kg/m^2.

Laboratory results revealed T 220 ng/dL (normal range, 240 to 800 ng/dL), LH 5 mIU/mL, FSH 6 mIU/mL, and prolactin 10 ng/mL.

What further work up is needed?
   A. MRI of the pituitary without contrast
   B. Evaluation for obstructive sleep apnea
   C. Ultrasound of the testes
   D. Repeat measurement of LH, FSH, and T levels after 10:00 AM

Answer: B (evaluation for obstructive sleep apnea)

Discussion (Case 3)

In addition to classic disorders that result in deficiencies of gonadotropin releasing hormone (GnRH), LH, FSH, or T, a common cause of borderline low T in a man with HTN, metabolic syndrome, and obesity is untreated sleep apnea (22–24). As the tongue falls back, oxygen levels drop, cortisol increases (contributing to insulin resistance and central weight redistribution), and catecholamines increase (contributing to worsening HTN). Obstructive sleep apnea (OSA) induces a small alteration in the GnRH pulse generator and there is also a change in SHBG with the central weight gain, and the total T level appears lower than the free T level. Patients with OSA have a risk of polycythemia, which is worsened if T therapy is given. It is unclear in controlled studies whether T levels normalize with treatment of OSA. However, with treatment, dietary changes, and lifestyle intervention, symptoms and signs will improve in some patients. If not, and if the patient fits the criteria of acquired hypogonadism, careful treatment with T therapy can be initiated after the OSA is treated with continuous positive airway pressure.

Case 4

A 58-year-old man with hyperlipidemia, hypertension, and coronary artery disease s/p /p stents 3 years ago, but with no current angina, presented with complaints of fatigue, decreased libido, and erectile dysfunction. Examination was pertinent for a BMI of 40 kg/m^2 and normal testicular size.

Laboratory results revealed T 220 ng/dL (normal range, 240 to 840 ng/dL), LH 6 mIU/mL, and FSH 7 mIU/mL.

Should this patient receive T therapy?

A. Yes

B. No

Answer: B (no)

Discussion (Case 4)

Earlier studies from the Baltimore Male Aging Study suggested that aging was associated with a low T level in up to 20% to 30% of patients (25). These studies were performed with no information on signs or symptoms or whether patients had hypogonadism. More careful exploration of the issue of age-related hypogonadism was undertaken by Wu *et al.*; they examined the incidence of age-related late-onset hypogonadism with specific criteria and use of a sensitive mass spectrometry T assay (6). Importantly, they reported that many men had symptoms but normal T levels, and conversely, many men had low T levels and no symptoms. The incidence of age-related hypogonadism with three symptoms and/or signs and low T level was only 2% to 3.5% of patients (not 20% to 30% of men) and increased with comorbid conditions, especially obesity. When BMI is modestly elevated, the total T level drops but the level of free T is still normal; with severe obesity, both levels drop. In a follow-up publication, men were instructed in diet and lifestyle; with substantial weight loss, the diagnosis of hypogonadism reversed (22).

Basaria *et al.* published the pivotal prospective investigation of whether high physiologic T levels could improve frailty in older men with comorbid conditions (26). The study

was halted at 24 weeks because of increased adverse cardiovascular events. During this time, the US Food & Drug Administration (FDA) published findings that many men were receiving T therapy without a diagnosis of hypogonadism and with a lack of hormone testing or follow-up laboratory testing. Two large epidemiologic studies suggested that men who received T therapy, especially after the age of 55 years, had increased risk of cardiovascular events (27, 28). This led the FDA to add a black box warning to testosterone preparations and insurance companies to add requirements for prior authorization (8).

Recently, the Testosterone Trials were published, which tried to recruit this subset of men to T therapy (29). Importantly, investigators screened 50,000 men and found 790 men with T levels <275 ng/dL with signs and symptoms, confirming that this disorder is rare—not common. Importantly, men with known causes of hypogonadism, CAD, benign prostatic hypertrophy, or depression were excluded. The administration of T gel to obtain mid-normal range for young men had very modest effects. Some improvements in erectile dysfunction, anemia, and depression were observed, but the major goal of improving strength or vitality was not achieved and there were no positive effects on cognition (30). Importantly, there was evidence of increased coronary plaque volume in older men receiving T therapy (31), which differed from prior reports of T therapy in older men with low or low-normal T levels on carotid intimal thickening and coronary calcium scores (32). There was a signal toward risk of polycythemia at 12 months, but no correlation with OSA was performed. No increased cardiac risk was observed in this selected cohort of patients.

A very recent review of Medicare databases suggests that men with CAD are receiving T therapy at the same rate as men without CAD risk for off-label use of T, suggesting a lack of response to FDA warnings in many parts of the United States (33). A cardiovascular risk trial is scheduled with ongoing recruitment, and a study in Australia to assess the effects of higher-dose T therapy to prevent diabetes is underway (34).

Taken together, there are data suggesting that T therapy in older men and in men with CAD risk for off-label use or for age-related hypogonadism may be of concern. T therapy in men with true hypogonadism at physiologic dosing may be appropriate. These men should not be denied physiologic T therapy because studies suggest that there is no excess risk in patients with true hypogonadism who are treated to physiologic T levels (35).

Case 4 (Continued)

The patient visited the local "low T clinic," where no additional laboratory values were checked, and he received nine T pellets. Repeat laboratory testing 3 weeks after placement of the pellets revealed T 1800 ng/dL, LH < 1.0 mIU/mL, FSH <1.0 mIU/mL, and Hct 58. He complained of some new chest pain with activity and worse snoring, but he reported having higher energy.

DISCUSSION: PHYSIOLOGIC VS PHARMACOLOGIC T THERAPY

For many years, the only type of T replacement therapy available was testosterone cypionate injection. The formulations result in a peak T level that exceeds the normal range and then decreases over various time intervals, depending on the type and dose (12). Patients noted highs and lows as well as an impact on mood, and compliance with injections has been variable. The new formulations of T patches and then various T gels administered to shoulders, under the arms, or in other locations were driven by a goal of removing the highs and lows. Absorption of the gel has been variable in individual patients and across populations, often because of lotion or soap on the skin, mode of administration, and concern of transfer to children or partner. Thus some have advocated for going back to injectable T but at lower, more frequent doses. Some advocate for giving the testosterone cypionate formulations subcutaneously rather than IM as approved, although no head-to-head pharmacologic studies have been published to date. To increase compliance, industry has created T pellets (implants), and testosterone undecanoate, which is a longer-term 3-month injectable, is used. The latter was initially refused by the US FDA because of concerns about lipid emboli, but it has been used in Europe for many years and was approved recently in the United States at a lower dose, with monitoring after each injection. These formulations return to a pattern of pharmacologic T therapy for several weeks after the administration of pellets or injections. The absolute levels of T can be extremely high in older men and if given at higher doses. In fact, some industry sponsors have suggested that these formulations are treatments for diabetes and obesity, most likely because of the pharmacologic dosing effects of anabolic T. Unfortunately, these formulations have not been extensively evaluated in older men or in those with CAD. Epidemiologic data suggest that injectable formulations of T therapy have higher cardiovascular risk than patch or gel formulations (10, 11). Long-term effects of pharmacologic T dosing (historically with testosterone cypionate formulations) include risk of polycythemia, edema, congestive heart failure, benign prostatic hypertrophy, and hypercoagulability (1, 2, 8, 36). Thus, in my opinion, depot and injectable formulations pose potential risk acutely in older patients. The potential long-term risk in younger populations and the exact degrees of risk remains to be evaluated. Physiologic T administration is optimal. Too little or too much T is a risk.

SUMMARY

- A patient with real hypogonadism has signs and symptoms, as well as low T levels with two morning laboratory measurements; an underlying cause can usually be identified.
- Common causes of acquired and often reversible low T include opioid narcotics, glucocorticoid injections, supplements, and untreated obstructive sleep apnea.

- When treating men with hypogonadism, they should be treated to physiologic (not pharmacologic) T levels, and the type of T therapy (topical vs injection, not pellets) should be considered.
- Before initiating T therapy, the risk/benefit should be considered, and during treatment, patients should be monitored for adverse effects.

References

1. Bhasin S, Brito JP, Cunningham GR, Hayes FJ, Hodis HN, Matsumoto AM, Snyder PJ, Swerdloff RS, Wu FC, Yialamas MA. Testosterone Therapy in Men With Hypogonadism: An Endocrine Society Clinical Practice Guideline. *J Clin Endocrinol Metab.* 2018;**103**(5):1715–1744.
2. Yeap BB, Grossmann M, McLachlan RI, Handelsman DJ, Wittert GA, Conway AJ, Stuckey BG, Lording DW, Allan CA, Zajac JD, Burger HG. Endocrine Society of Australia position statement on male hypogonadism (part 1): assessment and indications for testosterone therapy. *Med J Aust.* 2016;**205**(4):173–178.
3. Yeap BB, Wu FCW. Clinical practice update on testosterone therapy for male hypogonadism: contrasting perspectives to optimize care. *Clin Endocrinol (Oxf).* 2019;**90**(1):56–65.
4. Mangolim AS, Brito LAR, Nunes-Nogueira VS. Effectiveness of testosterone therapy in obese men with low testosterone levels, for losing weight, controlling obesity complications, and preventing cardiovascular events: protocol of a systematic review of randomized controlled trials. *Medicine (Baltimore).* 2018;**97**(17):e0482.
5. Travison TG, Vesper HW, Orwoll E, Wu F, Kaufman JM, Wang Y, Lapauw B, Fiers T, Matsumoto AM, Bhasin S. Harmonized reference ranges for circulating testosterone levels in men of four cohort studies in the United States and Europe. *J Clin Endocrinol Metab.* 2017;**102**(4):1161–1173.
6. Wu FC, Tajar A, Beynon JM, Pye SR, Silman AJ, Finn JD, O'Neill TW, Bartfai G, Casanueva FF, Forti G, Giwercman A, Han TS, Kula K, Lean ME, Pendleton N, Punab M, Boonen S, Vanderschueren D, Labrie F, Huhtaniemi IT; EMAS Group. Identification of late-onset hypogonadism in middle-aged and elderly men. *N Engl J Med.* 2010;**363**(2):123–135.
7. Camacho EM, Huhtaniemi IT, O'Neill TW, Finn JD, Pye SR, Lee DM, Tajar A, Bartfai G, Boonen S, Casanueva FF, Forti G, Giwercman A, Han TS, Kula K, Keevil B, Lean ME, Pendleton N, Punab M, Vanderschueren D, Wu FC; EMAS Group. Age-associated changes in hypothalamic-pituitary-testicular function in middle-aged and older men are modified by weight change and lifestyle factors: longitudinal results from the European Male Ageing Study. *Eur J Endocrinol.* 2013;**168**(3):445–455.
8. U.S. Food & Drug Administration. FDA Drug Safety Communication: FDA evaluating risk of stroke, heart attack and death with FDA-approved testosterone products. Available at: https://wayback.archive-it.org/7993/20170112031612/http://www.fda.gov/Drugs/DrugSafety/ucm383904.htm. Accessed 10 November 2018.
9. Yeap BB, Page ST, Grossmann M. Testosterone treatment in older men: clinical implications and unresolved questions from the Testosterone Trials. *Lancet Diabetes Endocrinol.* 2018;**6**(8):659–672.
10. Layton JB, Meier CR, Sharpless JL, Stürmer T, Jick SS, Brookhart MA. Comparative safety of testosterone dosage forms. *JAMA Intern Med.* 2015;**175**(7):1187–1196.
11. Wierman ME. Risks of different testosterone preparations: too much, too little, just right. *JAMA Intern Med.* 2015;**175**(7):1197–1198.
12. Shoskes JJ, Wilson MK, Spinner ML. Pharmacology of testosterone replacement therapy preparations. *Transl Androl Urol.* 2016;**5**(6):834–843.
13. Handelsman DJ. Testosterone and male aging: faltering hope for rejuvenation. *JAMA.* 2017;**317**(7):699–701.
14. Handelsman DJ. Pharmacoepidemiology of testosterone: curbing off-label prescribing. *Pharmacoepidemiol Drug Saf.* 2017;**26**(10):1248–1255.
15. Habib GS. Systemic effects of intra-articular corticosteroids. *Clin Rheumatol.* 2009;**28**(7):749–756.

16. Goel AP, Nguyen VH, Hamill-Ruth R. Use of a risk-stratification tool in identification of potential adrenal suppression preceding steroid injection therapy in chronic pain patients. *Pain Med.* 2015;**16**(12):2226–2234.

17. Friedly JL, Comstock BA, Heagerty PJ, Bauer Z, Rothman MS, Suri P, Hansen R, Avins AL, Nedeljkovic SS, Nerenz DR, Akuthota V, Jarvik JG. Systemic effects of epidural steroid injections for spinal stenosis. *Pain.* 2018;**159**(5):876–883.

18. Basaria S, Travison TG, Alford D, Knapp PE, Teeter K, Cahalan C, Eder R, Lakshman K, Bachman E, Mensing G, Martel MO, Le D, Stroh H, Bhasin S, Wasan AD, Edwards RR. Effects of testosterone replacement in men with opioid-induced androgen deficiency: a randomized controlled trial. *Pain.* 2015;**156**(2):280–288.

19. Rohayem J, Fricke R, Czeloth K, Mallidis C, Wistuba J, Krallmann C, Zitzmann M, Kliesch S. Age and markers of Leydig cell function, but not of Sertoli cell function predict the success of sperm retrieval in adolescents and adults with Klinefelter's syndrome. *Andrology.* 2015;**3**(5):868–875.

20. Seth A, Rajpal S, Penn RL. Klinefelter's syndrome and venous thrombosis. *Am J Med Sci.* 2013;**346**(2):164–165.

21. Vignozzi L, Corona G, Forti G, Jannini EA, Maggi M. Clinical and therapeutic aspects of Klinefelter's syndrome: sexual function. *Mol Hum Reprod.* 2010;**16**(6):418–424.

22. Camargo CA. Obstructive sleep apnea and testosterone. *N Engl J Med.* 1983;**309**(5):314–315.

23. Sandblom RE, Matsumoto AM, Schoene RB, Lee KA, Giblin EC, Bremner WJ, Pierson DJ. Obstructive sleep apnea syndrome induced by testosterone administration. *N Engl J Med.* 1983;**308**(9):508–510.

24. Shigehara K, Konaka H, Sugimoto K, Nohara T, Izumi K, Kadono Y, Namiki M, Mizokami A. Sleep disturbance as a clinical sign for severe hypogonadism: efficacy of testosterone replacement therapy on sleep disturbance among hypogonadal men without obstructive sleep apnea. *Aging Male.* 2018;**21**(2):99–105.

25. Harman SM, Metter EJ, Tobin JD, Pearson J, Blackman MR; Baltimore Longitudinal Study of Aging. Longitudinal effects of aging on serum total and free testosterone levels in healthy men. *J Clin Endocrinol Metab.* 2001;**86**(2):724–731.

26. Basaria S, Coviello AD, Travison TG, Storer TW, Farwell WR, Jette AM, Eder R, Tennstedt S, Ulloor J, Zhang A, Choong K, Lakshman KM, Mazer NA, Miciek R, Krasnoff J, Elmi A, Knapp PE, Brooks B, Appleman E, Aggarwal S, Bhasin G, Hede-Brierley L, Bhatia A, Collins L, LeBrasseur N, Fiore LD, Bhasin S. Adverse events associated with testosterone administration. *N Engl J Med.* 2010;**363**(2):109–122.

27. Vigen R, O'Donnell CI, Barón AE, Grunwald GK, Maddox TM, Bradley SM, Barqawi A, Woning G, Wierman ME, Plomondon ME, Rumsfeld JS, Ho PM. Association of testosterone therapy with mortality, myocardial infarction, and stroke in men with low testosterone levels. *JAMA.* 2013;**310**(17):1829–1836.

28. Finkle WD, Greenland S, Ridgeway GK, Adams JL, Frasco MA, Cook MB, Fraumeni JF Jr, Hoover RN. Increased risk of non-fatal myocardial infarction following testosterone therapy prescription in men. *PLoS One.* 2014;**9**(1):e85805.

29. Snyder PJ, Bhasin S, Cunningham GR, Matsumoto AM, Stephens-Shields AJ, Cauley JA, Gill TM, Barrett-Connor E, Swerdloff RS, Wang C, Ensrud KE, Lewis CE, Farrar JT, Cella D, Rosen RC, Pahor M, Crandall JP, Molitch ME, Cifelli D, Dougar D, Fluharty L, Resnick SM, Storer TW, Anton S, Basaria S, Diem SJ, Hou X, Mohler ER III, Parsons JK, Wenger NK, Zeldow B, Landis JR, Ellenberg SS; Testosterone Trials Investigators. Effects of testosterone treatment in older men. *N Engl J Med.* 2016;**374**(7):611–624.

30. Snyder PJ, Bhasin S, Cunningham GR, Matsumoto AM, Stephens-Shields AJ, Cauley JA, Gill TM, Barrett-Connor E, Swerdloff RS, Wang C, Ensrud KE, Lewis CE, Farrar JT, Cella D, Rosen RC, Pahor M, Crandall JP, Molitch ME, Resnick SM, Budoff M, Mohler ER III, Wenger NK, Cohen HJ, Schrier S, Keaveny TM, Kopperdahl D, Lee D, Cifelli D, Ellenberg SS. Lessons from the Testosterone Trials. *Endocr Rev.* 2018;**39**(3):369–386.

31. Budoff MJ, Ellenberg SS, Lewis CE, Mohler ER III, Wenger NK, Bhasin S, Barrett-Connor E, Swerdloff RS, Stephens-Shields A, Cauley JA, Crandall JP, Cunningham GR, Ensrud KE, Gill TM, Matsumoto AM, Molitch ME, Nakanishi R, Nezarat N, Matsumoto S, Hou X, Basaria S, Diem SJ, Wang C, Cifelli D, Snyder PJ. Testosterone treatment and coronary artery plaque volume in older men with low testosterone. *JAMA.* 2017;**317**(7):708–716.

32. Basaria S, Harman SM, Travison TG, Hodis H, Tsitouras P, Budoff M, Pencina KM, Vita J, Dzekov C, Mazer NA, Coviello AD, Knapp PE, Hally K, Pinjic E, Yan M, Storer TW, Bhasin S. Effects of testosterone administration for 3 years on subclinical atherosclerosis progression in older men with low or low-normal testosterone levels: a randomized clinical trial. *JAMA.* 2015;**314**(6):570–581.

33. Morden NE, Woloshin S, Brooks CG, Schwartz LM. Trends in testosterone prescribing for age-related hypogonadism in men with and without heart disease [published online ahead of print 28 December 2018]. *JAMA Intern Med.* doi:10.1001/jamainternmed.2018.6505.

34. Wittert G, Atlantis E, Allan C, Bracken K, Conway A, Daniel M, Gebski V, Grossmann M, Hague W, Handelsman DJ, Inder W, Jenkins A, Keech A, McLachlan R, Robledo K, Stuckey B, Yeap BB. Testosterone therapy to prevent type 2 diabetes mellitus in at-risk men (T4DM): design and implementation of a double-blind randomized controlled trial. *Diabetes Obes Metab.* 2019;1–9.

35. Shores MM, Biggs ML, Arnold AM, Smith NL, Longstreth WT Jr, Kizer JR, Hirsch CH, Cappola AR, Matsumoto AM. Testosterone, dihydrotestosterone, and incident cardiovascular disease and mortality in the cardiovascular health study. *J Clin Endocrinol Metab.* 2014;**99**(6):2061–2068.

36. Ponce OJ, Spencer-Bonilla G, Alvarez-Villalobos N, Serrano V, Singh-Ospina N, Rodriguez-Gutierrez R, Salcido-Montenegro A, Benkhadra R, Prokop LJ, Bhasin S, Brito JP. The efficacy and adverse events of testosterone replacement therapy in hypogonadal men: a systematic review and meta-analysis of randomized, placebo-controlled trials. *J Clin Endocrinol Metab.* 2018;**103**(5):1745–1754.

Fertility Considerations in Gender-Nonconforming Adolescents and Adults

M31
Presented, March 23–26, 2019

Jackie Gutmann, MD. Reproductive Medicine Associates of Philadelphia, King of Prussia, Pennsylvania 19406; and Department of Obstetrics and Gynecology, Thomas Jefferson University Hospital, Philadelphia, Pennsylvania 19107, E-mail: jackieg@rmaphiladelphia.com

CLINICAL SIGNIFICANCE

Gender nonconformity refers to the extent to which a person's gender identity, role, or expression differs from the cultural norms prescribed for people of a particular sex (1). Gender dysphoria refers to discomfort or distress caused by a discrepancy between a person's gender identity and that person's sex assigned at birth (2). Treatment is available to assist people with gender dysphoria in exploring their gender identity and finding a gender role with which they are comfortable. Both hormone and/or surgical therapy are available treatment options to facilitate social gender role transition as well as to allow the person to live in accordance with the gender experienced.

These interventions often have a negative effect on fertility. The World Professional Association of Transgender Health Standards of Care version 7 recommends that all health care professionals caring for persons with gender dysphoria should discuss reproductive options with patients prior to initiation of medical treatment (3).

Over time, awareness of the prevalence of persons identifying as gender nonconforming has increased dramatically, highlighting the importance of addressing fertility concerns in this population. When it was published in 1980, the 3rd edition of Diagnostic and Statistical Manual of Mental Disorders described the occurrence of gender identity disorder as "apparently rare" (4). More recently, the 5th edition of Diagnostic and Statistical Manual of Mental Disorders reported that the prevalence of male-to-female gender dysphoria was between 5 and 14 per 1000 adult males (0.5% to 1.4%) and between 2 and 3 per 1000 adult females (0.2% to 0.3%) for female-to-male gender dysphoria (5). It is unclear if the increase in prevalence is a true increase or simply a function of wider acceptance of people "coming out" as gender nonconforming. Recent data suggest that as many as approximately one in 200 adults in the United States self-identify as transgender (4). This underscores the importance of addressing fertility concerns in gender-nonconforming persons.

There is little research investigating the opinions of transgender persons regarding fertility preservation and parenting. However, what does exist suggests that if given the opportunity, many would consider gamete cryopreservation and would like to have the opportunity to have a biological child (6–8).

As simplistic as this may sound, at the time of this writing, three elements are required to achieve a pregnancy: oocytes, sperm, and uterus. The means by which an individual or couple builds their family will depend upon a number of factors, including the availability of gametes from the individual who has had or is planning a gender transition, whether they are partnered, and if so, the sex and available gametes (and potentially a uterus) of the individual with whom they are partnered. Although this discussion will focus on fertility and the use of assisted reproductive technologies to facilitate family building, there are other family-building pathways available (*e.g.*, adopting and fostering children). In addition, there will be individuals, both gender nonconforming and gender conforming, who elect child-free living.

BARRIERS TO OPTIMAL PRACTICE

It is apparent that the assertion that gender is not binary is receiving greater societal acceptance. This is in part evidenced by the fact that many professional societies, including the Endocrine Society, have published Committee Opinions and Clinical Practice Guidelines (9–11). It also seems that there is greater recognition that the fertility needs of gender-nonconforming individuals must be met, as evidenced by the recent World Professional Association of Transgender Health guidelines as well as the fact that fertility clinics are now providing information about transgender fertility care on their Web sites (12). Despite this, there is probably still reluctance in many situations for individuals to disclose their gender identity or for providers to have the will or tools necessary to address their transgender patients' fertility needs.

Many factors play a role in limiting patient access to fertility services, including lack of provider and patient education as well as cost, concerns related to the harvesting of gametes (masturbation for transwomen and invasiveness of oocyte cryopreservation cycle), and the desire to avoid a delay in initiating transition (13).

LEARNING OBJECTIVES

As a result of participating in this session, learners should be able to:
- Review the impact of hormone therapy and gender-affirming surgery on fertility
- Discuss options for oocyte or sperm banking prior to initiation of medical transition
- Describe fertility options after people have initiated hormone therapy and/or had some gender-affirming surgery

STRATEGIES FOR MANAGEMENT

Impact of Hormone Therapy and Gender-Affirming Surgery on Fertility: Transwomen

In transwomen, orchiectomy (with or without penectomy) will result in permanent infertility. Although amputation of the penis without orchiectomy will not result in sterility (sperm could be retrieved from the testes), these procedures are typically performed simultaneously.

The impact of estrogen therapy on testicular morphology and semen quality in transwomen is variable. Although some patients demonstrated severe involution of spermatogenesis as well as of Leydig cells, others maintained complete spermatogenesis with normal Leydig cell number (14). There are few data evaluating the return of testicular function after discontinuing estrogen therapy. Given the available data, one must presume that estrogen therapy in transwomen can result in substantial and potentially irreversible infertility.

Impact of Hormone Therapy and Gender-Affirming Surgery on Fertility: Transmen

In transmen, hysterectomy and oophorectomy would render the patient sterile. Hysterectomy alone allows use of a person's oocytes, although a gestational surrogate would be required to carry the pregnancy. Oophorectomy without hysterectomy, which is not commonly performed as a part of gender-affirming surgery, would allow an individual to carry a pregnancy but would require oocytes to come from another source (*e.g.*, a cisfemale partner or oocyte donor).

Masculinizing hormonal therapy typically causes amenorrhea, but generally does not result in depletion of oocytes (15). Although there are few data assessing oocyte function, there is a suggestion that increased androgen levels associated with gender-affirming hormonal therapy in transmen may adversely affect follicular development (16). More recently, histologic evaluation of ovarian tissue in transmen after >1 year of testosterone treatment demonstrated surprisingly normal cortical follicular distribution (13). Despite this reassuring information, transmen who intend to initiate hormone therapy should be counseled that their fertility may be compromised.

On the other hand, there are transmen who have conceived after having received or even while currently receiving testosterone therapy (17). Although some of these pregnancies were intended, many were not. Patients must be counseled that exogenous testosterone is not an adequate method of birth control and that given the possible adverse effects of exogenous testosterone on a developing fetus (especially if female), steps should be taken to avoid pregnancy. Although the study was not designed or powered to compare the risk of pregnancy-related complications in transmen with prior testosterone use, it seems that the rate of such complications is greater than in the general population. With respect to contraception, an intrauterine device would be an appropriate contraceptive method.

STRATEGIES FOR MAXIMIZING FERTILITY

Given the potential negative impact of gender-affirming hormone therapy and the definitive impact of gonadectomy, the ability to preserve gametes prior to the initiation of therapy is ideal. Unfortunately, this is not always possible. Gamete and embryo cryopreservation, as well as pregnancy, can be attempted after the initiation of hormone therapy.

Fertility Options: Transwomen

Fertility preservation options for transwomen include cryopreservation of sperm collected via ejaculation or cryopreservation of testicular tissue obtained by open biopsy or percutaneous aspiration. If hormone therapy has already been initiated, it must be discontinued for at least 3 months prior to attempting to collect a semen sample. It is possible that a longer time period will be required, and as noted earlier, normal sperm production after hormone therapy may never resume.

The cryopreservation of ejaculated sperm is the simplest and most reliable method of male fertility preservation. This option is only available to postpubertal individuals. The provider must be aware that postpubertal transwomen may find it difficult to masturbate to produce a semen sample for cryopreservation. This must be taken into consideration when counseling patients about fertility preservation options. The use of vibratory stimulation is available to facilitate collection. If collection is not possible via ejaculation, sperm can be obtained directly from the testicle, either by open biopsy or percutaneously via testicular sperm extraction.

After ejaculated sperm is cryopreserved, it is probable that storage in liquid nitrogen will maintain viability of the sperm indefinitely. Pregnancy using sperm stored for approximately 40 years has been reported (18). Depending on the sperm quality and assuming that the transwoman is partnered with a ciswoman (or any individual who has a uterus and ovaries), the cryopreserved sperm can be used for intrauterine insemination (IUI) or *in vitro* fertilization with intracytoplasmic sperm injection (IVF/ICSI). If the transwoman is partnered with a cisman or a partner who does not have a uterus and/or ovaries, or elects to parent without a partner, donor oocytes and/or a gestational surrogate will be necessary. Sperm obtained directly from the testicle will require IVF/ICSI.

Cryopreservation of testicular tissue obtained via testicular sperm extraction or biopsy is required in individuals who have not fully entered puberty prior to gonadal suppression and gender-affirming hormone therapy. This is considered experimental. To date, no pregnancies have been reported using cryopreserved testicular tissue from an immature testis (19).

Fertility Options: Transmen

Current fertility preservation options include cryopreservation of oocytes, embryos, or ovarian tissue. If hormone therapy has already been initiated, it must be discontinued prior to ovarian stimulation for oocyte retrieval. Typically, it would be appropriate to wait for at least one normal menstrual cycle (in the cycling patient). This often requires approximately 2 months.

With the advent of improved cryopreservation techniques, oocytes do not require fertilization before they are cryopreserved. This obviates the need for a partner or the use of donor sperm at the moment of the fertility preservation procedure. Technological improvements in oocyte cryopreservation have improved outcomes such that the success rate of oocyte cryopreservation has risen to the point that IVF pregnancy rates are similar to those achieved with fresh oocytes. Oocyte to embryo efficiency, however, may be somewhat less with cryopreserved oocytes (20).

Oocyte cryopreservation requires ovarian stimulation using gonadotropin therapy to mature multiple follicles. Monitoring the response to ovarian stimulation necessitates frequent blood work and ultrasounds, which are typically performed transvaginally. This process was shown to have a negative impact on gender dysphoria because the procedures involved are closely linked to their female assigned sex at birth (21). It is imperative that this is taken into consideration and may require some modification, including performing ultrasounds transabdominally. After ovarian follicles are adequately stimulated, which typically requires 9 to 12 days of subcutaneous injections, oocyte retrieval is performed. Next, the oocytes are vitrified, which is an ultra-rapid cryopreservation technique. Although oocyte cryopreservation is a relatively new procedure, it is probable (as it is with sperm) that oocytes can be cryopreserved indefinitely.

When the oocytes are ready to be used, they need to be warmed and then exposed to sperm. Because the zona pellucida hardens during the vitrification process, ICSI must be performed. The source of sperm could be a cismale partner or donor sperm. Next, the embryos are cultured in the IVF laboratory until they reach the blastocyst stage. A resulting embryo is then transferred into a uterus that has been appropriately prepared with hormones. The uterus could belong to the transman if he has not undergone hysterectomy, a cisfemale partner, or a gestational surrogate.

The process for obtaining oocytes for embryo cryopreservation is identical to that used for oocyte cryopreservation. After being obtained, oocytes are inseminated with sperm from a cismale partner, donor sperm, or perhaps from a transfemale partner. The embryos are cryopreserved after they reach the blastocyst stage. When they are ready to be used, typically a single embryo is thawed and transferred into an appropriate uterus. As with gametes, it is probable that embryos can be cryopreserved indefinitely. The longest known frozen human embryo to result in a successful birth was cryopreserved for approximately 24 years prior to use (22).

Cryopreservation of ovarian tissue obtained via laparoscopy is required in individuals who have not fully entered puberty prior to gonadal suppression and gender-affirming hormone therapy. This procedure is currently considered experimental. There are two reports of live births in patients who underwent ovarian tissue cryopreservation prior to menarche (19). In both cases, the tissue was transplanted into the pelvis of the patient. Additional research into *in vitro* maturation of oocytes and heterotopic ovarian tissue transplantation is ongoing.

MAIN CONCLUSIONS

Family-building options for gender-nonconforming individuals are dependent upon a host of factors. In all cases, sperm, oocytes, and a uterus are required to achieve a pregnancy. Available options are determined by whether gametes were cryopreserved prior to initiation of gender-affirming hormonal or surgical therapy; the possibility of obtaining gametes after initiation of medical therapy; and whether the individual has a partner and if so, the partner's biological sex. Table 1 lists many of the family-building options available to gender-nonconforming individuals, regardless of whether they have

Table 1. Representative Sample of Family-Building Options Available to Gender-Nonconforming Individuals

		Transman	Transwoman
Ciswoman		1. Ciswoman provides oocytes and uterus; donor sperm	1. Transwoman provides sperm; ciswoman provides oocytes and uterus
		2. Transman provides oocytes; ciswoman provides uterus; donor sperm	2. Ciswoman provides oocytes and uterus; donor sperm
		3. Transman provides uterus; ciswoman provides oocytes; donor sperm	
		4. Transman provides oocytes and uterus; donor sperm	
Cisman		1. Transman provides oocytes; cisman provides sperm; gestational surrogate provides uterus	1. Transwoman provides sperm; donor oocytes; gestational carrier provides uterus
		2. Cisman provides sperm; donor oocytes; gestational surrogate provides uterus	2. Cisman provides sperm; donor oocytes; gestational surrogate provides uterus
		3. Cisman provides sperm; traditional surrogate provides oocytes and uterus	3. Transwoman provides sperm; traditional surrogate provides oocytes and uterus
		4. Transman provides oocytes and uterus; cisman provides sperm	4. Cisman provides sperm; traditional surrogate provides oocytes and uterus

preserved gametes and/or still have testes or ovaries. The possibilities listed are not inclusive and presume that the gender-nonconforming individual is partnered with a cis-gendered individual who has functioning gonads or uterus, as appropriate. As stated previously, regardless of origin, making a baby in 2018 (and probably 2019) still requires oocytes, sperm, and a uterus.

CASE STUDIES

Typically, medical or scientific case presentations have right and wrong answers. This is not the case in the realm of family building. The decision to opt for one of many medically appropriate family-building options available not only depends on biological variables (source of oocytes, sperm, and uterus) but also on personal factors, including the desire for biological offspring and financial resources. That being said, there exist guiding principles that should be used when counseling gender-nonconforming persons.

Case 1

C.M., a 27-year-old transwoman, presented for sperm cryopreservation prior to initiating gender-affirming hormonal and surgical therapy. Eight vials of sperm were cryopreserved with a test thaw concentration of 32 million/mL and 65% motility. The morphology at the time of cryopreservation was normal at 7%, Strict Kruger.

Approximately 8 years later, C.M. and her (cisfemale) wife, L.M., are interested in initiating treatment. When discussing the couple's family-building plan, they note that they would like to have two children.

L.M. is a 36-year-old nulligravida with regular menses every 31 days. She has never tried to conceive and has no history of sexually transmitted infections. She is healthy, has not had any surgery, and does not take any medications. She does not smoke or drink, and her family history is noncontributory.

Question 1

The next step in the management of this patient is to:
  A. Assess ovarian reserve
  B. Assess uterotubal anatomy
  C. Prescribe prenatal vitamins
  D. All of the above

Discussion, Question 1

The correct answer is D, all of the above.

All individuals planning to carry a pregnancy should be taking 800 mcg of folic acid, which is contained in all prenatal vitamins, to reduce the risk of neural tube defects.

All patients attempting pregnancy, particularly as they age, should have an assessment of ovarian reserve because the information will help inform decision making. In this case, the couple would like to have two children, and it is probable that L.M. will be at least 38 years old when they attempt their

second pregnancy. If diminished reserve was suspected, more aggressive treatment might be recommended. Ovarian reserve testing would include determination of the level of anti–Müllerian hormone, which is made in the ovary and correlate with oocyte number and antral follicle count, which also correlates with oocyte number. Baseline (typically day 2, 3, or 4 of the cycle) FSH level, which is inversely correlated with likelihood of pregnancy, should also be obtained. It is noteworthy that age remains the most reliable predictor of likelihood of success.

It is important to document normal uterotubal anatomy prior to using a vial of sperm, particularly given that the supply is limited. Typically, uterotubal anatomy is assessed with hysterosalpingography, in which contrast is instilled under pressure into the uterus. If patent, the contrast will then fill the fallopian tubes and spill into the peritoneal cavity.

Case 1 (continued)

L.M. had a normal hysterosalpingogram, and ovarian reserve was good.

Question 2

Treatment options for this couple include:
  A. IUI without ovulation induction medication
  B. IUI with medication
  C. IVF/ICSI
  D. All of the above

Discussion, Question 2

The best answer is D, all of the above.

Given that L.M. is ovulatory and that the quality of the sperm is adequate, it would be reasonable to attempt IUI for two or three cycles. This could be with or without medication, although recent data suggest that ovulation induction does not increase the cycle fecundity rate. IVF/ICSI, which is more complex, more invasive, and significantly more expensive, offers the greatest likelihood of success. Given that there is a limited amount of sperm, this is also a reasonable alternative.

The likelihood of success with any fertility treatment is dependent upon female age, ovarian reserve testing results, quality of sperm, tubal patency, and treatment type. For this couple, the likelihood of success would be approximately 10% per IUI attempt and almost 50% for IVF/ICSI. Data for IVF results according to age are published by the Society for Assisted Reproductive Technology (23).

Cost varies across the country, and out-of-pocket costs depend upon insurance coverage. Many insurance plans will cover diagnostic testing, blood work, and ultrasounds associated with IUI. In the absence of coverage, out-of-pocket costs for monitoring and IUI generally range between $1000 and $2000. Although some states mandate IVF coverage and some companies provide such coverage independent of a state mandate, out-of-pocket costs for IVF (including medications) generally range from $13,000 to $20,000.

Case 1 (continued)

L.M. conceived in the second cycle of IUI (without taking any medications). Unfortunately, the pregnancy was lost at 7 weeks gestation. The couple underwent an additional cycle of IUI without success. Given that only five vials of sperm remained, the couple elected to proceed to IVF. They had a successful pregnancy and also had three embryos cryopreserved for later use. They returned 2 years later and achieved a pregnancy in the frozen embryo transfer cycle. Unfortunately, they subsequently divorced, and a legal battle ensued.

Case 2

S.B. is a 30-year-old amenorrheic transman who has been receiving testosterone treatment for approximately 5 years. He has had top surgery and is planning bottom surgery. He would like the opportunity to have a biological child. S.B. is healthy. His only medication is testosterone, and the only surgery he has had was a bilateral mastectomy.

S.B. is engaged to a 32-year-old cisfemale (A.S.), who has regular menses. She has no history of sexually transmitted infections and is healthy. She does not take any medications and has not had any surgery.

The couple would like to get pregnant in approximately 2 years.

Question 1

The next step in the management of this patient is:
  A. Ask the patient/couple to return for treatment when they are ready to get pregnant
  B. Initiate ovarian stimulation for the purpose of oocyte cryopreservation
  C. Discontinue testosterone, select a sperm donor, await menses, initiate ovarian stimulation, and cryopreserve embryos
  D. Discontinue testosterone, select a sperm donor, await menses, and begin a program of insemination of S.B.

Discussion, Question 1

The best answer is C, which is discontinue testosterone, select a sperm donor, await menses, initiate ovarian stimulation, and cryopreserve embryos.

It would be inappropriate to defer treatment because this would delay completion of S.B.'s transition and also continue to expose his oocytes to additional testosterone, which must be discontinued prior to initiating treatment. Patients who are discontinuing hormone therapy, especially testosterone, should be counseled that they will probably feel poorly until their own gonadal function returns.

Based on the history, there is no evidence that S.B. is interested in becoming pregnant. The most important question is whether oocytes or embryos should be cryopreserved. In this case, because the couple needs donor sperm, it is reasonable to cryopreserve embryos—a strategy that may have a

slightly higher likelihood of success. That being said, an argument could be made to cryopreserve oocytes so as not to commit them to the sperm donor.

Case 2 (continued)

S.B. discontinued testosterone and underwent ovarian stimulation and oocyte retrieval. The couple inseminated the oocytes with donor sperm from a commercial sperm bank. Six embryos were cryopreserved. S.B. reinitiated testosterone. The couple married, and A.S. underwent a program of IUI using the same sperm donor. She had a successful pregnancy in her third IUI. Two years later, A.S. underwent an embryo transfer of a single cryopreserved embryo. Although that pregnancy was lost, she conceived again with the next attempt and delivered a healthy baby. Their children are now 5 and 3 years old, and S.B. still takes testosterone but has not yet had oophorectomy and hysterectomy.

Case 3

J.T. is a 32-year-old transmale who had been on testosterone for 8 years, although had not been using testosterone for approximately 8 months. His menses were regular. He is otherwise healthy and takes no medication. His only surgery was a bilateral mastectomy.

He is married to T.T., who is a 37-year-old transfemale. T.T. had been taking estrogen intermittently for >10 years, but had been off of treatment for almost 1 year. A semen analysis was performed; the concentration was 800,000 million/mL and 22% motility. She is otherwise healthy, and her only surgery was breast implants. The couple was interested in pregnancy.

Question 1

What treatment options are available to this couple (choose all that apply)?
  A. J.T. undergoes insemination with T.T.'s sperm.
  B. J.T. undergoes insemination with donor sperm.
  C. J.T. undergoes ovarian stimulation and oocyte retrieval, IVF/ICSI is performed using T.T.'s sperm, and J.T. carries the pregnancy.
  D. J.T. undergoes ovarian stimulation and oocyte retrieval, IVF/ICSI is performed using T.T.'s sperm, and a gestational surrogate carries the pregnancy.

Discussion, Question 1

Answers B, C, and D are all viable options. Answer A is incorrect because T.T.'s sperm is not adequate for IUI.

In this situation, it was important to the couple to use T.T.'s sperm. J.T. elected to carry the pregnancy rather than using a gestational surrogate. The pregnancy was not considered high risk because J.T. was healthy, his uterine anatomy was normal, and he had not been taking hormones for almost 1 year. That being said, there are nonmedical challenges that may present when a man is pregnant.

Case 3 (continued)

J.T. underwent ovarian stimulation and oocyte retrieval, and the couple conceived in their third treatment cycle. They also have a single cryopreserved embryo. The pregnancy was uncomplicated, and the baby was delivered vaginally at term. J.T. received support from family, friends, and coworkers. Their son is now 3 years old. They are uncertain as to whether they want to grow their family.

References

1. Institute of Medicine. *The Health of Lesbian, Gay, Bisexual, and Transgender People: Building a Foundation for Better Understanding*. Washington, DC: The National Academies Press; 2011.
2. Coleman E, Bockting W, Botzer M, Cohen-Kettenis P, DeCuypere G, Feldman J, Fraser L, Green J, Knudson G, Meyer WJ, Monstrey S, Adler RK, Brown GR, Devor AH, Ehrbar R, Ettner R, Eyler E, Garofalo R, Karasic DH, Lev I, Mayer G, Meyer-Bahlburg H, Hall BP, Pfaefflin F, Rachlin K, Robinson B, Schechter S, Tangpricha V, van Trotsenburg M, Vitale A, Winter S, Whittle S, Wylie KR, Zucker K. Standards of care for the health of transsexual, transgender, and gender-nonconforming people, version 7. *Int J Transgenderism*. 2012;**13**(4):165–232.
3. American Psychiatric Association. *Diagnostic and Statistical Manual of Mental Disorders*, 3rd ed. Arlington, VA: American Psychiatric Press; 1980.
4. American Psychiatric Association. *Diagnostic and Statistical Manual of Mental Disorders*, 5th ed. Arlington, VA: American Psychiatric Press; 2013.
5. Zucker KJ. Epidemiology of gender dysphoria and transgender identity. *Sex Health*. 2017;**14**(5):404–411.
6. De Sutter P, Kira K, Verschoor A, Hotimsky A. The desire to have children and the 101 preservation of fertility in transsexual women. *Int J Transgend*. 2002;**6**(3).
7. Wierckx K, Van Caenegem E, Pennings G, Elaut E, Dedecker D, Van de Peer F, Weyers S, De Sutter P, T'Sjoen G. Reproductive wish in transsexual men. *Hum Reprod*. 2012;**27**(2):483–487.
8. Tornello SL, Bos H. Parenting intentions among transgender individuals. *LGBT Health*. 2017;**4**(2):115–120.
9. Hembree WC, Cohen-Kettenis PT, Gooren L, Hannema SE, Meyer WJ, Murad MH, Rosenthal SM, Safer JD, Tangpricha V, T'Sjoen GG. Endocrine treatment of gender-dysphoric/gender-incongruent persons: an Endocrine Society Clinical Practice Guideline. *J Clin Endocrinol Metab*. 2017;**102**(11):3869–3903.
10. Committee on Adolescent Health Care. Committee Opinion No. 685: Care for Transgender Adolescents. *Obstet Gynecol*. 2017;**129**(1):e11–e16.
11. Ethics Committee of the American Society for Reproductive Medicine. Access to fertility services by transgender persons: an Ethics Committee opinion. *Fertil Steril*. 2015;**104**(5):1111–1115.
12. Jin H, Dasgupta S. Disparities between online assisted reproduction patient education for same-sex and heterosexual couples. *Hum Reprod*. 2016;**31**(10):2280–2284.
13. Chen D, Matson M, Macapagal K, Johnson EK, Rosoklija I, Finlayson C, Fisher CB, Mustanski B. Attitudes toward fertility and reproductive health among transgender and gender-nonconforming adolescents. *J Adolesc Health*. 2018;**63**(1):62–68.
14. Schneider F, Kliesch S, Schlatt S, Neuhaus N. Andrology of male-to-female transsexuals: influence of cross-sex hormone therapy on testicular function. *Andrology*. 2017;**5**(5):873–880.
15. De Roo C, Lierman S, Tilleman K, Peynshaert K, Braeckmans K, Caanen M, Lambalk CB, Weyers S, T'Sjoen G, Cornelissen R, De Sutter P. Ovarian tissue cryopreservation in female-to-male transgender people: insights into ovarian histology and physiology after prolonged androgen treatment. *Reprod Biomed Online*. 2017;**34**(6):557–566.
16. Caanen MR, Soleman RS, Kuijper EA, Kreukels BP, De Roo C, Tilleman K, De Sutter P, van Trotsenburg MA, Broekmans FJ, Lambalk CB. Antimüllerian hormone levels decrease in female-to-male transsexuals using testosterone as cross-sex therapy. *Fertil Steril*. 2015;**103**(5):1340–1345.
17. Light AD, Obedin-Maliver J, Sevelius JM, Kerns JL. Transgender men who experienced pregnancy after female-to-male gender transitioning. *Obstet Gynecol*. 2014;**124**(6):1120–1127.
18. Szell AZ, Bierbaum RC, Hazelrigg WB, Chetkowski RJ. Live births from frozen human semen stored for 40 years. *J Assist Reprod Genet*. 2013;**30**(6):743–744.
19. Burns KC, Hoefgen H, Strine A, Dasgupta R. Fertility preservation options in pediatric and adolescent patients with cancer. *Cancer*. 2018;**124**(9):1867–1876.
20. Argyle CE, Harper JC, Davies MC. Oocyte cryopreservation: where are we now? *Hum Reprod Update*. 2016;**22**(4):440–449.
21. Armuand G, Dhejne C, Olofsson JI, Rodriguez-Wallberg KA. Transgender men's experiences of fertility preservation: a qualitative study. *Hum Reprod*. 2017;**32**(2):383–390.
22. Scutti S. (12/21/2017) The embryo is just a year younger than the mother who birthed her. CNN. Available at: https://www.cnn.com/2017/12/19/health/snowbaby-oldest-embryo-bn/index.html. Accessed 21 January 2019.
23. SART. Final cumulative outcome per egg retrieval cycle. Available at: https://www.sartcorsonline.com/rptCSR_PublicMultYear.aspx?reportingYear=2015. Accessed 21 January 2019.

Evaluation of the Infertile Couple: An Approach by a Couple of Endocrinologists

M37
Presented, March 23–26, 2019

Marcelle I. Cedars, MD. University of California San Francisco, San Francisco, California 94143, E-mail: marcelle.cedars@ucsf.edu

Bradley D. Anawalt, MD. University of Washington School of Medicine, Seattle, Washington 98195, E-mail: banawalt@medicine.washington

SIGNIFICANCE OF THE PROBLEM

Approximately one in eight couples has trouble conceiving or sustaining a pregnancy according to the Centers for Disease Control and Prevention 2006–2010 National Survey of Family Growth. In the United States, infertility is typically defined as the inability to conceive after 1 year, at which time an evaluation should begin. For women >35 years of age, evaluation is advised at 6 months. Although the percentage of women with infertility, and no living children, has increased largely due to the increasing age of first pregnancy, the overall percentage of women with infertility has been relatively stable over several decades. Although infertility is frequently considered a "women's disease," ~35% of couples will have both a male and female etiology of their infertility, with another 10% to 20% having a sole male factor as the identifiable cause.

Normal fertility requires a competent oocyte (requiring normal ovulatory function in the female), a functional sperm (requiring normal endocrinological function and spermatogenic capacity in the male), an anatomic capacity for sperm/egg interaction (functional cervix, uterus, and fallopian tubes in the female and functional vasa, epididymis, and penis in the man), and the capacity for implantation (endocrinological and anatomic uterine environment). Infertility or reduced fecundity (ability to produce a live born) can result from abnormalities in any of these areas. We are aware that today there are many ways to build a family and many types of families. Today we will focus on the endocrinological causes that prevent normal conception for men and women.

BARRIERS TO OPTIMAL PRACTICE

- Delay in attempts at pregnancy (increasing age of the female partner)
- Incomplete understanding of physiology of normal female and male reproductive function
- Cost and lack of access to fertility care, particularly due lack of insurance or underinsurance
- Perception that infertility is caused by the patient or couple (e.g., lifestyle choices such as delay in decision to conceive or exposure to sexually transmitted infections)
- Press/public focus on high tech treatments such as *in vitro* fertilization (IVF) (suggesting these expensive treatments are the only appropriate care and/or are so powerful they can overcome all factors, including age)

LEARNING OBJECTIVES

- Understand the evaluation of the infertile couple
  - ◦ Describe an approach to the anovulatory woman
  - ◦ Delineate the initial evaluation of a man with suspected infertility
- Select treatments that optimize patient physiology and reduce risk
- Summarize the likelihood of live births after treatment of infertility

STRATEGIES FOR DIAGNOSIS, MANAGEMENT, AND TREATMENT
Initial Evaluation of the Infertile Couple

Couples should begin an evaluation if they have not conceived after 1 year of active attempts. This assumes that the woman is having regular cycles and that there have been 12 "ovulatory, exposed" cycles. A woman who has had irregular cycles with long episodes of amenorrhea should begin an evaluation earlier because she is likely anovulatory. A women >35 years old should be evaluated for infertility after 6 months of unsuccessful active attempts.

Both members of an infertile couple should be evaluated, and the couple should be queried on whether they are having frequent (two to three times weekly) vaginal intercourse ("exposure"). A careful history should be taken for each member of the couple for causes of infertility, such as anovulation in the woman or hypogonadism in the man. If the female partner has a history suggestive of anovulation (e.g., fewer than six menstrual cycles per year) and the male partner's history and physical examination do not suggest a cause of infertility, then the evaluation should focus on identifying and treating the cause of anovulation; further evaluation of the man may be deferred.

Approach to Subfertile/Infertile Woman

The evaluation always begins with the woman, as women with normal fecundity usually conceive even with men who have subnormal reproductive function. The first approach to an infertile woman is to characterize the menstrual pattern. A history of regular, cyclic, predictable periods is associated with ovulation in >98% of cases. For women whose cycles are irregular and specifically those women with oligoamenorrhea, a careful history is important. This should begin with the onset of menses and the transition (if any) to irregularity. Additional questions should ascertain the presence or absence of symptoms of hypothyroidism, hyperprolactinemia, hypoestrogenism, and hyperandrogenism. These questions can guide the examination and laboratory investigation. Additionally, the history should focus on factors that would interfere with normal tubal function, such as a history of prior sexually transmitted infections, pelvic surgery, dysmenorrhea, or dyspareunia.

Physical examination of the woman should include assessment of vital signs (may point to thyroid or adrenal dysfunction), presence/absence of hyperandrogenism (hair growth, acne, and androgenic alopecia), thyromegaly, galactorrhea, and evidence of past and current estrogen (breast development and vaginal/cervical lubrication). A pelvic examination to feel the size and mobility of the uterus and any adnexal pain/tenderness should be performed. For those with unexplained infertility (no risk factors) or symptoms of endometriosis, a recto-vaginal examination can reveal uterosacral nodularity/tenderness that might further suggest this diagnosis. Laboratory testing for the anovulatory woman should include thyrotropin (TSH), prolactin, follicle-stimulating hormone (FSH), and estradiol. Additional testing of dehydroepiandrosterone sulfate, testosterone, and luteinizing hormone (LH) may be warranted in certain instances. All women should have an evaluation of ovarian reserve by either serum anti-Mullerian hormone (AMH) or ultrasound-guided antral follicle count.

The two most common causes of anovulation include polycystic ovary syndrome (PCOS), which is characterized by two of the following three: irregular cycles, hyperandrogenism and polycystic-appearing ovaries, and hypogonadotropic hypogonadism, which can be genetic, functional, or due to hypothyroidism or hyperprolactinemia.

For women with PCOS, screening should exclude dyslipidemia, fatty liver, and/or impaired glucose tolerance/diabetes, which may require further assessment, treatment, and/or weight loss prior to conception. For patients that are metabolically normal, ovulation induction is the first treatment approach. Agents that can be used include clomiphene citrate, metformin, and letrozole. Randomized controlled trials have identified letrozole as the most effective first-line treatment. Given intact feedback mechanisms in women with PCOS, only a short course of the "anti-estrogen" letrozole is enough to "jump start" the cycle by increasing FSH and allowing physiological response of the ovaries for development of the dominant follicle. Due to intact feedback from the hypothalamic-pituitary axis, most cycles are followed by ovulation of a single follicle, but a small risk (~5% to 8%) of multiple pregnancy is possible. About 85% of women with PCOS will conceive with these drugs.

For women with hypogonadotropic hypogonadism, the etiology of the low gonadotropins should be identified. Then, the primary source should be treated, including thyroid replacement or reduction in prolactin with dopamine agonists as appropriate. For women with Kallmann syndrome or functional hypothalamic amenorrhea, the ideal treatment is pulsatile administration of gonadotropin-releasing hormone (GnRH). This agent is not available in the United States, but it is under Food and Drug Administration review. Unless pulsatile GnRH becomes available, the standard treatment is the use of exogenous gonadotropins. Gonadotropin therapy is effective, but it is much more likely than GnRH therapy to be complicated by a high risk of multiple pregnancy and ovarian hyperstimulation because it acts directly on the ovaries. Women with hypogonadotropic hypogonadism seem to have a very narrow window between under- and over-response, making dosing quite difficult. Additionally, they typically have a high number of responsive follicles and are at high risk for multiple pregnancy.

Approach to the Subfertile/Infertile Man

Normal fertility in men requires three basic elements: the ability to produce normal sperm (normal germ cells), normal hormonal stimulation of spermatogenesis, and a patent, functional transportation system from the testes to ejaculation within the vagina. The ability to produce sperm requires normal germ cells and normal Leydig cell and Sertoli cell function (to generate high intratesticular testosterone concentrations and nurture spermatogenesis, respectively). LH and FSH are required for normal spermatogenesis, and patent and functional vasa deferentia and ejaculatory tract function are essential for normal delivery of sperm into the vaginal canal.

The evaluation for infertility in men includes a history and physical examination focusing on identifying causes of germ cell loss or absence (*e.g.*, alkylating chemotherapies), primary Leydig cell aplasia or destruction (*e.g.*, Klinefelter syndrome, which also causes germ cell destruction), hypogonadotropic hypogonadism (*e.g.*, due to pituitary tumor, hyperprolactinemia, Cushing syndrome, or androgenic anabolic steroid use), or abnormal sperm transportation (*e.g.*, absence or obstruction of the vasa deferentia or retrograde ejaculation). Any significant acute or chronic systemic medical illness may suppress spermatogenesis significantly due to suppression of the hypothalamopituitary axis or (less commonly) due to direct testicular effects.

The most important aspect of the physical examination is the examination of scrotal contents. Testicular volume is associated with spermatogenesis; very small testes (≤8 mL combined testicular volume) indicate low likelihood of spermatogenesis and is a poor prognostic sign for therapeutic effectiveness. Seminal fluid analysis should be performed in all men with suspected infertility, and many experts recommend measurement of serum testosterone, FSH, and LH in the initial evaluation, too.

A small percentage (<10%) of infertile men have medically treatable causes such as Kallmann syndrome or hypogonadotropic hypogonadism due to another cause. Gonadotropin replacement will improve spermatogenesis in most men with a combined testicular volume >8 mL. Human chorionic gonadotropin (hCG) therapy with or without recombinant human FSH therapy is the usual recommended therapy for men with infertility due to hypogonadotropic hypogonadism. Men with azoospermia without hypogonadotropic hypogonadism should be assessed for ejaculatory tract obstruction; they may have sperm that can be retrieved from the testes by surgical extraction. The treatment of infertility in men with oligospermia is controversial. Assisted reproductive technology is sometimes offered to such men.

MAIN CONCLUSIONS

The elements of the management of the infertile couple are the following:

- It is essential to evaluate members of an infertile couple.
- In the initial evaluation of an infertile couple, establishing whether the female partner is ovulating regularly is the most important question.

  - Young women that are ovulating will generally conceive with a subfertile male; restoration of ovulation in young women who are infertile will often result in conception for a couple.
  - Older women, especially those with diminished ovarian reserve, may have a shortened timeline for conception and should be managed more aggressively. They often require assisted reproductive technology to conceive after a short course of medical therapy and/or intrauterine insemination.
- Women with PCOS are best treated with weight reduction; if this fails to induce ovulation and/or the women is older, ovulation induction with letrozole is indicated.
- Women with hypogonadotropic hypogonadism should have the underlying cause corrected (hypothyroidism, hyperprolactinemia, or weight gain); for women with functional hypothalamic amenorrhea, ovulation induction with pulsatile GnRH is the most effective and physiological.
- Men who are suspected to be infertile should be evaluated with testicular volumetry, serum testosterone and gonadotropin measurement, and seminal fluid analysis.
- Most infertile men do not have a medically treatable cause.
- Men with obstructive azoospermia may have sperm that can be surgically extracted and used for assisted reproductive techniques for fertilization.

STRATEGIES FOR DIAGNOSIS, THERAPY, AND/OR MANAGEMENT: CASES
Case 1: A Young Couple That Consists of a Young Woman With Anovulation and Young Man With Decreased Spermatogenesis Are Having Trouble Conceiving

A couple presents for evaluation. The 28-year-old woman has had oligomenorrhea (fewer than six episodes of menstrual bleeding per year) since puberty. She has mild hirsutism and no history of prior conception. Her 32-year-old husband has no medical illnesses and no history of fathering a child. They have not been able to conceive after 9 months of trying to conceive (vaginal intercourse twice weekly without contraception).

The results of the examination of the woman are as follows (pertinent positives). Her body mass index (BMI) is 28 kg/m^2. The head, eyes, ears, nose, and throat (HEENT) exam reveals no thyromegaly. She has mild hirsutism on her chin and chest and acne on her face, chest, and back. Her waist circumference is 39 inches and she has hair up to her umbilicus. The pelvic exam reveals estrogenized mucus and no masses/tenderness. Her laboratory tests show normal TSH and prolactin levels.

What is the best course of management for this woman?

A. Advise them to keep trying to conceive and increase frequency to four times weekly
B. Measurement of serum AMH in the woman
C. Measurement of serum AMH in the woman and seminal fluid analysis for her husband
D. Trial of letrozole for the woman

Discussion
Answer: D
Although this couple does not meet the US definition of infertility (no conception after 1 year of trying), the woman is very likely anovulatory. Her history and examination indicate that she has PCOS, and a history of fewer than six menstrual cycles per year suggests that most, if not all, of her periods are anovulatory. Given the chronic oligo-anovulation, additional attempts at "trying" will have a very low likelihood for success. (Answer A is incorrect.) AMH will not add to the likely diagnosis of PCOS with anovulation and hyperandrogenism. (Answers B and C are incorrect.) Ovulation induction with the oral agent letrozole is most effective and the correct answer.

Some experts would evaluate this man with a seminal fluid analysis, but healthy young men are more than 90% likely to have a sperm in the ejaculate. Thus, the focus should be treatment of her chronic anovulation and not assessment of the man. All men with a risk factor for infertility, symptoms or signs of hypogonadism, or small testes should be assessed with measurement of serum testosterone and gonadotropins and seminal fluid analysis.

Your female patient calls your office the next day. Her husband was evaluated with a seminal fluid analysis that revealed no sperm.

Of the following, which is the best initial evaluation of the man?

A. Measurement of testicular volume and serum testosterone and gonadotropins
B. Measurement of serum testosterone, gonadotropins, and TSH
C. Measurement of serum testosterone, gonadotropins, TSH, prolactin, and ferritin
D. Measurement of serum testosterone, gonadotropins, TSH, prolactin, and ferritin and testicular ultrasound
E. Referral to an assisted reproductive technology expert for assessment of testicular biopsy for sperm harvesting for intracytoplasmic sperm injection

Discussion
Answer: A

As a general principle, seminal fluid analysis should be done two to three times because there is considerable day to day variation in sperm concentrations. In addition, seminal fluid analysis should be done after between 2 and 7 days of ejaculatory abstinence because sperm concentrations decline with shorter or longer intervals. With azoospermia (no sperm in the ejaculate), a repeat seminal fluid analysis will either show azoospermia or very few sperm.

Testicular volumes should also be assessed by Prader orchidometry. (The least expensive source of Prader orchidometers is through the Endocrine Society store.) Testicular volumes measured by Prader orchidometry are slightly smaller than values obtained by ultrasonography, but the values have a nearly linear correlation. Measurement of serum testosterone and gonadotropins is important to determine whether the man has primary or secondary hypogonadism. Men with high serum gonadotropins have primary hypogonadism and will not respond to medical therapy to increase spermatogenesis. Men with secondary hypogonadism will usually (80% to 85%) have improved spermatogenesis with gonadotropin replacement therapy. Total testicular volumes ≥ 10 mL suggest a much greater likelihood of response to gonadotropin replacement therapy. In men, subcutaneous administration of hCG and rhFSH is as safe as pulsatile subcutaneous GnRH therapy.

Answers B, C, and D are incorrect. Of the options offered, only testicular volume measurement by Prader orchidometry and measurement of serum testosterone and gonadotropin concentrations are part of the standard initial evaluation. Serum TSH is ordered if there is a clinical suspicion of thyroid dysfunction, and prolactin and ferritin are ordered if serum testosterone and gonadotropin concentrations suggest secondary hypogonadism. Testicular ultrasound is ordered if there is a testicular mass or suspicion of ejaculatory tract obstruction. Men should not be sent for possible assisted reproductive technology (answer E) until after an appropriate medical evaluation.

Case 2: A Couple That Consists of a 35-Year-Old Woman With Anovulation and a 31-Year-Old Man With Obstructive Azoospermia Are Having Trouble Conceiving

A couple presents to the office with 5 months of infertility. The 35-year-old female partner has not had a menstrual cycle since she stopped oral contraceptive pills 5 months ago. Her 31-year-old partner is healthy and has no significant medical history and no risk factors for infertility. The woman has always been thin and was a competitive athlete in her teens and twenties. She cycled regularly after puberty but became amenorrheic in high school. She has been on oral contraceptive pills since that time.

The results of the examination of the woman are as follows (pertinent positives). Her pulse is 54 and BMI is 18 kg/m^2. The HEENT exam reveals normal thyroid. She has no hirsutism or acne. The pelvic exam reveals a pale atrophic vaginal mucosa and no cervical mucus. The bimanual examination reveals no pelvic masses/tenderness and a small uterus. The laboratory tests show normal prolactin and TSH, FSH = 3.6, and estradiol = 10 (ultrasensitive assay).

The results of the examination of the man are as follows. He has normal vital signs, his BMI is 33 kg/m^2, and he is well virilized. The HEENT exam reveals a normal thyroid. He has a normal penis, testes that are 20 mL bilaterally with no masses, and no palpable vasa deferentia. The laboratory tests show normal serum testosterone, LH, and FSH, and his seminal fluid reveals azoospermia.

For this woman, which of the following would be the best treatment to improve her fertility?
- A. Pulsatile GnRH therapy
- B. Letrozole
- C. Anastrozole
- D. Recombinant FSH and hCG
- E. Referral to an assisted reproductive technology expert for assessment of ovarian biopsy and IVF

Discussion
Answer: A

Based on this history and laboratories, this patient has hypogonadotropic hypogonadism. This is likely functional in nature. She should be queried about her diet and exercise patterns, and she should be counseled that a slightly higher body weight might be useful for ovulation. However, the appropriate medical treatment is to replace the missing hormone, GnRH. The patient would not be expected to respond to aromatase inhibitors or clomiphene since her serum estradiol is already low. FSH and hCG can be given, but the risk for ovarian hyperstimulation and multiple pregnancy is high in a young, likely otherwise fertile woman, so careful management is required by an experienced provider. Ovarian biopsy would not be indicated, and IVF is reserved for circumstances when single follicular development is not achieved with exogenous gonadotropin and pulsatile GnRH therapy is not available.

For this man, which of the following tests would be the most useful test to determine the cause of his infertility?
- A. Serum AMH
- B. Serum karotype
- C. Testicular ultrasound
- D. Testicular biopsy

Discussion
Answer: C

This man with normal testicular volumes, no palpable vasa deferentia, and normal serum gonadotropins and azoospermia likely has obstructive azoospermia. Infertility due to obstructive azoospermia can be successfully treated with testicular biopsy for sperm extraction followed by fertilization of an ovum with assisted reproductive techniques. Testicular ultrasound (preferably transrectal ultrasound) would confirm obstruction and absence of vasa deferentia. Absence of the vasa deferentia strongly suggests cystic fibrosis. Men may present with infertility and congenital absence of the vasa deferentia as the sole manifestations of a mutation of the cystic fibrosis gene. Such men are offered genetic counseling before undergoing fertility treatment.

AMH is made by the Sertoli cells in men. Serum AMH has an inverse relationship to serum AMH and tends to be low in men with defects in spermatogenesis. It is likely to be normal in this man, and serum AMH never makes a definitive diagnosis of the cause of male infertility. (Answer A is wrong.) This man does not have features of Klinefelter syndrome, and a serum karyotype will not be useful (answer B). Testicular biopsy would be useful for potential sperm extraction should this man opt for treatment of obstructive azoospermia, but the diagnosis of cystic fibrosis in this man would be made by genetic testing. (Answer D is wrong.)

Recommended Reading

Anawalt BD. Approach to male infertility and induction of spermatogenesis. *J Clin Endocrinol Metab.* 2013;**98**(9):3532–3542.

Caroppo E, Colpi EM, Gazzano G, Vaccalluzzo L, Scroppo FI, D'Amato G, Colpi GM. Testicular histology may predict the successful sperm retrieval in patients with non-obstructive azoospermia undergoing conventional TESE: a diagnostic accuracy study. *J Assist Reprod Genet.* 2017;**34**(1):149–154.

Cissen M, Bensdorp A, Cohlen BJ, Repping S, de Bruin JP, van Wely M. Assisted reproductive technologies for male subfertility. *Cochrane Database Syst Rev.* 2016;**2**:CD000360.

Dumont A, Dewailly D, Plouvier P, Catteau-Jonard S, Robin G. Comparison between pulsatile GnRH therapy and gonadotropins for ovulation induction in women with both functional hypothalamic amenorrhea and polycystic ovarian morphology. *Gynecol Endocrinol.* 2016;**32**(12): 999–1004.

Goodman NF, Cobin RH, Futterweit W, Glueck JS, Legro RS, Carmina E; American Association of Clinical Endocrinologists (AACE). American College of Endocrinology (ACE); Androgen Excess and PCOS Society (AES): guide to best practices in the evaluation and treatment of polycystic ovary syndrome – Part 1. *Endocr Pract.* 2015;**21**:1291–1300.

Goodman NF, Cobin RH, Futterweit W, Glueck JS, Legro RS, Carmina E; American Association of Clinical Endocrinologists (AACE). American College of Endocrinology (ACE); Androgen Excess and PCOS Society: Clinical Review: guide to the best practices in the evaluation and treatment of polycystic ovary syndrome – Part 2. *Endocr Pract.* 2015; **21**:1415–1426.

Gordon CM, Ackerman KE, Berga SL, Kaplan JR, Mastorakos G, Misra M, Murad MH, Santoro NF, Warren MP. Functional hypothalamic amenorrhea: an Endocrine Society clinical practice guideline. *J Clin Endocrinol Metab.* 2017;**102**(5):1413–1439.

Gunn DD, Bates GW. Evidence-based approach to unexplained infertility: a systematic review. *Fertil Steril.* 2016;**105**(6):1566–1574.e1.

Legro RS, Barnhart HX, Schlaff WD, Carr BR, Diamond MP, Carson SA, Steinkampf MP, Coutifaris C, McGovern PG, Cataldo NA, Gosman GG, Nestler JE, Giudice LC, Leppert PC, Myers ER; Cooperative Multicenter Reproductive Medicine Network. Clomiphene, metformin, or both for infertility in the polycystic ovary syndrome. *N Engl J Med.* 2007; **356**(6):551–566.

Legro RS, Brzyski RG, Diamond MP, Coutifaris C, Schlaff WD, Casson P, Christman GM, Huang H, Yan Q, Alvero R, Haisenleder DJ, Barnhart KT, Bates GW, Usadi R, Lucidi S, Baker V, Trussell JC, Krawetz SA, Snyder P, Ohl D, Santoro N, Eisenberg E, Zhang H; NICHD Reproductive Medicine Network. Letrozole versus clomiphene for infertility in the polycystic ovary syndrome. *N Engl J Med.* 2014;**371**(2):119–129.

Ribeiro MA, Gameiro LF, Scarano WR, Briton-Jones C, Kapoor A, Rosa MB, El Dib R. Aromatase inhibitors in the treatment of oligozoospermic or azoospermic men: a systematic review of randomized controlled trials. *JBRA Assist Reprod.* 2016;**20**(2):82–88.

Shoshany O, Abhyankar N, Mufarreh N, Daniel G, Niederberger C. Outcomes of anastrozole in oligozoospermic hypoandrogenic subfertile men. *Fertil Steril.* 2017;**107**(3):589–594.

Showell MG, Mackenzie-Proctor R, Brown J, Yazdani A, Stankiewicz MT, Hart RJ. Antioxidants for male subfertility. *Cochrane Database Syst Rev.* 2014;**12**(12):CD007411.

Smith JF, Walsh TJ, Turek PJ. Ejaculatory duct obstruction. *Urol Clin North Am.* 2008;**35**(2):221–227, viii.

Stokes VJ, Anderson RA, George JT. How does obesity affect fertility in men - and what are the treatment options? *Clin Endocrinol (Oxf).* 2015; **82**(5):633–638.

Sunderam S, Kissin DM, Crawford SB, Folger SG, Jamieson DJ, Barfield WD; Centers for Disease Control and Prevention (CDC). Assisted reproductive technology surveillance--United States, 2011. *MMWR Surveill Summ.* 2014;**63**(10):1–28.

Tranoulis A, Laios A, Pampanos A, Yannoukakos D, Loutradis D, Michala L. Efficacy and safety of pulsatile gonadotropin-releasing hormone therapy among patients with idiopathic and functional hypothalamic amenorrhea: a systematic review of the literature and a meta-analysis. *Fertil Steril.* 2018;**109**(4):708.e8–719.e8.

What's New in Anabolic Steroid and SARMS Abuse?

M38
Presented, March 23–26, 2019

Richard J. Auchus, MD, PhD. Metabolism, Endocrinology, and Diabetes/Internal Medicine and Pharmacology, University of Michigan and Ann Arbor VA Medical Center, Ann Arbor, Michigan 48109, E-mail: rauchus@med.umich.edu

SIGNIFICANCE OF THE CLINICAL PROBLEM

Anabolic-androgen steroid (AAS) abuse has been prevalent among elite athletes since the 1950s. The organized, state-sponsored East German androgen doping program exemplifies the early years of AAS abuse: clandestine and limited, with the medical community largely oblivious to the phenomenon. Since then, the scope of the problem has grown dramatically and taken on several facets. AAS doping remains prevalent in elite and professional sports despite sophisticated antidoping programs for the simple fact that AAS are very inexpensive and effective performance-enhancing substances. More relevant to the practicing endocrinologist, the majority of AAS users are not elite athletes but recreational athletes, bodybuilders, or nonathletes who take these drugs to acquire a larger and more muscular physique more than to improve sports performance.

It is estimated that there are 3 million AAS users in the United States today. With a population of 328 million, that is 1/1,000, about the prevalence of primary hyperparathyroidism and more than all patients with HIV and type 1 diabetes mellitus combined. Hardly any of these are elite or professional athletes. It is also estimated that 6% of US high school students have experimented with AAS, and rates are similar in other developed countries. Most of these users simply want to look "buff," but in an important subset of men and boys, the use is driven from an underlying distorted body image. This condition is known as "muscle dysmorphia" or "reverse anorexia nervosa." These men perceive themselves as being "too small," when in fact they are large and muscular by normative standards. They exercise and diet compulsively, and they are paradoxically uncomfortable removing their shirts in public for embarrassment of their perceived scrawny physique. AAS use increases their size, and withdrawal feeds into their abnormal perception of body image, thus perpetuating AAS use.

Chronic AAS use causes hypothalamic-pituitary-gonadal axis suppression, infertility, acne, and, with oral androgens, dyslipidemia. Less well-defined or predictable side effects include mood changes and irritability or outright manic behavior, prostate enlargement, polycythemia, and cardiovascular complications. The evidence supporting increased venous thrombosis, atherosclerosis, cardiovascular events, or cerebrovascular events is controversial and limited, although reports of relatively young and otherwise healthy men having these complications without other likely cause raise concern. Strong evidence has accumulated that AAS users develop a hypertrophic, restrictive cardiomyopathy, particularly among current users. Women who take androgens also experience breast atrophy, clitoral enlargement, hirsutism, menstrual irregularities and infertility, and voice deepening. Some women who chronically use AAS develop painful polycystic ovaries. A large cohort of chronic AAS users is now reaching middle age, and the consequences of prior AAS and its impact on common age-related morbidities will become more apparent in coming years.

Finally, much like renegade pain clinics fueling the opiate epidemic, charlatan physicians are fueling the AAS epidemic with the indiscriminate prescription of testosterone for men who do not meet the FDA-approved indication for therapy: a low testosterone in association with a causative medical condition. These men are now committed to lifelong testosterone replacement and unknown complications. Furthermore, AAS and selective androgen receptor modulators (SARMs) are widely available on the internet without prescription, although the purity and integrity of these preparations are highly variable.

BARRIERS TO OPTIMAL PRACTICE
- The paucity of good clinical studies about AAS abuse
- Limited training in AAS abuse in residency and fellowship programs
- Reluctance of AAS patients to engage doctors or participate in clinical research
- Plethora of drugs and regimens, easily accessed on the internet and dubious quality
- No funding from National Institutes of Health for AAS abuse

LEARNING OBJECTIVES
As a result of participating in this session, learners should be able to:
- Compare anabolic steroid use patterns for elite athletes and recreational users
- List common sources of androgens and SARMs for illicit acquisition
- Review the data on cardiovascular complications of androgen doping

STRATEGIES FOR DIAGNOSIS AND MANAGEMENT
It is generally not difficult to identify an AAS user when a man presents for medical attention due to a complication from their habit, but it is often difficult to identify the average user in public. As a general rule, AAS users vigorously deny their

practice to the point of absurdity, similar to the sagas of Floyd Landis, Marion Jones, and Barry Bonds. AAS use is the leading, and perhaps only, diagnosis in a young man with atrophic testes, suppressed gonadotropins and testosterone, and bulky musculature. Commercial laboratories that offer urine AAS testing include NMS Laboratories, Aegis® Sciences, and now also ARUP Laboratories and Quest Diagnostics™; however, the ethics of ordering such testing without informing the patient is questionable.

It is difficult to establish rapport with these patients when they are not forthcoming with information and have no motivation to change their habits. Acknowledging the value of fitness and exercise is a starting point. The "scare tactic" warning of AAS side effects rarely works in these men unless they are presenting specifically for one of these complications. A matter-of-fact and direct but firm approach tends to make progress, but goals and the role of the endocrinologist need to be established early.

If discontinuation is desired, which is rarely the case, then switching to testosterone with a clearly defined taper and no refills prescribed without follow-up visits is the only way to stay on trajectory. Users will always want to take more and to taper more slowly, but the plan needs to be firm and agreed upon, much like narcotic withdrawal agreements. Switching to human chorionic gonadotropin (hCG) injections and/or clomiphene or aromatase inhibitors once physiologic dosing is achieved will stimulate endogenous testosterone production. The Leydig cells respond to hCG after just a few doses despite prior AAS use; however, hCG does not drive the central components of the axis to recover. Clomiphene and aromatase inhibitors relieve the negative feedback of estrogens and might help to stimulate gonadotropin production. Beyond these general statements, little is known about the best dosing and monitoring regimens for these patients. Sperm will not be found in the ejaculate for at least 4 months and often never recovers.

MAIN CONCLUSIONS/POINTS OF INTEREST/CLINICAL PEARLS

- AAS abuse is widespread, and most users are not professional or elite athletes.
- Prior or current AAS abuse is a common cause of infertility and testosterone insufficiency.
- AAS abusers do not trust the medical profession, except for charlatan physicians who indiscriminately prescribe AAS for personal profit.
- Optimal strategies for medically supervised AAS withdrawal and recovery of testicular function are not known.
- Long-term consequences of chronic AAS use are not known.

CASE DISCUSSIONS
Case 1
A 27-year-old white male presents for evaluation of azoospermia with his wife. She does much of the talking while he

paces impatiently. They have been married for 2 years and have had unprotected intercourse several times a week, but she has not conceived. She has regular monthly menses and no medical problems. His libido is strong, or as his wife describes "hard to control." He served in the military for 14 months but was dishonorably discharged after insubordination with his commanding officer. He has held various short-term jobs since then but spends 2 to 3 hours weightlifting four times a week. He is a very picky eater and uses a variety of supplements, which he did not bring.

Physical Examination
The patient's blood pressure is 160/90, heart rate 85, weight 283 lbs, height 5'10", and body fat by bioimpedance 4%. The patient is a muscular, irritable man wearing a heavy sweatshirt that he is reluctant to remove. He has a 2/4 holosystolic cardiac murmur, pustular acne on his back, firm sterile abscesses on thighs and buttocks, shaved pubic hair, testes <4 mL bilateral, normal circumcised phallus, and no varicocele.

Laboratory Data
The patient's testosterone is <20 ng/dL, LH <0.1 IU/L, and FSH <0.3 IU/L. His prolactin, thyroid function tests, and cortisol are all normal. His hematocrit is 58%. The results of the semen analysis are as follows: 1.2 mL, fructose positive, and no sperm on spun specimen.

Questions
1. What is the most likely cause of his infertility?
    A. Klinefelter syndrome
    B. Pituitary tumor
    C. AAS use
    D. Narcotic use
    E. Vas deferens obstruction
2. How would you approach the patient?
3. What treatment would you recommend?

Answers
1. C.
2. The approach was discussed above. I will share some of the approaches I have taken, and the audience will be asked to share theirs.
3. As discussed above, the patient has to relinquish control of treatment to the endocrinologist. If he is not willing to do so, there is no physician-patient relationship as a basis for management.

Case 2
A 46-year-old white male presents to your office to establish care for hypogonadism. Growth and puberty were normal, and he fathered three children with this wife, the youngest being

15 years old. He is an avid cyclist, and 3 years ago he noticed that he "just could not hit the times he used to." He felt that something was wrong and saw a "Men's Health Clinic," which was not covered by his insurance. The clinic practitioners did a wide battery of serum and saliva testing, and he was told that his problem was "low testosterone" due to "idiopathic hypogonadotropic hypogonadism." He was treated with Androgel 1.62%, at first two pumps per day. He states that he immediately felt markedly better with more energy, although his cycling times only improved slightly. After 8 months, he started to notice fatigue again and returned to the clinic, where his dose was increased to three pumps and then 6 months later four pumps per day. He lost his job a year later, claiming that there were "conflicts at work" and that he had a "false-positive drug test." He can no longer afford to see the clinic, and he has insurance from his wife's job, so he is asking you to refill his scripts. He is also asking for you to fill out a therapeutic use exemption application so he can comply with USA Cycling's RaceClean Program that prohibits the use of performance-enhancing substances without a medical indication.

Physical Examination

The patient's blood pressure is 144/88, heart rate 56, weight 185 lbs, and height 5′9″. The patient is a lean, muscular man with rushed speech. He has normal strength, hyperactive reflexes, fine tremor, and dilated pupils. He has normal thyroid and sinus bradycardia. His testicles are 6 mL and soft bilateral.

Laboratory Data

The patient's testosterone is 1,220 ng/dL with SHBG 27 mmol/L, LH <0.1 IU/L, FSH <0.3 IU/L, and hematocrit 54%.

Questions

1. Does his prescription meet the Food and Drug Administration (FDA)–approved indication for testosterone therapy?
   A. Yes
   B. No
2. Is he doping?
   A. Yes
   B. No
3. Are you going to refill his script and support his therapeutic use exemption application?

Answers

1. B.
2. A.

3. Testosterone doping among recreational athletes is under-recognized as a form of medically condoned doping and drug abuse, due to charlatan physicians who profit from these patients. As a community, endocrinologists need more protection and resources to deal with these drug abusers and their addictions. There are subtle clues that he has moved on to abusing other drugs as well.

Recommended Reading

Baggish AL, Weiner RB, Kanayama G, Hudson JI, Lu MT, Hoffmann U, Pope HG, Jr. Cardiovascular toxicity of illicit anabolic-androgenic steroid use. *Circulation.* 2017;**135**(21):1991–2002.

Goldman AL, Pope HG, Jr, Bhasin S. The health threat posed by the hidden epidemic of anabolic steroid use and body image disorders among young men [published online ahead of print 17 September 2018]. *J Clin Endocrinol Metab.* doi:10.1210/jc.2018-01706.

Kanayama G, Brower KJ, Wood RI, Hudson JI, Pope HG, Jr. Anabolic-androgenic steroid dependence: an emerging disorder. *Addiction.* 2009;**104**(12):1966–1978.

Kanayama G, Brower KJ, Wood RI, Hudson JI, Pope HG, Jr. Treatment of anabolic-androgenic steroid dependence: Emerging evidence and its implications. *Drug Alcohol Depend.* 2010;**109**(1-3):6–13.

Kanayama G, Hudson JI, DeLuca J, Isaacs S, Baggish A, Weiner R, Bhasin S, Pope HG, Jr. Prolonged hypogonadism in males following withdrawal from anabolic-androgenic steroids: an under-recognized problem. *Addiction.* 2015;**110**(5):823–831.

Kanayama G, Pope HG, Jr. History and epidemiology of anabolic androgens in athletes and non-athletes. *Mol Cell Endocrinol.* 2018;**464**:4–13.

Kaufman MJ, Janes AC, Hudson JI, Brennan BP, Kanayama G, Kerrigan AR, Jensen JE, Pope HG, Jr. Brain and cognition abnormalities in long-term anabolic-androgenic steroid users. *Drug Alcohol Depend.* 2015;**152**: 47–56.

Pope HG, Jr, Khalsa JH, Bhasin S. Body image disorders and abuse of anabolic-androgenic steroids among men. *JAMA.* 2017;**317**(1): 23–24.

Pope HG, Jr, Kouri EM, Hudson JI. Effects of supraphysiologic doses of testosterone on mood and aggression in normal men: a randomized controlled trial. *Arch Gen Psychiatry.* 2000;**57**(2):133–140, discussion 155–156.

Pope HG, Jr, Wood RI, Rogol A, Nyberg F, Bowers L, Bhasin S. Adverse health consequences of performance-enhancing drugs: an Endocrine Society scientific statement. *Endocr Rev.* 2014;**35**(3):341–375.

Snyder PJ, Bhasin S, Cunningham GR, Matsumoto AM, Stephens-Shields AJ, Cauley JA, Gill TM, Barrett-Connor E, Swerdloff RS, Wang C, Ensrud KE, Lewis CE, Farrar JT, Cella D, Rosen RC, Pahor M, Crandall JP, Molitch ME, Cifelli D, Dougar D, Fluharty L, Resnick SM, Storer TW, Anton S, Basaria S, Diem SJ, Hou X, Mohler ER III, Parsons JK, Wenger NK, Zeldow B, Landis JR, Ellenberg SS; Testosterone Trials Investigators. Effects of testosterone treatment in older men. *N Engl J Med.* 2016;**374**(7):611–624.

Van Wagoner RM, Eichner A, Bhasin S, Deuster PA, Eichner D. Chemical composition and labeling of substances marketed as selective androgen receptor modulators and sold via the Internet. *JAMA.* 2017;**318**(20): 2004–2010.

Wood RI, Johnson LR, Chu L, Schad C, Self DW. Testosterone reinforcement: intravenous and intracerebroventricular self-administration in male rats and hamsters. *Psychopharmacology (Berl).* 2004;**171**(3):298–305.

Challenging Cases in the Endocrine Management of Gender Dysphoria and Gender Incongruence

M49
Presented, March 23-26, 2019

Stephen M. Rosenthal, MD. Department of Pediatrics, Division of Pediatric Endocrinology, University of California, San Francisco, San Francisco, California 94143, E-mail: stephen.rosenthal@ucsf.edu

Micol S. Rothman, MD. Department of Medicine, Division of Endocrinology, University of Colorado School of Medicine, Aurora, Colorado 80045, E-mail: micol.rothman@ucdenver.edu

Joshua D. Safer, MD, FACP. Center for Transgender Medicine and Surgery, Mount Sinai Health and Icahn School of Medicine at Mount Sinai, New York, New York 10029, E-mail: jsafer0115@gmail.com

SIGNIFICANCE OF THE CLINICAL PROBLEM

It is well documented that gender-nonconforming individuals face many barriers to optimal health and may avoid seeking needed medical care (1). Despite the recent increased awareness of transgender health, the 2015 US Transgender Survey, which included 27,715 respondents from all 50 US states, reported that 33% of respondents had a negative experience with a health care provider and 23% did not seek medical care because of fears about mistreatment. In addition, 55% of those respondents who sought coverage for transition-related surgery and 25% of those who sought coverage for hormones in the past year were denied (2). Data from the 22 states that asked about transgender identity in the 2015 U.S. Behavioral Risk Factor Surveillance System revealed that transmen were 2.5 times more likely than cismen and almost four times more likely than ciswomen to lack health care coverage (3). Respondents also reported difficulty in finding providers with knowledge of transgender care and are frequently placed in the position of having to educate their health care team. Creating a welcoming environment for patients includes, but is not limited to, provider and staff education, identifying and using patients' preferred names and pronouns, being mindful of protected health information on paper and electronic forms, and establishing gender-neutral facilities.

With their detailed knowledge of hormone physiology and treatment, endocrinologists are uniquely positioned to provide gender-affirming hormone therapy. A 2017 Mayo Clinic and Endocrine Society (ES) Web-based anonymous survey of endocrinology fellowship program directors, with a response rate just higher than 50%, found that 72% of respondents provided teaching on transgender health topics, but 94% indicated that fellowship training in transgender health is important. Of the practicing US medical doctor members of the ES who responded to the same survey (only a 6% response rate), 80% had treated a transgender patient, but 81% had never received formal training in transgender health management (4). These results indicate that competence among endocrinologists needs to increase, especially as the number of patients being referred to endocrinologists rises. Similar themes have emerged with respect to care for transgender youth/adolescents. A 2015 survey of members of the Pediatric Endocrine Society and of the Society for Adolescent Health and Medicine (combined response rate of 21.9%; n = 475) revealed that principal barriers to provision of transgender-related care were lack of the following: adequate training, exposure to transgender patients, available qualified mental health providers, and insurance reimbursement (5).

BARRIERS TO OPTIMAL PRACTICE

Multiple barriers to care exist, including difficulty in accessing care and lack of insurance coverage for gender-affirming hormone therapy and surgery. Of note, none of the recommended medical interventions are labeled for use in gender incongruent and gender dysphoric adolescents, further complicating access to care. Patients may be well informed about options that are not discussed in guidelines and may ask about use of medications that the practicing endocrinologist is not accustomed to prescribing. In addition, some unknowns about the long-term outcomes of patients who receive gender-affirming hormone therapy may add to a provider's discomfort with prescribing.

LEARNING OBJECTIVES

As a result of participating in this session, learners should be able to:

- Identify barriers to care in the treatment of gender-nonconforming patients
- Use the ES guidelines to initiate gender-affirming hormone therapy
- Recognize challenging clinical situations where best practices are not yet known
- Be familiar with long-term data in the field to date, as well as areas that require further research

STRATEGIES FOR DIAGNOSIS, THERAPY, AND/OR MANAGEMENT

The current World Professional Association for Transgender Health (WPATH) and ES guidelines state that the criteria for initiating gender-affirming hormone therapy in adults require persistent and well-documented gender dysphoria and gender incongruence, age of majority and capacity to consent, and that mental health concerns (if present) be reasonably well controlled. Importantly, studies have shown decreases in anxiety and depression in patients after initiation of gender-affirming hormone therapy, and these conditions are certainly not considered contraindications to hormonal treatment. It is also important to note that previous iterations of the ES Clinical Practice Guidelines (CPG) and the WPATH Standards of Care have required real-life experience, but more recent guidelines do not state this as a requirement for initiating gender-affirming hormone therapy. Both the ES and WPATH specify a need for persistent, consistent transgender identity before the initiation of hormone therapy.

On the basis of pioneering work from the Netherlands, the care of transgender youth has been primarily informed by CPG from the ES and cosponsoring organizations and by the Standards of Care from the WPATH. These documents endorse the use of pubertal blockers in gender dysphoric and gender incongruent adolescents using GnRH agonists at Tanner Stage 2 of pubertal development (testicular volume ≥ 4 mL for assigned males at birth; initial stage of breast budding for assigned females at birth). In addition to reaching early puberty, ES criteria for initiation of pubertal blockers include the following: adolescents must meet diagnostic criteria for gender dysphoria and gender incongruence (optimally determined by a qualified mental health gender specialist), any coexisting medical or psychosocial concerns that could interfere with treatment have been addressed, and the adolescent has requested treatment and provided informed assent and the parents or legal guardians have provided informed consent.

GnRH agonists, which are considered fully reversible treatments, pause puberty in this clinical setting. As a result, GnRH agonists provide additional time for gender identity exploration without the pressure of continued pubertal progression and prevent irreversible development of secondary sex characteristics associated with the puberty that is not aligned with the person's gender identity. Such undesired physical changes include prominent Adam's apple, lowered voice, male bone configuration, and potentially tall stature in assigned males at birth. In assigned females at birth, undesired physical changes include breast development, female body habitus, and potentially short stature. Although GnRH agonists are the preferred option for pubertal suppression, this treatment is costly and often inaccessible. Other options for pubertal suppression include depot and oral progestins.

Adolescents who continue to meet the criteria for gender incongruence and gender dysphoria may request phenotypic transition with sex steroids. The most recent version of the ES CPG recommends initiating treatment "using a gradually increasing dose schedule after a multidisciplinary team of medical and mental health professionals has confirmed the persistence of gender dysphoria/gender incongruence and sufficient mental health capacity to give informed consent, which most individuals have by age 16 years." An important change in the current ES CPG is the acknowledgment that there may be compelling reasons to start sex hormone treatment before the age of 16 years in some adolescents with gender incongruence and gender dysphoria.

Typically, the goal of transfeminine treatment is to lower testosterone levels into the female range without resorting to significantly supraphysiologic doses of estrogens. Multiple options for estrogen therapies exist, as noted in the guidelines cited below. Estrogen can be given via an oral, transdermal, or intramuscular route. Transdermal delivery may have an advantage in avoiding first-pass metabolism and stimulation of clotting factors in the liver and is often the treatment route of choice for older individuals. GnRH agonists are also used at times to block production of testosterone; however, these must be given as an injection and can be costly, as noted above. Antiandrogens are often used as an adjunct to estrogen treatment to block the action of testosterone. The antiandrogen of choice in the United States is spironolactone because of its long-term safety profile, arising from its 50-year history as a potassium-sparing diuretic for treatment of hypertension. Higher doses of spironolactone are used to block testosterone than are required for blood pressure control. Often, up to 200 mg/d is used (in divided doses if needed for the patient to tolerate). Cyproterone acetate is not available in the United States, but is used in other parts of the world and probably acts as a more potent testosterone suppressant.

Estradiol levels are expected to increase when using estradiol-based preparations. However, estradiol levels will not reflect the use of conjugated estrogens or ethinyl estradiol. Ethinyl estradiol is no longer recommended for routine use in gender-affirming hormone therapy because it has been associated with adverse events. It is expected that testosterone levels will decline with all types of estrogen therapy. The ES guidelines suggest that estradiol levels should not exceed a peak of 100 to 200 pg/mL and that testosterone levels should be suppressed to less than 50 ng/dL. The ES guidelines also suggest that patients should be evaluated approximately every 3 months (i.e., with dose changes) for the first year with measurements of serum estradiol and testosterone, with the addition of potassium surveillance if receiving spironolactone. Thereafter, assessments and laboratory testing can be done once or twice per year in a stable patient.

For patients with gender incongruence and gender dysphoria who want to pursue masculinizing therapy, testosterone is the mainstay. It is typically given via injection with weekly or every other week dosing. Testosterone can also be administered via transdermal gel or patch depending on patient preference, compliance, insurance coverage, and cost. Testosterone undecanoate has been widely used in Europe for many years. It was introduced in the United States several years ago, but requires a Risk Evaluation and Mitigation

Strategy program due to concerns about pulmonary oil microembolism and anaphylaxis, thereby limiting its use. A GnRH agonist or progestins (via oral delivery, injection, or intrauterine device placement) have been used when menses have persisted beyond the first 6 to 12 months of therapy.

As serum testosterone levels rise, estradiol and gonadotropin levels become suppressed. The ES guidelines suggest aiming for a testosterone level midway between injections of 400 to 700 ng/mL or peaks and troughs inside the physiologic range. The ES guidelines advise monitoring levels approximately every 3 months for the first year (*i.e.*, with dose changes) and then once or twice yearly going forward. The recommendation for routine monitoring of estradiol levels was removed in the 2017 ES guidelines.

The hematocrit level will frequently increase with testosterone therapy and may necessitate a dose reduction or use of alternative agents. Other etiologies of an elevated hematocrit level, such as obstructive sleep apnea and tobacco use, should be investigated. Changes in the lipid profile, with increases in serum triglycerides and low-density lipoprotein cholesterol with concomitant decreases in high-density lipoprotein cholesterol, have been observed. The ES guidelines suggest checking hemoglobin and hematocrit levels at baseline, approximately every 3 months for the first year of testosterone therapy (*i.e.*, with dose changes), and then once or twice yearly. The ES guidelines suggest measuring weight, blood pressure, and lipids at regular intervals.

Age-appropriate primary care and cancer screening should be provided to all patients. It is important to note that cancer screening should be done on the basis of the organs present, *e.g.*, breast, cervix, or prostate.

Although some of the long-term health effects remain unknown, the largest trials to date have reported increased risk of venous thromboembolism (VTE) in transfeminine patients. A recent US study [Study of Transition, Outcomes and Gender (STRONG) cohort], consisting of 6,456 Kaiser Permanente members, reported a higher incidence of VTE among transwomen compared with cisgender patients. Transfeminine participants had a higher incidence of VTE, with 2- and 8-year risk differences of 4.1 (95% CI, 1.6 to 6.7) and 16.7 (95% CI, 6.4 to 27.5) per 1000 persons relative to cisgender men and 3.4 (95% CI, 1.1 to 5.6) and 13.7 (95% CI, 4.1 to 22.7) relative to cisgender women (6). This should not serve as a reason to deny patients gender-affirming hormone therapy, but should be discussed with patients in the context of risks and benefits before initiation of therapy. Among transmasculine patients in the study, there were no significant differences in events relative to the reference populations.

With respect to transgender adolescents, recommended medical treatments have potential adverse effects. The use of GnRH agonists in early pubertal gender-dysphoric adolescents may lead to impaired bone mineralization and compromised fertility, as well as unclear effects on brain development, body mass index (BMI), and body composition. A small number of short-term studies have thus far evaluated potential adverse effects of gender-affirming sex hormones in transgender adolescents. No changes in blood pressure, BMI standard deviation score, lean body mass percentage, or fat percentage were observed in a study of transgender females treated for 1 to 3 years, primarily with gradually increasing doses of 17β-estradiol (7). Hyperprolactinemia was observed in one individual who had received high-dose ethinyl estradiol treatment to limit statural growth (7). In a separate study, following treatment with testosterone in transgender males, there was an increase in BMI and in hemoglobin/hematocrit levels (supraphysiologic hematocrit levels were observed in 4% of individuals) and a decrease in high-density lipoprotein cholesterol levels; no abnormalities were seen in blood pressure, renal and liver function studies, or HbA$_{1c}$ levels (8). Further prospective studies focused on long-term safety and efficacy are necessary to optimize GnRH agonist treatment and gender-affirming sex hormone use in gender-dysphoric and gender-incongruent adolescents.

It should be noted that clinicians more frequently see patients who identify as nonbinary, *i.e.*, not as transmen or transwomen, but along the transmasculine/transfeminine continuum. There are no data to guide the initiation and maintenance of hormone therapy in such patients. However, the authors have some clinical experience in this area, which will be discussed in the case studies. It is anticipated that WPATH Standards of Care Version 8 (in press) will also provide clinicians with some guidance in this area.

Cases
Case 1
A 16-year-old transman has been taking testosterone for 9 months. He is troubled by ongoing uterine bleeding. His BMI is 32 kg/m^2.

Current regimen: 90 mg testosterone weekly

Laboratory results: Total testosterone 810 ng/dL, estradiol 83 pg/mL, LH < 1

Which of the following is least likely to help?

A. Intrauterine levonorgestrel
B. Adjustment of testosterone dose
C. GnRH agonist
D. Aromatase inhibitor

Answer: C

Inducing amenorrhea is a goal for many transmasculine patients because ongoing bleeding can be a source of dysphoria. In most patients, bleeding will stop in 1 to 6 months with the use of testosterone alone because testosterone leads to endometrial atrophy. At times, adjusting the testosterone dose can help. With this patient's testosterone level and LH suppression, a lower dose may decrease aromatase activity. In the case of ongoing bleeding, we generally advise an ultrasound to evaluate for structural issues and to assess the lining. In a patient with ongoing bleeding, estrogen is typically avoided because of concerns about feminizing effects; however, progestogens are on option. Oral norethindrone is often used as first line in the United States, but injectable, intradermal, and intrauterine devices can all be considered. Concerns about the use of these agents include lipid and mood effects, and in the case of long-term injectable treatment, bone density. Other options include GnRH agonists to block FSH and LH production. However, because this patient's LH level is already suppressed, there may not be additional benefit. In obese patients, increased peripheral aromatization to estradiol can be an issue, and there have been case reports of treatment with aromatase inhibitors. We advise caution in this area because of the profound effect seen on bone with use of these agents in other populations, *i.e.*, postmenopausal women with breast cancer. Some patients may ultimately pursue having a hysterectomy after evaluating the risks and benefits and having a discussion regarding future fertility and family planning.

Case 2

A 54-year-old transwoman veteran with a history of hypertension and ongoing tobacco use is seen for follow up on her gender-affirming hormone therapy. She has been on hormone therapy for 2 years. Her current regimen is estradiol patch 2 × 0.100-mcg patches twice weekly and spironolactone 100 mg daily. Her blood pressure is well controlled on an angiotensin-converting enzyme inhibitor. She is also taking a selective serotonin reuptake inhibitor. She has the following questions. 1) I read about bicalutamide on the Internet, and some people like it more than spironolactone—can I try it? 2) Can you give me more information about progesterone for breast growth? 3) My patches irritate my skin. Can I switch to injections?

Bloodwork results: Estradiol 105 pg/mL, testosterone 35 ng/mL. Normal potassium level and liver panel.

Which of the following are true?

A. Progesterone has been shown to improve breast development in transwomen.
B. Bicalutamide has been associated with increases in liver enzymes in cis men treated for prostate cancer.
C. The ES guidelines advise never to use injectable estrogen.
D. Injectable estrogen can help transwomen develop breasts more quickly than oral estrogen.

Answer: B

Patients often have questions about medications that are not well studied. There are no data to support the routine use of progesterone in transwomen for breast growth. One study that evaluated different hormone protocols (with and without progesterone) did not find a difference in rates of requests for breast augmentation among the various protocols (9). Injectable estrogen does not speed up breast development and although it is not generally recommended as first-line therapy in the United States, it is included in the ES guidelines. Although bicalutamide (an androgen receptor antagonist used in the treatment of prostate cancer) has been associated with

increased liver enzymes, patients may ask about its use. Although a recent study showed some improvement in hirsutism in a group of ciswomen with polycystic ovary syndrome treated with an oral contraceptive pill plus bicalutamide (10), we are not aware of any data on using this agent as part of a gender-affirming hormone therapy regimen.

Case 3

A 21-year-old college senior, who was recorded as female at birth, identifies as nonbinary and prefers they pronouns. They have questions about testosterone. They report that they do have dysphoria related to their breasts and bind frequently. They are wondering if they could undergo top surgery/mastectomy and some initiation of testosterone therapy. They are worried about testosterone and male pattern hair loss and do not want to "go all the way."

What are ES recommendations for top surgery?

A. This patient identifies as nonbinary and should not be considered for top surgery.
B. This patient could be considered for top surgery, but only after 1 year of receiving hormones.
C. Hormones are not an absolute requirement for top surgery.
D. This patient is too young to consider top surgery, regardless of hormone use.

Answer: C

ES guidelines note that 1 year of gender-affirming hormone therapy is generally required for surgery, unless the therapy is not desired or is medically contraindicated. In addition, ES guidelines specifically state that the timing for breast surgery should be determined on the basis of the individual patient's physical and mental health status, without a specific age requirement.

This case will serve to discuss the medical and surgical treatment of patients who present as nonbinary.

Several guidelines are referenced above and serve as key reviews on this topic (11–13). Portions of this handout also appear in an upcoming review chapter (14).

References
1. Safer JD, Coleman E, Feldman J, Garofalo R, Hembree W, Radix A, Sevelius J. Barriers to healthcare for transgender individuals. *Curr Opin Endocrinol Diabetes Obes.* 2016;**23**(2):168–171.
2. Vokes T, Lentle B. The ISCD and vertebral fractures. *J Clin Densitom.* 2016;**19**(1):5–7.
3. Nokoff NJ, Scarbro S, Juarez-Colunga E, Moreau KL, Kempe A. Health and cardiometabolic disease in transgender adults in the United States: Behavioral Risk Factor Surveillance System 2015. *J Endocr Soc.* 2018;**2**(4):349–360.
4. Davidge-Pitts C, Nippoldt TB, Danoff A, Radziejewski L, Natt N. Transgender health in endocrinology: current status of endocrinology fellowship programs and practicing clinicians. *J Clin Endocrinol Metab.* 2017;**102**(4):1286–1290.
5. Vance SR Jr, Halpern-Felsher BL, Rosenthal SM. Health care providers' comfort with and barriers to care of transgender youth. *J Adolesc Health.* 2015;**56**(2):251–253.
6. Getahun D, Nash R, Flanders WD, Baird TC, Becerra-Culqui TA, Cromwell L, Hunkeler E, Lash TL, Millman A, Quinn VP, Robinson B,

Roblin D, Silverberg MJ, Safer J, Slovis J, Tangpricha V, Goodman M. Cross-sex hormones and acute cardiovascular events in transgender persons: a cohort study. *Ann Intern Med.* 2018; **169**(4):205–213.

7. Hannema SE, Schagen SEE, Cohen-Kettenis PT, Delemarre-van de Waal HA. Efficacy and safety of pubertal induction using 17β-estradiol in transgirls. *J Clin Endocrinol Metab.* 2017;**102**(7):2356–2363.

8. Jarin J, Pine-Twaddell E, Trotman G, Stevens J, Conard LA, Tefera E, Gomez-Lobo V. Cross-sex hormones and metabolic parameters in adolescents with gender dysphoria. *Pediatrics.* 2017;**139**(5): e20163173.

9. Wierckx K, Gooren L, T'Sjoen G. Clinical review: breast development in trans women receiving cross-sex hormones. *J Sex Med.* 2014;**11**(5): 1240–1247.

10. Moretti C, Guccione L, Di Giacinto P, Simonelli I, Exacoustos C, Toscano V, Motta C, De Leo V, Petraglia F, Lenzi A. Combined oral contraception and bicalutamide in polycystic ovary syndrome and severe hirsutism: a double-blind randomized controlled trial. *J Clin Endocrinol Metab.* 2018;**103**(3):824–838.

11. Deutsch MB, ed. Guidelines for the primary and gender-affirming care of transgender and gender nonbinary people. 2nd ed. Available at: http://transhealth.ucsf.edu/pdf/Transgender-PGACG-6-17-16.pdf. Accessed 6 August 2018.

12. Hembree WC, Cohen-Kettenis PT, Gooren L, Hannema SE, Meyer WJ, Murad MH, Rosenthal SM, Safer JD, Tangpricha V, T'Sjoen GG. Endocrine treatment of gender-dysphoric/gender-incongruent persons: an Endocrine Society Clinical Practice Guideline. *J Clin Endocrinol Metab.* 2017;**102**(11):1–35.

13. World Professional Association for Transgender Health. WPATH Standards of Care V.7. Available at: https://www.wpath.org/media/cms/Documents/SOC%20v7/SOC%20V7_English.pdf. Accessed 6 August 2018.

14. Rothman MS, Iwamoto SJ. Gender-affirming treatment of adults with gender incongruence and gender dysphoria. In: McDermott MT, ed. *Endocrine Secrets.* 7th ed. Philadelphia: Elsevier Saunders; 2019 (in press).

Premature Menopause: Etiology and Optimal Hormone Replacement Therapy

M57
Presented, March 23–26, 2019

Cynthia A. Stuenkel, MD. Division of Endocrinology, Department of Medicine, University of California, San Diego, School of Medicine, La Jolla, California 92093, E-mail: castuenkel@ucsd.edu

Sarah L. Berga, MD. Division of Reproductive Endocrinology and Infertility, Department of Obstetrics and Gynecology, University of Utah School of Medicine, Salt Lake City, Utah 84132, E-mail: sarah.berga@hsc.utah.edu

SIGNIFICANCE OF THE CLINICAL PROBLEM
Definition
Spontaneous premature menopause (age < 40 years), also referred to as primary ovarian insufficiency (POI), is often conceptualized as an isolated loss of ovarian function. However, this notion requires updating. There is not only a wide spectrum of presentation, but also an emergent understanding that the causes are many and that different etiologies are associated with different, but important, health consequences. Thus, POI may be a harbinger of significant health risks associated with more than just loss of ovarian function.

The nomenclature used to describe declining ovarian function resulting from loss of oocytes varies and reflects in part the multiplicity of etiologies that range from exposure to chemotherapeutic agents for treatment of cancer to premature loss of oocytes from known genetic and autoimmune causes to surgical removal to unexplained causes (1). Premature menopause is defined as the onset of menopause (*i.e.,* the cessation of cyclic ovarian function because of oocyte depletion or oophorectomy) before age 40 years. The American College of Obstetricians and Gynecologists defines POI as a spectrum of declining ovarian reserve and reduced fecundity and defines overt ovarian insufficiency as loss of ovarian function in women age <40 years who display elevated follicle-stimulating hormone (FSH) and amenorrhea (2). Premature spontaneous menopause differs from surgical menopause in etiology, presentation, physiology, and long-term sequelae. Although the former involves only the loss of oocytes and follicles from the ovarian cortex, the latter entails complete loss of ovarian function. This includes the loss of androgen-producing theca and stromal compartments that would otherwise continue to secrete androgens that could then be aromatized to estrogens in response to tonically elevated luteinizing hormone (LH) levels. POI is estimated to occur in 1% of women, with early menopause (ages 40 to 45 years) affecting ~5% of women, although the rate of POI in Sweden may be closer to 2% (3). A recent study by Jiao *et al.* (4) of 955 women with POI demonstrated that the three main etiologies for spontaneous POI are genetic, autoimmune, and idiopathic, with more than half being idiopathic and 10% to 15% being genetic. Genetic causes are more common in women who present with primary versus secondary amenorrhea. More than 80 candidate genes have been identified (5). Desai and Rajkovic (6) reported that of 44 genomic loci associated with POI, 29 were DNA damage response genes. In 2018, the *BRCA2* mutation was reported as a cause of POI in two sisters with 46,XX genotype (7); *BRCA* is important for DNA repair. The authors emphasized the need to screen affected individuals not only for POI but also for cancers. In the study by Jiao *et al.* (4), the most common autoimmune conditions in women with autoimmune POI were thyroiditis, psoriasis, and rheumatoid arthritis. Ovarian inflammation resulting from autoimmunity may be transient and difficult to detect (8). Screening for thyroid and adrenal antibodies is important for predicting concomitant autoimmune conditions (5). Epidemiological studies suggest that POI is associated with shorter lifespan, increased risk for diabetes mellitus, and increased risk for cardiovascular disease, but causality has not been established. Although earlier menopause may be a marker for accelerated aging, menopause *per se* has been suggested to accelerate aging and to be slowed by appropriate hormone replacement therapy (9, 10).

Clinical Overview
At a minimum, premature loss of ovarian function, both sex steroid production and fertility, is associated with the classical albeit protean and variable symptoms of menopause, grief response because of unanticipated loss of fertility, and the long-term consequences of premature reduction in endogenous sex steroids: bone loss, cardiovascular risk, cognitive decline, and neurological sequelae. It may also be associated with premature aging, cancers, and autoimmune conditions. Additional signs and symptoms may reflect the specific etiology contributing to premature menopause. Although an increasing number of factors have been identified that can contribute to premature menopause (Table 1), comprehensive genetic screening for possible and established causes is not widely available, and therefore, the precise etiology often remains unknown.

BARRIERS TO OPTIMAL PRACTICE
- Delay in time from onset of symptoms/signs to clinical diagnosis and therapeutic intervention
- Lack of prospective, longitudinal, observational cohort studies

Table 1. Premature Menopause: Etiologies

Iatrogenic
Pelvic surgery
Oophorectomy
Hysterectomy
Cancer therapy
Chemotherapy
Radiation therapy
Immune therapies
Cyclophosphamide
Spontaneous
Idiopathic 90%
Genetic
Turner's syndrome XO
Fragile X premutation carrier
Translocations long arm X chromosome (15%-30% familial)
BRCA1 and *BRCA2* mutations
Autoimmune
Autoimmune polyglandular syndromes
FSH receptor mutation
Metabolic
Galactosemia
Environmental risks
Tobacco

- Absence of large, long-term randomized trials to determine optimal preparation, route of administration, dose, duration, and clinical outcome of hormone therapy in this population
- Screening for and treating associated concomitant conditions

LEARNING OBJECTIVES

As a result of participating in this session, learners should be able to:

- Implement a logical diagnostic evaluation to identify common etiologies of premature menopause
- Detect and treat associated medical conditions
- Outline options for hormone therapy preparation, dose, duration, and suggested monitoring
- Counsel regarding fertility options

STRATEGIES/DIAGNOSIS, THERAPY, AND/OR MANAGEMENT

A common challenge for practitioners who make the diagnosis of POI is providing appropriate and comprehensive care. POI has many causes and therefore many concomitant conditions. Loss of ovarian function alone has many sequelae, including mood disorders, sleep disruption, fatigue, vasomotor symptoms, and low libido, in addition to menstrual irregularities. Practitioners may be perplexed by the constellation of symptoms in young women that are unexpected, and this may lead to delays in diagnosing, treating, and counseling as well as to misattribution. Women with POI may have their symptoms incorrectly attributed to anxiety or depressive disorders, stress, and other etiologies of reproductive hormonal imbalances before the correct diagnosis is established. This delay in diagnosis and treatment contributes to psychological suffering and frustration, as well as possible negative medical sequelae of prolonged estrogen deficiency (11).

Formal criteria allow for the diagnosis of POI after >3 months of amenorrhea in a woman with previous regular menstrual cycles in the presence of FSH in the postmenopausal range on two separate measurements at least 1 month apart. However, given intermittent ovarian function, POI may present as menstrual irregularity and elevated gonadotropins with preserved ovarian function. Recent studies suggest that antimullerian hormone (AMH) is a good marker of ovarian reserve and contributes to diagnosing the spectrum of POI (11). Studies show as much as a 10-fold variation in oocyte endowment from woman to woman at any age (12). Because a number of processes can contribute to premature menopause (5), a straightforward diagnostic approach is recommended (Table 2).

The approach to patient management in women with POI focuses on hormone therapy, discussing options for family building, and delineating concurrent conditions specific to cause. Hormone therapy for the patient with POI can truly be regarded as hormone replacement therapy. The choice of hormone therapy is guided by the etiology and extent of the loss of ovarian function and the current desire for fertility (Table 3). For women with POI (idiopathic, autoimmune polyglandular syndrome, or FMR1 premutation), 100 μg transdermal estradiol (TD E2) is often recommended as treatment of choice (2, 11, 13, 14). Although estradiol levels fluctuate in ovulatory cycles from a low in the early follicular phase to a high in the preovulatory phase, the mean physiological

Table 2. Premature Menopause: Diagnostic Workup

Laboratory evaluation
HCG
FSH, LH, estradiol, progesterone
Prolactin
TSH
Thyroid peroxidase antibodies
AMH
Additional testing
FMR1 (fragile X) premutation
Karyotype
Antiadrenal antibodies (21-hydroxylase)
DHEAS
Ovarian ultrasound
Antral follicle count

Table 3. Premature Menopause: Options for Therapy

Contraception
Oral contraceptives
May be more socially acceptable to young women but higher dose than required; suppression of IGF-1 compromises bone benefit
Levonorgestrel IUD
Provides endometrial protection and contraception
Hormone therapy
Preparation
Select per usual medical criteria
Transdermal preferred
Oral therapies acceptable
Dose
Higher than postmenopausal recommendations
Transdermal E2 100-μg patch
17-B E2 1–2 mg orally once daily
CEE 0.625–1.25 mg orally once daily
Progestogen if uterus
Micronized progesterone
100 mg/d continuously
200 mg/d 12 days per month sequentially
Medroxyprogesterone acetate
2.5–5 mg/d continuously
10 mg/d 12 days per month sequentially
Route of administration
Personal preference and usual medical criteria
Duration
Advised to age of anticipated menopause, then reassess annually
Fertility
Advise that course can be unpredictable
5%–10% chance of conception and pregnancy
If conception desired, counsel about donor oocytes and confine MHT to estradiol and progesterone to avoid teratotoxicity
Evaluate AMH, antral follicle count at baseline
Assisted reproductive therapy options
Autologous
Egg retrieval and freezing
IVF
Egg or embryo donation

circulating concentration of estradiol in ovulatory women during midreproductive years is ~100 to 110 pg/mL and serves as a physiological benchmark for titrating estradiol administration (15). In most women of normal height and weight, a TD E2 patch delivering 100 μg/d closely approximates endogenous estrogen (estradiol and estrone) levels in ovulatory women. However, in women with surgical menopause, customary estradiol levels may not completely mitigate

symptoms. Dose titration may be required, and androgen therapy may be needed. With transdermal therapy, the increased estradiol/estrone ratio seen with oral estradiol formulations is avoided. A more physiological approach may reduce risk and increase effectiveness. For instance, although oral estrogen suppresses insulin-like growth factor (IGF)-1, transdermal does not and thus may enhance bone formation. For women with concurrent diabetes or migraine headaches (a frequent component of FMR1 premutation syndrome), transdermal therapy is thought to be safer (13, 14). Women with a uterus require concurrent progestogen therapy. Options for continuous progestogen administration include micronized progesterone 100 mg/d or medroxyprogesterone acetate 2.5 to 5 mg/d or a progestin-releasing intrauterine device (IUD) (2). If fertility is desired, TD E2 with micronized progesterone (MP) is safer, because both are identical to the hormones produced by the ovaries and placenta before and during gestation. Whether a progestin is administered continuously or sequentially for 12 to 14 d/mo at a higher dose would depend on patient preference, time since diagnosis (sequential might be more acceptable initially), and fertility considerations. Cyclic progestin exposure typically leads to withdrawal bleeding, whereas continuous progestin exposure may lead to amenorrhea or unpredictable spotting and bleeding. Benefits of progestin-releasing IUDs include contraception and low rates of unpredictable spotting.

The question of whether oral contraceptive therapy is an appropriate replacement option merits consideration. A frequently cited statistic is that because of occasional spontaneous resumption of ovarian function, women with POI have a 5% to 10% chance of spontaneous pregnancy (16). For those accepting the possibility of pregnancy, a cyclical regimen with TD E2 and MP is advised. A missed withdrawal bleed warrants a pregnancy test (16). For those desiring contraception, an alternative approach to oral contraception would be continuous TD E2 with a levonorgestrel IUD (2).

Because POI can be diagnosed in women decades younger than the average age of menopause, experts universally agree that in the absence of contraindications, hormone therapy should be continued at least until the age of anticipated natural menopause (age 51 years) and then reassessed (13, 14, 16). From a risk standpoint, young women are considered to be at much lower baseline risk for cardiovascular events than those in the Women's Health Initiative (ages 50 to 79 years at enrollment), so although precise estimates have not been determined in clinical trials, long-duration therapy is thought to be safe for women with POI, and omission of ovarian hormone replacement is proposed to increase long-term health burden (17).

Fertility options for women with POI include oocyte and embryo donation, both of which allow women and their partners to fully experience pregnancy, delivery, and lactation. Rapid progress in techniques of oocyte cryopreservation for women with cancer facilitates the availability of this option to women at risk for POI (5). Resulting embryos could also be screened before implantation to determine if they harbor the same and other germ line mutations. Depending on markers of ovarian reserve, women with FMR1 premutation could consider egg banking, because POI will ultimately arise in one in five carriers. Women with POI resulting from known genetic causes such as 45,XO are also at risk for cardiac anomalies and aneurysms. Concurrent health conditions must be investigated and their impact on pregnancy estimated before oocyte or embryo donation is initiated.

MAIN CONCLUSIONS

- The primary etiology of nonsurgical premature menopause/POI is reduced follicle count.
- The causes of follicular depletion are many; a full evaluation will aid in delineating significant concomitant conditions such as autoimmune hypoadrenalism or hypothyroidism or components of FMR1 premutation syndrome.
- Surgical menopause differs significantly from POI (follicular depletion syndromes) in that androgen levels are reduced in women who have undergone bilateral oophorectomy.
- Hormone therapy should be offered and tailored to individual preferences and underlying etiology of POI.
- The advent of oocyte cryopreservation has facilitated third-party reproduction, and it should be discussed with women presenting with POI who are open to this option.
- Autologous oocyte harvest and banking in women before cancer therapies and those determined to have FMR1 premutation with adequate ovarian reserve are an option.

CASES WITH QUESTIONS AND ANSWERS
Case 1

A 29-year-old G0 was diagnosed with POI when she was referred from her primary care provider after a year of amenorrhea thought to be secondary to marathon training. In addition to a lack of menstrual cycles, the patient had also sought relief for anxiety symptoms characterized by what she described as panic attacks, mostly awakening her from sleep. She noted that sex had become a bit uncomfortable, and she wondered if that might be due to the change in condoms her boyfriend is using. Menarche was at age 12 years, and she described regular monthly menstrual cycles until her late 20s when she noticed she was missing an occasional period. On her examination, she appeared fit and in overall good health. Her body mass index was 24 kg/m^2 and had been stable since college. The rest of her examination was normal.

On laboratory evaluation, a pregnancy test was negative, prolactin was normal, thyrotropin (TSH) was elevated at 27 mIU/L, and LH and FSH were both in the menopausal range. Estradiol was <40 pg/mL. Karyotype was 46,XX without evidence of FMR1 premutation. On subsequent testing, antibodies

to 21-hydroxlylase were elevated, cosyntropin stimulation test was normal, and thyroid peroxidase antibodies were positive. Type 1 interferon autoantibodies were negative. The patient was started on levothyroxine therapy at 100 μg/d with normalization of TSH.

When learning that her diagnosis of POI was likely associated with an autoimmune polyendocrine syndrome, she decided that conception was a desired option and was informed that 5% to 10% of women in her situation ovulate and conceive. She was started on an estradiol 100-μg transdermal patch and cycled with micronized progesterone at 200 mg for 12 d/mo. She was advised to have a pregnancy test if she failed to bleed as scheduled.

If she decided to switch to oral estradiol therapy versus transdermal, her thyroid replacement dose would likely:
- A. Stay the same because of no change in thyroid binding globulin (TBG)
- B. Decrease because of reduction in TBG
- C. Increased because of increase in TBG
- D. Increased because of decrease in TBG

Answer: C

Given the positive 21-hydroxylase antibodies, the best approach to monitoring adrenal function would be to:
- A. 8 AM cortisol every 6 months
- B. Salivary cortisol at bedtime every 3 months
- C. Cosyntropin test every 12 months
- D. ACTH determination annually

Answer: C

If she decides she is no longer open to the possibility of pregnancy, optimal contraception would include:
- A. Oral contraceptive pills
- B. Vaginal contraceptive ring
- C. Levonorgestrel IUD
- D. Medroxyprogesterone injection

Answer: C

Given the constellation of this patient's endocrine disorders (history of autoimmune thyroid disease, POI, and 21-hydroxlylase antibodies), she meets criteria for an autoimmune polyendocrine syndrome, likely APS-2 (18). This syndrome has a prevalence of 1:1000 and requires hormone replacement for all affected systems with added surveillance for development of other associated conditions. Women with treated hypothyroidism may need to increase thyroxine replacement after initiation of oral estrogen therapy, because the increase in TBG leads to a decrease in free T$_4$. If she were to change to TD E2 therapy, TSH should be rechecked in 6 weeks, and the dose of thyroxine replacement could likely be reduced. Given the elevation of 21-hydroxylase antibodies, surveillance would include an annual cosyntropin test. The patient should be cautioned about symptoms of adrenal insufficiency particularly in the setting of a concurrent illness. The choice of contraceptive is driven by both efficacy and the hypothesis that high doses of estrogen suppress IGF-1 and compromise bone formation. Given that women with POI might not have yet achieved peak bone mass, expert opinion prefers TD E2 therapy. Cyclical progestins will not be adequate to suppress ovulation, so another method of contraception is necessary. The levonorgestrel IUD provides both endometrial protection and contraception.

Case 2

After a weekend discussion with friends, a 27-year-old G0 medical student decides to explore the option of freezing her eggs. She still has a year of school with residency training to follow. She is not currently in a relationship, and she is concerned that waiting will compromise her fertility. She presents to a reproductive endocrinologist at her institution and is advised to have a number of screening tests to assess ovarian reserve and genetic risks. She reports menarche at age 12 years, with normal menstrual cycles. She had a levonorgestrel IUD placed several years ago, and since that time, her menstrual cycles have been lighter. She takes escitalopram for anxiety and allergy medicines for seasonal symptoms and mild asthma. She has a history of rare migraine with aura since high school. Physical examination reveals a healthy young woman with normal secondary sexual characteristics. External genitalia and bimanual examination are normal.

Laboratory evaluation on day 3 of the menstrual cycle includes LH of 2.3 mIU/mL (normal range, 1.9-12.5 mIU/mL), FSH of 4 mIU/mL (normal range, 2.5-10.2 mIU/mL), and AMH of 2.7 ng/mL (normal range, 1-3.5 ng/mL). Transvaginal ultrasound confirmed normal pelvic anatomy and antral follicle count of eight (normal range, six to 10).Genetic testing (confirmed by a second laboratory) revealed a fragile X premutation with 30 repeats and two AGG interruptions on allele 1 and 56 repeats with zero interruptions on allele 2.

What is the best way to advise a newly diagnosed FMR1 premutation carrier who currently reports normal menstrual cycles?

  A. Advise that her genetic status increases her risk of POI (one in five carriers)
  B. Schedule annual AMH and antral follicle count to monitor ovarian reserve
  C. Encourage her to move ahead with plans for egg banking
  D. Counsel that in vitro fertilization with embryo screening for fragile X is available
  E. All of the above
  Answer: E

If this patient develops POI, the optimal hormone therapy will be:
  A. Oral estradiol and MP
  B. Oral conjugated equine estrogen and medroxyprogesterone acetate
  C. Transdermal estradiol and micronized progesterone
  D. Oral contraceptive therapy
  Answer: C

Appreciation of the clinical spectrum of disorders associated with FMR1 premutation has recently evolved. FMR1 mutations refer to an expansion of the CGG repeat on the FMR1 gene. The normal CGG range of repeats is six to 44; those with 55 to 200 repeats have the premutation associated with POI, and those with >200 repeats have fragile X syndrome (19). Prevalence estimates for the premutation in women range between one in 148 and one in 204 (19). As diagnoses are made in the setting of egg banking and fertility evaluations, endocrinologists may need to address concerns of young women with normal menstrual cycles who face a one in five likelihood of developing POI (19). Associated medical challenges in women with the premutation include hypertension and thyroid disease, migraines, emotional disorders (anxiety), and cognitive (executive function) challenges (19). At advanced ages, adults with the premutation can develop tremor/ataxia syndrome (20). Clear guidelines for monitoring reproductive status in carriers has not been established, but we recommend education of patients to report menstrual irregularities promptly. No strategies have been identified to slow the process of follicular atresia, whereas prospective annual monitoring of AMH and/or antral follicle count could detect progressive decline in ovarian reserve and anticipate early estrogen therapy. In this patient, genetic screening of embryos after in vitro fertilization of harvested eggs would be an option. Given the patient's history of migraines with aura, transdermal hormone therapy is recommended (13, 14).

Case 3

A 35-year-old G2P2 *BRCA1* carrier recently completed risk-reducing bilateral oophorectomy. She has been surprised by the intensity of her symptoms and is struggling with hot flashes, sleep deprivation, and keeping up with her two small children. She belongs to a national support group called FORCE where many *BRCA* mutation carriers acknowledge receiving menopausal hormone therapy after prophylactic oophorectomy both for symptom relief as well as for health preservation (heart, bone, brain). She has contemplated, but not yet scheduled, bilateral mastectomy. Mammography and MRI have been negative. She wonders what you recommend for symptom relief. Can she safely take hormone therapy? The best options to relieve menopausal symptoms in women with *BRCA* mutation include:

  A. Cognitive behavior therapy or hypnosis
  B. Venlafaxine 75 mg extended-release per day or gabapentin 300 to 900 mg daily
  C. Estradiol 50-μg transdermal patch with progesterone 100 mg/d for 12 days each month
  D. Conjugated equine estrogens 0.625 mg/d alone
  E. Individualized decision making regarding risks and benefits
  Answer: E

Women with *BRCA* gene mutations who elect risk-reducing oophorectomy often do so before age 40 years (21). As such, there is a concern that, whereas at reduced risk for ovarian and breast cancers, these patients may be at increased risk for long-term sequelae of premature estrogen deficiency. A number of groups have advised in favor of hormone replacement therapy (22–24), although observational data suggesting safety from the standpoint of breast cancer are sparse, and clinical trials have not been conducted. A recent observational study reported a decrease in breast cancer for women receiving 7 years of estrogen alone therapy, with an increased risk in those receiving therapies including progestogens (25), a pattern reminiscent of the breast cancer findings from the Women's Health Initiative (26). Furthermore, the risk of endometrial cancer in women with *BRCA* mutations may paradoxically increase with progesterone therapy (25). Therefore, in the absence of clear evidence, it seems most reasonable to take an individualized approach and temper recommendations for hormone replacement based upon age and ovarian status, uterine status, and breast status. For the patient who has also elected bilateral mastectomy and hysterectomy, hormone therapy is simplified, because estrogen alone is adequate and likely to be, but not proven, safer.

References

1. Welt CK. Primary ovarian insufficiency in adolescents and young women. *Clin Endocrinol (Oxf)*. 2008;**68**:499–509.
2. American College of Obstetricians and Gynecologists. Hormone therapy in primary ovarian insufficiency. Committee Opinion Number 698. May 2017. *Obstet Gynecol*. 2017;**129**(5):e134–e141.
3. Lagergren K, Hammar M, Nedstrand E, Bladh M, Sydsjö G. The prevalence of primary ovarian insufficiency in Sweden; a national register study. *BMC Womens Health*. 2018;**18**(1):175.
4. Jiao X, Zhang H, Ke H, Zhang J, Cheng L, Liu Y, Qin Y, Chen Z-J. Premature ovarian insufficiency: phenotypic characterization within different etiologies. *J Clin Endocrinol Metab*. 2017;**102**(7):2281–2290.
5. Rossetti R, Ferrari I, Bonomi M, Persani L. Genetics of primary ovarian insufficiency. *Clin Genet*. 2017;**91**(2):183–198.
6. Desai S, Rajkovic A. Genetics of reproductive aging from gonadal dysgenesis through menopause. *Semin Reprod Med*. 2017;**35**(2):147–159.
7. Weinberg-Shukron A, Rachmiel M, Renbaum P, Gulsuner S, Walsh T, Lobel O, Dreifuss A, Ben-Moshe A, Zeligson S, Segel R, Shore T, Kalifa R, Goldberg M, King MC, Gerlitz O, Levy-Lahad E, Zangen D. Essential role of *BRCA2* in ovarian development and function. *N Engl J Med*. 2018;**379**(11):1042–1049.
8. Silva CA, Yamakami LY, Aikawa NE, Araujo DB, Carvalho JF, Bonfá E. Autoimmune primary ovarian insufficiency. *Autoimmun Rev*. 2014;**13**(4-5):427–430.
9. Levine ME, Lu AT, Chen BH, Hernandez DG, Singleton AB, Ferrucci L, Bandinelli S, Salfati E, Manson JE, Quach A, Kusters CD, Kuh D, Wong A, Teschendorff AE, Widschwendter M, Ritz BR, Absher D, Assimes TL, Horvath S. Menopause accelerates biological aging. *Proc Natl Acad Sci USA*. 2016;**113**(33):9327–9332.
10. Lin J, Kroenke CH, Epel E, Kenna HA, Wolkowitz OM, Blackburn E, Rasgon NL. Greater endogenous estrogen exposure is associated with longer telomeres in postmenopausal women at risk for cognitive decline. *Brain Res*. 2011;**1379**:224–231.
11. Sullivan SD, Sarrel PM, Nelson LM. Hormone replacement therapy in young women with primary ovarian insufficiency and early menopause. *Fertil Steril*. 2016;**106**(7):1588–1599.
12. Cui L, Qin Y, Gao X, Lu J, Geng L, Ding L, Qu Z, Zhang X, Chen ZJ. Antimüllerian hormone: correlation with age and androgenic and metabolic factors in women from birth to postmenopause [published correction appears in *Fertil Steril*. 2018;**109**(5):942]. *Fertil Steril*. 2016;**105**(2):481–5.e1.
13. Stuenkel CA, Davis SR, Gompel A, Lumsden MA, Murad MH, Pinkerton JV, Santen RJ. Treatment of symptoms of the menopause: an Endocrine Society clinical practice guideline. *J Clin Endocrinol Metab*. 2015;**100**(11):3975–4011.
14. The NAMS 2017 Hormone Therapy Position Statement Advisory Panel. The 2017 hormone therapy position statement of the North American Menopause Society. *Menopause*. 2017;**24**(7):728–753.
15. Berga SL. Systemic benefits of cyclic ovarian function. *J Soc Gynecol Investig*. 2001;**8**(1, Suppl):S3–S6.
16. American College of Obstetricians and Gynecologists. Primary ovarian insufficiency in adolescents and young women. Committee Opinion Number 605. July 2014 (Reaffirmed 2016).
17. Faubion SS, Kuhle CL, Shuster LT, Rocca WA. Long-term health consequences of premature or early menopause and considerations for management. *Climacteric*. 2015;**18**(4):483–491.
18. Husebye ES, Anderson MS, Kämpe O. Autoimmune polyendocrine syndromes. *N Engl J Med*. 2018;**378**(12):1132–1141.
19. Wheeler A, Raspa M, Hagerman R, Mailick M, Riley C. Implications of the *FMR1* Premutation for children, adolescents, adults, and their families. *Pediatrics*. 2017;**139**(Suppl 3):S172–S182.
20. Man L, Lekovich J, Rosenwaks Z, Gerhardt J. Fragile X-Associated diminished ovarian reserve and primary ovarian insufficiency from molecular mechanisms to clinical manifestations. *Front Mol Neurosci*. 2017;**10**:290.
21. Hartmann LC, Lindor NM. The role of risk-reducing surgery in hereditary breast and ovarian cancer. *N Engl J Med*. 2016;**374**(5):454–468.
22. American College of Obstetricians and Gynecologists. Hereditary breast and ovarian cancer syndrome. ACOG Practice Bulletin Number 182, September 2017. *Obstet Gynecol*. 2017;**130**:e110–e126.
23. Birrer N, Chinchilla C, Del Carmen M, Dizon DS. Is hormone replacement therapy safe in women with a BRCA mutation? A systematic review of the contemporary literature. *Am J Clin Oncol*. 2018;**41**(3):313–315.
24. Vaz-Luis I, Partridge AH. Exogenous reproductive hormone use in breast cancer survivors and previvors. *Nat Rev Clin Oncol*. 2018;**15**(4):249–261.
25. Kotsopoulos J, Gronwald J, Karlan BY, Huzarski T, Tung N, Moller P, Armel S, Lynch HT, Senter L, Eisen A, Singer CF, Foulkes WD, Jacobson MR, Sun P, Lubinski J, Narod SA; Hereditary Breast Cancer Clinical Study Group. Hormone replacement therapy after oophorectomy and breast cancer risk among BRCA1 mutation carriers. *JAMA Oncol*. 2018;**4**(8):1059–1065.
26. Manson JE, Chlebowski RT, Stefanick ML, Aragaki AK, Rossouw JE, Prentice RL, Anderson G, Howard BV, Thomson CA, LaCroix AZ, Wactawski-Wende J, Jackson RD, Limacher M, Margolis KL, Wassertheil-Smoller S, Beresford SA, Cauley JA, Eaton CB, Gass M, Hsia J, Johnson KC, Kooperberg C, Kuller LH, Lewis CE, Liu S, Martin LW, Ockene JK, O'Sullivan MJ, Powell LH, Simon MS, Van Horn L, Vitolins MZ, Wallace RB. Menopausal hormone therapy and health outcomes during the intervention and extended poststopping phases of the Women's Health Initiative randomized trials. *JAMA*. 2013;**310**(13):1353–1368.

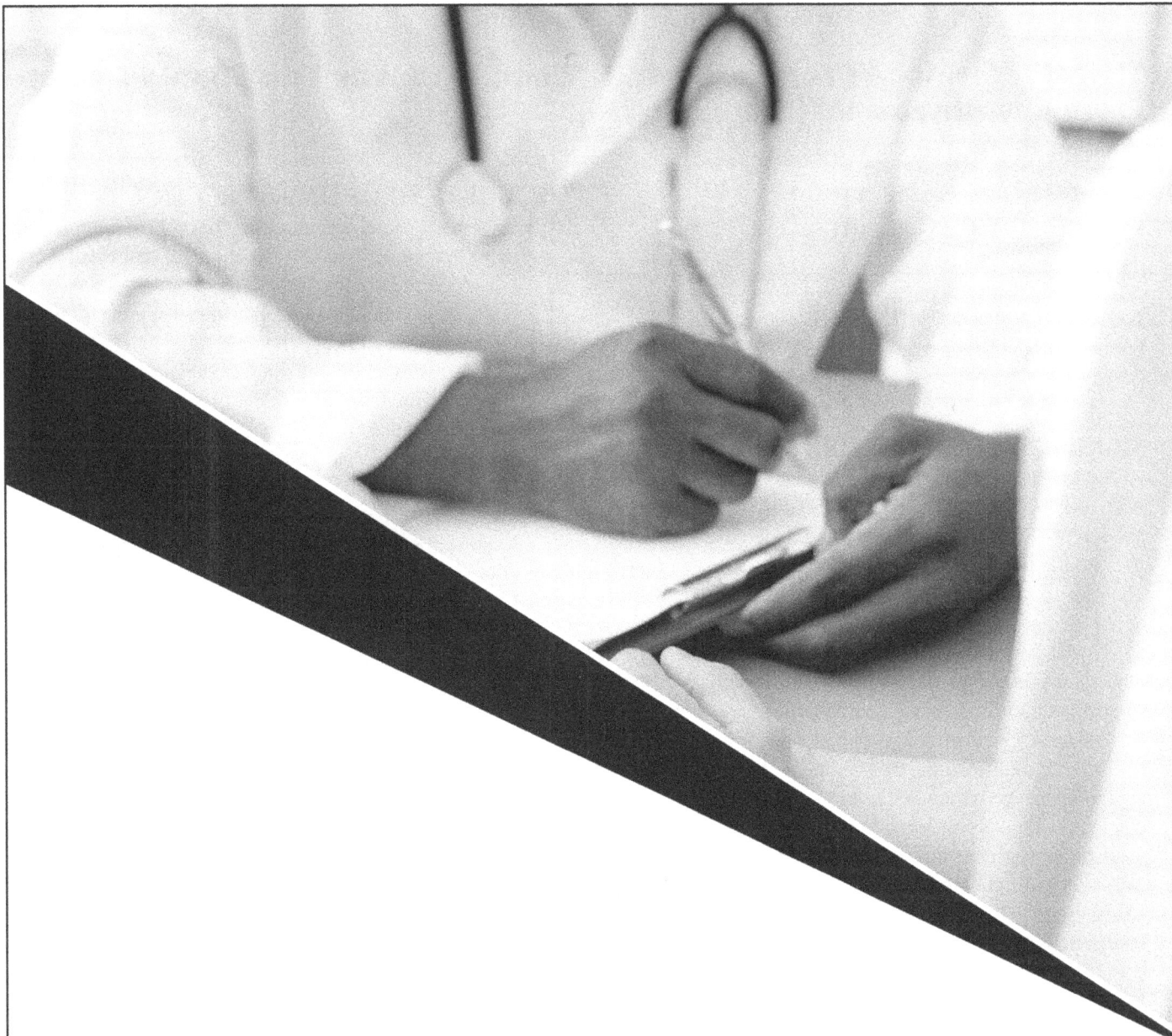

THYROID

Thyroid Hormone Preparations: If, When, and Why You Should Deviate From Levothyroxine

M10
Presented, March 23–26, 2019

Jacqueline Jonklaas, MD, PhD. Division of Endocrinology, Georgetown University, Washington, DC 20007, E-mail: jonklaaj@georgetown.edu

SIGNIFICANCE OF THE CLINICAL PROBLEM

Hypothyroidism is a common endocrine problem affecting ~5% to 15% of adults (1). Because hypothyroidism generally has no cure, the vast majority of treated individuals will need to continue thyroid hormone (TH) preparations indefinitely. The goal of treatment with TH is to reverse the biochemical abnormalities and signs and symptoms of hypothyroidism (2). Given that hypothyroidism does not resolve without treatment, the efficacy of therapy is of paramount importance to patients and physicians. Desiccated thyroid extract (DTE) derived from animal thyroid glands was the original treatment for hypothyroidism until the 1970s, when prescription of synthetic levothyroxine (LT_4) increased, subsequently becoming the most frequently used therapy (3). The paradigms used for prescribing and monitoring therapy have become well standardized based on a long experience with the use of LT_4 therapy. LT_4 is one of the most commonly prescribed medications in the United States (4).

Since the 1990s, there has been interest in synthetic combination therapy employing both LT_4 and liothyronine (LT_3). This interest has been spurred by the fact that some patients do not feel completely well while taking LT_4 alone (5, 6), along with the knowledge that the normally functioning thyroid gland produces both thyroxine (T_4) and triiodothyronine (T_3). Fourteen randomized, controlled studies of synthetic combination therapy (LT_4/LT_3) have been conducted (2, 7–9). A few of these have shown improved health-related quality of life or neurocognitive function, but most have not shown such benefit (2, 7–9). Some studies have shown patient preference for LT_4/LT_3 (10–14). One trial of DTE showed no improvement in quality of life or neurocognitive functioning but did show some patient preference (15). Physicians treating patients with hypothyroidism currently face a quandary because of a strong and persistent patient interest in both synthetic combination therapy (LT_4/LT_3) and DTE (5), but failure of clinical studies testing LT_4/LT_3 or DTE to show a benefit with respect to patient health-related quality of life, performance, or neurocognitive functioning. The current state of knowledge leaves physicians uncertain of the balance between the benefits and risks of combination therapy. In addition, if combination therapy is pursued, the optimal approach to monitoring and adjusting therapy is uncertain.

BARRIERS TO OPTIMAL PRACTICE

- Uncertainty regarding choosing the optimal treatment for hypothyroidism based on the ability of that treatment to fully reverse hypothyroidism
- Inadequate understanding of the underpinning for patient dissatisfaction with LT_4 therapy
- Understanding the conflicting data regarding biochemical euthyroidism based on normal thyrotropin (TSH) and patient dissatisfaction with LT_4 therapy
- Determining whether low T_3 levels or presence of deiodinase or TH transporter polymorphisms are responsible for patient dissatisfaction with LT_4 therapy
- Appreciating the heterogeneity of LT_4/LT_3 trials that have already been conducted
- Understanding the conflicting results of LT_4/LT_3 trials
- Developing better patient-centered outcomes that can be used to design better trials of LT_4/LT_3 and/or DTE
- Determining the long-term benefits and risks of LT_4/LT_3 or DTE therapy

LEARNING OBJECTIVES

As a result of participating in this session, learners should be able to:

- Discuss the standard-of-care treatment of hypothyroidism
- Discuss the knowledge gap regarding combination therapy for hypothyroidism
- Understand the evidence for and against combination therapy with T_3-containing products

STRATEGIES FOR DIAGNOSIS, THERAPY, AND/OR MANAGEMENT

Diagnosis

Alternative therapies other than LT_4 may be considered when an individual does not feel well or fully restored to health while receiving LT_4 therapy. It is crucial to rule out other causes of the patient's poor quality of life, other than inadequate therapy for hypothyroidism. This is especially important because the symptoms of hypothyroidism are nonspecific and overlap with symptoms of other conditions (16). Patients with unresolved symptoms may be more likely to be screened for hypothyroidism, and in fact, many patients suspected of having hypothyroidism do not have this diagnosis, despite their symptoms (17). In addition, patients with hypothyroidism may also have more comorbid conditions than the general population (18), and their symptoms may be associated with these conditions. It is also possible that autoimmunity *per se* affects quality of life. Therefore, a thorough investigation for other causes that merit treatment is essential before embarking on a trial of alternative therapies.

In addition, although there are suggestive data about dissatisfaction with LT_4 and response to combination therapy being associated with type 2 deiodinase genotype (better response in patients who are Ala/Ala homozygotes), the data are conflicting and not confirmed in prospective studies (19, 20). Therefore, even if such a polymorphism is identified in a patient, it is not yet clear that the patient would be more likely to respond favorably to combination therapy. Moreover, low T_3 levels while taking LT_4 do not predict response to combination therapy (21).

Therapy and Management
If a trial of combination therapy is embarked upon, it must be considered that although trials of such therapy have shown some patient preference, when taken together these trials have not shown improvement in other parameters. Health-related quality of life or mood was studied in 13 trials. Superiority of combination therapy on multiple measures was shown in two trials (11, 13), superiority of combination therapy on a minority of measures was seen in two trials (22, 23) (with superiority shown at 3 months but not at 12 months in the longer trial) (22), and no superiority of combination therapy was seen in nine trials. Neurocognitive functioning was studied in 10 trials. Superiority of combination therapy on multiple measures was seen in one trial (11), superiority of combination therapy on a minority of measures was observed in one trial (12), and no superiority of combination therapy was detected in eight trials. Treatment preference was studied in five blinded, cross-over design trials. Combination therapy was preferred in four trials (10–13) of 128 patients. In contrast, no treatment preference between groups was seen in one trial of 101 patients (24). Treatment preference was studied in two blinded, parallel design trials. Combination therapy was preferred in one trial of 130 patients (14). However, no preference was seen in another trial of 573 patients (22). Similarly, in the one randomized controlled study of DTE (15), DTE therapy did not result in a significant improvement in quality of life, although multiple different parameters were assessed. DTE resulted in modest weight loss (3 lbs; ~2%), and preference for extract was associated with weight loss.

In addition, the trials of synthetic combination therapy were all heterogeneous with respect to their dosing regimens (actual dose and frequency of dose) and the biochemical end points achieved, thus providing little guidance to the prescribing physician. Doses approximating a physiological ratio are recommended in guidelines (25). However, higher doses of T_3 are often requested by patients. If therapy is initiated, it is not known which parameters should be monitored and whether simply TSH should be monitored, or whether FT_4 and T_3 levels should be monitored as well. T_3 levels may be problematic because these peak considerably after taking LT_3 (26) and so may pose a problem with respect to being used to adjust LT_3 therapy. Although toxicity of combination therapy has generally not been reported, adverse effects with long-term therapy have not been investigated, and the best means of monitoring for cardiac or skeletal adverse effects has not been established. Furthermore, little is known about LT_3 therapy in those who are older, those with chronic medical conditions, children, or men. The financial cost of combination therapy is likely to be higher for both the patient and the medical system compared with LT_4 therapy. These are all important considerations, because recent data suggest that physicians are prescribing combination therapy more frequently than in the past (27, 28).

These safety concerns are further accentuated if a trial of DTE is being considered. Not only are there fewer controlled data about such therapy, but the occurrence of T_3 thyrotoxicosis has been clearly documented as well.

MAIN CONCLUSIONS
More research is sorely needed to understand why some patients prefer combination therapy. Additional randomized controlled clinical trials need to be conducted focusing on the subgroups thought most likely to benefit from combination therapy. Such groups might include, for example, those who have the Thr92Ala polymorphisms, those who are unhappy while taking LT_4 and in whom other causes of dissatisfaction have not been identified, and those who have undergone thyroidectomy. Pregnant women should be excluded from such trials. Furthermore, such trials should employ physiological dosing and be of longer duration than prior trials. Careful power calculations should be performed so that any future studies conducted have adequate power to answer the questions being asked. Standardized patient-reported outcomes need to be included among the end points of these future studies, and rigorous monitoring for adverse effects should occur. When available, sustained-release T_3 should also be studied.

Meanwhile, until such results are available, if a trial of combination therapy is pursued for an individual patient, it should be pursued with careful monitoring. If there is no perceived benefit after a reasonable period of time, the therapy should be discontinued, and care should be taken to avoid LT_3 dose escalation that results in sustained supraphysiological T_3 levels.

CASES
Case 1
Vignette
A 29-year-old woman with Hashimoto's hypothyroidism is taking 100 μg LT_4. She is frustrated because she is gaining weight despite regular exercise, is tired throughout the day, and has poor memory and work performance. Physical examination suggests she is clinically euthyroid. Her body mass index (BMI) and laboratory values are as follows: BMI, 25 kg/m² (normal range, 18.5 to 24.9 kg/m²); TSH, 3.9 mIU/L (normal range, 0.4 to 4.0 mIU/L); free T_4, 1.3 ng/dL (normal

range, 0.8 to 1.8 ng/dL); and total T$_3$, 75 ng/dL (normal range, 80 to 180 ng/dL).

Questions: Which Would You Do?
A. Continue current LT$_4$
B. Increase LT$_4$ dose
C. Add 2.5 µg of LT$_3$ twice daily and reduce LT$_4$
D. Add 2.5 µg of LT$_3$ twice daily to current LT$_4$
E. Replace LT$_4$ with thyroid extract (*e.g.*, armour thyroid)
F. Replace LT$_4$ with LT$_3$ as single therapy

Potential Answers and Discussion
Answers given by American Thyroid Association (ATA) members during a survey:
A. Continue current LT$_4$: 14.6%
B. Increase LT$_4$ dose: 63.6%
C. Add 2.5 µg of LT$_3$ twice daily and reduce LT$_4$: 3%
D. Add 2.5 µg of LT$_3$ twice daily to current LT$_4$: 17.4%
E. Replace LT$_4$ with thyroid extract (*e.g.*, armour thyroid): 1.1%
F. Replace LT$_4$ with LT$_3$ as single therapy: 0.3%

Case 2
Vignette
A 29-year-old woman with Hashimoto's hypothyroidism is taking 100 µg of LT$_4$. She is frustrated because she is gaining weight despite regular exercise, is tired throughout the day, and has poor memory and work performance. She requests combination therapy. Physical examination suggests she is clinically euthyroid. Her BMI and laboratory values are as follows: BMI, 25 kg/m^2 (normal range, 18.5 to 24.9 kg/m^2); TSH, 2.2 mIU/L (normal range, 0.4 to 4.0 mIU/L); free T$_4$, 1.3 ng/dL (normal range, 0.8 to 1.8 ng/dL); and total T$_3$, 75 ng/dL (normal range, 80 to 180 ng/dL).

Questions: Which Would You Do?
A. Continue current LT$_4$
B. Increase LT$_4$ dose
C. Add 2.5 µg of LT$_3$ twice daily and reduce LT$_4$
D. Add 2.5 µg of LT$_3$ twice daily to current LT$_4$
E. Replace LT$_4$ with thyroid extract (*e.g.*, armour thyroid)
F. Replace LT$_4$ with LT$_3$ as single therapy

Potential Answers and Discussion
Answers given by ATA members during a survey:
A. Continue current LT$_4$: 32%
B. Increase LT$_4$ dose: 9.9%
C. Add 2.5 µg of LT$_3$ twice daily and reduce LT$_4$: 33.9%
D. Add 2.5 µg of LT$_3$ twice daily to current LT$_4$: 17.9%
E. Replace LT$_4$ with thyroid extract (*e.g.*, armour thyroid): 6.3%
F. Replace LT$_4$ with LT$_3$ as single therapy: 0.0%

Case 3
Vignette
A 29-year-old woman with Hashimoto's hypothyroidism is taking 100 µg of LT$_4$. She is frustrated because she is gaining weight despite regular exercise, is tired throughout the day, and has poor memory and work performance. She previously participated in a study that showed she had a genetic problem with converting T$_4$ to T$_3$. She requests combination therapy. Physical examination suggests she is clinically euthyroid. Her BMI and laboratory values are as follows: BMI, 25 kg/m^2 (normal range, 18.5 to 24.9 kg/m^2); TSH, 2.2 mIU/L (normal range, 0.4 to 4.0 mIU/L); free T$_4$, 1.3 ng/dL (normal range, 0.8 to 1.8 ng/dL); and total T$_3$, 75 ng/dL (normal range, 80 to 180 ng/dL).

Questions: Which Would You Do?
A. Continue current LT$_4$
B. Increase LT$_4$ dose
C. Add 2.5 µg of LT$_3$ twice daily and reduce LT$_4$
D. Add 2.5 µg of LT$_3$ twice daily to current LT$_4$
E. Replace LT$_4$ with thyroid extract (*e.g.*, armour thyroid)
F. Replace LT$_4$ with LT$_3$ as single therapy

Potential Answers and Discussion
Answers given by ATA members during a survey:
A. Continue current LT$_4$: 16.5%
B. Increase LT$_4$ dose: 6.9%
C. Add 2.5 µg of LT$_3$ twice daily and reduce LT$_4$: 41.6%
D. Add 2.5 µg of LT$_3$ twice daily to current LT$_4$: 28.7%
E. Replace LT$_4$ with thyroid extract (*e.g.*, armour thyroid): 3.3%
F. Replace LT$_4$ with LT$_3$ as single therapy: 3.0%

References
1. Taylor PN, Albrecht D, Scholz A, Gutierrez-Buey G, Lazarus JH, Dayan CM, Okosieme OE. Global epidemiology of hyperthyroidism and hypothyroidism. *Nat Rev Endocrinol.* 2018;**14**(5):301–316.
2. Jonklaas J, Bianco AC, Bauer AJ, Burman KD, Cappola AR, Celi FS, Cooper DS, Kim BW, Peeters RP, Rosenthal MS, Sawka AM; American Thyroid Association Task Force on Thyroid Hormone Replacement. Guidelines for the treatment of hypothyroidism: prepared by the american thyroid association task force on thyroid hormone replacement. *Thyroid.* 2014;**24**(12):1670–1751.
3. Taylor RL, Kaufmann S. Trends in classification usage in the mental retardation literature. *Ment Retard.* 1991;**29**(6):367–371.
4. Kantor ED, Rehm CD, Haas JS, Chan AT, Giovannucci EL. Trends in prescription drug use among adults in the United States from 1999-2012. *JAMA.* 2015;**314**(17):1818–1831.
5. Peterson SJ, Cappola AR, Castro MR, Dayan CM, Farwell AP, Hennessey JV, Kopp PA, Ross DS, Samuels MH, Sawka AM, Taylor PN, Jonklaas J, Bianco AC. An online survey of hypothyroid patients demonstrates prominent dissatisfaction. *Thyroid.* 2018;**28**(6):707–721.
6. Saravanan P, Chau WF, Roberts N, Vedhara K, Greenwood R, Dayan CM. Psychological well-being in patients on 'adequate' doses of l-thyroxine: results of a large, controlled community-based questionnaire study. *Clin Endocrinol (Oxf).* 2002;**57**(5):577–585.
7. Escobar-Morreale HF, Botella-Carretero JI, Morreale de Escobar G. Treatment of hypothyroidism with levothyroxine or a combination of

levothyroxine plus L-triiodothyronine. *Best Pract Res Clin Endocrinol Metab.* 2015;**29**(1):57–75.

8. Grozinsky-Glasberg S, Fraser A, Nahshoni E, Weizman A, Leibovici L. Thyroxine-triiodothyronine combination therapy versus thyroxine monotherapy for clinical hypothyroidism: meta-analysis of randomized controlled trials. *J Clin Endocrinol Metab.* 2006;**91**(7): 2592–2599.

9. Ma C, Xie J, Huang X, Wang G, Wang Y, Wang X, Zuo S. Thyroxine alone or thyroxine plus triiodothyronine replacement therapy for hypothyroidism. *Nucl Med Commun.* 2009;**30**(8):586–593.

10. Bunevicius R, Jakuboniene N, Jurkevicius R, Cernicat J, Lasas L, Prange AJ Jr. Thyroxine vs thyroxine plus triiodothyronine in treatment of hypothyroidism after thyroidectomy for Graves' disease [published correction appears in Endocrine. 2014;45(1):161]. *Endocrine.* 2002;**18**(2):129–133.

11. Bunevicius R, Kazanavicius G, Zalinkevicius R, Prange AJ Jr. Effects of thyroxine as compared with thyroxine plus triiodothyronine in patients with hypothyroidism. *N Engl J Med.* 1999;**340**(6):424–429.

12. Escobar-Morreale HF, Botella-Carretero JI, Gómez-Bueno M, Galán JM, Barrios V, Sancho J. Thyroid hormone replacement therapy in primary hypothyroidism: a randomized trial comparing L-thyroxine plus liothyronine with L-thyroxine alone. *Ann Intern Med.* 2005; **142**(6):412–424.

13. Nygaard B, Jensen EW, Kvetny J, Jarløv A, Faber J. Effect of combination therapy with thyroxine (T4) and 3,5,3′-triiodothyronine versus T4 monotherapy in patients with hypothyroidism, a double-blind, randomised cross-over study. *Eur J Endocrinol.* 2009;**161**(6): 895–902.

14. Appelhof BC, Fliers E, Wekking EM, Schene AH, Huyser J, Tijssen JG, Endert E, van Weert HC, Wiersinga WM. Combined therapy with levothyroxine and liothyronine in two ratios, compared with levothyroxine monotherapy in primary hypothyroidism: a double-blind, randomized, controlled clinical trial. *J Clin Endocrinol Metab.* 2005; **90**(5):2666–2674.

15. Hoang TD, Olsen CH, Mai VQ, Clyde PW, Shakir MK. Desiccated thyroid extract compared with levothyroxine in the treatment of hypothyroidism: a randomized, double-blind, crossover study. *J Clin Endocrinol Metab.* 2013;**98**(5):1982–1990.

16. Jonklaas J. Persistent hypothyroid symptoms in a patient with a normal thyroid stimulating hormone level. *Curr Opin Endocrinol Diabetes Obes.* 2017;**24**(5):356–363.

17. Bould H, Panicker V, Kessler D, Durant C, Lewis G, Dayan C, Evans J. Investigation of thyroid dysfunction is more likely in patients with high psychological morbidity. *Fam Pract.* 2012;**29**(2):163–167.

18. Peterson SJ, McAninch EA, Bianco AC. Is a normal TSH synonymous with "euthyroidism" in levothyroxine monotherapy? *J Clin Endocrinol Metab.* 2016;**101**(12):4964–4973.

19. Panicker V, Saravanan P, Vaidya B, Evans J, Hattersley AT, Frayling TM, Dayan CM. Common variation in the DIO2 gene predicts baseline psychological well-being and response to combination thyroxine plus triiodothyronine therapy in hypothyroid patients. *J Clin Endocrinol Metab.* 2009;**94**(5):1623–1629.

20. Wouters HJ, van Loon HC, van der Klauw MM, Elderson MF, Slagter SN, Kobold AM, Kema IP, Links TP, van Vliet-Ostaptchouk JV, Wolffenbuttel BH. No effect of the Thr92Ala polymorphism of deiodinase-2 on thyroid hormone parameters, health-related quality of life, and cognitive functioning in a large population-based cohort study. *Thyroid.* 2017;**27**(2):147–155.

21. Medici BB, la Cour JL, Michaelsson LF, Faber JO, Nygaard B. Neither baseline nor changes in serum triiodothyronine during levothyroxine/ liothyronine combination therapy predict a positive response to this treatment modality in hypothyroid patients with persistent symptoms. *Eur Thyroid J.* 2017;**6**(2):89–93.

22. Saravanan P, Simmons DJ, Greenwood R, Peters TJ, Dayan CM. Partial substitution of thyroxine (T4) with tri-iodothyronine in patients on T4 replacement therapy: results of a large community-based randomized controlled trial. *J Clin Endocrinol Metab.* 2005;**90**(2):805–812.

23. Valizadeh M, Seyyed-Majidi MR, Hajibeigloo H, Momtazi S, Musavinasab N, Hayatbakhsh MR. Efficacy of combined levothyroxine and liothyronine as compared with levothyroxine monotherapy in primary hypothyroidism: a randomized controlled trial. *Endocr Res.* 2009;**34**(3):80–89.

24. Walsh JP, Shiels L, Lim EM, Bhagat CI, Ward LC, Stuckey BG, Dhaliwal SS, Chew GT, Bhagat MC, Cussons AJ. Combined thyroxine/ liothyronine treatment does not improve well-being, quality of life, or cognitive function compared to thyroxine alone: a randomized controlled trial in patients with primary hypothyroidism. *J Clin Endocrinol Metab.* 2003;**88**(10):4543–4550.

25. Wiersinga WM, Duntas L, Fadeyev V, Nygaard B, Vanderpump MP. 2012 ETA guidelines: the use of L-T4 + L-T3 in the treatment of hypothyroidism. *Eur Thyroid J.* 2012;**1**(2):55–71.

26. Saravanan P, Siddique H, Simmons DJ, Greenwood R, Dayan CM. Twenty-four hour hormone profiles of TSH, free T3 and free T4 in hypothyroid patients on combined T3/T4 therapy. *Exp Clin Endocrinol Diabetes.* 2007;**115**(4):261–267.

27. Jonklaas J, Tefera E, Shara N. Physician choice of hypothyroidism therapy: influence of patient characteristics. *Thyroid.* 2018;**28**(11): 1416–1424.

28. Jonklaas J, Tefera E, Shara N. Prescribing therapy for hypothyroidism: influence of physician characteristics [published online ahead of print 30 October 2018]. *Thyroid.* doi:10.1089/thy.2018.0369.

Molecular Markers Guiding Intervention and Treatment

M21
Presented, March 23–26, 2019

Sarah E. Mayson, MD. Division of Endocrinology, Metabolism and Diabetes, University of Colorado School of Medicine, Aurora, Colorado 80045, E-mail: sarah.mayson@ucdenver.edu

Michael W. Yeh, MD, FACS. Section of Endocrine Surgery, David Geffen School of Medicine, University of California, Los Angeles, Los Angeles, California 90095, E-mail: myeh@mednet.ucla.edu

SIGNIFICANCE OF THE CLINICAL PROBLEM

Thyroid nodules are present in up to 50% of the adult population. Because ~95% of thyroid nodules are benign, the avoidance of unnecessary surgery (overtreatment) is important. At the same time, the clinician must detect and appropriately target clinically significant thyroid cancers for surgical management and potentially adjuvant therapies. The establishment of a tissue diagnosis via fine-needle aspiration (FNA) biopsy represents the first step in evaluating most thyroid nodules. Morphologic cytology yields benign results in 70% of cases, malignant results in 5% to 10% of cases, and indeterminate results in the remaining 20% to 25% of cases. The underlying malignancy rate in indeterminate thyroid nodules (Bethesda III or IV) is 10% to 40% (1). Since 2012, various molecular profiling platforms have emerged to provide further diagnostic information in indeterminate thyroid nodules. These tests have the potential to add value to patient care by permitting the avoidance of diagnostic hemithyroidectomy and potentially guiding the extent of initial surgery.

BARRIERS TO OPTIMAL PRACTICE

- Incomplete understanding of the performance characteristics and limitations of existing molecular profiling tests, especially in light of rapid evolution in technology
- Institutional or practice pattern variation in the underlying prevalence of malignancy in indeterminate thyroid nodules

LEARNING OBJECTIVES

As a result of participating in this session, learners should be able to:

- Articulate the performance characteristics [sensitivity, specificity, positive predictive value (PPV), negative predictive value (NPV)] of the most commonly used molecular testing platforms for indeterminate thyroid nodules
- Understand how the prevalence of malignancy and noninvasive follicular thyroid neoplasm with papillary-like nuclear features (NIFTP) in a given population may influence the PPV and NPV of molecular diagnostic tests
- Review what is known about the long-term outcomes of conservatively managed thyroid nodules with indeterminate cytopathology and negative molecular diagnostic testing

STRATEGIES FOR DIAGNOSIS, THERAPY, AND/OR MANAGEMENT

Performance Characteristics of Diagnostic Tests

Test sensitivity is defined as the proportion of patients with a disease testing positive for that disease (true positives); specificity is the proportion without a disease testing negative (true negatives). PPV refers to the proportion of positive tests that are true positives, whereas NPV is the proportion of negative tests that are true negatives. Sensitivity and specificity are inherent properties of a given diagnostic test, whereas PPV and NPV are affected by the population prevalence of the disease. PPV decreases and NPV increases with lower disease prevalence; the converse is true when prevalence rises. Molecular diagnostic tests with high sensitivity and NPV are generally used as rule-out tests, whereas those with high specificity and PPV are used as rule-in tests.

Thyroid Cytopathology Reporting and Estimates of Malignancy Risk

Molecular testing is currently performed only on indeterminate thyroid nodules. The Bethesda System for Reporting Thyroid Cytopathology (TBSRTC) was first proposed in 2007 and later revised in 2017 to standardize terminology used to report thyroid cytopathology and reflect updated studies regarding the malignant potential of certain follicular thyroid tumors (1, 2). Using this system, thyroid FNA samples are classified into one of six cytologic categories [I, nondiagnostic; II, benign; III, atypia of undetermined significance or follicular lesion of undetermined significance (AUS/FLUS); IV, follicular neoplasm or suspicious for follicular neoplasm (FN/SFN); V, suspicious for malignancy; or VI, malignant], each of which has a corresponding risk of malignancy. Benign and malignant cytologic results in TBSRTC are highly accurate, with a 0% to 3% risk of malignancy in the benign category and 94% to 99% risk in the malignant category. Bethesda categories III through V are considered indeterminate and assigned to specimens demonstrating varying degrees of cytologic and/or architectural atypia (Table 1).

The updated 2017 Bethesda system reflects validation studies documenting malignancy rates that differed from those TBSRTC had initially established (3). As shown in Table 1, a higher risk of malignancy is now predicted for

Table 1. TBSRTC in 2009 and 2017 With Updated Risks of Malignancy

TBSRTC Diagnostic Category	2009 TBSRTC (2) Predicted ROM (%)	Bongiovanni (3) Observed ROM (%)	2017 TBSRTC (1) Predicted ROM (%)	
			NIFTP Nonmalignant	NIFTP Malignant
I. Nondiagnostic	1–4	9–32	5–10	5–10
II. Benign	0–3	1–10	0–3	0–3
III. AUS/FLUS	~5–15	6–48	6–18	10–30
IV. SFN/FN	15–30	14–34	10–40	25–40
V. Suspicious for malignancy	60–75	45–60	45–60	50–75
VI. Malignant	97–99	94–100	94–96	97–99
Abbreviation: ROM, risk of malignancy.				

thyroid nodules with AUS/FLUS (III) or FN/SFN (IV) cytopathology, whereas the risk of malignancy associated with Bethesda V cytology is slightly lower (1). Because the PPV and NPV of each molecular test hinge on the prevalence of malignancy in the population being evaluated, the higher risk of malignancy associated with Bethesda III and IV cytopathologies would have the potential to decrease the NPV and increase the PPV of a given test.

Substantial site-to-site variability in the malignancy rates of thyroid nodules with indeterminate cytology (especially Bethesda III and V) has been documented (4). It is therefore recommended that each institution or region calculate its own malignancy rates for each of the Bethesda categories. Institutional or regional malignancy rates should ideally be based on a 3- to 5-year average, because year-to-year variability in malignancy rates, particularly with indeterminate cytopathology readings, has also been documented (Bethesda III, range 8% to 38%; Bethesda IV, range 0% to 42%) (5).

Impact of NIFTP on Thyroid Cytopathology and Molecular Testing

Described in 2016, NIFTP is a nonmalignant thyroid tumor that possesses the characteristic nuclear features of papillary thyroid carcinoma but is associated with a very low risk of adverse outcomes (6). Before 2016, these lesions were classified as a form of the follicular variant of papillary thyroid cancer, but now, NIFTP tumors are more aptly thought of as premalignant. The change in nomenclature better reflects their indolent clinical behavior and discourages overtreatment. However, the introduction of NIFTP further complicates the interpretation of thyroid cytopathology. The estimated risk of malignancy associated with each of the Bethesda indeterminate (III to V) and malignant categories is affected by whether NIFTP tumors are considered malignant. For example, the estimated risk of malignancy associated with AUS/FLUS cytology is 10% to 30% if NIFTP is counted as a malignant tumor, but it decreases to 6% to 18% after NIFTP is excluded (1).

The introduction of NIFTP as a nonmalignant entity lowers the risk of malignancy predicted by a positive molecular test result. For example, a retrospective study of 384 thyroid nodules with indeterminate cytology at a single institution demonstrated a decrease in the PPV of the Afirma gene expression classifier (GEC) test from 42% to 24% for Bethesda III and 23% to 13% for Bethesda IV nodules after NIFTP cases were reclassified as nonmalignant (7). It is important to note that the newest molecular tests [Afirma genomic sequencing classifier (GSC) and ThyroSeq v3] were intentionally trained to classify NIFTP as positive (8–10). This would effectively triage NIFTP tumors to surgical excision, which is in keeping with current management recommendations for these tumors with malignant potential. However, because the prevalence of NIFTP among surgically resected thyroid nodules with indeterminate cytology and positive molecular test results is relatively high (44% in a pragmatic randomized trial comparing ThyroSeq v2 and Afirma GEC tests), a conservative surgical approach (lobectomy) is recommended for most thyroid nodules in this setting (11).

Currently Available Molecular Tests for Indeterminate Thyroid Nodules

Afirma GSC

Technology. The Afirma GSC principally uses mRNA expression patterns to risk stratify indeterminate nodules as benign or suspicious. Next-generation sequencing data are used to generate gene expression counts, identify variants, detect fusion pairs, and calculate loss-of-heterozygosity statistics. After the detection of parathyroid tissue and medullary thyroid carcinomas, BRAF mutations and RET/PTC fusions are detected and classified as malignant upstream of the core classifier. The remaining follicular thyroid neoplasms then enter the core classifier, which utilizes machine learning algorithms to distinguish between benign and malignant lesions. One important development between the GSC and the prior-generation GEC is improved specificity in the discernment of Hurthle cell lesions. The Hurthle cell classifier examines mitochondrial genes and chromosomal-level loss-of-heterozygosity statistics to permit a greater fraction of nonneoplastic Hurthle cell lesions to be correctly classified as benign (9).

Clinical Performance and Validation. The clinical performance of Afirma GSC was described in a large-scale (N = 191), industry-sponsored, multicenter, blinded validation study published in May 2018 (9). The prevalence of malignancy in the tested population was 24% among Bethesda III and IV nodules. The sensitivity and specificity of the GSC were 91% and 68%, respectively. The PPV and NPV were 47% and 96%, respectively.

Workflow. FNA material is immediately placed in a proprietary collection microtubule. Samples may be stored at room temperature for up to 72 hours. Thereafter, the samples should be frozen and transported on ice. Because only a minority of FNAs yield an indeterminate result, many samples collected as an additional pass during initial FNA may end up not being used. Furthermore, the practical issue of storing samples and then retrieving/sending select samples out for analysis may be a challenge depending on how a given clinical center is structured. Some centers have consequently elected to bring patients with indeterminate cytologic results back to perform a second FNA dedicated to molecular testing. Clinical centers that use Afirma GSC have the option of performing morphologic cytopathology locally or sending samples to a centralized facility for processing (Thyroid Cytopathology Partners).

ThyroSeq v3

Technology. The ThyroSeq v3 genomic classifier uses next-generation sequencing to analyze DNA and mRNA. It assesses five classes of genetic alterations in 112 thyroid cancer–related genes: point mutations, insertions/deletions, gene fusions, copy number alterations, and gene expression alterations. Similar to other molecular testing platforms, the logical flow begins with the detection of parathyroid cells, C cells, and nonthyroidal cells. The remaining follicular thyroid lesions enter the genomic classifier. Each genetic alteration is assigned a weight of 0 to 2 based on the strength of its association with thyroid cancer. The genomic classifier score is then calculated using a formula that considers the weight, number, and type of alterations (8).

Clinical Performance and Validation. The clinical performance of ThyroSeq v3 was described in a large-scale (N = 232), non–industry-sponsored, multicenter, blinded validation study published in November 2018 (10). The prevalence of cancer or NIFTP was 28%. The sensitivity and specificity of ThyroSeq v3 were 94% and 82%, respectively. The PPV and NPV were 66% and 97%, respectively.

Workflow. FNA material is immediately placed in a proprietary collection vial. Samples may be stored at room temperature for no more than 3 hours and in a refrigerator for no more than 24 hours. Thereafter, samples should be frozen and shipped on ice. The workflow and storage issues associated with ThyroSeq v3 are similar to those encountered with Afirma GSC.

ThyGenX/ThyraMIR

Technology. ThyGenX/ThyraMIR is a duplex assay. The first stage, ThyGenX, uses next-generation sequencing to detect five mutations and three gene fusions. Nodules harboring *BRAF* V600E mutations or clonal *RET/PTC1* or *RET/PTC3* mutations are classified as malignant. The remaining nodules then enter the second stage, ThyraMIR, which measures expression levels of 10 miRNAs and assesses malignancy risk using a proprietary algorithm.

Clinical Performance and Validation. The clinical performance of ThyGenX/ThyraMIR was described in a moderately sized (N = 109), industry-sponsored, multicenter, retrospective study published in 2015 (12). The prevalence of malignancy was 32%. The sensitivity and specificity were 89% and 85%, respectively. The PPV and NPV were 78% and 94%, respectively. In September 2018, Interpace Diagnostics launched a new molecular testing product, ThyGeNEXT, that has yet to be clinically validated.

Workflow. Because ThyGenX/ThyraMIR analyzes DNA and miRNA, both of which are stable molecules, specimen handling and storage are less critical. One option is to obtain FNA material and place it in a proprietary preservative vial. Alternatively, nucleic acid may be isolated from routinely prepared formalin-fixed histopathology or alcohol-fixed cytopathology slides. This may confer a workflow advantage.

Studies Comparing Performance of Molecular Tests

In June 2018, Livhits *et al.* (11) published a prospective, single-center, unblinded, non–industry-sponsored, pragmatic clinical trial comparing the performance of Afirma GEC and ThyroSeq v2 (N = 159). Primary end points were number of diagnostic thyroidectomies avoided, specificity, and PPV (Fig. 1). The prevalence of malignancy was 14%. Diagnostic thyroidectomy was avoided in 39% of patients tested with Afirma GEC and 62% of patients tested with ThyroSeq v2. The specificity of Afirma GEC was 66%, in comparison with 91% for ThyroSeq v2. The PPV of Afirma GEC was 39%, in comparison with 57% for ThyroSeq v2.

In October 2018, Livhits *et al.* (13) presented an identically designed prospective trial comparing the clinical performance of Afirma GSC and ThyroSeq v3. Although the results were preliminary, both tests displayed incremental improvements in PPV, with ThyroSeq v3 demonstrating nonsignificantly higher specificity and PPV compared with Afirma GSC. A comparison of molecular tests is summarized in Table 2.

MAIN CONCLUSIONS

- Each molecular diagnostic test has inherent strengths, weaknesses, and limitations, which must be taken into consideration during use in clinical practice. The sensitivity of current generation tests is high, ranging from 89% to 94%, making them all well suited to rule out malignancy. Specificity is lower and varies more widely, from 68% to 85%.

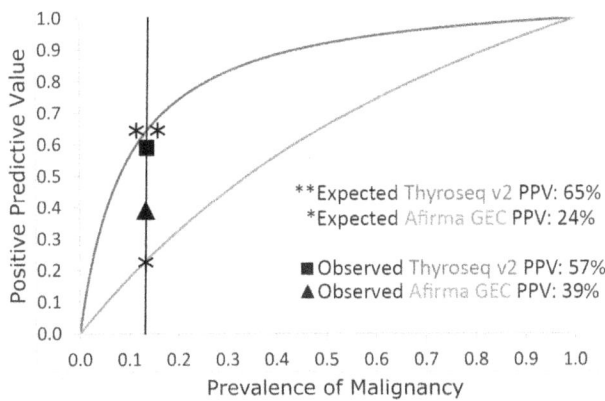

Figure 1. PPV varies with the prevalence of malignancy in the tested population: a comparison of Afirma GEC and ThyroSeq v2 performance. Adapted with permission from Livhits MJ, Kuo EJ, Leung AM, et al. Gene expression classifier vs targeted next-generation sequencing in the management of indeterminate thyroid nodules. *J Clin Endocrinol Metab.* 2018;103(6):2261–2268.

- The NPV and PPV of molecular diagnostic tests are influenced by population malignancy rates, which should ideally be determined in a site-specific manner.
- Indeterminate thyroid nodules with benign/negative molecular tests results are generally observed in clinical practice. Long-term follow-up studies reveal that surgical excision rates remain low over time, and the rate of malignancy in nodules that are excised is reassuringly low (as illustrated in Case 3).

CASES
Case 1
Molecular Test Performance in Indeterminate Thyroid Nodules With Low- to Intermediate-Risk Sonographic Patterns
A 66-year-old woman presents with an incidentally discovered right thyroid nodule. She is euthyroid without risk factors for thyroid cancer. Ultrasound reveals a 2-cm isoechoic, well-demarcated nodule without contralateral nodules or abnormal lymph nodes. FNA reveals AUS (Bethesda III), and molecular testing with ThyroSeq v3 is positive for an *NRAS* mutation, conferring a 50% risk of malignancy.

What is the most appropriate next step in management? What is the breakdown of histopathology findings in *RAS*-positive indeterminate thyroid nodules?

Discussion
RAS mutations (*HRAS*, *NRAS*, *KRAS*) comprise the majority of alterations found among ThyroSeq v2 positive results. Nodules with isolated *RAS* mutations are almost equally likely to be benign thyroid adenomas, NIFTP tumors, or thyroid cancers (11, 17). In the presence of low- to intermediate-risk sonographic features, isolated *RAS*-positive nodules may be managed with active surveillance or thyroid lobectomy. Indeterminate thyroid nodules with positive molecular testing results and American Thyroid Association (ATA) high-risk sonographic features are likely to be malignant and should be managed accordingly (18).

Case 2
Molecular Test Performance in Hurthle Cell Nodules
A 42-year-old woman presents with a 2-year history of an asymptomatic 3-cm right thyroid nodule. She has no risk factors for thyroid cancer. Ultrasound reveals a hypoechoic solid nodule measuring $3.1 \times 2.8 \times 1.6$ cm in the right thyroid lobe with well-defined regular margins consistent with the ATA intermediate-suspicion pattern. No contralateral nodules or abnormal lymph nodes are noted. Serum thyrotropin was 3.0 μU/mL (3.0 mU/L). FNA shows FLUS with a Hurthle cell predominance (Bethesda III). The Afirma GEC test yields a suspicious result.

What management would you recommend for this patient? What is the performance of Afirma GEC in Hurthle cell nodules?

Table 2. Comparative Performance of Molecular Diagnostic Tests Used in Evaluation of Thyroid Nodules With Indeterminate Cytopathology

Molecular Test	TBSRTC	Sensitivity (%)	Specificity (%)
167 mRNA GEC (Afirma GEC) (14)[ab]	III–V	92	52
Seven-gene panel (ThyroSeq v0) (15)[b]	III–V	61	98
19-gene panel (ThyroSeq v2) (16)[b]	III	91	92
	IV	90	93
Eight-gene panel/miRNA GEC (ThyGenX/ThyraMIR) (12)	III–IV	89	85
RNAseq panel (Afirma-GSC) (9)	III–IV	91	68
112-gene panel (ThyroSeq v3 GC) (10)[a]	III–IV	94	82

Abbreviation: RNAseq, RNA sequencing.
[a] Blinded, prospective multicenter trial.
[b] Independent clinical validation studies available.

Discussion

Afirma GEC carries a low specificity in the diagnosis of Hurthle cell lesions (9). That is, Hurthle cell lesions are often categorized as GEC suspicious but have a low rate of malignancy on surgical excision (19). Therefore, the management of such patients should be determined based on the likelihood of malignancy predicted by the patient's clinical risk factors, ultrasound findings, and cytopathology results. In the case described, the most appropriate next step in management would be to perform a repeat FNA for cytology, given that repeat FNA will yield a definitive diagnosis in most cases (20). However, if diagnostic surgery were to be pursued, a lobectomy would be strongly recommended. Refinements were made in the new Afirma GSC to address the low specificity of GEC with Hurthle cell lesions (as described under Afirma GSC technology). A subanalysis of 26 Hurthle cell neoplasms in the GSC clinical validation study demonstrated a significant improvement in the specificity of the test (59%) without any change in sensitivity (89%) (9). The specificity of ThyroSeq v3 in Hurthle cell nodules was evaluated in the recently published multicenter clinical validation study. The study cohort included 49 Hurthle cell nodules (10 malignant, 39 benign). With 13 of 39 histologically benign lesions testing falsely positive, the calculated specificity of ThyroSeq v3 is 67% for Hurthle cell nodules (compared with 82% for the study cohort overall) (10).

Case 3
Long-Term Clinical Behavior of Thyroid Nodules With Negative Molecular Testing

A 66-year-old man underwent ultrasound-guided FNA biopsy and molecular testing of his 2-cm left thyroid nodule 1 year ago. Cytopathology revealed an FN (Bethesda IV), and Afirma GEC testing was benign. The patient opted to pursue clinical and ultrasound surveillance, given the negative molecular test result. Today his neck examination is stable, and a repeat ultrasound also demonstrates unchanged size and appearance of the nodule.

What is the natural history of GEC-benign thyroid nodules? What proportion demonstrate growth over time? What is the likelihood that the nodule will require surgical intervention? How common is thyroid malignancy in resected nodules?

Discussion

Longer-term follow-up studies of thyroid nodules with indeterminate cytology and negative Afirma GEC testing have generally been reassuring. Surgical excision rates are low overall (5% to 7%), and malignancy is uncommon (5, 21). In a multicenter follow-up study of 546 GEC-benign thyroid nodules, 18% of nodules underwent surgical resection, and only 1.8% were malignant (22). Angell *et al.* (21) demonstrated that the growth of GEC-benign nodules was comparable to that of nodules with benign cytology (~8% of nodules in each

group grew by >20% in two dimensions) after a median follow up of 13 months. Deaver *et al.* (5) found that size remained stable in a majority (>70%) of nodules after a median follow-up of 46 months for Bethesda III and 62 months for Bethesda IV nodules (5). Overall these data support the safety of clinical and sonographic surveillance as an alternative to surgery in the management of thyroid nodules with indeterminate cytology but benign GEC testing.

Case 4
Molecular Test Result With Multiple Mutations

A 56-year-old man presents with a 2.5-cm thyroid nodule. FNA is suspicious for FN (Bethesda IV), and ThyroSeq v3 reveals mutations in both *NRAS* and TERT, conferring a 95% risk of malignancy. Sonographically, this is a solitary, slightly hypoechoic, well-demarcated nodule with an ATA intermediate-risk appearance and normal lymph nodes.

What is the most appropriate next step in management? What is the biological behavior of thyroid tumors harboring multiple mutations?

Discussion

Thyroid tumors harboring mutated *BRAF* plus TERT or *RAS* plus TERT combinations are almost always malignant. Furthermore, thyroid cancers with these mutations are highly aggressive, exhibiting increased rates of recurrence and disease-specific death (23, 24). Although the tumor in this case did not exhibit high-risk sonographic features, the molecular profile supersedes other clinical features in this instance. This patient is best managed with total thyroidectomy, with or without neck dissection, followed by radioactive iodine ablation. Histopathology revealed poorly differentiated thyroid carcinoma of follicular origin.

References

1. Cibas ES, Ali SZ. The 2017 Bethesda System for reporting thyroid cytopathology. *Thyroid.* 2017;**27**(11):1341–1346.
2. Cibas ES, Ali SZ. The Bethesda System for reporting thyroid cytopathology. *Thyroid.* 2009;**19**(11):1159–1165.
3. Bongiovanni M, Spitale A, Faquin WC, Mazzucchelli L, Baloch ZW. The Bethesda System for Reporting Thyroid Cytopathology: a meta-analysis. *Acta Cytol.* 2012;**56**(4):333–339.
4. Alexander EK, Schorr M, Klopper J, Kim C, Sipos J, Nabhan F, Parker C, Steward DL, Mandel SJ, Haugen BR. Multicenter clinical experience with the Afirma gene expression classifier. *J Clin Endocrinol Metab.* 2014;**99**(1):119–125.
5. Deaver KE, Haugen BR, Pozdeyev N, Marshall CB. Outcomes of Bethesda categories III and IV thyroid nodules over 5 years and performance of the Afirma gene expression classifier: A single-institution study. *Clin Endocrinol (Oxf).* 2018;**89**(2):226–232.
6. Nikiforov YE, Seethala RR, Tallini G, Baloch ZW, Basolo F, Thompson LD, Barletta JA, Wenig BM, Al Ghuzlan A, Kakudo K, Giordano TJ, Alves VA, Khanafshar E, Asa SL, El-Naggar AK, Gooding WE, Hodak SP, Lloyd RV, Maytal G, Mete O, Nikiforova MN, Nosé V, Papotti M, Poller DN, Sadow PM, Tischler AS, Tuttle RM, Wall KB, LiVolsi VA, Randolph GW, Ghossein RA. Nomenclature revision for encapsulated follicular variant of papillary thyroid carcinoma: a paradigm shift to

reduce overtreatment of indolent tumors. *JAMA Oncol.* 2016;**2**(8): 1023–1029.

7. Hang JF, Westra WH, Cooper DS, Ali SZ. The impact of noninvasive follicular thyroid neoplasm with papillary-like nuclear features on the performance of the Afirma gene expression classifier. *Cancer Cytopathol.* 2017;**125**(9):683–691.

8. Nikiforova MN, Mercurio S, Wald AI, Barbi de Moura M, Callenberg K, Santana-Santos L, Gooding WE, Yip L, Ferris RL, Nikiforov YE. Analytical performance of the ThyroSeq v3 genomic classifier for cancer diagnosis in thyroid nodules. *Cancer.* 2018;**124**(8):1682–1690.

9. Patel KN, Angell TE, Babiarz J, Barth NM, Blevins T, Duh QY, Ghossein RA, Harrell RM, Huang J, Kennedy GC, Kim SY, Kloos RT, LiVolsi VA, Randolph GW, Sadow PM, Shanik MH, Sosa JA, Traweek ST, Walsh PS, Whitney D, Yeh MW, Ladenson PW. Performance of a genomic sequencing classifier for the preoperative diagnosis of cytologically indeterminate thyroid nodules. *JAMA Surg.* 2018;**153**(9):817–824.

10. Steward DL, Carty SE, Sippel RS, Yang SP, Sosa JA, Sipos JA, Figge JJ, Mandel S, Haugen BR, Burman KD, Baloch ZW, Lloyd RV, Seethala RR, Gooding WE, Chiosea SI, Gomes-Lima C, Ferris RL, Folek JM, Khawaja RA, Kundra P, Loh KS, Marshall CB, Mayson S, McCoy KL, Nga ME, Ngiam KY, Nikiforova MN, Poehls JL, Ringel MD, Yang H, Yip L, Nikiforov YE. Performance of a multigene genomic classifier in thyroid nodules with indeterminate cytology: A prospective blinded multicenter study [published online ahead of print 8 November 2018]. *JAMA Oncol.* doi:10.1001/jamaoncol.2018.4616.

11. Livhits MJ, Kuo EJ, Leung AM, Rao J, Levin M, Douek ML, Beckett KR, Zanocco KA, Cheung DS, Gofnung YA, Smooke-Praw S, Yeh MW. Gene expression classifier vs targeted next-generation sequencing in the management of indeterminate thyroid nodules. *J Clin Endocrinol Metab.* 2018;**103**(6):2261–2268.

12. Labourier E, Shifrin A, Busseniers AE, Lupo MA, Manganelli ML, Andruss B, Wylie D, Beaudenon-Huibregtse S. Molecular testing for miRNA, mRNA, and DNA on fine-needle aspiration improves the preoperative diagnosis of thyroid nodules with indeterminate cytology. *J Clin Endocrinol Metab.* 2015;**100**(7):2743–2750.

13. Livhits MJ, Zhu C, Du L, Leung AM, Rao J, Levin M, Douek ML, Beckett KR, Cheung DS, Gofnung Y, Yeh MW. Genomic sequencing classifier versus Thyroseq v3 in the management of indeterminate thyroid nodules: a randomized clinical trial. Presented at: 88th Annual Meeting of the American Thyroid Association; 3–7 October 2018; Washington, DC.

14. Alexander EK, Kennedy GC, Baloch ZW, Cibas ES, Chudova D, Diggans J, Friedman L, Kloos RT, LiVolsi VA, Mandel SJ, Raab SS, Rosai J, Steward DL, Walsh PS, Wilde JI, Zeiger MA, Lanman RB, Haugen BR. Preoperative diagnosis of benign thyroid nodules with indeterminate cytology. *N Engl J Med.* 2012;**367**(8):705–715.

15. Nikiforov YE, Ohori NP, Hodak SP, Carty SE, LeBeau SO, Ferris RL, Yip L, Seethala RR, Tublin ME, Stang MT, Coyne C, Johnson JT, Stewart AF, Nikiforova MN. Impact of mutational testing on the diagnosis and management of patients with cytologically indeterminate thyroid nodules: a prospective analysis of 1056 FNA samples. *J Clin Endocrinol Metab.* 2011;**96**(11):3390–3397.

16. Nikiforova MN, Wald AI, Roy S, Durso MB, Nikiforov YE. Targeted next-generation sequencing panel (ThyroSeq) for detection of mutations in thyroid cancer. *J Clin Endocrinol Metab.* 2013;**98**(11): E1852–E1860.

17. Marcadis AR, Valderrabano P, Ho AS, Tepe J, Swartzwelder CE, Byrd S, Sacks WL, Untch BR, Shaha AR, Xu B, Lin O, Ghossein RA, Wong RJ, Marti JL, Morris LGT. Interinstitutional variation in predictive value of the ThyroSeq v2 genomic classifier for cytologically indeterminate thyroid nodules. *Surgery.* 2019;**165**(1):17–24.

18. Wang MM, Beckett KR, Douek ML, Masamed R, Patel MK, Tseng CH, Yeh MW, Leung AM, Livhits MJ. Role of molecular testing in cytologically indeterminate, sonographically suspicious thyroid nodules. Presented at: 88th Annual Meeting of the American Thyroid Association; 3–7 October 2018; Washington, DC.

19. Brauner E, Holmes BJ, Krane JF, Nishino M, Zurakowski D, Hennessey JV, Faquin WC, Parangi S. Performance of the Afirma gene expression classifier in Hürthle cell thyroid nodules differs from other indeterminate thyroid nodules. *Thyroid.* 2015;**25**(7):789–796.

20. Haugen BR, Alexander EK, Bible KC, Doherty GM, Mandel SJ, Nikiforov YE, Pacini F, Randolph GW, Sawka AM, Schlumberger M, Schuff KG, Sherman SI, Sosa JA, Steward DL, Tuttle RM, Wartofsky L. 2015 American Thyroid Association management guidelines for adult patients with thyroid nodules and differentiated thyroid cancer: The American Thyroid Association Guidelines Task Force on Thyroid Nodules and Differentiated Thyroid Cancer. *Thyroid.* 2016;**26**(1): 1–133.

21. Angell TE, Frates MC, Medici M, Liu X, Kwong N, Cibas ES, Kim MI, Marqusee E. Afirma benign thyroid nodules show similar growth to cytologically benign nodules during follow-up. *J Clin Endocrinol Metab.* 2015;**100**(11):E1477–E1483.

22. Angell TE, Maurer R, Chen AC, Deaver KE, Endo M, Marshall CB, Mayson SE, Nabhan F, Ro K, Sipos JA, Yeh MW, Livhits MJ. Multicenter follow up and outcomes of Afirma GEC benign thyroid nodules. Presented at: 88th Annual Meeting of the American Thyroid Association; 3–7 October 2018; Washington, DC.

23. Song YS, Lim JA, Choi H, Won JK, Moon JH, Cho SW, Lee KE, Park YJ, Yi KH, Park DJ, Seo JS. Prognostic effects of TERT promoter mutations are enhanced by coexistence with BRAF or RAS mutations and strengthen the risk prediction by the ATA or TNM staging system in differentiated thyroid cancer patients. *Cancer.* 2016;**122**(9):1370–1379.

24. Liu R, Bishop J, Zhu G, Zhang T, Ladenson PW, Xing M. Mortality risk stratification by combining BRAF V600E and TERT promoter mutations in papillary thyroid cancer: genetic duet of BRAF and TERT promoter mutations in thyroid cancer mortality [published online ahead of print 1 September 2016]. *JAMA Oncol.* doi:10.1001/jamaoncol.2016.3288.

Evaluation and Treatment of Thyroid Nodules and Differentiated Thyroid Carcinoma in Children and Adolescents

M22
Presented, March 23–26, 2019

Andrew J. Bauer, MD. Pediatric Thyroid Center, Children's Hospital of Philadelphia, Philadelphia, Pennsylvania 19104; and Perelman School of Medicine, University of Pennsylvania, Philadelphia, Pennsylvania 19104, E-mail: bauera@chop.edu

Herbert Chen, MD, FACS. Department of Surgery, University of Alabama at Birmingham, Birmingham, Alabama 35233; and American Association of Endocrine Surgeons, Lexington, Kentucky 40507, E-mail: hchen@uabmc.edu

SIGNIFICANCE OF THE CLINICAL PROBLEM

Approximately 1% to 2% of pediatric patients have a thyroid nodule noted on physical examination (PE), and up to 18% have a thyroid abnormality (cyst or nodule) on ultrasound (US). For a majority of patients, there is no identifiable etiology; however, multiple factors are associated with increased risk for developing a nodule and/or thyroid cancer, the most common being previous history of exposure to radiation for treatment of a nonthyroid malignancy.

Over the last decade, the annual incidence of pediatric thyroid carcinoma has steadily increased. The increase in the number of adolescent patients diagnosed with thyroid cancer has followed similarly reported data in adults. Although the greatest increase has been in tumors between 0.5 and 1 cm, there has been an increase in the diagnosis of tumors across all sizes, suggesting that the increased use of imaging is not solely responsible for the increasing trend.

BARRIERS TO OPTIMAL PRACTICE

- The low incidence and typically indolent clinical course of disease pose significant challenges to optimizing and individualizing care.
- The low incidence of disease is associated with a decreased opportunity to develop medical and surgical expertise. At the same time, nonportability of insurance and cost limit the ability of patients to travel to centers with greater expertise. This leads to wide variability in the approach to diagnosis and treatment and an increased risk of complications.

LEARNING OBJECTIVES

After this Meet the Professor session, participants will be able to:

- Identify the incidence and risk factors associated with the development of thyroid nodules and thyroid cancer in children and adolescents
- Incorporate the pediatric-specific issues into the development of an age-appropriate evaluation and treatment plan
- Discuss benefits and risks of thyroid surgery
- Develop an understanding of patient-specific data used to stratify medical and surgical treatments

STRATEGIES FOR DIAGNOSIS, THERAPY, AND/OR MANAGEMENT
Patients at Increased Risk

The most common risk factors for developing thyroid nodules and thyroid cancer include:

- Familial predisposition
  Nonsyndromic: not associated with a clinical phenotype or an increased risk of developing other tumors
  Syndromic: associated with a clinical phenotype and an increased risk of developing other tumors [eg, PTEN hamartoma syndrome (PHTS), DICER1-related syndrome, familial adenomatous polyposis, Carney complex, and multiple endocrine neoplasia type 2]
- Previous exposure to ionizing radiation: radiation used to treat a non–thyroid-related malignancy, repeated exposure to diagnostic radiologic imaging, or environmental (nuclear power plant accident or ambient)

A majority of patients are diagnosed with differentiated thyroid cancer (DTC) after discovery of an asymptomatic nodule or persistent cervical lymphadenopathy with no identifiable risk factors. For patients in the high-risk categories, there is disagreement and variation in practice with regard to if and when surveillance USs should be performed. Those in favor of screening refer to an increased risk of thyroid malignancy within these subpopulations, with an interest in identifying the cancer at an earlier state of metastasis, when less aggressive treatment may be sufficient to achieve remission. Those against surveillance raise concern over the potential for an increased number of procedures performed to detect a small number of clinically significant thyroid malignancies as well as the potential for patients with indolent cancers, which may not have been associated with clinically significant disease over their lifetime, to be subjected to treatment; ~10% of us will die as a result of old age and be found to have had an incidental, indolent thyroid cancer on autopsy.

Familial Nonmedullary Thyroid Carcinoma

Familial nonmedullary thyroid carcinoma is defined by the presence of two or more first-degree relatives with a history of DTC. There are conflicting data as to if, when, and with what frequency family members should undergo surveillance thyroid US screening. With some evidence of anticipation (ie, earlier development of thyroid cancer in succeeding generations), it is reasonable that the first US be performed during early adolescence.

Genetic Syndromes

PHTS, DICER1 pleuropulmonary blastoma syndrome, familial adenomatous polyposis, and Carney complex syndrome are the most frequent syndromes associated with an increased risk of thyroid nodules and DTC (Table 1). Multiple endocrine neoplasia type 2 is the syndrome associated with an increased risk for developing medullary thyroid cancer (MTC). In pediatrics, ≥75% of MTCs are associated with germ line mutations in the *RET* proto-oncogene (in adults, ≥75% of MTCs are sporadic). Details on individual risk and timing of surveillance can be found in GeneReviews (http://www.ncbi.nlm.nih.gov/books/NBK1116/).

Nonthyroid Childhood Malignancies

For survivors of nonthyroid childhood malignancies, there is a 10- to 18-fold increased incidence of developing thyroid carcinoma, with a latency range of 5 to 35 years. Within this cohort, younger age at the time of exposure and female sex are both associated with an increased risk for and shorter latency in development of thyroid nodules and thyroid cancer. The amount of radiation exposure also affects risk, with lower doses associated with a fairly linear relationship between dose and risk up to ~18 Gy. Within this group of patients, annual PE of the thyroid should be instituted with the first 3 years postexposure, with consideration of annual thyroid US surveillance starting 3 to 5 years postexposure.

Autoimmune Thyroid Disease

There seems to be an increased risk of thyroid nodules in patients with autoimmune thyroid disease. However, there are mixed reports regarding whether there is an increased risk of thyroid cancer. Thyroid US should be considered if there is thyroid gland asymmetry, suspicion of a nodule based on PE, or asymmetric persistent lymphadenopathy, particularly in the mid to lower neck (levels III and IV). Thyroid US should also be considered during evaluation for definitive treatment of autoimmune hyperthyroidism (Graves' disease), because there is an increased risk of malignancy in nodular Graves' disease. Interpreting thyroid US in the setting of autoimmune thyroid disease may be challenging, because the tissue typically has a patchy or focal nodular (cobblestoned) appearance. This may make it difficult to determine if a region is a nodule or a pseudonodule (an area of irregularity associated with the autoimmune process), increasing the chances that fine-needle aspiration (FNA) biopsy will need to be performed. Viewing the area in video cine mode and with color Doppler is essential in determining if the area is a nodule or a pseudonodule.

Evaluation
US

Thyroid US is an inexpensive and noninvasive method for evaluating and screening for thyroid nodules. US can detect lesions as small as 2 to 3 mm and provides information on the size, location, echogenicity, blood flow, multiplicity, and potential involvement of regional lymph nodes. There are several systems that may be used to stratify which nodules should undergo FNA, including the American Thyroid Association (ATA) thyroid nodule sonographic pattern system and the American College of Radiology Thyroid Imaging Reporting and Data System (TI-RADS). Both of these systems have been validated in pediatrics and are being increasingly incorporated into clinical practice. For TI-RADS, thyroid nodule composition, echogenicity, shape, margin, and presence of echogenic foci are the scorable features. Size is an added component, with a decreasing diameter to perform FNA associated with increasing features concerning for malignancy. Blood flow on Doppler imaging is not considered an actionable feature; however, the presence of cervical lymphadenopathy is important and may

Table 1. Molecular Genetics of Pediatric Thyroid Cancer

Oncogene	Increased Risk of DTC	Increased Risk of Invasive Disease
BRAF	Yes	Adults (high risk)
		Pediatrics (moderate risk)
RET-PTC fusion	Yes	Yes (high risk)
NTRK fusion	Yes	Yes (high risk)
BRAF fusion	Yes	Pediatrics (yes; limited data)
DICER1, RAS	Yes, but also found in benign disease (NIFTP and FA)	No; may be associated with dedifferentiated disease (uncommon in pediatrics)

Adapted with permission from Bauer AJ. Molecular genetics of thyroid cancer in children and adolescents. *Endocrinol Metab Clin North Am.* 2017;46(2):389–403.
Abbreviations: FA, follicular adenoma; NIFTP, noninvasive follicular thyroid neoplasm with papillary-like nuclear features.

overrule the likelihood of thyroid malignancy in nodules that would otherwise be considered too small to pursue FNA. Additional important points to remember:

- If a thyroid nodule is found, US examination of the lateral neck is a critical step to help determine the malignant potential of a thyroid lesion.
- Within pediatrics and young adults, a diffusely infiltrative form of papillary thyroid carcinoma (PTC; diffuse sclerosing variant PTC) presents with a large, heterogeneous gland, scattered microcalcifications (snowstorm), hyperemia, and lateral neck lymphadenopathy. This may occupy half of or the entire gland. There is no distinct nodule on US.
- Cystic composition is the single most reliable feature to predict a low-risk lesion (>50% to 75% cystic).

FNA Biopsy

FNA biopsy is the most efficient method for determining the malignant potential of a thyroid nodule. Conscious sedation for younger children and anxiolytics for adolescents are appropriate and recommended. Distraction techniques may also be attempted rather than using sedation. US guidance and bedside confirmation of sample adequacy decrease the rate of inadequate sampling. In patients with multinodular disease, FNA should be performed on nodules that display different echogenic features; the largest nodule may not be the most concerning for malignancy. FNA of concerning lateral neck lymph nodes allows for appropriate surgical planning. A thyroglobulin (Tg) level obtained from saline washout of the FNA needle can aid in diagnosing lymph node metastasis if the cytology is equivocal. The Bethesda System for Reporting Thyroid Cytopathology (TBSRTC) is the most commonly used system to define the risk of malignancy from FNA samples.

Similar to adults, up to 20% to 30% of pediatric and young adult patients or more will have indeterminate cytology, and the risk of malignancy in pediatric patients with indeterminate cytology seems to be higher than that in the adult-based TBSRTC. The presence of an oncogene driver mutation or fusion increases the likelihood that the nodule is malignant. Gene expression or sequencing classifiers and miRNA panels have not been adequately studied in pediatrics and should not be used in patients <21 years of age.

Other Methods of Evaluation

Radioiodine Scan. In general, thyroid radioisotope scans are not helpful in distinguishing benign from malignant disease. Although there is a lower incidence of malignancy in functional (warm or hot) nodules, there are reports of PTC being associated with autonomous nodules and toxic multinodular goiter.

In practice, radioiodine scans should be performed only when screening laboratories reveal suppressed thyrotropin (TSH) and the US reveals a thyroid nodule. The uptake and scan may be used to confirm autonomous function; however, because of the risk of malignancy, lobectomy should be considered

over radioactive iodine (RAI) ablation for hot thyroid nodules. FNA may be used to aid in this decision.

FDG-PET. There have been multiple studies in adult patients with thyroid cancer exploring the potential utility of fluorodeoxyglucose–positron emission tomography (FDG-PET) to identify metastatic disease. Unfortunately, there is significant overlap between standard uptake values for benign and malignant disease. In pediatric patients, the increased incidence of non–thyroid-related cervical adenopathy further complicates the interpretation of FDG-PET. Therefore, FDG-PET should not be a routine test in determining the malignant potential of a thyroid nodule in a child or adolescent.

Alternatively, if FDG-PET is performed for evaluation of nonthyroid malignancy and there is incidental uptake noted within the thyroid, thyroid US and FNA should be considered as the next steps in the evaluation. Approximately 40% of these lesions are ultimately found to be malignant.

Last, for the uncommon pediatric patient with non–RAI-avid disease, FDG-PET may be used to find persistent metastatic disease not discovered by US or axial imaging.

Surgery

Preoperative Staging for Surgery (Bethesda Categories V and VI)

Careful and deliberate US investigation of the neck should be a routine part of the preoperative evaluation, with the highest incidence of lymph node metastasis found in cervical levels VI (central neck) followed by III, IV, and II (depending on location of the thyroid nodule, upper vs lower pole of the thyroid lobe).

Features that are diagnostic and/or concerning for metastatic disease to lymph nodes include:

Concerning	Diagnostic
Rounded shape	Peripheral blood flow on Doppler
Increased echogenicity	Microcalcifications
Absent fatty hilum	Cystic changes

For patients with extensive lymphadenopathy, neck CT with contrast or MRI may be considered to more thoroughly evaluate deep regions of the neck as well as the aerodigestive track.

Preoperative screening for evidence of pulmonary metastasis may also be considered, but it rarely has an impact on the decision over the initial surgical approach. Routine chest x-ray has low sensitivity to detect metastatic disease, because a majority of pediatric patients with pulmonary disease have micronodular (1 to 3 mm per lesion) metastases.

Surgical Approach

Total thyroidectomy (TT) is the procedure of choice for a majority of pediatric patients if the FNA result is suspicious (risk of malignancy >75%) or consistent with malignancy (>98% risk of malignancy). Up to 20% to 25% of patients will have occult bilateral disease not detected on US, with multiple studies showing a higher risk of recurrence and subsequent need for second procedures when less than TT is performed. Prophylactic central neck dissection, either ipsilateral or bilateral, can be considered for most patients secondary to the increased rate of lymph node metastasis. In adults, a randomized prospective trial did not show any benefit and was associated with a significantly higher complication rate with the addition of a central neck dissection. Therefore, in adults, routine prophylactic central neck dissection is typically not performed. In pediatrics, there is ongoing discussion on the clinical benefit of prophylactic central neck dissection. The 2015 ATA pediatric guidelines recommend prophylactic central neck dissection in an effort to help define the invasive behavior of disease and to stratify which patients may or may not benefit from RAI therapy. With the addition of more recent data from South Korea (Jeon *et al.*), patients with five or fewer lymph nodes displaying micrometastases are considered to have a high likelihood of surgical remission (ATA low risk for persistent postsurgical disease), whereas patients with more than five lymph nodes or extrathyroidal extension are at increased risk of persistent postsurgical disease (ATA moderate risk). Lateral neck dissection should only be pursued if suspicious lymph nodes are identified on the preoperative staging US.

Lobectomy may be considered for patients when FNA of a solitary nodule reveals a follicular lesion of undetermined significance (pediatric risk of malignancy, 15% to 20%) or follicular neoplasm (pediatric risk of malignancy, 30% to 40%). The advantage to performing less aggressive surgery is a lower surgical complication risk and avoidance of lifelong thyroid hormone replacement. The disadvantage is the potential need for completion thyroidectomy if the final histology reveals invasive PTC or follicular thyroid carcinoma (FTC). For patients found to have encapsulated noninvasive follicular variant PTC, lobectomy without completion thyroidectomy may be adequate to achieve surgical remission. If less aggressive surgical intervention is pursued, the risks and benefits of less aggressive surgery must be discussed with the family.

Risk of Surgical Complications

The most common complications after thyroidectomy are transient or permanent hypoparathyroidism and damage to the recurrent laryngeal nerve (RLN). Complications can be markedly reduced by referral to a high-volume thyroid surgeon, a surgeon who performs ≥30 thyroid surgeries annually. Within this setting, the risk of permanent hypothyroidism should be <3% to 4%, and the risk of permanent laryngeal nerve damage <1% to 2%.

Several studies have been shown that the incidence of symptomatic hypocalcemia after thyroidectomy can be reduced using a PTH protocol. Obtaining intraoperative PTH or postoperative PTH in the postanesthesia care unit can be used to predict patients at risk for hypoparathyroidism, allowing early initiation of calcitriol and calcium therapy. With the

modernization of these and other surgical practices, there is at least one thyroid surgery center that has safely performed lobectomy and thyroidectomy as outpatient procedures for most adolescents and adults. Many surgeons have advocated for use of RLN monitoring. Several studies, including a large randomized prospective trial, have shown that the use of the intraoperative nerve monitor does not reduce incidence of nerve injury; however, the use of RLN monitoring can reduce the catastrophic risk of bilateral RLN damage by alerting the surgeon in real time to unilateral RLN signal loss and affording an altered, less aggressive dissection to the contralateral side.

Radioiodine Therapy

Individual patient risk and postoperative staging data should be used to determine which patients may benefit from RAI treatment. The 2015 ATA pediatric guidelines provide detail on the use of postsurgical RAI as well as surveillance and additional RAI therapy for patients with evidence of persistent disease (regional and pulmonary).

Patients with solitary disease confined to the thyroid (T1 or T2) and no evidence of lymph node metastasis (N0) are considered to be ATA low risk for postsurgical disease. These patients can be followed with postoperative TSH-suppressed Tg every 3 to 4 months to determine if and/or when additional staging would be indicated. A thyroid US at 6 to 12 months should be obtained as part of the surveillance process.

Patients with evidence of extrathyroidal extension, extensive central neck lymph node metastasis (fewer than five lymph nodes with PTC), lateral neck lymph node metastasis (N1b), and distant metastasis (most commonly to the lungs) are considered ATA moderate to high risk for persistent postsurgical disease. These patients should undergo postoperative assessment (staging) to define the location and extent of disease. Postoperative staging includes a TSH-stimulated Tg and a diagnostic whole-body scan (DxWBS), preferably using iodine-123 (^{123}I). Patients are placed on a low-iodine diet, and thyroid hormone is withdrawn ~2 weeks before the DxWBS. To optimize RAI uptake, TSH must be >30 μIU/mL. The TSH-stimulated Tg and the DxWBS data are then used to determine if RAI is appropriate, as well as the delivered activity (dose) of radioiodine (^{131}I) therapy. Dosing can be empiric, using standard adult dosing adjusted based on weight (kg) and data from the DxWBS, or determined by dosimetry.

If the TSH-stimulated Tg (anti-Tg negative) is undetectable and there is no evidence of uptake on DxWBS, RAI may not be of any benefit. For all patients who receive RAI therapy, a post-treatment scan should be obtained 5 to 7 days after ^{131}I administration to take advantage of the increased sensitivity to localize metastatic disease not noted on the lower-dose DxWBS. The addition of single-photon emission CT (SPECT)/CT to the RAI WBS should be considered to anatomically define the location of RAI uptake in less common or unexpected locations.

Long-Term Follow-Up

The mainstay of long-term therapy is TSH suppression. PE with laboratory surveillance [TSH, free T_4, Tg, and anti-Tg antibody (TgAb)] is typically performed at 3-month intervals, with neck US performed every 6 to 12 months. With the incorporation of ultrasensitive Tg assays, the trend of Tg and/or TgAb is a sensitive marker for disease status. After initial treatment, the Tg nadir may not be achieved for 12, 15, 18, or more months. With this in mind, if the Tg trend is decreasing, and there is no evidence of persistent disease on PE and neck US, continued surveillance is indicated. If the Tg plateaus and or increases, repeat neck US should be performed to look for evidence of persistent surgically resectable disease. Noncontrast chest CT should be considered if the neck US is negative. If neither the US nor CT reveal an explanation for the Tg, repeat TSH-stimulated Tg and DxWBS should be considered. The most common locations of persistent or recurrent PTC are the neck, followed by lung and then bone; in FTC, lung and/or bone may be more frequent than the neck. Although there are no data showing an absolute relationship between the Tg level and the degree of disease burden, higher levels are frequent in patients with pulmonary metastasis. In selected patients, hybrid imaging using SPECT with CT allows for optimal anatomic localization of disease if uptake is in an unexpected location or if additional surgical resection is being considered.

Up to one third of patients with pulmonary metastasis develop persistent stable disease that may not show progression. This is determined after a second RAI treatment where the Tg level does not decrease and repeat radiologic imaging (noncontrast chest CT) continues to show persistent disease. In these patients, repeat RAI therapy does not seem to offer any benefit. These patients should be followed with serial noncontrast chest CT, and if there is evidence of anatomic progression, repeat RAI could be attempted. Alternatively, systemic therapy using a tyrosine kinase inhibitor or targeted therapy could be considered based on the extent of disease. Every year, there are newer, more effective drugs being introduced into clinical practice. Consultation with a provider with experience in treating pediatric patients with progressive RAI-refractory disease is critical to determining the timing, medication (often based on somatic mutation analysis), dosing, and surveillance plan for adverse reactions as well as response to therapy.

MAIN CONCLUSIONS/POINTS OF INTEREST/CLINICAL PEARLS

Long-term survival for childhood thyroid cancer is excellent, even in children with extensive cervical neck lymph node metastasis as well as pulmonary metastasis. However, although cancer-specific mortality is low, the risk of treatment complications and the risk of recurrence are higher compared with adults with similar disease. Therefore, using disease-specific mortality as a metric is not informative in an effort to stratify treatment of DTC in pediatrics. Our goal must be focused on improving disease-free survival and optimizing individualized therapy to decrease the risk of complications. The formation of regional pediatric thyroid centers capable of providing the full spectrum of medical and surgical resources for evaluation and care will aid efforts to decrease potential short- and long-term complications for children and adolescents with thyroid nodules and/or thyroid cancer. Great strides in care and quality of life can be achieved with the formation of a national pediatric consortium comprising a community of regional centers combined with patient-driven advocacy (eg, Thyroid Cancer Survivors' Association; http://www.thyca.org).

CASES

Case 1

An 11.5-year-old girl presents with 5-kg weight loss associated with purposeful diet modification and increased exercise. On examination, her primary care provider notes increased baseline heart rate (103 beats/min) and an enlarged thyroid. Thyroid function tests are ordered and reveal a TSH of 0.02 mIU/L (normal range, 0.5 to 4.3 mIU/L), T_3 of 2.5 ng/mL (normal range, 0.8 to 2.1 ng/mL), and free T_4 of 2.6 ng/dL (normal range, 0.9 to 1.4 ng/dL). Her medical history and her family history are noncontributory. She is referred to pediatric endocrinology for further evaluation.

What test would you order to delineate the diagnosis? Are there advantages to one test over the other?

A. TSH-receptor antibody
B. Thyroid-stimulating immunoglobulin (TSI)
C. Thyroid US
D. ^{131}I or ^{123}I uptake and scan

Results reveal an elevated TSI of 271% (<129%) and 52.9% uptake at 24 hours (<30%). Methimazole is started at 20 mg twice daily (0.6 mg/kg per day; 67 kg).

Follow-up examination 3 months after initial presentation is concerning for asymmetrically enlarged lymph nodes in the right lateral neck. Thyroid US is ordered and reveals multiple, solid hypoechoic nodules in the right lobe (one ~1- × 0.8- × 1.3-cm hypoechoic nodule in the posterior aspect of the right lobe is shown) with enlarged, rounded lymph nodes in right and left lateral neck at levels II, III, and IV, with increased echogenicity, no microcalcifications, and peripheral flow on Doppler imaging (one large abnormal lymph node between the right carotid artery and jugular vein is shown).

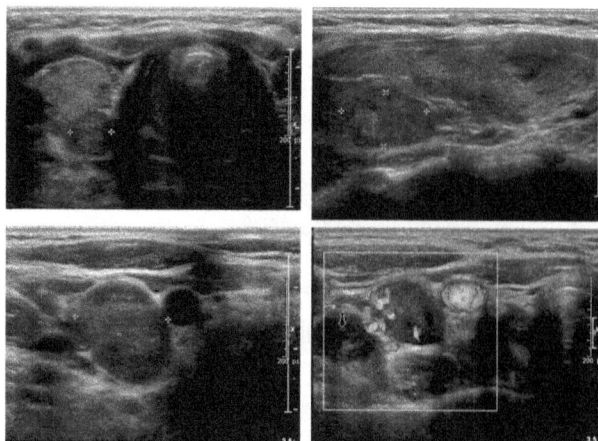

What diagnostic test would you perform next?

A. Thyroid uptake and scan (^{131}I or ^{123}I)

B. Core biopsy of the right thyroid nodule and lateral lymph node

C. FNA biopsy of the right thyroid nodule and lateral lymph node

D. Excisional or wedge biopsy of a right lateral lymph node

FNA biopsy is consistent with PTC with metastasis to the right and left lateral neck.

Would you consider additional preoperative imaging? If so, which of the following would you obtain?

A. Chest x-ray

B. Noncontrast chest CT

C. Neck CT

D. Neck MRI

Neck MRI is complete and confirms the presence of bilateral, lateral neck, pretracheal, submandibular, and superior mediastinal lymph node metastasis without evidence of aerodigestive or vascular invasion.

TT and central, bilateral, lateral neck dissection are performed and multifocal and bilateral PTC with tall-cell features, extrathyroidal extension, extensive lymphovascular invasion, and metastasis to the central and lateral neck lymph nodes with extracapsular invasion into soft tissue (T3N1bMx) is found.

Four weeks after surgery, the patient is placed on a low-iodine diet and thyroid hormone withdrawal. ^{123}I DxWBS reveals diffuse pulmonary disease as well as two areas of increased uptake in the neck. US of these two cervical foci shows a postoperative right-sided hematoma or seroma and a persistent 1.3- × 0.7- × 0.5-cm left-sided lymph node with evidence of PTC metastasis. TSH is 147.5 mIU/L, and Tg is 2613 ng/mL; anti-Tg is undetectable.

Would you proceed with radioiodine therapy or pursue resection of the persistent left-sided pathologic lymph node?

Would you use empiric dosing adjusted for age, weight, and persistent disease or use dosimetry to calculate the administered radioiodine activity?

The patient is administered 94.5 mCi of ^{131}I (3497 Mbq). Post-RAI treatment scan reveals no additional lesions. The patient is placed on TSH-suppressive therapy, and TSH-suppressed Tg levels are followed every 3 months.

How would you follow her persistent cervical disease?

How would you follow her lung disease?

When would you repeat a TSH-stimulated Tg and a DxWBS?

When would you consider repeat administration of RAI?

Case 2

A 12-year-old boy presents with a 2.3-cm left thyroid nodule. He is otherwise healthy without any other notable medical history. There is no family history of thyroid disease. PE is normal except for the palpable thyroid nodule on the left. TSH is normal. US reveals a solid left 2/3-cm mass without any other thyroid lesions.

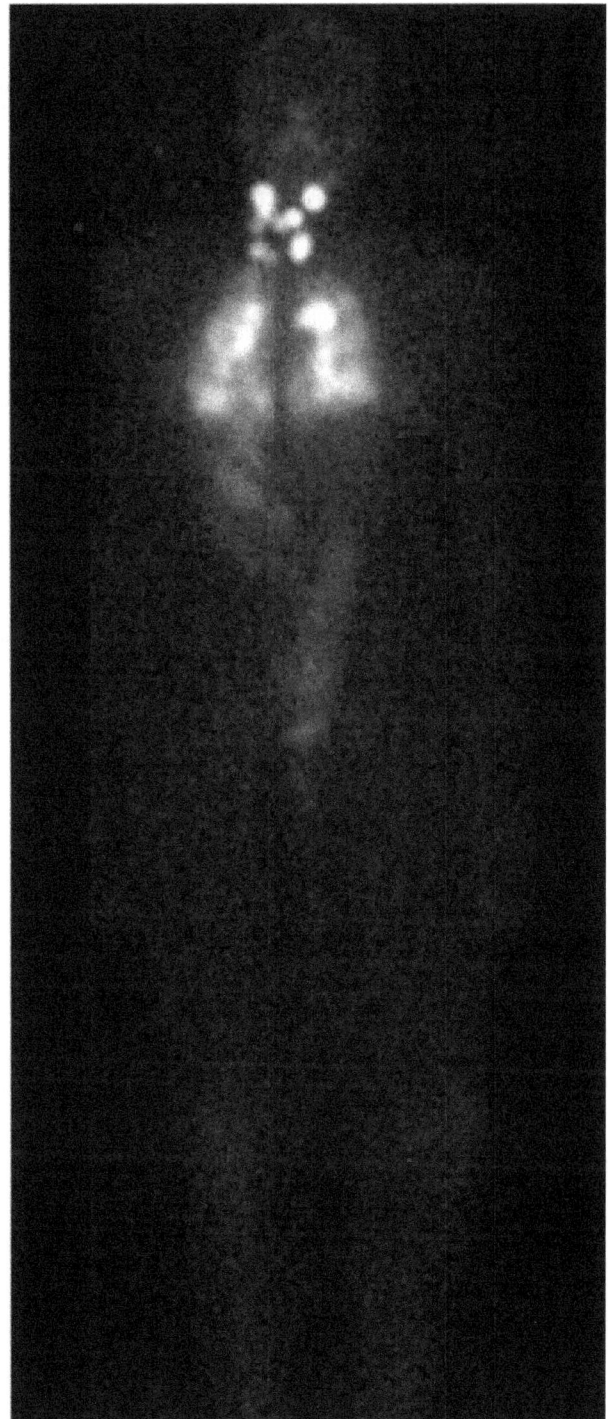

FNA of the thyroid nodules reveals a follicular lesion of undetermined significance (Bethesda III).

Because the FNA result was reported under the TBSRTC as indeterminate (follicular lesion of undetermined significance or follicular neoplasm), would you consider ordering either of the tests listed below? Are there data to support their use in pediatrics?

A. Oncogene panel

B. Gene expression classifier panel

C. MiRNA panel

After a discussion of the surgical options, the patient undergoes a left thyroid lobectomy as an outpatient procedure. Surgery is uncomplicated. He is seen with his parents in the postoperative clinic 10 days later. The final pathology is a PTC of 2.3 cm. There is no extrathyroidal invasion, and the margins are negative.

What is your next recommendation?

Recommended Reading

Biko J, Reiners C, Kreissl MC, Verburg FA, Demidchik Y, Drozd V. Favourable course of disease after incomplete remission on (131)I therapy in children with pulmonary metastases of papillary thyroid carcinoma: 10 years follow-up. *Eur J Nucl Med Mol Imaging.* 2011; **38**(4):651–655.

Carter Y, Chen H, Sippel RS. An intact parathyroid hormone-based protocol for the prevention and treatment of symptomatic hypocalcemia after thyroidectomy. *J Surg Res.* 2014;**186**(1):23–28.

Clement SC, Kremer LCM, Verburg FA, Simmons JH, Goldfarb M, Peeters RP, Alexander EK, Bardi E, Brignardello E, Constine LS, Dinauer CA, Drozd VM, Felicetti F, Frey E, Heinzel A, van den Heuvel-Eibrink MM, Huang SA, Links TP, Lorenz K, Mulder RL, Neggers SJ, Nieveen van Dijkum EJM, Oeffinger KC, van Rijn RR, Rivkees SA, Ronckers CM, Schneider AB, Skinner R, Wasserman JD, Wynn T, Hudson MM, Nathan PC, van Santen HM. Balancing the benefits and harms of thyroid cancer surveillance in survivors of Childhood, adolescent and young adult cancer: recommendations from the international Late Effects of Childhood Cancer Guideline Harmonization Group in collaboration with the PanCareSurFup Consortium. *Cancer Treat Rev.* 2018;**63**: 28–39.

Demidchik YE, Demidchik EP, Reiners C, Biko J, Mine M, Saenko VA, Yamashita S. Comprehensive clinical assessment of 740 cases of surgically treated thyroid cancer in children of Belarus. *Ann Surg.* 2006;**243**(4):525–532.

Francis GL, Waguespack SG, Bauer AJ, Angelos P, Benvenga S, Cerutti JM, Dinauer CA, Hamilton J, Hay ID, Luster M, Parisi MT, Rachmiel M, Thompson GB, Yamashita S; American Thyroid Association Guidelines Task Force. Management guidelines for children with thyroid nodules and differentiated thyroid cancer. *Thyroid.* 2015;**25**(7):716–759.

Gannon AW, Langer JE, Bellah R, Ratcliffe S, Pizza J, Mostoufi-Moab S, Cappola AR, Bauer AJ. Diagnostic accuracy of ultrasound with color flow Doppler in children with thyroid nodules. *J Clin Endocrinol Metab.* 2018;**103**(5):1958–1965.

Gupta A, Ly S, Castroneves LA, Frates MC, Benson CB, Feldman HA, Wassner AJ, Smith JR, Marqusee E, Alexander EK, Barletta J, Doubilet

PM, Peters HE, Webb S, Modi BP, Paltiel HJ, Kozakewich H, Cibas ES, Moore FD Jr, Shamberger RC, Larsen PR, Huang SA. A standardized assessment of thyroid nodules in children confirms higher cancer prevalence than in adults. *J Clin Endocrinol Metab.* 2013;**98**(8): 3238–3245.

Hay ID, Gonzalez-Losada T, Reinalda MS, Honetschlager JA, Richards ML, Thompson GB. Long-term outcome in 215 children and adolescents with papillary thyroid cancer treated during 1940 through 2008. *World J Surg.* 2010;**34**(6):1192–1202.

Jarzab B, Handkiewicz Junak D, Włoch J, Kalemba B, Roskosz J, Kukulska A, Puch Z. Multivariate analysis of prognostic factors for differentiated thyroid carcinoma in children. *Eur J Nucl Med.* 2000;**27**(7):833–841.

Jeon MJ, Kim YN, Sung TY, Hong SJ, Cho YY, Kim TY, Shong YK, Kim WB, Kim SW, Chung JH, Kim TH, Kim WG. Practical initial risk stratification based on lymph node metastases in pediatric and adolescent differentiated thyroid cancer. *Thyroid.* 2018;**28**(2):193–200.

Mallick R, Asban A, Chung S, Hur J, Lindeman B, Chen H. To admit or not to admit? Experience with outpatient thyroidectomy for Graves' disease in a high-volume tertiary care center. *Am J Surg.* 2018;**216**(5): 985–989.

Martinez-Rios C, Daneman A, Bajno L, van der Kaay DCM, Moineddin R, Wasserman JD. Utility of adult-based ultrasound malignancy risk stratifications in pediatric thyroid nodules. *Pediatr Radiol.* 2018;**48**(1): 74–84.

Padovani RP, Robenshtok E, Brokhin M, Tuttle RM. Even without additional therapy, serum thyroglobulin concentrations often decline for years after total thyroidectomy and radioactive remnant ablation in patients with differentiated thyroid cancer. *Thyroid.* 2012;**22**(8): 778–783.

Sawka AM, Thabane L, Parlea L, Ibrahim-Zada I, Tsang RW, Brierley JD, Straus S, Ezzat S, Goldstein DP. Second primary malignancy risk after radioactive iodine treatment for thyroid cancer: a systematic review and meta-analysis. *Thyroid.* 2009;**19**(5):451–457.

Tessler FN, Middleton WD, Grant EG, Hoang JK, Berland LL, Teefey SA, Cronan JJ, Beland MD, Desser TS, Frates MC, Hammers LW, Hamper UM, Langer JE, Reading CC, Scoutt LM, Stavros AT. ACR Thyroid Imaging, Reporting and Data System (TI-RADS): white paper of the ACR TI-RADS Committee. *J Am Coll Radiol.* 2017; **14**(5):587–595.

Tuggle CT, Roman SA, Wang TS, Boudourakis L, Thomas DC, Udelsman R, Ann Sosa J. Pediatric endocrine surgery: who is operating on our children? *Surgery.* 2008;**144**(6):869–877, discussion 877.

Verburg FA, Reiners C, Hänscheid H. Approach to the patient: role of dosimetric RAI Rx in children with DTC. *J Clin Endocrinol Metab.* 2013; **98**(10):3912–3919.

Thyroid Storm and Myxedema Coma*

M29
Presented, March 23–26, 2019

Henry B. Burch, MD. Division of Diabetes, Endocrinology and Metabolic Diseases, National Institute of Diabetes and Digestive and Kidney Disease, National Institutes of Health, Bethesda, Maryland 20892, E-mail: henry.burch@nih.gov

THYROID STORM: SIGNIFICANCE OF THE CLINICAL PROBLEM

Thyroid storm is a life-threatening manifestation of severe thyrotoxicosis, characterized by a systemic decompensation and ~10% mortality. Multiple factors determine the devolution of uncomplicated thyrotoxicosis into thyroid storm, including age, comorbidity, rapidity of onset, and the presence or absence of a precipitating event. Thyroid storm is triggered when the cumulative effect of these factors surpasses a patient's ability to maintain adequate metabolic, thermoregulatory, and cardiovascular compensatory mechanisms. The high morbidity and mortality associated with thyroid storm requires both early recognition and a steadfast commitment to an aggressive multifaceted therapeutic intervention.

BARRIERS TO OPTIMAL PRACTICE

Early recognition and a commitment to an aggressive multifaceted treatment approach are essential to patient survival, yet thyroid storm is often not immediately recognized and may be confused for other acute presentations, such as severe infection or sepsis, psychosis, or primary cardiovascular event. Undertreatment in the early stages of thyroid storm.

LEARNING OBJECTIVES

As a result of participating in this session, learners should be able to
- Review the diverse clinical presentations of thyroid storm
- Compare and contrast current empiric methods for making the diagnosis of thyroid storm
- Review the multipronged management of thyroid storm
- Discuss measures to prevent thyroid storm

STRATEGIES FOR DIAGNOSIS AND MANAGEMENT OF THYROID STORM

Making the Diagnosis of Thyroid Storm

Laboratory parameters have little value in distinguishing uncomplicated thyrotoxicosis from thyroid storm. A diagnostic point scale was proposed by Burch and Wartofsky in 1993 to distinguish uncomplicated thyrotoxicosis from impending or established thyroid storm (1, 2) (Table 1). The Burch-Wartofsky Point Scale (BWPS) is an empirically derived system that incorporates three principal observations in patients with thyroid storm, including (i) the continuum of end organ dysfunction, (ii) the high variability of individual patient presentation, and (iii) the high mortality associated with a missed diagnosis. An additional empirically defined diagnostic system was proposed by the Japanese Thyroid Association (JTA) in 2012 (3). The JTA system uses combinations of clinical features to assign patients to the diagnostic categories thyroid storm 1 (TS1) or thyroid storm 2 (TS2). Data comparing these two diagnostic systems suggest an overall agreement, but the JTA system has a tendency toward underdiagnosis using the JTA categories of TS1 and TS2, compared with a BWPS ≥45. For example, in a recent study of 25 patients with a clinical diagnosis of thyroid storm, the BWPS was ≥45 in 20 patients and 25 to 44 in the remaining 5, but these latter 5 patients (20%) were not identified using the JTA system (4). In the same series, among 125 patients hospitalized with a clinical diagnosis of compensated thyrotoxicosis but not in thyroid storm, 27 (21.6%) had a BWPS ≥45 and 21 (16.8%) were either TS1 or TS2, suggesting similar rates of overdiagnosis with these two systems. However, an additional 50 patients (40%) hospitalized with a clinical diagnosis of thyrotoxicosis without thyroid storm would have been diagnosed as having impending thyroid storm by the BWPS, which reinforces that a BWPS in the 25 to 44 range does not replace clinical judgment in the selection of patients for aggressive therapy. Finally, in a study including 28 patients diagnosed with thyroid storm based on clinical presentation and the BWPS, 1 patient had a BWPS of 45 but did not meet JTA criteria for thyroid storm (5).

CASE SUBJECT

A 57-year-old woman diagnosed with Graves' disease 2 months earlier presents to the emergency department with fever, nausea/vomiting, and palpitations occurring 1 week after running out of methimazole.

Her medical history includes Graves' disease. Her current medications are methimazole 30 mg daily (ran out 1 week ago) and atenolol 50 mg daily (ran out 1 week ago). She smokes one pack of tobacco per day. Her physical examination shows a temperature of 102.7°F and pulse 124 bpm. The eye exam revealed a clinical activity score = 3, no proptosis, and normal extraocular movement. The thyroid has a diffuse goiter with bruit. Her lungs have bibasilar rales. She has a tremor in an extremity. Her Mini-Mental State Examination score is 25/30.

Table 1. BWPS for Thyroid Storm

Criteria	Points
Thermoregulatory dysfunction	
Temperature (°F)	
99.0–99.9	5
100.0–100.9	10
101.0–101.9	15
102.0–102.9	20
103.0–103.9	25
≥104.0	30
Cardiovascular dysfunction	
Tachycardia	
100–109	5
110–119	10
120–129	15
130–139	20
≥140	25
Atrial fibrillation	
Absent	0
Present	20
Congestive heart failure	
Absent	0
Mild (pedal edema)	5
Moderate (basilar rales)	10
Severe (pulmonary edema)	20
GI dysfunction	
Absent	0
Moderate (diarrhea, abdominal pain, nausea/vomiting)	10
Severe (jaundice)	20
Central nervous system disturbance	
Absent	0
Mild (agitation)	10
Moderate (delirium, psychosis, extreme lethargy)	20
Severe (seizure, coma)	30
Precipitant history	
Negative	
Positive	10
Total scores	
>45	Thyroid storm
25–44	Pending thyroid storm
<25	Storm unlikely

The treatment of an impending or established thyroid storm is directed at each therapeutically accessible point in the thyroid hormone synthetic, secretory, and peripheral action pathways. Concurrently, aggressive intervention is directed at the reversal of ongoing or incipient decompensation of normal homeostatic mechanisms (Table 2). Reproduced with permission from Burch HB, Wartofsky L. Life-threatening thyrotoxicosis: thyroid storm. *Endocrinol Metab Clin North Am.* 1993;22(2):263–277.

The results of her laboratory tests are as follows: free T_4 >7 ng/dL (0.8 to 1.8 ng/dL), free T_3 12.1 ng/mL (2.0 to 4.4 ng/mL), thyrotropin (TSH) 0.001 mU/L, and total bilirubin 1.5 mg/dL (0.2 to 1.2 mg/dL). Her ECG shows sinus tachycardia. Her chest X-ray shows cephalization of flow and interstitial edema.

Table 2. Thyroid Storm: Drugs and Doses

Drug	Dosing	Comment
Propylthiouracil	500–1000 mg load, then 250 mg every 4 hours	Inhibits new hormone synthesis
		Blocks T_4-to-T_3 conversion
		Alternate drug: methimazole 60–80 mg daily
Propranolol	60–80 mg every 4 hours	Consider invasive monitoring
		Blocks T_4-to-T_3 conversion in high doses
		Alternate drug: esmolol infusion
Iodine (saturated solution of potassium iodide)	Five drops (0.25 mL or 250 mg) orally every 6 hours	Start 1 hour after antithyroid drugs
		Inhibits new hormone synthesis
		Blocks thyroid hormone release
		Alternate drug: Lugol's solution
Hydrocortisone	300 mg IV load, then 100 mg every 8 hours	May block T_4-to-T_3 conversion
		Prophylaxis against relative adrenal insufficiency
		Alternate drug: dexamethasone

Questions

1. Does this patient meet diagnostic criteria for thyroid storm?
2. How would you manage this patient?
3. How would you prevent future events?

References

1. Burch HB, Wartofsky L. Life-threatening thyrotoxicosis. Thyroid storm. *Endocrinol Metab Clin North Am.* 1993;**22**(2):263–277.
2. Warnock AL, Cooper DS, Burch HB. Life threatening thyrotoxicosis. Thyroid storm and adverse effects of antithyroid drugs. In: Matfin G, ed. *Endocrine and Metabolic Medical Emergencies.* Washington, DC: Endocrine Press, John Wiley and Sons Ltd; 2018: 110–126.
3. Akamizu T, Satoh T, Isozaki O, Suzuki A, Wakino S, Iburi T, Tsuboi K, Monden T, Kouki T, Otani H, Teramukai S, Uehara R, Nakamura Y, Nagai M, Mori M; Japan Thyroid Association. Diagnostic criteria, clinical features, and incidence of thyroid storm based on nationwide surveys. *Thyroid.* 2012;**22**(7):661–679.
4. Angell TE, Lechner MG, Nguyen CT, Salvato VL, Nicoloff JT, LoPresti JS. Clinical features and hospital outcomes in thyroid storm: a retrospective cohort study. *J Clin Endocrinol Metab.* 2015;**100**(2):451–459.
5. Swee DS, Chng CL, Lim A. Clinical characteristics and outcome of thyroid storm: a case series and review of neuropsychiatric derangements in thyrotoxicosis. *Endocr Pract.* 2015;**21**(2):182–189.

*The views expressed in this manuscript are those of the authors and do not reflect the official policy of the National Institutes of Health, the Department of Health and Human Services, or the United States Government. The author is an employee of the U.S. Government. This work was prepared as part of the author's official duties. Title 17 U.S.C. 105 provides the "Copyright protection under this title is not available for any work of the United States Government." Title 17 U.S.C. 101 defines a U.S. Government work as a work prepared by an employee of the U.S. Government as part of that person's official duties. The author certifies that all individuals who qualify as authors have been listed; each has participated in the conception and design of this work, the analysis of data (when applicable), the writing of the document, and/or the approval of the submission of this version; that the document represents valid work; that if the author used information derived from another source, he obtained all necessary approvals to use it and made appropriate acknowledgments in the document; and that the author takes public responsibility for it.

Thyroid Storm and Myxedema Coma*

M29
Presented, March 23–26, 2019

Joanna Klubo-Gwiezdzinska, MD, PhD, MHSc. Metabolic Disease Branch, National Institute of Diabetes and Digestive and Kidney Diseases, National Institutes of Health, Bethesda, Maryland 20814, E-mail: joanna. klubo-gwiezdzinska@nih.gov

MYXEDEMA COMA: SIGNIFICANCE OF THE CLINICAL PROBLEM

Myxedema coma is a life-threatening manifestation of severe hypothyroidism, but fortunately it is rare, with an incidence of 0.22 per million/y (1, 2). It occurs usually in elderly women with a history of long-standing hypothyroidism, neck surgery, or therapy with radioactive iodine and is exacerbated by a precipitating event. The mortality rate remains very high, ranging from 20% to 30%, although it has significantly improved compared with historical cohorts, where the death rate was as high as 60% to 80% (1, 2). Early diagnosis and intensive multifaceted care addressing multiorgan failure are critical in management of patients with myxedema coma.

BARRIERS TO OPTIMAL PRACTICE

Due to its rarity, myxedema coma tends to be underdiagnosed among patients admitted to the hospital. In fact, one of the studies documented that half of myxedema coma patients were missed during the initial stay in the emergency department (3). Any delay in diagnosis and implementation of appropriate therapy increases the likelihood of a fatal outcome. Myxedema coma is associated with complications affecting multiple organs, including but not limited to depressed hypoxic respiratory drive and ventilatory response to hypercapnia, cardiogenic

Table 1.   Clinical Manifestations of Myxedema Coma

System	Manifestations
Thermoregulation	Hypothermia, as low as 80°F (26.7°C)
Central nervous system and psychiatric manifestations	Unconsciousness, altered orientation, cerebellar signs (poorly coordinated purposeful movements of the hands and feet, ataxia, adiadochokinesia), poor memory and recall, amnesia, seizures including status epilepticus, depression, paranoia, hallucinations ("myxedema madness")
Respiratory system	Hypoventilation due to depressed hypoxic respiratory drive and ventilatory response to hypercapnia, partial obstruction of the upper airways caused by edema of the tongue or vocal cords, decreased tidal volume secondary to pleural effusion or ascites
Cardiovascular system	Cardiogenic shock due to impaired cardiac contractility or cardiac tamponade caused by the accumulation of fluid rich in mucopolysaccharides within the pericardial sac, arrhythmias (bradycardia, varying degrees of atrio-ventricular blocks, prolonged Q-T interval, which can result in torsades de pointes)
Renal manifestations	Hyponatremia due to impaired water diuresis caused by reduced delivery of water to the distal nephron, decreased GFR and renal plasma flow, atony of the urinary bladder with retention of large residual urine volumes, renal failure often as a result of underlying rhabdomyolysis
GI system	Gastric atony, impaired peristalsis, even paralytic ileus due to mucopolysaccharide infiltration and edema of the muscularis and neuropathic changes, ascites, GI bleeding secondary to an associated coagulopathy
Hematological manifestations	Higher risk of bleeding caused by coagulopathy related to an acquired von Willebrand syndrome (type 1) and decreases in factors V, VII, VIII, IX, and X or disseminated intravascular coagulation associated with sepsis; granulocytopenia predisposing to severe infections; microcytic anemia secondary to hemorrhage, or a macrocytic anemia caused by vitamin B12 deficiency
Metabolic manifestations	Hypoglycemia, hypercholesterolemia
Skin	Dry, cold skin, edema

The laboratory workup may reveal hypoxemia, hypercapnia, lactic acidosis, anemia, hyponatremia, hypoglycemia, hypercholesterolemia, high serum creatine kinase concentrations, an elevated creatinine, and a decreased GFR. Most patients have low serum free thyroxine (FT_4) and high serum TSH; however, the degree of TSH elevation does not correlate with the severity of symptoms. The TSH level can even be low or normal, due to nonthyroidal illness ("euthyroid sick" syndrome, presence of central hypothyroidism, or TSH-lowering effects of medications such as steroids, dopamine, or dobutamine). Myxedema coma, as a true medical emergency, requires a multifaceted approach to treatment in a critical care setting. The summary of medical management of this life-threatening condition is summarized in Table 2. (See also reference [1].)

shock, severe hyponatremia, kidney failure due to rhabdo-myolysis, and gastrointestinal (GI) bleeding due to coagulop-athy, which, along with a necessity of appropriate management of the precipitating event, may pose a therapeutic challenge.

LEARNING OBJECTIVES

As a result of participating in this session, learners should be able to
- Review the clinical presentation of myxedema coma
- Recognize key features, enabling appropriate and timely diagnosis

- Summarize implementation of an appropriate management plan addressing multiorgan failure
- Discuss pros and cons of therapy with levothyroxine alone or levothyroxine combined with triiodothyronine

STRATEGIES FOR DIAGNOSIS, THERAPY, AND/OR MANAGEMENT

The key clinical features enabling appropriate diagnosis of myxedema coma are altered mental status and hypothermia in a patient with a history of a precipitating event such as cold exposure (winter months), infection, drugs (*e.g.*, diuretics

Table 2. Treatment of Patients With Myxedema Coma

Presentation	Treatment
Hypothyroidism	Large initial IV dose of 300–500 μg T_4, if no response add T_3; or initial IV dose of 200–300 μg T_4 plus 10–25 μg T_3
Airways and ventilation	The maintenance of patent airways is the single most important supportive measure. Mechanical ventilation is usually required during the first 36–48 hours.
	Patients should not be extubated prematurely and before full consciousness is attained.
Hypothermia	Blankets or increased room temperature, no active rewarming
	Too aggressive warming may cause peripheral vasodilatation, which may exacerbate hypotension or shock.
Hypotension	Hydrocortisone 100 mg every 6–8 hours
	Fluids administered cautiously as 5% to 10% glucose in 0.5 N sodium chloride if hypoglycemia is present, or as isotonic normal saline if hyponatremia is present
	Vasopressors as needed
Hyponatremia	Severe symptomatic acute hyponatremia (105–120 mmol/L) requires administration of a small amount of hypertonic saline (50–100 mL 3% sodium chloride over 10–15 minutes), to increase sodium concentration by ~2–6 mmol/L. The increase of the Na concentration by 4–6 mmol/L is sufficient to reverse the most serious manifestations of hyponatremia (4).
	In patients with chronic hyponatremia, the correction should not exceed 10–12 mmol/L in 24 hours or 18 mmol/L in 48 h.
	After achieving a sodium level of >120 mmol/L, restriction of fluids and treatment of hypothyroidism and relative adrenal insufficiency
	Vaptans for euvolemic and hypervolemic hyponatremia
Kidney failure	Dialysis if needed
General supportive measures	Treatment of underlying problems: infection, congestive heart failure, GI bleeding
	The dosage of specific medications may need to be modified based on their altered distribution and slowed metabolism in myxedema.

Administration of thyroid hormone is essential; however, one of the most controversial aspects of the management of myxedema coma is which thyroid hormone preparation to give (T_4 or T_3) and what dose is optimal. The administration of high doses carries the risk of precipitating potentially fatal tachycardias or myocardial infarction, but a low dose may be unable to reverse the pathophysiology underlying this extreme form of hypothyroidism. Treatment with T_4 may be less effective due to impaired conversion of T_4 into T_3 in myxedema coma, but treatment with T_3 may expose tissues, specifically the myocardium, to unexpectedly high levels of thyroid hormone. There is a consensus regarding the initial IV route of administration, as GI absorption of thyroid hormones might be impaired (1–5). Typically, a large initial IV loading dose of 300 to 500 μg T_4 is suggested to saturate the binding site on thyroxine-binding globulin, transthyretin, and albumin, followed by daily doses of 1.6 μg/kg (initially IV, and orally when feasible). Larger doses have been associated with increased mortality (5). If there is no response within 24 hours, addition of T_3 is recommended. An alternative scheme is an initial IV dose of 200 to 300 μg T_4 plus 10 to 25 μg T_3, followed by 2.5 to 10 μg T_3 every 8 hours, depending on the patient's age and presence of cardiovascular risk factors. Upon clinical improvement, T_3 is discontinued and a daily oral T_4 replacement dose is maintained. The American Thyroid Association guidelines for the treatment of hypothy-roidism recommend "an initial loading dose of levothyroxine (200 to 400 μg IV) and IV glucocorticoid administration (strong recommendation, low-quality evidence) (6). Additional administration of IV liothyronine in a loading dose of 5 to 20 μg can be considered (weak recommendation, low-quality of evidence)" (6). (See also reference [1].)

or sedatives), trauma, stroke, heart failure, or GI bleeding. Myxedema coma as an end-stage manifestation of hypothyroidism is associated with clinical manifestations affecting multiple organ systems. The clinical signs and symptoms of myxedema coma are summarized in Table 1.

MAIN CONCLUSIONS

Myxedema coma is a medical emergency requiring early diagnosis and a multifaceted approach to treatment in a critical care setting. The key diagnostic pearls are altered mental status, hypothermia, and sometimes a precipitating event in a patient with a history of hypothyroidism, previous neck surgery, or therapy with radioactive iodine. The most important therapeutic measures are protection of airways in a patient with altered mental status, appropriate therapy of the underlying precipitating event, management of multiorgan failure in a critical care setting, and IV replacement of thyroid hormones preceded by steroid administration (Table 2). The optimal regimen for thyroid hormone replacement is unknown and may consist of IV levothyroxine or IV combination therapy with levothyroxine and triiodothyronine.

CASE SUBJECT

A 70-year-old female is admitted to the emergency department with pneumonia, bradycardia with first-degree atrioventricular block, and somnolence lasting for the past 24 hours. Past medical history is significant for Graves' disease treated with radioactive iodine several years ago, hypertension, and hyperlipidemia. Current medications include lisinopril, hydrochlorothiazide, and simvastatin. Physical exam reveals a somnolent, disoriented woman, with cold, dry skin, blood pressure of 85/50 mm Hg, heart rate of 48 bpm, temperature of 35°C, shallow breathing (12 breaths/min), crackles involving the right lower lobe of the lungs, and swelling of the face and lower extremities. Laboratory results reveal a white blood cell count 18,000/μL with left shift, hemoglobin 11.8 g/dL, platelets 350,000/μL, Na 122 mmol/L, K 3.8 mmol/L, glucose 60 mg/dL, creatinine 1.6 mg/dL, glomerular filtration rate (GFR) 45 mL/min/1.73 m^2, creatine kinase 10,000 IU/mL, TSH 35 mIU/mL, and free T_4 0.4 ng/dL (N 0.9 to 1.6 ng/dL). The arterial blood gas is significant for respiratory acidosis.

Questions

1. What is the false statement regarding this patient?
   A. The most likely etiology of the patient's symptoms is severe untreated hypothyroidism/myxedema coma.
   B. The treatment should consist of intubation/mechanical ventilation, wide spectrum antibiotics for pneumonia, hydrocortisone IV, and levothyroxine IV.
   C. Myxedema coma as the cause of the patient's presentation is unlikely, given that the TSH level is only 35 mIU/mL, and with myxedema coma, TSH levels are always above 100 mIU/mL.
   D. The patient is at risk for developing GI bleeding.

E. Pneumonia is the most likely precipitating event leading to the acute decompensation.

Correct answer: C

2. Hyponatremia in myxedema coma is caused by
   A. Increased serum antidiuretic hormone (ADH) levels and decreased water diuresis
   B. Increases serum ADH levels and increased water diuresis
   C. Decreased serum ADH levels and increased water diuresis
   D. Decreased serum ADH levels and decreased water diuresis
   E. Myxedema coma is never associated with hyponatremia.

Correct answer: A

3. What is the most likely etiology of kidney failure in this patient?
   A. Rhabdomyolysis
   B. Hypotension
   C. Use of diuretics
   D. None of the above
   E. A, B, and C

Correct answer: E

References

1. Klubo-Gwiezdzinska J, Wartofsky L. Thyroid emergencies. *Med Clin North Am.* 2012;**96**(2):385–403.
2. Ono Y, Ono S, Yasunaga H, Matsui H, Fushimi K, Tanaka Y. Clinical characteristics and outcomes of myxedema coma: analysis of a national inpatient database in Japan. *J Epidemiol.* 2017;**27**(3):117–122.
3. Chen YJ, Hou SK, How CK, Chern CH, Lo HC, Yen DH, Huang CI, Lee CH. Diagnosis of unrecognized primary overt hypothyroidism in the ED. *Am J Emerg Med.* 2010;**28**(8):866–870.
4. Verbalis JG, Goldsmith SR, Greenberg A, Korzelius C, Schrier RW, Sterns RH, Thompson CJ. Diagnosis, evaluation, and treatment of hyponatremia: expert panel recommendations. *Am J Med.* 2013;**126**(10, Suppl 1):S1–S42.
5. Ridgway EC, McCammon JA, Benotti J, Maloof F. Acute metabolic responses in myxedema to large doses of intravenous l-thyroxine. *Ann Intern Med.* 1972;**77**:549–556.
6. Jonklaas J, Bianco AC, Bauer AJ, Burman KD, Cappola AR, Celi FS, Cooper DS, Kim BW, Peeters RP, Rosenthal MS, Sawka AM; American Thyroid Association Task Force on Thyroid Hormone Replacement. Guidelines for the treatment of hypothyroidism: prepared by the American Thyroid Association Task Force on Thyroid Hormone Replacement. *Thyroid.* 2014;**24**(12):1670–1751.

Thyroid Cancer: When Is Lobectomy Not Enough?

M50
Presented, March 23–26, 2019

Bryan R. Haugen, MD. Department of Medicine, Division of Endocrinology, University of Colorado School of Medicine, Aurora, Colorado 80045, E-mail: bryan.haugen@ucdenver.edu

Julie Ann Sosa, MA, MD. Department of Surgery, University of California at San Francisco, San Francisco, California 94143, E-mail: julie.sosa@ucsf.edu

SIGNIFICANCE OF THE CLINICAL PROBLEM

Thyroid cancer is the fastest-increasing cancer in the United States, with incidence up by >300% over the last 30 years (1). It is the fifth-leading cancer diagnosis in US women. It is anticipated that thyroid cancer will overtake colorectal cancer and uterine cancer to become the third-most common cancer diagnosis in US women by 2020. There is growing evidence that thyroidectomy in patients with papillary thyroid cancer (PTC), the most common thyroid cancer diagnosis, has higher complication rates compared with lobectomy, even among high-volume surgeons, and some patients may not do well while receiving levothyroxine therapy after thyroidectomy. The decision regarding which patients with a PTC cytologic diagnosis should undergo lobectomy vs thyroidectomy remains a major gap in our patient care and patient outcomes.

BARRIERS TO OPTIMAL PRACTICE

Due to the indolent nature of the disease, patients have to be followed for decades to account for predictors of survival when considering lobectomy vs thyroidectomy for treatment of PTC. In addition, because differentiated thyroid cancer (DTC) is generally not a mortal disease, there is a paucity of death events, making mortality as an outcome a challenging measure. The number of patients who are needed in a study cohort is often prohibitively high, and the cost of following a study cohort over many decades is not feasible.

As a result, ongoing controversies include the following:
- Active surveillance vs thyroid lobectomy for papillary microcarcinomas
- Thyroid lobectomy vs total thyroidectomy for low-risk DTC
- Molecular testing vs diagnostic surgery for indeterminate thyroid nodules
- Thyroid surgery alone vs thyroidectomy plus prophylactic central lymph node dissection for patients with DTC and without clinical or radiographic evidence of metastatic disease

LEARNING OBJECTIVES

As a result of participating in this session, learners should be able to:
- Understand recommendations regarding extent of surgery for low-risk DTC from the American Thyroid Association guidelines for the management of thyroid nodules and DTC
- Apply the primary data and evidence underlying the American Thyroid Association guidelines for the management of low-risk DTC

STRATEGIES FOR DIAGNOSIS, THERAPY, AND/OR MANAGEMENT

The primary guiding principles used in development of the 2015 American Thyroid Association Management Guidelines for Adult Patients with Thyroid Nodules and Differentiated Thyroid Cancer were to keep the guidelines question-based, making recommendations on the basis of the highest quality of evidence possible while trying to be helpful to clinicians caring for patients with thyroid nodules and DTC (2). The striking, increasing incidence of DTC and the low, stable mortality rate also had a substantial influence on our deliberations, especially where the evidence was of lower quality.

The recommendation (35B) that addresses surgical approach to the majority of patients who have intrathyroidal PTC is probably the most changed, controversial, and misunderstood. This recommendation states that either thyroidectomy or lobectomy is a reasonable surgical approach for patients with 1- to 4-cm DTC without evidence of extrathyroidal extension or clinically apparent lymph node disease on preoperative examination or imaging. This is a strong recommendation with moderate-quality evidence from large database studies. A majority of the studies show that overall survival and disease-free survival are not negatively affected by lobectomy compared with thyroidectomy (3–10), although a minority of studies showed that thyroidectomy has a better outcome (11, 12). Despite the preponderance of moderate-quality evidence in support of a lobectomy for these patients, the task force chose a bit more of a conservative path recommending either a thyroidectomy or lobectomy, leaving the thyroidectomy option in place to enable radioiodine therapy or to enhance follow-up on the basis of disease features and/or patient preferences. It is also recommended that these patients have a careful neck ultrasound to assess for other thyroid nodules, extrathyroidal extension, and any abnormal lymph nodes. The feedback that we have received suggests that many people believe that we have a strong preference for lobectomy in patients with 1- to 4-cm DTC. Although the literature may support this approach, we did leave open the option for a lobectomy or thyroidectomy for these patients. Interestingly, this is a strong recommendation, which would be defined as "most clinicians should offer this course of action." However, the recommended course of action is either a lobectomy or thyroidectomy—not supporting one approach over the other. We left this as a strong recommendation to alert clinicians to give serious consideration to a lobectomy because this is a substantial departure from previous guidelines recommendations. Interestingly, this is somewhat "back to the future," because lobectomy was a recommended approach for these patients decades ago. We believe that if and when this specific recommendation is more widely adopted, surgical outcomes and quality of life will be improved for many of these low-risk patients.

MAIN CONCLUSIONS

Patients with DTC, most of whom have received fine-needle aspiration results that are diagnostic or suspicious for PTC, can be considered for lobectomy as a primary surgical approach. Moderate-quality evidence from multiple database and large single-center noncontrolled studies suggests that patients with 1- to 4-cm DTC can be considered for lobectomy. Tumor-specific considerations include the location of the tumor, evidence for extrathyroidal extension, presence of nodules in the ipsilateral lobe, and presence of abnormal lymph nodes. Patient-specific considerations include preoperative dependence on thyroid hormone as well as addressing the patient's concerns regarding their disease and therapies. It is also important to have a cohesive treatment team that is comfortable with managing and monitoring patients after lobectomy.

Case 1

A 53-year-old woman noted a right neck lump. Neck ultrasound revealed a suspicious right 2.4-cm thyroid nodule. She has no specific symptoms. No extrathyroidal extension or abnormal lymph nodes were seen. The left lobe had no nodules. The primary surgical approach to be considered should be:

A. Thyroidectomy with a prophylactic central neck dissection
B. Thyroidectomy alone
C. Thyroidectomy or lobectomy (correct answer)
D. Lobectomy alone

Case 2

A 55-year-old man noted a right neck lump. Neck ultrasound revealed a 4.3-cm thyroid nodule; it is asymptomatic, and the patient is risk averse. There are no pathologic lymph nodes. Outside ultrasound-guided fine-needle aspiration revealed benign findings. Reinterpretation of the cytology is Bethesda III–atypia of undetermined significance. A 1-cm thyroid nodule with a linear calcification is seen in the contralateral lobe. The next step should be:

A. Total thyroidectomy
B. Right thyroid lobectomy

C. Repeat biopsy of the right-sided thyroid nodule with molecular testing
D. Biopsy of the left thyroid nodule (correct answer)

Case 3

A 36-year-old woman underwent a comprehensive annual check-up, including a neck ultrasound, in China. A 1.1-cm very posterior nodule was identified in the right thyroid lobe, abutting the trachea, with microcalcifications; biopsy is consistent with PTC. There are no contralateral nodules or pathologic lymphadenopathy. The patient is anxious about the potential diagnosis but does not want a neck scar. The appropriate next step would be:

A. Observation
B. Transoral thyroidectomy
C. Right thyroid lobectomy
D. Right thyroid lobectomy or total thyroidectomy (correct answer)

References

1. Lim H, Devesa SS, Sosa JA, Check D, Kitahara CM. Trends in thyroid cancer incidence and mortality in the United States, 1974-2013. *JAMA.* 2017;**317**(13):1338–1348.
2. Haugen BR, Alexander EK, Bible KC, Doherty GM, Mandel SJ, Nikiforov YE, Pacini F, Randolph GW, Sawka AM, Schlumberger M, Schuff KG, Sherman SI, Sosa JA, Steward DL, Tuttle RM, Wartofsky L. 2015 American Thyroid Association Management Guidelines for Adult Patients with Thyroid Nodules and Differentiated Thyroid Cancer: The American Thyroid Association Guidelines Task Force on Thyroid Nodules and Differentiated Thyroid Cancer. *Thyroid.* 2016;**26**(1): 1–133.
3. Haigh PI, Urbach DR, Rotstein LE. Extent of thyroidectomy is not a major determinant of survival in low- or high-risk papillary thyroid cancer. *Ann Surg Oncol.* 2005;**12**(1):81–89.
4. Barney BM, Hitchcock YJ, Sharma P, Shrieve DC, Tward JD. Overall and cause-specific survival for patients undergoing lobectomy, near-total, or total thyroidectomy for differentiated thyroid cancer. *Head Neck.* 2011;**33**(5):645–649.
5. Vaisman F, Shaha A, Fish S, Michael Tuttle R. Initial therapy with either thyroid lobectomy or total thyroidectomy without radioactive iodine remnant ablation is associated with very low rates of structural disease recurrence in properly selected patients with differentiated thyroid cancer. *Clin Endocrinol (Oxf).* 2011;**75**(1):112–119.
6. Mendelsohn AH, Elashoff DA, Abemayor E, St John MA. Surgery for papillary thyroid carcinoma: is lobectomy enough? *Arch Otolaryngol Head Neck Surg.* 2010;**136**(11):1055–1061.
7. Nixon IJ, Ganly I, Patel SG, Palmer FL, Whitcher MM, Tuttle RM, Shaha A, Shah JP. Thyroid lobectomy for treatment of well differentiated intrathyroid malignancy. *Surgery.* 2012;**151**(4):571–579.
8. Matsuzu K, Sugino K, Masudo K, Nagahama M, Kitagawa W, Shibuya H, Ohkuwa K, Uruno T, Suzuki A, Magoshi S, Akaishi J, Masaki C, Kawano M, Suganuma N, Rino Y, Masuda M, Kameyama K, Takami H, Ito K. Thyroid lobectomy for papillary thyroid cancer: long-term follow-up study of 1,088 cases. *World J Surg.* 2014; **38**(1):68–79.
9. Adam MA, Pura J, Gu L, Dinan MA, Tyler DS, Reed SD, Scheri R, Roman SA, Sosa JA. Extent of surgery for papillary thyroid cancer is not associated with survival: an analysis of 61,775 patients. *Ann Surg.* 2014;**260**(4):601–605, discussion 605–607.
10. Adam MA, Pura J, Goffredo P, Dinan MA, Hyslop T, Reed SD, Scheri RP, Roman SA, Sosa JA. Impact of extent of surgery on survival for papillary thyroid cancer patients younger than 45 years. *J Clin Endocrinol Metab.* 2015;**100**(1):115–121.

11. Bilimoria KY, Bentrem DJ, Ko CY, Stewart AK, Winchester DP, Talamonti MS, Sturgeon C. Extent of surgery affects survival for papillary thyroid cancer. *Ann Surg.* 2007;**246**(3):375–381, discussion 381–384.

12. Hay ID, Grant CS, Bergstralh EJ, Thompson GB, van Heerden JA, Goellner JR. Unilateral total lobectomy: is it sufficient surgical treatment for patients with AMES low-risk papillary thyroid carcinoma? *Surgery.* 1998;**124**(6):958–964, discussion 964–966.

Interactive Interpretation of Thyroid Ultrasound

M58
Presented, March 23–26, 2019

Jennifer Sipos, MD. Division of Endocrinology, The Ohio State University, Columbus, Ohio 43210, E-mail: jennifer.sipos@osumc.edu

Susan Mandel, MD. Perelman School of Medicine, University of Pennsylvania, Philadelphia, Pennsylvania 19104, E-mail: susan.mandel@uphs.upenn.edu

SIGNIFICANCE OF THE PROBLEM

Thyroid nodules are a common clinical entity. Although the exact prevalence is unknown, up to 70% of patients may harbor a thyroid nodule (1). The majority of such nodules are benign; however, the 10% to 15% risk of malignancy in any given nodule is high enough to necessitate further evaluation (2,3). It is not possible to perform fine-needle aspiration (FNA) of all nodules identified, however. Fortunately, many nodules may be accurately triaged based on their sonographic appearance alone. There are several sonographic classification systems currently in use that assist the clinician in categorizing each nodule, assigning a malignancy risk, determining the need for FNA, and providing surveillance parameters.

The two most commonly used sonographic stratification systems are the pattern-based classification system of the American Thyroid Association (ATA) (4) and the points-based system created by the American College of Radiology Thyroid Imaging, Reporting and Data System (ACR TI-RADS) (5).

BARRIERS TO OPTIMAL PRACTICE

- The ability to differentiate benign and malignant thyroid nodules based on their sonographic pattern
- Various ultrasound risk-stratification systems exist, at times providing conflicting recommendations regarding the optimal classification and intervention thresholds for the same nodule

LEARNING OBJECTIVES

As a result of participating in this session, learners should be able to:

- Characterize nodules based on their sonographic appearance
- Assign nodules to the appropriate risk category of the ATA and ACR TI-RADS ultrasound classification systems

Table 1. ATA Sonographic Risk Stratification of Thyroid Nodules

Sonographic Pattern	Ultrasound Features	Estimated Risk of Malignancy (%)	FNA Cutoff	Surveillance
Benign	Simple cysts (no solid component)	<1	No FNA	Not required
Very low suspicion	Spongiform or partially cystic nodule without any ultrasound features in low-, intermediate-, or high-suspicion patterns	<3	FNA ≥2 cm or observation	Not required but if desired, repeat ultrasound at ≥24 mo
Low suspicion	Isoechoic or hyperechoic solid nodule, or partially cystic nodule with eccentric solid areas, without high-risk features[a]	5–10	FNA ≥1.5 cm	Repeat ultrasound at 12–24 mo
Intermediate suspicion	Hypoechoic solid nodule with smooth margins without high-risk features[a]	10–20	FNA ≥1.0 cm	Repeat ultrasound at 12–24 mo
High risk	Solid hypoechoic nodule or solid hypoechoic component of a partially cystic nodule with ≥1 of the following features: irregular margins (infiltrative or microlobulated), microcalcifications, taller than wide shape, rim calcifications with small extrusive soft tissue component, evidence of ETE	>70–90	FNA ≥1.0 cm	Repeat ultrasound and FNA within 12 mo

Adapted under a Creative Commons BY-NC license from Haugen BR, Alexander EK, Bible KC, et al. 2015 American Thyoid Association management guidelines for adult patients with thyroid nodules and differentiated thyroid cancer. *Thyroid.* 2016; 26(1):1–133.
Abbreviation: ETE, extrathyroidal extension.
[a] High-risk features include irregular margins (infiltrative or microlobulated), microcalcifications, taller than wide shape, rim calcifications with small extrusive soft tissue component, and evidence of ETE.

- Outline the thresholds for FNA and surveillance scans for each classification system

STRATEGIES FOR DIAGNOSIS, THERAPY, AND MANAGEMENT

The ATA ultrasound stratification system (Table 1) uses pattern-based classification to assign a malignancy risk to each nodule (4). This approach is beneficial for clinicians because of its ease of recognition and its improved interobserver agreement when compared with identification of individual sonographic features (6,7). Furthermore, the sensitivity of individual sonographic features is insufficient to reliably rule out the likelihood of malignancy (4). One limitation of this system is that not all nodules may be captured with these five patterns, such as isoechoic nodules with a suspicious sonographic feature. However, these atypical nodules represent a small minority of all lesions seen in clinical practice.

The ACR TI-RADS (Tables 2 and 3) uses a points-based system to categorize the malignancy risk of thyroid nodules (5). A higher point tally is associated with a greater likelihood of malignancy and a corresponding lower threshold for FNA. Widely used by radiologists, this classification system has the advantage of providing guidance for nodules of all types. Although the risk of malignancy for each category overlaps with those seen in the ATA classification, the ACR TI-RADS thresholds for FNA of

nodules corresponding to low- and intermediate-risk nodules is higher.

CASES WITH QUESTIONS AND ANSWERS
Case 1

A 58-year-old woman presents with a palpable 2-cm right-sided nodule. There are no compressive symptoms. Her thyrotropin level is normal, and she denies family history of thyroid cancer or personal history of radiation exposure. An ultrasound of the neck demonstrates a 1.4- × 1.4- × 2.1-cm nodule. What is the ATA risk classification of this nodule?

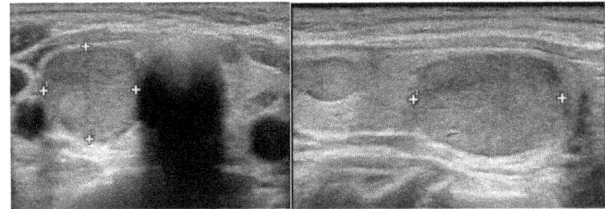

A. Benign
B. Very low risk
C. Low risk
D. Intermediate risk
E. High risk

Table 2. ACR-TIRADS Thyroid Nodule Sonographic Characterization and Scoring

Composition	Echogenicity	Shape	Margin	Echogenic Foci
Cystic 0	Anechoic 0	Wider than tall 0	Smooth 0	None 0
Spongiform 0	Hyperisoechoic 1	Taller than wide 3	Ill-defined 0	Comet tails 0
Mixed 1	Hypoechoic 2		Lobulated/irregular 2	Macrocalcifications 1
Mostly solid or completely solid 2	Very hypoechoic 3		ETE 3	Peripheral/rim 2
				Punctate 3

Abbreviation: ETE, extrathyroidal extension.

Table 3. Individual Sonographic Features and Associated Points: ACR TI-RADS Classification

Points	Description	Malignancy Risk (%)	FNA Threshold	Surveillance[a]	Repeat Ultrasound
0	TR1: benign	<2	No FNA	None	None
2	TR2: not suspicious	<2	No FNA	None	None
3	TR3: mildly suspicious	5	FNA ≥2.5 cm	Follow if ≥1.5 cm	1, 3, and 5 y
4–6	TR4: moderately suspicious	5–20	FNA ≥1.5 cm	Follow if ≥1.0 cm	1, 2, 3, and 5 y
≥7	TR5: highly suspicious	>20	FNA ≥1.0 cm	Follow if ≥0.5 cm	Annually for 5 y

Abbreviation: TR, TIRADS risk score.
[a] Necessity of surveillance for nodules below each threshold is unclear.

Answer: D (intermediate risk)

The nodule is mildly hypoechoic with regular (smooth) margins. It lacks any suspicious sonographic features such as irregular margins (infiltrative or microlobulated), microcalcifications, taller than wide shape, rim calcifications with small extrusive soft tissue component, or evidence of extrathyroidal extension. The risk of malignancy in such nodules is 10% to 20%. The threshold for FNA in this nodule is 1.0 cm.

Case 2

A 24-year-old man is referred for evaluation of a new neck mass. It has been present for 4 months and has not responded to a course of oral antibiotics. An ultrasound of the neck reveals the following nodule.

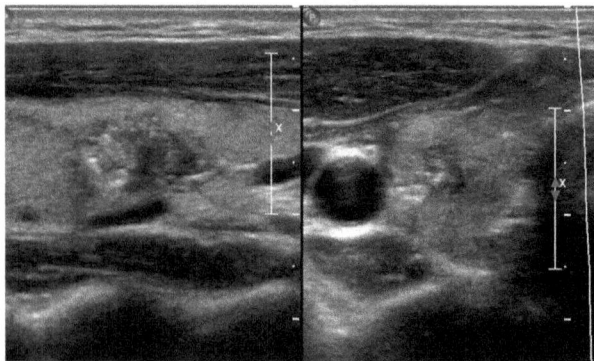

What is the ACR TI-RADS score for this nodule?
A. TR1
B. TR2
C. TR3
D. TR4
E. TR5

Answer: E (TR5)

This nodule has 10 points: mostly solid (two), hypoechoic (two), taller than wide (three), irregular/lobulated margins (two), and macrocalcifications (one). It is a high-risk nodule with a ≥20% risk of malignancy, probably much higher given all of the suspicious sonographic features. In addition, this patient had abnormal-appearing lymph nodes in the lateral neck. When abnormal nodes are identified, these may require aspiration with measurement of thyroglobulin in the needle washout.

Case 3

A 78-year-old woman presents for evaluation of incidentally noted thyroid nodules during carotid Doppler examination. She denies any symptoms and has a normal thyrotropin level.

Her ultrasound is shown below.

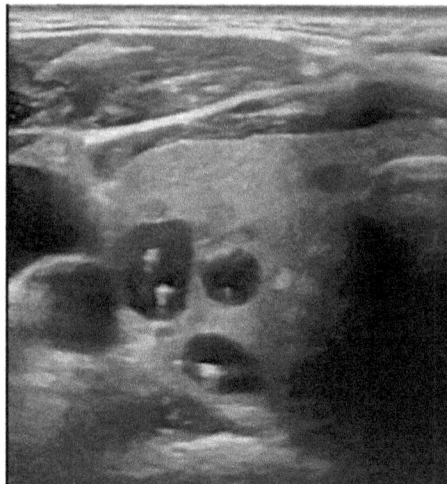

Which nodule should be biopsied?
A. The largest nodule
B. All of them
C. None of them

Answer: C (none of them)

These nodules are all benign colloid nodules. They do not require aspiration unless they are causing compressive symptoms. Small nodules such as these are highly unlikely to result in compressive symptoms. Larger cystic nodules may be aspirated to relieve compressive symptoms. The areas of hyperechogenicity in these nodules represent the comet-tail sign, which is a very reassuring finding in association with a cystic nodule lacking any other suspicious sonographic features. These are not calcifications. Nodules such as these do not require surveillance imaging.

Case 4

A 66-year-old woman presents for evaluation of a thyroid nodule noted incidentally on a computed tomography scan of the neck obtained after a recent motor vehicle accident. She denies any compressive symptoms, radiation exposure, or family history of thyroid cancer.

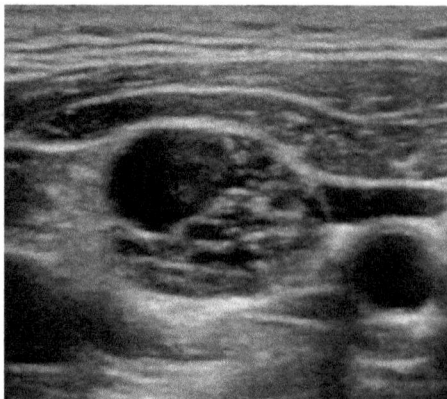

What is the ATA classification of this nodule?
A. Benign
B. Very low risk
C. Low risk
D. Intermediate risk
E. High risk

Answer: B (very low risk)

This nodule has a spongiform pattern and a very low risk of malignancy. As such, these nodules do not require FNA but may be considered for aspiration if >2 cm.

The hyperlucent areas noted in this nodule do not represent microcalcifications. These areas result from posterior acoustic enhancement along the back wall of a minute cyst. These are not suspicious findings and do not increase the risk associated with this nodule.

CONCLUSIONS

Thyroid nodules are highly prevalent but have a low overall risk of malignancy. The risk of malignancy of the individual nodule can be further delineated based on its sonographic appearance. Characterization of each nodule is critical for appropriately triaging the lesion for FNA and surveillance imaging.

References

1. Mazzaferri EL. Management of a solitary thyroid nodule. *N Engl J Med.* 1993;**328**(8):553–559.
2. Yang J, Schnadig V, Logrono R, Wasserman PG. Fine-needle aspiration of thyroid nodules: a study of 4703 patients with histologic and clinical correlations. *Cancer.* 2007;**111**(5):306–315.
3. Yassa L, Cibas ES, Benson CB, Frates MC, Doubilet PM, Gawande AA, Moore FD Jr, Kim BW, Nosé V, Marqusee E, Larsen PR, Alexander EK. Long-term assessment of a multidisciplinary approach to thyroid nodule diagnostic evaluation. *Cancer.* 2007;**111**(6):508–516.
4. Haugen BR, Alexander EK, Bible KC, Doherty GM, Mandel SJ, Nikiforov YE, Pacini F, Randolph GW, Sawka AM, Schlumberger M, Schuff KG, Sherman SI, Sosa JA, Steward DL, Tuttle RM, Wartofsky L. 2015 American Thyroid Association Management Guidelines for Adult Patients with Thyroid Nodules and Differentiated Thyroid Cancer: The American Thyroid Association Guidelines Task Force on Thyroid Nodules and Differentiated Thyroid Cancer. *Thyroid.* 2016;**26**(1):1–133.
5. Tessler FN, Middleton WD, Grant EG, Hoang JK, Berland LL, Teefey SA, Cronan JJ, Beland MD, Desser TS, Frates MC, Hammers LW, Hamper UM, Langer JE, Reading CC, Scoutt LM, Stavros AT. ACR Thyroid Imaging, Reporting and Data System (TI-RADS): White Paper of the ACR TI-RADS Committee. *J Am Coll Radiol.* 2017;**14**(5):587–595.
6. Russ G, Royer B, Bigorgne C, Rouxel A, Bienvenu-Perrard M, Leenhardt L. Prospective evaluation of Thyroid Imaging Reporting and Data System on 4550 nodules with and without elastography. *Eur J Endocrinol.* 2013;**168**(5):649–655.
7. Cheng SP, Lee JJ, Lin JL, Chuang SM, Chien MN, Liu CL. Characterization of thyroid nodules using the proposed Thyroid Imaging Reporting and Data System (TI-RADS). *Head Neck.* 2013;**35**(4):541–547.

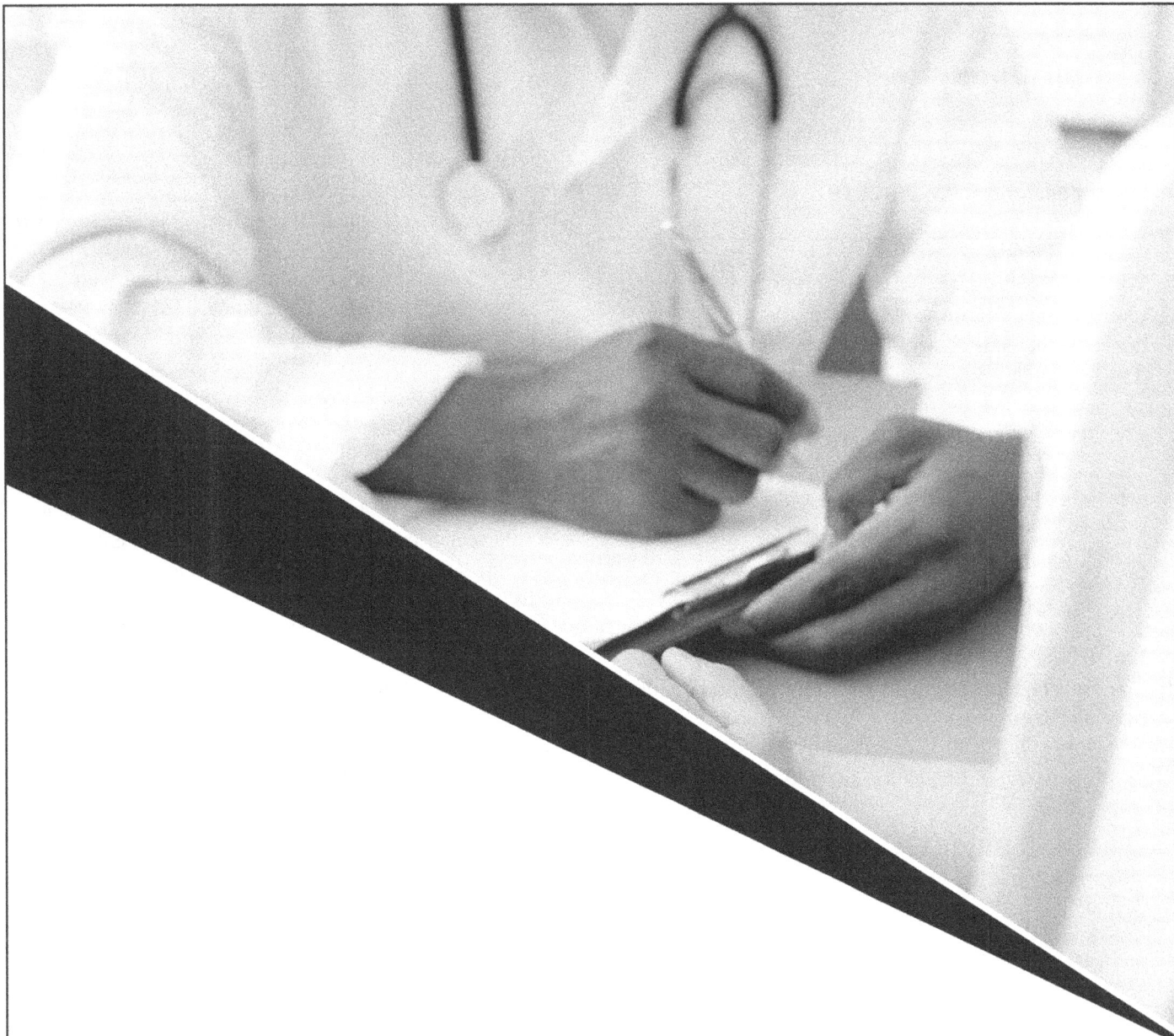

MISCELLANEOUS

E-Mail Consults

M40
Presented, March 23–26, 2019

William F. Young, Jr., MD. Division of Endocrinology, Diabetes, Metabolism, and Nutrition, Department of Internal Medicine, Mayo Clinic, Rochester, Minnesota 55905, E-mail: young.william@mayo.edu

SIGNIFICANCE OF THE CLINICAL PROBLEM
This is an atypical Meet the Professor (MTP) session. We are not addressing a specific topic or problem; but rather, this session will be a demonstration of the types of adrenal-related patient management questions clinicians are challenged with every day.

BARRIERS TO OPTIMAL PRACTICE
Unfortunately, many patients with adrenal disorders do not conveniently fit with what is written in clinical practice guidelines. Guidelines are frequently based on the ideal world—a place not frequently visited by most patients.

LEARNING OBJECTIVES
As a result of participating in this session, learners should be able to:
- Recognize common clinical questions about adrenal disorders from clinicians in practice
- Discuss commonsense approaches to difficult adrenal management issues
- Illustrate the challenges of providing useful guidance in an environment of limited information

STRATEGIES FOR DIAGNOSIS, THERAPY, AND/OR MANAGEMENT
The focus of this MTP session is all about the diagnosis, treatment, and overall management of patients who either have or are suspected to have adrenal disorders. At the time of writing this syllabus, I have answered 7572 e-mails from clinicians in the United States and around the world. Typically the e-mail question is based on diagnostic and management issues of a single patient. It occurred to me in 2006 that I should start saving these e-mail queries. The first e-mail I saved was 29 January 2006 with the subject line title "need more help, again!"

In 2006, I saved 76 e-mail questions into an Outlook folder titled "E-mail Consults." The numbers of e-mails saved to this folder have increased each year: 665 in 2017 and 663 in 2018 (through 18 November 2018). During the MTP session, we will "mine" this Outlook e-mail consult folder for challenging adrenal cases and situations and discuss approaches to address the conundrums presented.

Here is a typical e-mail consult:

Hi Dr. Young,

I wondered if I could run a case by you. I have a patient with a 1.5-cm adrenal adenoma 3 HU, urine normetanephrine, total metanephrines, and norepinephrine 2 to 3.5 times the upper limit of normal, but he is on Adderall, Abilify, Vyvanse, and Wellbutrin and is unable to be off these meds for 2 weeks for retesting. I was planning to have him check a serum chromogranin A level and possibly an MIBG (metaiodobenzylguanidine) scan, but would these meds also interfere with the scan results? Anything else you might suggest? Thanks so much in advance!

In circumstances where the case is quite complicated or high risk, or I am uneasy about the validity or completeness of the information provided, I will start my e-mail answer with "I can't give any formal treatment recommendations without seeing the patient, but generally we would…" And I will conclude my e-mail comments with "This general information should not be viewed as patient-specific diagnostic or treatment information. Specific recommendations can be made only after a face-to-face consult with the patient."

MAIN CONCLUSIONS
It is impossible for clinical practice guidelines to cover all clinical presentations and confounding factors. Seeking limited guidance with curbside phone calls or e-mail communications can be very helpful in steering clinical management.

Recommended Reading
Canu L, Van Hemert JAW, Kerstens M, Hartman RP, Khanna A, Kraljevic I, Kastelan D, Badiu C, Ambroziak U, Tabarin A, Haissaguerre M, Buitenwerf E, Visser A, Mannelli M, Arlt W, Chortis V, Bourdeau I, Gagnon N, Buchy M, Borson-Chazot F, Deutschbein T, Fassnacht M, Hubalewska Dydejczyk HA, Motyka M, Rzepka E, Casey RT, Challis BG, Quinkler M, Vroonen L, Spyroglou A, Beuschlein F, Lamas C, Young WF, Bancos I, Timmers HJLM. CT characteristics of pheochromocytoma—relevance for the evaluation of adrenal incidentaloma [published online ahead of print 31 October 2018]. *J Clin Endocrinol Metab.* doi:10.1210/jc.2018-01532.

Funder JW, Carey RM, Mantero F, Murad MH, Reincke M, Shibata H, Stowasser M, Young WF, Jr. The management of primary aldosteronism: case detection, diagnosis, and treatment: an Endocrine Society clinical practice guideline. *J Clin Endocrinol Metab.* 2016;**101**(5): 1889–1916.

Hamidi O, Young WF, Jr, Iñiguez-Ariza NM, Kittah NE, Gruber L, Bancos C, Tamhane S, Bancos I. Malignant pheochromocytoma and paraganglioma: 272 patients over 55 years. *J Clin Endocrinol Metab.* 2017; **102**(9):3296–3305.

Hurtado MD, Cortes T, Natt N, Young WF, Jr, Bancos I. Extensive clinical experience: hypothalamic-pituitary-adrenal axis recovery after adrenalectomy for corticotropin-independent cortisol excess. *Clin Endocrinol (Oxf).* 2018;**89**(6):721–733.

Kim DH, Kwon HJ, Ji SA, Jang HR, Jung SH, Kim JH, Kim JH, Lee JE, Huh W, Kim YG, Kim DJ, Oh HY. Risk factors for renal impairment revealed after unilateral adrenalectomy in patients with primary aldosteronism. *Medicine (Baltimore)*. 2016;**95**(27):e3930.

Kramers BJ, Kramers C, Lenders JW, Deinum J. Effects of treating primary aldosteronism on renal function. *J Clin Hypertens (Greenwich)*. 2017; **19**(3):290–295.

Lenders JW, Duh QY, Eisenhofer G, Gimenez-Roqueplo AP, Grebe SK, Murad MH, Naruse M, Pacak K, Young WF, Jr; Endocrine Society. Pheochromocytoma and paraganglioma: an Endocrine Society clinical practice guideline. *J Clin Endocrinol Metab*. 2014;**99**(6):1915–1942.

Shariq OA, Bancos I, Cronin PA, Farley DR, Richards ML, Thompson GB, Young WF, Jr, McKenzie TJ. Contralateral suppression of aldosterone at adrenal venous sampling predicts hyperkalemia following adrenalectomy for primary aldosteronism. *Surgery*. 2018;**163**(1): 183–190.

Strajina V, Al-Hilli Z, Andrews JC, Bancos I, Thompson GB, Farley DR, Lyden ML, Dy BM, Young WF, McKenzie TJ. Primary aldosteronism: making sense of partial data sets from failed adrenal venous sampling-suppression of adrenal aldosterone production can be used in clinical decision making. *Surgery*. 2018;**163**(4):801–806.

Vanderveen KA, Thompson SM, Callstrom MR, Young WF, Jr, Grant CS, Farley DR, Richards ML, Thompson GB. Biopsy of pheochromocytomas and paragangliomas: potential for disaster. *Surgery*. 2009;**146**(6): 1158–1166.

Young WF Jr. Clinical practice. The incidentally discovered adrenal mass. *N Engl J Med*. 2007;**356**(6):601–610.

Young WF Jr. Diagnosis and treatment of primary aldosteronism: practical clinical perspectives [published online ahead of print 25 September 2018]. *J Intern Med*. doi:10.1111/joim.12831.

NOTES